Forensic Neuropsychology

Forensic Neuropsychology

A SCIENTIFIC APPROACH

EDITED BY

Glenn J. Larrabee

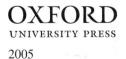

OXFORD
UNIVERSITY PRESS
2005

OXFORD
UNIVERSITY PRESS

Oxford University Press, Inc., publishes works that further
Oxford University's objective of excellence
in research, scholarship, and education.

Oxford   New York
Auckland   Cape Town   Dar es Salaam   Hong Kong   Karachi
Kuala Lumpur   Madrid   Melbourne   Mexico City   Nairobi
New Delhi   Shanghai   Taipei   Toronto

With offices in
Argentina   Austria   Brazil   Chile   Czech Republic   France   Greece
Guatemala   Hungary   Italy   Japan   Poland   Portugal   Singapore
South Korea   Switzerland   Thailand   Turkey   Ukraine   Vietnam

Copyright © 2005 by Oxford University Press, Inc.

Published by Oxford University Press, Inc.
198 Madison Avenue, New York, New York 10016
www.oup.com

Oxford is a registered trademark of Oxford University Press

Library of Congress Cataloging-in-Publication Data
Forensic neuropsychology : a scientific approach / [edited by] Glenn J. Larrabee.
p. ; cm.
Includes bibliographical references.
ISBN-13 978-0-19-515899-1
ISBN 0-19-515899-7
1. Forensic neuropsychology.   I. Larrabee, Glenn J.
[DNLM: 1. Forensic Medicine.   2. Neuropsychology.   3. Brain Injuries.   W 700 F71503 2005]
RA1147.5.F675   2005
614'.15—dc22   2004050061

9 8 7 6 5 4 3 2 1

Printed in the United States of America
on acid-free paper

To my wife, Jan, and my son, Zack, for their love and support.

Preface

Forensic neuropsychology, the use of neuropsychology to address legal questions, has grown in an exponential fashion since my first publication in this area (Larrabee, 1990). Any current issue of the *Archives of Clinical Neuropsychology* is likely to contain a publication on some aspect of forensic neuropsychology. *The Clinical Neuropsychologist*, now the official journal of the American Academy of Clinical Neuropsychology, contains "Forensic Applications," a separate section devoted solely to forensic neuropsychology. Presently, forensic referrals represent the primary source of income for private practitioners (Sweet, Moberg, & Suchy, 2000).

My experience over the last 15 years has been consistent with the experience of my colleagues in that the majority of my forensic work arose initially in the civil courts in the context of personal injury litigation. Over time, forensic issues diversified; I have been asked to render expert opinions in probate court matters such as capacity to execute a valid last will and testament. I have also been asked to render expert opinions in criminal matters, assisting the court in addressing questions of whether a defendant possesses the competency to proceed to trial or whether a defendant was not responsible, as a result of neuropsychological deficit, for the alleged crime.

As my forensic practice grew, I became increasingly aware of how we, as neuropsychologists, are uniquely trained to address issues that arise in the context of legal questions. Obviously, neuropsychological data can provide information regarding the damages someone may have sustained as the result of a traumatic brain injury or neurotoxic exposure. In addition, our training in the evaluation of language, memory, intellectual, and problem solving skills provides us with unique skills that allow us to assist the court in addressing both civil and criminal competencies and legal responsibilities.

I have also followed the burgeoning literature in forensic neuropsychology and quickly came to appreciate the importance of working closely with representatives of the legal system to gain a better appreciation of the questions I was asked to address. Forensic practice requires high standards because the forensic neuropsychologist must act in an ethical, scientific, and nonbiased manner. In other words, as experts we are seekers of and advocates for the scientific truth, based on our training and experience, rather than advocates for or against a particular client's legal interests.

Addressing legal questions is a complex endeavor. Damages in a civil personal injury lawsuit are not fully addressed by the scores a litigant obtains on a neuropsychological evaluation; rather, these scores must be integrated with the medical history preceding and following the alleged injury, as well as integrated with the litigant's developmental, social, educational, and occupational history. Competencies are not answered by a diagnosis of dementia or amnesia, but rather by the person's ability to perform specific tasks indicative of possessing the legal competency at issue. An elderly person may possess testamentary capacity despite the presence of dementia. Similarly, a criminal defendant may possess competency to proceed to trial despite demonstrating significant impairments on neuropsychological testing.

The present book, *Forensic Neuropsychology: A Scientific Approach*, is the result of my perception of the need for a text that reflects the growth of the field of forensic neuropsychology, including the expansion of neuropsychology into areas of competencies and responsibilities, and the complexity of the issues that forensic neuropsychologists are asked to address. All of us who do forensic neuropsychology are aware of the increasing legal scrutiny of our qualifications to offer expert opinions.

Neuropsychologists and forensic experts in other specialties are well aware of the *Daubert v. Merrell Dow* (1993) decision mandating use of principles that have a sound scientific basis. Consequently, I have chosen to emphasize the science of neuropsychology by focusing on the basic principles of scientific reasoning, hypothesis testing, and diagnostic decision making in the first chapter, "A Scientific Approach to Forensic Neuropsychology."

Science represents both a way of investigating problems and the accumulation of knowledge in a particular area of study, such as neuropsychology. This highlights the need for up-to-date reviews of areas particularly pertinent to the practice of forensic neuropsychology. These reviews are authored by neuropsychologists who have conducted empirical research in the different topic areas and include my chapters "Assessment of Malingering" and "Mild Traumatic Brain Injury" as well as the chapters "Moderate and Severe Traumatic Brain Injury," by Sherer and Madison, "Forensic Aspects of Pediatric Traumatic Brain Injury," by Donders, "Neurotoxic Injury," by Bolla, and "Functional Neuroimaging in Forensic Neuropsychology," by Ricker. Also of interest in this group of chapters, and particularly important in respect to differential diagnosis, is the chapter by Binder, "Forensic Assessment of Medically Unexplained Symptoms."

Marson and Hebert provide a good demonstration of the application of scientific research in addressing, in their chapter "Assessing Civil Competencies in Older Adults With Dementia: Consent Capacity, Financial Capacity, and Testamentary Capacity," various competencies in the elderly. Denney comprehensively addresses criminal forensic neuropsychology in his two chapters, "Criminal Forensic Neuropsychology and Assessment of Competency" and "Criminal Responsibility and Other Criminal Forensic Issues." Grote incorporates both the recently published "Ethical Principles of Psychologists and Code of Conduct" and the Health Insurance Portability and Accountability Act (HIPAA) in his chapter, "Ethical Practice of Forensic Neuropsychology." Greiffenstein (a neuropsychologist) and Cohen (an attorney) provide a comprehensive overview of the effective practice of forensic neuropsychology in their chapter, "Neuropsychology and the Law: Principles of Productive Attorney–Neuropsychologist Relations."

Forensic neuropsychology is an exciting and challenging area of neuropsychology. My collaborators and I hope that we have provided a useful reference for both neuropsychologists and attorneys who seek neuropsychological expertise in the legal arena.

I gratefully acknowledge the assistance of several individuals whose contributions have helped see this work to completion. First, I acknowledge the assistance of Bridgette O'Brien, B.S., who helped read and proof the contents of the entire volume. Her attention to detail was invaluable. Next, I am most appreciative of the contributions of Kristin Wright, B.A., who set up the database and assisted in the statistical analyses for my research cited in my chapter on malingering. Patricia Reynolds, M.L.S., and Inez Tamanaha, M.L.S., of the Bishopric Medical Library at Sarasota Memorial Hospital in Florida, were most helpful in providing articles for the three chapters I prepared for the current volume. Last, Paul R. Lees-Haley, Ph.D., provided an informative review of my chapters covering the scientific approach, assessment of malingering, and mild traumatic brain injury.

REFERENCES

Daubert v. Merrell Dow, 509 U.S. 579 (1993).

Larrabee, G. J. (1990). Cautions in the use of neuropsychological evaluation in legal settings. *Neuropsychology, 4*, 239–247.

Sweet, J. J., Moberg, P. J., & Suchy, Y. (2000). Ten-year follow-up survey of clinical neuropsychologists: Part II. Private practice and economics. *The Clinical Neuropsychologist, 14*, 479–495.

Contents

Contributors

Laurence M. Binder, Ph.D., ABPP-Cn., independent practice, Beaverton, Oregon, and Departments of Neurology and Psychiatry, Oregon Health and Sciences University, Portland, Oregon

Karen I. Bolla, Ph.D., Departments of Neurology, Psychiatry and Behavioral Sciences, and Environmental Health Sciences, Johns Hopkins University School of Medicine and Bloomberg School of Public Health, Baltimore, Maryland

Larry Cohen, J.D., Ph.D., private practice attorney, Phoenix, Arizona

Robert L. Denney, Psy.D., ABPP-Cn., Fp., ABPN, U.S. Medical Center for Federal Prisoners and Forest Institute of Professional Psychology, Springfield, Missouri

Jacobus Donders, Ph.D., ABPP-Cn., Rp., Mary Free Bed Rehabilitation Hospital, Grand Rapids, Michigan

Manfred F. Greiffenstein, Ph.D., ABPP-Cn., Psychological Systems Inc., Royal Oak, Michigan

Christopher Grote, Ph.D., ABPP-Cn., Department of Psychology, Rush-Presbyterian–St. Luke's Medical Center, Chicago, Illinois

Katina Hebert, M.S., Department of Psychology, University of Alabama, Tuscaloosa, Alabama

Glenn J. Larrabee, Ph.D., ABPP-Cn., independent practice, Sarasota, Florida

Charlene F. Madison, Ph.D., Nexus Health Systems and University of Houston, Houston, Texas

Daniel C. Marson, J.D., Ph.D., Department of Neurology and Alzheimer's Disease Research Center, University of Alabama at Birmingham, Birmingham, Alabama

Joseph H. Ricker, Ph.D., ABPP-Cn., Rp., Department of Physical Medicine and Rehabilitation, University of Pittsburgh, Pittsburgh, Pennsylvania

Mark Sherer, Ph.D., ABPP-Cn., Methodist Rehabilitation Center, and Departments of Neurology and Psychiatry, University of Mississippi Medical Center, Jackson, Mississippi

Forensic Neuropsychology

1

A Scientific Approach
to Forensic Neuropsychology

GLENN J. LARRABEE

This book emphasizes a scientific approach to the practice of forensic neuropsychology: the application of neuropsychology to legal issues that arise in both civil and criminal legal proceedings. In certain circumstances, neuropsychological deficits have a direct bearing on legal issues, for example, in establishment of damages in a personal injury case (see chapters 4 and 6–9, this volume). In other settings, a person may have impaired neuropsychological test scores, but the impairment alone does not provide the answer to the legal issue; for example, an older person may have dementia, but still possess competency to execute a valid will (chapter 11, this volume); a person facing criminal charges may have neuropsychological impairment, but still be found competent to stand trial and be responsible for the criminal act (chapters 12 and 13, this volume).

Greiffenstein and Cohen (chapter 2) discuss issues related to the admissibility of expert neuropsychological testimony related to *Frye v. United States* (1923) and to *Daubert v. Merrell Dow* (1993), legal standards that emphasize acceptability of a particular scientific methodology by ones' peers and standards that mandate a particular methodology meet scientific principles, such as possessing a known error rate, and the potential to be falsified or discredited (cf. Popper, 1959).

WHAT IS SCIENCE?

The goals of the empirical natural sciences include exploration, description, explanation, and prediction of worldly occurrences or phenomena (Badia & Runyon, 1982; Hempel, 1966; Kerlinger, 1973). Science is concerned with things that can be publicly observed and tested as opposed to metaphysical explanations (Kerlinger, 1973).

Science differs from pseudoscience in a number of ways (Lilienfeld, Lynn, & Lohr, 2003). Some of the features of pseudoscience include overuse of ad hoc hypotheses to immunize claims from falsification; evasion of peer review; absence of self-correction; and emphasis on confirmation rather than refutation. Regarding this last point, Lilienfeld et al. (2003) cited the physicist Feynman (1985), who maintained that the essence of science is a bending over backward to prove oneself wrong. Referencing Popper (1959) and Meehl (1978), Lilienfeld et al. noted that scientists ideally subject their claims to grave risk of refutation, contrasted with pseudoscientists, who tend to seek only confirming evidence for their claims. Because a determined advocate for a particular pseudoscientific position can find at least some supportive evidence for essentially any claim, Lilienfeld et al. described this confirmatory hypothesis testing strategy as "an inefficient means of rooting out error in one's web of beliefs" (p. 7).

The basic aim of science is explanation, and the explanations offered by science are theories (Kerlinger, 1973). More formally specified, theories are sets of concepts, definitions, and propositions that present a systematic view of phenomena by specifying relations among variables, with the purpose of explaining and predicting the phenomena (Kerlinger, 1973). Kerlinger further defined research as "systematic, controlled, empirical, and critical investigation of hypothetical propositions about the presumed relations among rational phenomena" (p. 11).

Science is hypotheticodeductive (Badia & Runyon, 1982; Hempel, 1966; Kerlinger, 1973). A hypothesis represents a conjectural statement or tentative proposition about the relation between two or more variables, for example, between duration of coma and memory test performance 1-year status post–traumatic brain injury (TBI). The scientist than deduces the consequences of the hypothesis he or she has formulated (e.g., those brain-injured subjects with shorter durations of coma will perform better on memory testing than will those with longer durations of coma).

A long tradition in psychology is the Fisherian tradition of specifying a hypothesis for a given relationship (e.g., between coma and memory test performance), which is then contrasted with a hypothesis of no effect, otherwise known as the *null hypothesis* (Kerlinger, 1973; Meehl, 1978). Meehl criticized the null hypothesis testing approach as responsible for the slow progress of "soft psychology," resulting in "a disturbing absence of that cumulative character that is so impressive in disciplines like astronomy, molecular biology, and genetics" (p. 807). As Meehl noted, the null hypothesis, taken literally, is always false. He recommended the Popperian approach (Popper, 1959) of subjecting hypotheses to grave danger of refutation with *modus tollens*: "If p, then q; not q, therefore not p." In this manner, theories or hypotheses that survive the most attempts at refutation are the best-supported theories.

In his 1978 article, Meehl did specify "five noble traditions in clinical psychology," two of which are directly relevant to the practice of clinical and forensic neuropsychology: (a) descriptive clinical psychiatry (for the discipline of neuropsychology, descriptive behavioral neurology can also be included) and (b) psychometric assessment. Arguably, both of these "noble traditions" have led to an accumulation of information in clinical psychology in general, and neuropsychology in particular, contributing to the cumulative nature of knowledge in these disciplines that Meehl found lacking in comparisons of the "soft" science of psychology with the "hard" sciences such as astronomy.

A SCIENTIFIC APPROACH TO NEUROPSYCHOLOGICAL EVALUATION

Conducting a neuropsychological evaluation and making a neuropsychological diagnosis regarding the presence of brain damage can be conceptualized as a scientific endeavor. The scientific endeavor includes formulation of hypotheses that are then checked for support or, better yet, subjected to attempts at refutation. The formulation of various different hypotheses corresponds to formulation of differential diagnoses. More specifically, in a particular civil forensic case seeking damage for an alleged TBI, alternative hypotheses could include (a) neuropsychological deficits secondary to TBI; (b) no evidence for any neuropsychological deficits; (c) neuropsychological deficits secondary to a preexisting condition such as learning disability, hypertension, or dementia; (d) neuropsychological deficits secondary to a psychiatric condition that is related or unrelated to the accident in question; or (e) neuropsychological deficits secondary to malingering.

The appropriate use of logical and scientific reasoning in performing a forensic evaluation is critical to avoid committing diagnostic errors. At present, there is a growing problem of overdiagnosis of neuropsychological deficits in legal settings because of failure to analyze cases critically and scientifically (Faust, Ziskin, & Hiers, 1991; Larrabee, 1990, 2000b; Russell, 1990; Wedding & Faust, 1989). This failure frequently results in inadequate differential diagnosis (Binder, 1997).

Faulty logic commonly leads to diagnostic error. E. Miller (1983) noted the argument "if damage to structure X is known to produce a decline on Test T, it is tempting to argue that any new subject or group of subjects having a relatively poor performance on T must have a lesion at X" is the same as the argument "because a horse meets the test of being a large animal with four legs, then any newly encountered large animal with four legs is a horse" (p. 131). Larrabee (1990, 2000b) extended E. Miller's (1983) example to the diagnostic decision of "brain damage" versus "no brain damage": If brain-damaged subjects perform poorly on neuropsychological tests, then any new person who performs poorly on neuropsychological tests must be brain damaged.

As Russell (1990) and Russell and Kolitz-Russell (2003) observed, neuropsychological tests are measures of cognitive abilities rather than tests of brain damage. Consequently, neuropsychological test performance can be poor for many reasons other than brain damage, including limited cooperation or inattentiveness caused by fatigue, pain, discomfort, medication effects, substance abuse, learning disability, psychiatric diagnosis, or poor motivation (Binder, 1997; Larrabee, 1990).

Faust and colleagues have written extensively about sources of error and bias in clinical decision making (Faust, 1989; Faust & Nurcombe, 1989; Faust et al., 1991; Wedding & Faust, 1989). Failure to consider base rate information can be a major factor in misdiagnosis. The term *base rate* refers to the frequency with which something occurs; for example, if 5 in 100 persons with mild traumatic brain injury (MTBI) suffer persisting neuropsychological deficits, the base rate is 5%. Lack of awareness of base rates and biases such as confirmation bias or hindsight bias can lead to the formation of illusory correlations or "seeing" relationships that do not exist (Wedding & Faust, 1989).

The original work on illusory correlations was conducted by the Chapmans (Chapman & Chapman, 1967), who presented psychology undergraduates with human figure drawings accompanied by randomly paired symptom statements (e.g., "suspiciousness" would appear in association with accented eyes as frequently as it appeared in association with nonaccented eyes). Despite the absence of systematic relationships in the data, the psychology students attributed diagnostic "signs" to the relationships they had assumed existed in the first place (e.g., associating accented eyes in human figure drawings with "suspiciousness"). Chapman and Chapman commented that the erroneously reported correlations corresponded to associative connections between symptoms and drawing characteristics (formed by their research subjects), as well as to what their subjects *expect to see* before they actually observed. Essentially, the Chapman and Chapman research subjects demonstrated both a failure to consider base rates as well as a confirmation bias (i.e., seeing what they expected to see).

Chapman and Chapman (1969) further demonstrated the presence of illusory correlations based on the judgments of practicing clinicians. As shown by Kurtz and Garfield (1978), the bias toward forming illusory correlation could not be overcome, even when subjects were provided with special pretraining against illusory correlations.

The diagnostic significance of base rate data is further underscored by the investigation by Lees-Haley and Brown (1993), who tabulated the frequency of so-called neuropsychological complaints in two groups of subjects: (a) 50 outpatients from a group family practice clinic and (b) 170 litigants filing personal injury claims for emotional distress or industrial stress, with no known history of head injury, toxic exposure, seizure disorder, or neuropsychological impairment and without any claim for central nervous system (CNS) injury (non-CNS litigants). Symptoms commonly thought of as indicative or "diagnostic" of TBI and neurotoxic exposure occurred frequently in the medical controls (MCs) and non-CNS litigants. For example, "difficulty concentrating" was reported by 26% of MCs and 78% of non-CNS litigants; "headache" was reported by 62% of MCs and 88% of non-CNS litigants; and "irritability" was reported by 38% of MCs and 77% of non-CNS litigants.

The data presented by Lees-Haley and Brown (1993) highlighted significant problems with the sensitivity and specificity of common neuropsychological symptom checklists. *Sensitivity* refers to the frequency or rate of occurrence of a finding among patients with the condition in question, whereas *specificity* refers to the frequency of negative test results among patients who do not have the illness or condition in question (Baldessarini, Finklestein, & Arana, 1983). If the base rate of a symptom used to diagnose concussion such as headache in non-CNS samples is ignored, this would lead to misdiagnosis of brain damage or dysfunction in 62% of MCs and 88% of non-CNS litigants based on the data compiled by Lees-Haley and Brown.

Faust et al. (1991) and Wedding and Faust (1989) discussed two major types of bias in clinical judgment and decision making: hindsight bias and confirmation bias. *Hindsight bias* is the tendency to believe, once the outcome of an event is known, that the outcome could have been more easily predicted than is actually the case. Thus, knowing about an event through clinical history (e.g., a blow to the head in an automobile accident) leads clinicians to believe they can predict the outcome of the event and diagnose neuropsychological deficits consistent with TBI.

Hindsight bias can be closely associated with confirmation bias, which has been discussed as the tendency to seek confirming evidence at the expense of ignoring disconfirming evidence for a set of diagnostic hypotheses. In confirmation bias, initial hypotheses are subjected to preferential analysis, so that the clinician is much more lenient or accepting of information supporting the initial hypothesis and more critical and less accepting of information contradicting the initial hypothesis, demonstrating a propensity toward asymmetric error costs (Trope, Gervey, & Liberman, 1997). Moreover, Trope et al. observed that persons are more likely to terminate hypothesis testing prematurely once they receive information supporting their described hypothesis. Although it is tempting to attribute confirmation bias to the emphasis on null hypothesis testing in psychological research (cf. Meehl, 1978), confirmation bias may represent a common judgment error in human decision making (cf. Trope et al., 1997).

I previously described an example of confirmation bias in a litigant alleging TBI (Larrabee, 2000b). In this case, it was questionable that the litigant ever struck her head (she claimed she did; records did not substantiate this claim). Nonetheless, the litigant had no loss of consciousness, posttraumatic amnesia, history of acute focal neurological signs, or abnormal neurological findings, yet she was diagnosed as suffering brain damage on the basis of a Wechsler Memory Scale–Revised (WMS-R; Wechsler, 1987) Attention Concentration Index (AC) of 75. The psychologist in this case selectively ignored the WMS-R General Memory Index (GM) of 129, which not only contradicted the presence of brain damage, but also was highly inconsistent with the patient's AC of 75. It is logically and clinically inconsistent that a person with impaired attention at the 5th percentile could have memory function at the 97th percentile. Actually, the 54-point GM minus AC difference score had a probability of malingering greater than .99 based on Mittenberg, Azrin, Millsaps, and Heilbronner's (1993) research on detection of malingered head trauma using atypical patterns of performance on the WMS-R.

Wedding and Faust (1989) provided a number of strategies that can be employed to reduce biases in clinical judgment, beginning with the recommendation that the clinician know the literature on human judgment. Trope et al. (1997) provided a concise review of human judgment and decision making. The Wedding and Faust article also reviewed relevant literature on judgment, decision making, and clinical versus actuarial prediction. Wedding and Faust recommended avoiding prematurely abandoning useful decision-making rules by starting with the most valid information, listing alternative diagnostic options and seeking evidence for each, and systematically listing disconfirmatory information. Consideration of disconfirmatory information is particularly important for reducing confirmation bias. Wedding and Faust noted that neuropsychologists frequently make up lists of test findings that support particular hypotheses, but recommended also listing all data that argue *against* these hypotheses.

Along these lines, I (Larrabee, 2000b) found it useful to frame hypothetical questions such as, "What kind of brain damage causes poor performance on the Category Test (Reitan & Wolfson, 1993), California Verbal Learning Test-II (Delis, Kramer, Kaplan, & Ober, 2000), and Finger Tapping (Reitan & Wolfson, 1993), with above-average performance on the Wisconsin Card Sorting Test (Heaton, Chelune, Talley, Kay, & Curtiss, 1993), Verbal Selective Reminding Test (Buschke, 1973; Hannay & Levin, 1985; Larrabee, Trahan, & Levin, 2000), Trail Making B (Army Individual Test Battery, 1944), and the Grooved Pegboard (Lafayette Instrument, P.O. Box 5729, Lafayette, IN)?" Indeed, to counter the diagnostic bias to find brain impairment when there is none (cf. Russell, 1990; Wedding & Faust, 1989), the neuropsychologist should first list all evidence suggesting no evidence for brain impairment (e.g., clinical history of no loss of consciousness or posttraumatic amnesia, normal magnetic resonance imaging scan, normal performance on sensitive tests such as Trail Making B and Verbal Selective Reminding).

I suggested a four-component consistency analysis in neuropsychological decision making (Larrabee, 1990, 1992, 1997, 2000b):

1. Are the data consistent within and between neuropsychological domains?
2. Is the neuropsychological profile consistent with the suspected etiologic condition?
3. Are the neuropsychological data consistent with the documented severity of injury?
4. Are the neuropsychological data consistent with the subject's behavioral presentation?

The data to be considered in this consistency analysis include a detailed and extensive interview, detailed record review, and extensive and redundant neuropsychological test measures within each of several functional domains, including language, perception, sensorimotor function, attention/information processing, psychomotor speed, verbal and visual learning and memory, intelligence and problem solving, and motivation and personality.

The clinical interview is conducted prior to testing and yields information about the subject's recollection of the original injury or trauma (e.g., head injury, toxic exposure, hypoxic event); subsequent symptoms and change in symptoms over time; other health care providers the subject has seen; and the procedures, diagnoses, and treatments the subject has received. This information, when cross-checked against the medical records for accuracy, provides an informal clinical assessment of the subject's memory function. In the specific case of closed head injury, detailed questioning about the events leading up to and following the accident (e.g., where the person was headed prior to the accident, the time the accident occurred, recall of events from the scene of the accident, diagnostic procedures in the hospital) can be compared to the medical records and allows a retrospective determination of the presence and duration of posttraumatic amnesia. Detailed interviewing about the events of the accident also allows the opportunity to evaluate for the presence/absence of the arousal or distress that could indicate potential for posttraumatic stress disorder. A background interview covering early development, nuclear family, school experiences, occupational history, marital history, prior personal and family medical history, substance abuse, and prior litigation and criminal history must also be conducted. The data from this interview are then checked and validated against medical, school, work, and criminal records.

Following completion of the interview, record review, and collection of the neuropsychological test data, the consistency analysis is conducted. First, analysis of the consistency within and between domains should be conducted. Within domains, a person who performs poorly on Wechsler Memory Scale, Third Edition (WMS-III; Wechsler, 1997) Mental Control should not perform above average on the Paced Auditory Serial Addition Test (Gronwall, 1977); a person who performs poorly on Trail Making A should not perform normally on Trail Making B; a person with very poor performance on Finger Tapping should not have normal Grooved Pegboard Performance. Between domains, a subject with very poor attention should not perform normally on memory tests; a person with borderline scores on intelligence and problem solving should not have superior memory function.

Second, the neuropsychological test score profile should be consistent with established patterns for known disorders such as amnesia or dementia. In my experience, litigants with neuropsychological deficits typically do not present with test patterns that suggest focal neurobehavioral disorders such as aphasia or neglect; rather, litigants either present with a pattern of test results suggestive of amnesia (i.e., specific impairment in memory functions, with other neuropsychological functions essentially preserved) or dementia (i.e., impairment in memory as well as in other neuropsychological functions, typically intelligence and problem-solving skills). Patients with true amnestic disturbance do not perform poorly on the Wechsler Adult Intelligence Scale, Third Edition (WAIS-III; Wechsler, 1997) Digit Span, Arithmetic, or Digit Symbol; although patients with dementia may perform poorly on Digit Span, Arithmetic, or Digit Symbol, they do not perform at above-average levels on complex problem-solving tasks such as WAIS-III Block Design or the Category Test.

This general principle also applies to awareness of test profile patterns that could indicate the presence of a preexisting condition. I (Larrabee, 1990) previously described a case of misdiagnosis in which a psychologist diagnosed left hemisphere brain damage in a patient with an alleged MTBI (no loss of consciousness or posttraumatic amnesia, normal neuroradiological findings) who had reduced right-hand motor functions, lower Verbal IQ relative to Performance IQ, and poor verbal memory. The psychologist did not consider evidence of learning disability verified through school records and the effects of peripheral injury to the right upper extremity (with evidence suggesting functional overlay). These neglected factors provided a much more compelling interpretation of the subject's performance than the original diagnosis of left hemisphere brain damage.

The third consistency requirement is that level of neuropsychological test performance should be consistent with the severity of injury. This can be considered as biological severity "indexing" or "referencing" (Larrabee, 1990, 1997, 2000b). Dikmen, Machamer, Winn, and Temkin (1995) provided 1-year outcome data for varying degrees of head trauma severity, ranging from subjects who could follow a doctor's commands within 1 hour to persons who took longer than 1 month to follow a doctor's commands following a TBI. Consequently, a litigant who was briefly unconscious at the scene of the accident, who recalls transportation to the hospital, and who has a Glasgow Coma Scale (GCS) of 15 (i.e., is oriented, follows commands, eyes open spontaneously), no focal neurological signs, and normal magnetic resonance imaging scan of the brain should not perform on neuropsychological tests at a level equivalent to that produced by subjects who have sustained 2 weeks of coma following their TBI.

Rohling, Meyers, and Millis (2003) provided a statistical methodology, based on the Rohling interpretive method of deriving an overall test battery mean (OTBM; L. S. Miller & Rohling, 2001), that allows for an analysis of neuropsychological data as a function of head injury severity. The methodology proposed by Rohling et al. (2003) yields essentially identical results when based on an expanded Halstead-Reitan Battery (HRB; Reitan & Wolfson, 1993) such as that used by Dikmen et al. (1995), as well as when based on a battery employing standard measures of motor function, attention, processing speed, verbal and visual memory, and intellectual and problem-solving skills (the Meyers Short Battery; Volbrecht, Meyers, & Kaster-Bundgaard, 2000).

Finally, test performance should be compared to other aspects of a subject's behavior. A person who has good memory in the clinical interview, demonstrated by accurate recall of doctors seen, evaluations, and treatments and validated by cross-checking the actual medical records, should not perform in a significantly impaired fashion on formal memory testing. I previously described two examples of this type of inconsistency (Larrabee, 2000b). One case of alleged MTBI accurately analyzed his current Wechsler Adult Intelligence Scale–Revised (WAIS-R; Wechsler, 1981) Digit Symbol performance as superior to testing conducted 2 years earlier, showing evidence of excellent memory, yet the subject performed very poorly on all memory tests administered by the author. Another subject with alleged MTBI performed on memory tests at a level similar to that associated with Alzheimer's disease (AD), yet on the second day of examination noticed that the clock had been removed from the wall of the examining suite.

Hill (1965) presented nine factors that should be considered before moving from the observation of an *association* between a particular environmental condition and a particular disease, to inferring that the environmental condition is related to *causation* of that disease. Although the factors posited by Hill are particularly relevant to inferring causation in neurotoxicology, certain of those factors are also related to other traumatic CNS events.

The first of Hill's (1965) factors is the *strength* of the association, which he illustrated by describing the association between lung cancer and smoking. In particular, the strength of association was demonstrated by the dose–response relationship between number of cigarettes smoked per day and increased incidence of lung cancer.

Hill's (1965) second factor is the *consistency* of the association, that is, if the association has been repeatedly observed by different persons, in different places, circumstances, and times. The example used by Hill was the increased incidence of cancer of the lung and nasal sinuses among nickel refiners in South Wales, found by Hill as well as by other investigators. When a change was instituted in the refining process, not a single person working after the change was made developed cancer of the nose. An example relevant to neuropsychology is the repeated observation that memory impairment and slowed information-processing speed are common long-term residual effects of severe closed head trauma.

Third is Hill's (1965) factor of *specificity*; that is, the association between disease and environment is only seen in specific subjects exposed to a specific environment. If the association between the environment and disease is limited to specific workers and to particular sites and types of disease and there is no association between the work and other fatal illnesses, there clearly is a strong argument supporting causation. Hill's principle of specificity is perhaps the most difficult to satisfy in neuropsychology given the nonspecific nature of symptomatic complaints (cf. Lees-Haley & Brown, 1993) and the fact that deficits in attention, memory, and executive functions can be seen in a variety of neurobehavioral disorders. The process of careful differential diagnosis advocated in this section is particularly essential because of the low specificity of these complaints and performance patterns.

Hill's (1965) fourth causal factor, *temporality*, refers to the temporal contingency between the environmental factor and development of disease. In one recent case of mine, memory complaints were present before the accident in question; indeed, there was a closer temporal relationship between the preaccident memory complaints and the accident than there was for onset of memory complaints following the accident.

Fifth is Hill's (1965) *biological gradient* or dose–response curve. Of course, this is related to Hill's first principle of strength, as well as to my recommendation to analyze data, particularly for cases of closed head injury, in relation to the severity of initial trauma, referred to as biological indexing or referencing (Larrabee, 1990; also see Rohling et al., 2003). Bolla discusses the importance of analyzing dose–response in chapter 9, this volume.

Hill's (1965) sixth factor, *plausibility*, refers to the biological plausibility of the purported causal relationship. Bolla provides additional discussion of biological plausibility in chapter 9 on neurotoxic injury in this volume. As she argues, if several animal studies show that a particularly high level of exposure to a specific chemical does not produce any health effects in animals, then there is little reason to suspect that health effects would be produced in humans at a lower level.

The seventh causal factor posited by Hill (1965) is that of *coherence*. Hill stated that the cause-and-effect interpretation of data should not seriously conflict with the natural history and biology of a particular disease or disorder. An example of a failure to consider this principle is the interpretation of severe memory impairment as indicative of sequelae of uncomplicated MTBI when this is *not* characteristic of the natural history of MTBI (see chapter 7, this volume).

Hill's (1965) eighth factor, *experiment*, allows for demonstration of a causal relationship between environment and disease by manipulating an environmental factor and then evaluating the results. For example, taking some preventive action that consequently lowers the incidence of the disease, such as reducing dust in the workplace and finding a reduction in a particular disease. Experiment or quasi-experiment can provide the strongest evidence for the causation hypothesis. Chapters 7 and 9 in this volume discuss the importance of careful control of competing variables in research on the outcome of MTBI and neurotoxic injury, respectively.

Analogy is Hill's (1965) ninth factor for demonstrating a causal association. As an example, Hill noted that, given the known effects of thalidomide and rubella on fetal development, doctors would be prepared to accept slighter but similar evidence regarding another drug or another viral disease in pregnancy.

Hill (1965) pointed out that none of his nine factors can bring indisputable evidence for or against a cause–effect hypothesis, and none can be required as a sine qua non. Moreover, formal tests of significance cannot provide the answers to the nine factors, although these statistical tests can remind the investigator of the effects that chance can create; beyond that, statistics contribute nothing to the proof of the cause–effect hypothesis.

In summarizing Hill's points as they relate to neuropsychological decision making as well as the consistency analysis I advocate, everything must make "neuropsychological sense" (Larrabee, 1990; Stuss, 1995). When significant departures from Hill's principles are observed or inconsistencies appear in the neuropsychological data, diagnoses other than the injury or illness alleged by the litigant must be considered, including the possibility of invalid test performance.

CLASSIFICATION STATISTICS IN
NEUROPSYCHOLOGICAL DIAGNOSIS

Similar to clinical psychology research in general, neuropsychological research has relied primarily on null hypothesis significance testing. Such testing can yield statistically significant mean differences between reference groups on a given dependent variable that do not necessarily either reflect a clinically meaningful finding or provide clinically useful information (Woods, Weinborn, & Lovejoy, 2003). In contrast, classification accuracy statistics do provide information diagnostically important in individual clinical use (Baldessarini et al., 1983; Glaros & Kline, 1988; Meehl & Rosen, 1955).

Traditional classification accuracy statistics include sensitivity, specificity, hit rates, predictive values, and odds ratios (Baldessarini et al., 1983; Glaros & Kline, 1988; Ivnik et al., 2001; Woods et al., 2003). As defined in this chapter, sensitivity refers to the proportion of patients with a given disorder who show a characteristic of interest (i.e., an impaired neuropsychological test score), defined as True positives/(True positives + False negatives). Specificity refers to the proportion of control subjects or some other reference sample without the characteristic of interest (i.e., who have nonimpaired neuropsychological test scores), defined as True negatives/(True negatives + False positives). A *hit rate* index describes the total proportion of accurately classified cases, (True positives + True negatives)/*N*.

It is not uncommon that when cutting scores are derived to define sensitivity, specificity, and hit rate, these cutting scores are based on equal sample sizes of persons (a) with a given disorder, such as TBI, and (b) those without the given disorder, such as normal or nonneurological medical orthopedic patient control subjects (cf. Dikmen et al., 1995). This essentially sets the base rate or frequency of occurrence of the disorder at 50%, which may not be the actual base rate in the total population (also see Baldessarini et al., 1983). Predictive value statistics do take into account the population base rate of the disorder in question. Theoretically, sensitivity and specificity are independent of the base rate or prevalence of illness in the population tested (Baldessarini et al., 1983). Positive predictive power (PPP; also referred to as positive predictive value, PPV) is the ratio of true positive scores to total positive scores: True positive/(True positive + False positive). PPP reflects the probability of the *presence* of a disease or disorder given a positive test finding. Negative predictive power (NPP; also referred to as negative predictive value, NPV) is the ratio of true negatives to total negative scores, True negatives/(True negatives + False negatives), and reflects the probability of the *absence* of a disease or disorder given a negative test finding.

Odds ratios or likelihood ratios reflect the likelihood that a person who achieves an impaired test score has the disorder of interest in comparison to an individual who performs within normal limits (Ivnik et al., 2001). Per Woods et al. (2003) and Ivnik et al. (2001), the odds ratio is computed as [(True positive)(True negative)]/[(False positive)(False negative)]. Obviously, sensitivity, specificity, and odds ratios are dependent on the setting of a particular cutting score for the determination of abnormality. PPP and NPP are dependent on sensitivity, specificity, *and* prevalence of the condition of interest.

By plotting true-positive rates and false-positive rates for different cutting scores on a particular test, the receiver operating characteristic (also known as the relative operating characteristic) of the test can be determined (Hsaio, Bartko, & Potter, 1989; Swets, 1973). The area under the curve generated by the different cutting scores and their associated true-positive and false-positive rates give the overall diagnostic efficiency of the test, with an upper limit of 1.0 (perfect diagnostic accuracy) and a lower limit of 0.50 (chance).

Baldessarini et al. (1983) provided the formula for computing PPP and NPP. Sensitivity is represented as x; specificity is represented as y; prevalence (base rate) is represented as p.

$$PPP = [(p)(x)]/[(p)(x) + (1 - p)(1 - y)].$$
$$NPP = [(1 - p)(y)]/[(1 - p)(y) + (p)(1 - x)].$$

Baldessarini et al. (1983) provided an example demonstrating the effect of prevalence/base rate on PPP and NPP from a study employing the dexamethasone suppression test as an indicator of the presence of major depression. In the original study sample, 100 depressed patients were compared to 100 neurotic patients, creating a prevalence/base rate of depression of 50%. Of the 100 depressed patients, 70 were identified as depressed (true positives), and 30 were misidentified (false negatives), giving a sensitivity of 70. Of the 100 neurotic patients, 5 tested positive for depression (false negatives), whereas 95 tested negative for depression, yielding a specificity of 95%. In the original derivation sample, the PPP was 70 (true positive)/(70 true positive + 5 false positive), which equals 70/75 or 93.3%. Similarly, derived via the formula, [(0.5)(0.7)]/[(0.5)(0.7) + (1 - 0.5)(1 - 0.95)], PPP is 93.3%. NPP is (95 true negative) + (30 false negative), which equals 95/125 or 76.0%. Also, derived via the formula, NPP is [(1 - 0.5)(0.95)]/[(1 - 0.5)(0.95) + (0.5)(1 - 0.7)] = 0.76 or 76%.

Baldessarini et al. (1983) demonstrated the effect of change in prevalence/ base rate of depression on PPP and NPP for the test of depression. Moving from the derivation study in which the base rate of major depressive disorder was 50% to a general psychiatric practice in which the base rate of major depressive disorder was 10%, but keeping sensitivity at 70% and specificity at 95%, reduces PPP to 12.3%, but increases NPP to 99.7%.

Baldessarini et al. (1983) demonstrated a reciprocal relationship between PPP and NPP as a function of prevalence/base rate, with sensitivity and specificity held constant. At low prevalence/base rates, a negative test result is more likely to be true than a positive result. This results in a loss of PPP moving from an artificial setting in test populations with a high prevalence of an illness or condition of interest into more realistic clinical settings. The converse is true of NPP as a function of prevalence/base rate, with sensitivity and specificity held constant. Thus, at high prevalence/base rates, a positive test result is more likely to be true than a negative test result.

When prevalence/base rate is held constant, PPP is affected more by changes in specificity, that is, when the rate of false positives is low. Conversely, NPP is highest when sensitivity is high, that is, when the rate of false negatives is low (Baldessarini et al., 1983).

The overall accuracy of a test cutting score is a function of the positive and negative base rates in the population as well as the positive and false-positive rates associated with the cutting score (Meehl & Rosen, 1955). The ratio of the positive base rate P to the negative base rate Q must be greater than the ratio of the false-positive rate p_2 to the true-positive rate p_1, or $P/Q > p_2/p_1$. Stated otherwise (Gouvier, 1999), the combined error rate of a test must be smaller than the base rate of the condition that the test is designed to detect.

As reviewed by Woods et al. (2003), classification statistics, particularly those related to PPP, NPP, and odds ratios, are underused in neuropsychological research. Indeed, in their review of five prominent neuropsychology journals published during the years 2000 and 2001, only 31% of neuropsychology articles published indices of sensitivity, with fewer than 3% reporting predictive values or risk ratios.

Two studies in which I have been involved provide a further perspective on PPP and NPP. In the first, Binder, Rohling, and Larrabee (1997) determined 5% prevalence of chronic persisting neuropsychological deficit following MTBI. Assuming sensitivity of 80% and specificity of 88% for neuropsychological tests (using the Heaton, Grant, & Matthews, 1991, data, and an Average Impairment Rating cut score of T score = 39), PPP for neuropsychological detection of persisting impairment following MTBI was .26, with NPP at .99, at the base rate of 5%. Thus, a clinician is more likely to be correct when diagnosing no persisting impairment in MTBI.

I (2003) developed a five-variable algorithm for detection of malingering based on atypical (for moderate or severe TBI) performance on any two (or three) variables, including Benton Visual Form Discrimination (Benton, Sivan, Hamsher, Varney, & Spreen, 1994), Finger Tapping, Reliable Digit Span (Greiffenstein, Baker, & Gola, 1994), Wisconsin Card Sorting Failure to Maintain Set, and the Lees-Haley Fake Bad Scale (Lees-Haley, English, & Glenn, 1991). Based on a positive score (i.e., in the malingering range) on any two of the five indicators, sensitivity for detection of definite or probable malingered neurocognitive dysfunction (Slick, Sherman, & Iverson, 1999) was .878 and specificity (for correct detection of moderate/severe TBI, neurological or psychiatric patients) was .944. Using a base rate of malingering of 40% in litigated minor head injury (Larrabee, 2003; Mittenberg, Patton, Canyock, & Condit, 2002), PPP for this formula was .913, with NPP of .921.

SCIENTIFIC STATUS OF NEUROPSYCHOLOGICAL TESTING

This section provides a brief overview of general issues related to the scientific status of neuropsychological test procedures. This is by no means an exhaustive review, and the reader is directed to more comprehensive reviews, including the widely referenced texts by Lezak, Howieson, and Loring (2004) and Spreen and Strauss (1998).

The discipline of neuropsychology in America dates to the 1940s and 1950s with the establishment of laboratories by Arthur Benton, Ward Halstead, and Ralph Reitan (Reitan & Wolfson, 1996; Tranel, 1996). During this same time period, laboratories were formed by Zangwill in England and Hécaen in France, and Luria had initiated his investigations in Russia (Soviet Union) (Hécaen & Albert, 1978; Luria, 1966; McFie, 1975). As currently practiced, neuropsychology has benefited from psychometric influences (e.g., principles of test construction, methodology for determining reliability and validity), developments in experimental psychology (e.g., signal detection methodology; information-processing models), and behavioral neurology (Larrabee & Crook, 1988; Lezak et al., 2004; Milberg, Hebben, & Kaplan, 1996).

Psychological and neuropsychological testing has established validity, comparable to the validity of tests used in clinical medicine (Meyer et al., 2001). A meta-analytic review by Zakzanis, Leach, and Kaplan (1999) demonstrated varying patterns of effect sizes for measures of verbal and performance skill, attention, memory, cognitive flexibility/abstraction, and manual dexterity as a function of different neurobehavioral disorders such as AD, frontotemporal dementia, Parkinson's disease, multiple sclerosis, Huntington's disease and as a function of psychiatric disorders such as schizophrenia and major depressive disorder. Neuropsychological testing of adults is accepted by neurologists as "established," with Class II evidence and Type A recommendation, and was found by the Therapeutics and Technology Assessment Subcommittee of the American Academy of Neurology (AAN) to be appropriate for a wide range of neurological disorders, including TBI, cerebrovascular disease, Parkinson's disease, HIV encephalopathy, multiple sclerosis, epilepsy, and neurotoxic exposure ("Assessment: Neuropsychological Testing of Adults," 1996). In particular, the AAN views neuropsychological documentation as critical in cases where litigation concerns the presence of cognitive impairment ("Assessment: Neuropsychological Testing," 1996). Although some have questioned certain conclusions reached by the Technology and Therapeutics Subcommittee (Reynolds, 2001), "These criticisms aside, the AAN report does make a positive contribution to the field of neuropsychology and concludes by recommending that neuropsychological assessment of adults has value to neurologists in particular circumstances" (p. 200).

Some have stated that certain fixed battery neuropsychological test procedures such as the HRB or Luria Nebraska Neuropsychological Battery (LNNB; Golden, Purisch, & Hammeke, 1985) are the only acceptably validated procedures for use in forensic neuropsychology (Hom, 2003; McKinzey, 2000). In contrast, a survey by Lees-Haley, Smith, Williams, and Dunn (1996) found, in a review of 100 forensic neuropsychological evaluations conducted in 20 states and in the province of Ontario, Canada, that the HRB and LNNB were rarely used. Lees-Haley et al. found that only 10% used the LNNB, and approximately 21% used the HRB, contrasted with 75% that used the WAIS-R, 68% that used the Minnesota Multiphasic Personality Inventory (MMPI; Hathaway & McKinley, 1983)/MMPI-2 (Butcher, Dahlstrom, Graham, Tellegen, & Kaemmer, 1989), and 51% that used the WMS (Wechsler, 1945) and WMS-R. These percentages make it difficult to argue that fixed batteries are the standard of practice in forensic settings.

Recommendations for the use of the HRB or LNNB over other neuropsychological procedures are not supported by empirical studies that have compared both batteries to the WAIS (Wechsler, 1955), WAIS-R, or Auditory Verbal Learning Test (Rey, 1964). Based on WAIS IQ scores and global impairment scores for the HRB and LNNB, Kane, Parsons, and Goldstein (1985) found essentially equivalent classification of brain damage versus control subjects. Sherer, Scott, Parsons, and Adams (1994) also found that the WAIS-R and HRB were equivalent in sensitivity to the presence of brain damage.

Chelune (1982) attributed the equivalent sensitivity to brain damage of the HRB and LNNB to the variance these procedures share with WAIS IQ. The equivalent sensitivity of the WAIS/WAIS-R and HRB for brain damage is further understood as a function of shared underlying (neuro)psychological constructs of (a) visuospatial reasoning and problem solving, (b) attention/concentration, and (c) psychomotor speed (Larrabee, 2000a; Leonberger, Nicks, Larrabee, & Goldfader, 1992).

Memory is only weakly assessed on the original LNNB (Larrabee, Kane, Schuck, & Francis, 1985) and is not assessed at all on the HRB (Leonberger et al., 1992). This explains why J. B. Powell, Cripe, and Dodrill (1991) found that the Auditory Verbal Learning Test, particularly Trial 5, was more sensitive than any other single test on the HRB, as well as more sensitive than the HRB Impairment Index, in discriminating normal subjects from a group of subjects with a variety of neurological disorders.

Dikmen et al. (1995), in their study of long-term sequence of TBI, found that the two most sensitive tests (i.e., the first tests to pick up, as a function of head trauma severity, differences in performance 1-year status postinjury) were the Verbal Selective Reminding Test and Trail Making B for the head-injured subjects who took between 1 and 24 hours to follow commands. The HRB Impairment Index did not show differences in 1-year outcome until TBI severity reached 25 hours to 6 days of coma (with coma defined by time to follow commands). Last, Rohling et al. (2003) found that a flexible battery, employing a core set of tests of language, spatial judgment, motor and tactile function, verbal and visual learning and memory, and intelligence and problem solving, showed the same dose–response association with head injury severity found by Dikmen et al. (1995), who used an HRB augmented by the WAIS and memory procedures such as the Verbal Selective Reminding test.

As demonstrated by Rohling et al. (2003), what is important in conducting neuropsychological evaluation is that the examination, using standardized and validated tests, should cover the key areas of neuropsychological function. These core neuropsychological functions include language, perceptual/spatial ability, sensorimotor function (particularly manual motor function), attention and information processing, psychomotor speed, verbal and visual learning and memory, intellectual and problem-solving skills, academic functions, personality, and motivation ("Assessment: Neuropsychological Testing of Adults," 1996; Larrabee, 2000a; Lezak et al., 2004; Spreen & Strauss, 1998; Zakzanis et al., 1999).

Multiple measures are recommended for each of the above areas of function; for example, Finger Tapping, Grip Strength (Reitan & Wolfson, 1993), and the Grooved Pegboard can be used to assess manual motor function. This recommendation goes counter to Wedding and Faust's (1989) recommendation to avoid reliance on highly intercorrelated measures. Wedding and Faust argued that, to the extent tests are redundant, using a second test merely remeasures what the first test does, and diagnostic or predictive accuracy is minimally increased. This observation is certainly true if and only if the clinician's sole concern was the reliability and validity of test scores. However, this is not the case in clinical and forensic neuropsychology, for which the reliability and validity of the individual participant's performance is also at issue (see chapter 4 on malingering). Thus, inclusion of multiple measures of each domain, some easier, some more difficult, allows analysis of within-domain consistency of performance.

As an example employing multiple measures of motor function, Greiffenstein, Baker, and Gola (1996) studied patients with severe TBI who also had unambiguous motor abnormalities on standard neurological examination and found these subjects had different patterns of motor performance on Finger Tapping, Grip Strength, and the Grooved Pegboard test, in comparison to the motor performance patterns of litigants with persistent post-concussion syndrome. The patients with severe TBI performed less well on the Grooved Pegboard relative to Finger Tapping and Grip Strength, whereas the litigants with persistent postconcussion syndrome showed the opposite pattern, performing better on the Grooved Pegboard in comparison to Finger Tapping and Grip Strength.

Some have argued for predicting expected levels of neuropsychological test performance based on estimated premorbid IQ (Tremont, Hoffman, Scott, &

Adams, 1998). This approach is only applicable if there is a correlation of a particular neuropsychological test with IQ; even then, there can be considerable regression to the mean, particularly if there is no preexisting IQ test, and IQ itself must be estimated (Larrabee, 2000a). For example, Tremont et al. (1998) found that the Category Test correlated .5 with Full Scale IQ (FIQ). In someone for whom preinjury testing was unavailable but who actually had a "true" premorbid IQ of 130, the estimated premorbid IQ based on a multiple R of .60 (Barona, Reynolds, & Chastain, 1984) would be 118 (1.2 SD above the mean). If the expected Category Test score was then estimated on the basis of this estimated IQ, the predicted Category Test score would be .5 × 1.2 or .6 SD above the mean, for a T-score equivalent of 56 (standard error of estimate of 8.66) or an IQ-equivalent score of 109 (standard error of estimate of 12.99).

Estimated premorbid IQ scores themselves have large standard errors of estimate (SEEs) when based on demographic factors (Barona et al., 1984; range of SEE is 12 to 13 IQ points). The size of the SEE can be reduced using current function measures such as the Wechsler Test of Adult Reading (WTAR), in combination with demographic factors, but the WTAR itself must be estimated based on demographic factors to ensure the score has not been affected by brain dysfunction (Psychological Corporation, 2001). Although the WTAR can be useful for estimating premorbid IQ, it is not useful for predicting premorbid memory function (Psychological Corporation, 2001).

Some have advocated using performance on current IQ subtests that are resistant to effects of cerebral dysfunction (i.e., "hold" tests) or picking the highest subtest scores on current IQ testing (the "best performance method"; see Lezak et al., 2004) to estimate premorbid IQ. Krull, Scott, and Sherer (1995) and Scott, Krull, Williamson, Adams, and Iverson (1997) have developed a procedure for predicting premorbid IQ that combines demographic information with current performance on the Vocabulary and Picture Completion subtests of the WAIS-R, the Oklahoma Premorbid Intelligence Estimate (OPIE).

B. D. Powell, Brossart, and Reynolds (2003) compared the OPIE procedure to Barona et al.'s (1984) demographic estimation of premorbid IQ in both normal and clinical patients and found that the OPIE was less sensitive (i.e., predicted lower premorbid IQ) in the clinical sample. This is not unexpected because the OPIE ignores regression to the mean effects and contaminates the predictor (Vocabulary and Picture Completion subtests) with the criterion (IQ; i.e., the Vocabulary and Picture Completion subtests are used to predict IQ, which is also based partly on the Vocabulary and Picture Completion subtests).

Finally, performance on WAIS-R subtests such as Vocabulary or Picture Completion that are thought to be less sensitive to the effects of brain damage can still be affected by brain dysfunction. Specifically, Larrabee, Largen, and Levin (1984) found that using performance on hold or best-performance WAIS subtests to estimate premorbid IQ underestimated premorbid level of function by a full standard deviation or more for subjects who had mild-to-moderate AD compared to WAIS IQ scores produced by normal controls matched on age, education, and gender. Although coworkers and I (Larrabee et al., 1984) did not employ Vocabulary in our investigation, the Information subtest mean for the AD patients was 3.0 age-scaled score points lower than that of the age-, education-, and gender-matched controls, with the Picture Completion subtest mean falling 5.44 age-scaled score points lower for the AD patients.

The point of the discussion is that estimation of premorbid neuropsychological ability is a risky enterprise. In my opinion, the clinician is better off using neuropsychological test procedures that have been carefully standardized on the basis of relevant demographic factors such as age, education, and gender (cf. Heaton et al., 1991, but note the concerns of Fastenau, 1998). By evaluating and adjusting for demographic factors related to test performance during test norming and development, essentially the test procedures are precorrected for premorbid level of function. In this vein, Heaton, Taylor, and Manly (2003) developed demographically corrected norms for the WAIS-III and WMS-III. Review of preinjury standardized test scores is also helpful for establishing the level of preinjury function, but provides information typically related to academic achievement and less often to intellectual level of function.

As discussed in this chapter, the actual neuropsychological data must be interpreted in the context of other data using appropriate scientific judgment and reasoning. Use of a large number of tests can result in abnormal scores in entirely normal individuals. In an expanded HRB consisting of 40 scores, only 10% of Heaton et al.'s (1991) normal adults produced no scores falling at a T-score of ≤ 39 (defined as abnormal). The group median in Heaton et al.'s normal adult sample was 4 abnormal scores of 40, and 45% of the sample had anywhere from 5 to 20 scores falling at $T \leq 39$.

Ingraham and Aiken (1996) presented an empirical approach to determine abnormality in test batteries with multiple measures; for example, in a battery with 30 scores in which the criterion is 3 tests falling at 1 SD below the mean, the probability is nearly .90 that this will occur by chance. Note that Ingraham and Aiken based their computations on *independent* scores, which is likely not the case in an actual test battery. Ingraham and Aiken argued that correlated scores reduce the likelihood of abnormal findings; hence, the probabilities are likely somewhat overestimated.

Determination of abnormalities in performance based on test score variability depends on the range of variability in normal subjects, which can be quite large. Schretlen, Munro, Anthony, and Pearlson (2003) studied the maximum range between a normal subject's highest and lowest scores on 32 z-transformed scores derived from 15 neuropsychological tests. The smallest maximum difference was 1.6 *SD*, with the largest maximum difference 6.1 *SD*. Again, knowledge of the literature pertaining to patterns of performance in different neurobehavioral disorders and use of the judgment strategies recommended in this chapter can reduce the risk of making an erroneous conclusion of deficit, when the pattern of performance is actually the result of nonpathological normal variability or random factors.

SUMMARY

This chapter reviewed scientific factors relevant to the practice of forensic neuropsychology. The scientific method was reviewed, including the hypothetico-deductive approach, with particular emphasis on the importance of seeking disconfirming evidence to strengthen both scientific and diagnostic hypotheses. Factors related to diagnostic error were reviewed, including faulty use of logic, illusory correlation, hindsight bias, and confirmation bias. Recommendations for effective diagnostic formulations aimed at reducing judgmental bias were made, and statistics relevant to diagnostic decision making were reviewed, including discussion of base rates, sensitivity, specificity, and positive and negative predictive power. Finally, general issues relevant to neuropsychological testing in forensic settings were considered.

The remainder of this book expands on the science of forensic neuropsychology. All of the contributors are actively involved in empirical research in neuropsychology and are respected and well-known scientist/clinicians. The cumulative aspect of science is represented by chapters that present up-to-date reviews of major areas of concern, including assessment of malingering (chapter 4), acquired brain damage in children (chapter 6), MTBI (chapter 7), moderate-to-severe TBI (chapter 8), neurotoxic injury (chapter 9), and functional neuroimaging (chapter 5).

The special circumstances in which the scientist/clinician must effectively communicate results to attorneys and the court is covered in chapter 2. Issues pertinent to civil and criminal competencies and criminal responsibilities are addressed in chapters 11–13. In particular, chapter 11 demonstrates a cutting-edge scientific approach to the assessment of competencies in the elderly. Chapter 10 provides a new perspective on somatoform stress disorders that is important in performing differential diagnosis of litigants/defendants, and the ethics of appropriate forensic practice are addressed in chapter 3.

ACKNOWLEDGMENT

I acknowledge the assistance of Bridgette O'Brien in the preparation of this chapter.

REFERENCES

Army Individual Test Battery. (1944). *Manual of directions and scoring*. Washington, DC: War Department. Adjutant General's Office.

Assessment: Neuropsychological testing of adults. Considerations for neurologists. Report of the Therapeutics and Technology Assessment Subcommittee of the American Academy of Neurology. (1996). *Neurology, 47*, 592–599.

Badia, P., & Runyon, R. P. (1982). *Fundamentals of behavioral research*. Reading, MA: Addison-Wesley.

Baldessarini, R. J., Finklestein, S., & Arana, G. W. (1983). The predictive power of diagnostic tests and the effect of prevalence of illness. *Archives of General Psychiatry, 40*, 569–573.

Barona, A., Reynolds, C. R., & Chastain, R. (1984). A demographically based index of premorbid intelligence for the WAIS-R. *Journal of Consulting and Clinical Psychology, 52*, 885–887.

Benton, A. L., Sivan, A. B., Hamsher, K. deS., Varney, N. R., & Spreen, O. (1994). *Contributions to neuropsychological assessment. A clinical manual* (2nd ed.). New York: Oxford University Press.

Binder, L. M. (1997). A review of mild head trauma. Part II: Clinical implications. *Journal of Clinical and Experimental Neuropsychology, 19*, 432–457.

Binder, L. M., Rohling, M. L., & Larrabee, G. J. (1997). A review of mild head trauma. Part I: Meta-analytic review of neuropsychological studies. *Journal of Clinical and Experimental Neuropsychology, 19*, 421–431.

Buschke, H. (1973). Selective reminding for analysis of memory and learning. *Journal of Verbal Learning and Verbal Behavior, 12*, 543–550.

Butcher, J. N., Dahlstrom, W. G., Graham, J. R., Tellegen, A., & Kaemmer, B. (1989). *Minnesota Multiphasic Personality Inventory-2 (MMPI-2). Manual for administration and scoring*. Minneapolis: University of Minnesota Press.

Chapman, L. J., & Chapman, J. P. (1967). Genesis of popular but erroneous psychodiagnostic observations. *Journal of Abnormal Psychology, 72*, 193–204.

Chapman, L. J., & Chapman, J. P. (1969). Illusory correlation as an obstacle to the use of valid psychodiagnostic signs. *Journal of Abnormal Psychology, 74*, 271–280.

Chelune, G. J. (1982). A reexamination of the relationship between the Luria-Nebraska and Halstead-Reitan Batteries: Overlap with the WAIS. *Journal of Consulting and Clinical Psychology, 50*, 578–580.

Daubert v. Merrell Dow, 509 U.S. 579 (1993).

Delis, D. C., Kramer, J. H., Kaplan, E., & Ober, B. A. (2000). *CVLT-II. California Verbal Learning Test. Second edition. Adult version*. San Antonio, TX: The Psychological Corporation.

Dikmen, S. S., Machamer, J. E., Winn, H. R., & Temkin, N. R. (1995). Neuropsychological outcome at 1-year post head injury. *Neuropsychology, 9*, 80–90.

Fastenau, P. S. (1998). Validity of regression-based norms: An empirical test of the comprehensive norms with older adults. *Journal of Clinical and Experimental Neuropsychology, 20*, 906–916.

Faust, D. (1989). Data integration in legal evaluations: Can clinicians deliver on their premises? *Behavioral Sciences and the Law, 7*, 469–483.

Faust, D., & Nurcombe, B. (1989). Improving the accuracy of clinical judgement. *Psychiatry, 52*, 197–208.

Faust, D., Ziskin, J., & Hiers, J. B. (1991). *Brain damage claims*: *Coping with neuropsychological evidence* (Vol. 1). Los Angeles: Law and Psychology Press.

Feynman, R. P. (with R. Leighton). (1985). *Surely you're joking, Mr. Feynman*: *Adventures of a curious character.* New York: Norton.

Frye v. United States (D.C. Cir. 1923) 293 F. 1013.

Glaros, A. G., & Kline, R. B. (1988). Understanding the accuracy of tests with cutting scores: The sensitivity, specificity, and predictive value model. *Journal of Clinical Psychology, 44*, 1013–1023.

Golden, C. J., Purisch, A. D., & Hammeke, T. A. (1985). *Luria-Nebraska Neuropsychological Battery*: *Forms I and II.* Los Angeles: Western Psychological Services.

Gouvier, W. D. (1999). Base rates and clinical decision making in clinical neuropsychology. In J. J. Sweet (Ed.), *Forensic neuropsychology. Fundamentals and practice* (pp. 27–37). Lisse, The Netherlands: Swets and Zeitlinger.

Greiffenstein, M. F., Baker, W. J., & Gola, T. (1994). Validation of malingered amnesia measures with a large clinical sample. *Psychological Assessment, 6*, 218–224.

Greiffenstein, M. F., Baker, W. J., & Gola, T. (1996). Motor dysfunction profiles in traumatic brain injury and post-concussion syndrome. *Journal of the International Neuropsychological Society, 2*, 477–485.

Gronwall, D. M. A. (1977). Paced auditory serial addition task: A measure of recovery from concussion. *Perceptual and Motor Skills, 44*, 367–373.

Hannay, H. J., & Levin, H. S. (1985). Selective Reminding Test: An examination of the equivalence of four forms. *Journal of Clinical and Experimental Neuropsychology, 7*, 251–263.

Hathaway, S. R., & McKinley, J. C. (1983). *The Minnesota Multiphasic Personality Inventory manual.* New York: The Psychological Corporation.

Heaton, R., Taylor, M. J., & Manly, J. (2003). Demographic effects and use of demographically corrected norms with the WAIS-III and WMS-III. In D. S. Tulsky, D. H. Saklofske, G. J. Chelune, R. K. Heaton, R. J. Ivnik, R. Bornstein, et al. (Eds.), *Clinical interpretation of the WAIS-III and WMS-III* (pp. 181–210), San Diego, CA: Academic Press.

Heaton, R. K., Chelune, G. J., Talley, J. L., Kay, G. G., & Curtiss, G. (1993). *Wisconsin Card Sorting Test manual. Revised and expanded.* Odessa, FL: Psychological Assessment Resources.

Heaton, R. K., Grant, I., & Matthews, C. G. (1991). *Comprehensive norms for an expanded Halstead-Reitan Battery*: *Demographic corrections, research findings, and clinical applications.* Odessa, FL: Psychological Assessment Resources.

Hécaen, H., & Albert, M. L. (1978). *Human neuropsychology.* New York: Wiley.

Hempel, C. G. (1966). *Philosophy of natural science.* Englewood Cliffs, NJ: Prentice-Hall.

Hill, A. B. (1965). The environment and disease. Association and causation. *Proceedings of the Royal Society of Medicine, 58*, 295–300.

Hom, J. (2003). Forensic neuropsychology: Are we there yet? *Archives of Clinical Neuropsychology, 18*, 827–845.

Hsiao, J. K., Bartko, J. J., & Potter, W. Z. (1989). Diagnosing diagnoses. Receiver operating characteristic methods and psychiatry. *Archives of General Psychiatry, 46*, 664–667.

Ingraham, L. J., & Aiken, C. B. (1996). An empirical approach to determining criteria for abnormality in test batteries with multiple measures. *Neuropsychology, 10*, 120–124.

Ivnik, R. J., Smith, G. E., Cerhan, J. H., Boeve, B. F., Tangalos, E. G., & Peterson, R. C. (2001). Understanding the diagnostic capabilities of cognitive tests. *The Clinical Neuropsychologist, 15*, 114–124.

Kane, R. L., Parsons, O. A., & Goldstein, G. (1985). Statistical relationships and discriminative accuracy of the Halstead-Reitan, Luria-Nebraska, and Wechsler IQ scores in the identification of brain damage. *Journal of Clinical and Experimental Neuropsychology, 7*, 211–233.

Kerlinger, F. N. (1973). *Foundations of behavioral research* (2nd ed.). New York: Holt, Rinehart, and Winston.

Krull, K. R., Scott, J. G., & Sherer, M. (1995). Estimation of premorbid intelligence from combined performance and demographic variables. *The Clinical Neuropsychologist, 9*, 83–88.

Kurtz, R. M., & Garfield, S. L. (1978). Illusory correlation: A further exploration of Chapman's paradigm. *Journal of Consulting and Clinical Psychology, 46*, 1009–1015.

Larrabee, G. J. (1990). Cautions in the use of neuropsychological evaluation in legal settings. *Neuropsychology, 4*, 239–247.

Larrabee, G. J. (1992). Interpretive strategies for evaluation of neuropsychological data in legal settings. *Forensic Reports, 5*, 257–264.

Larrabee, G. J. (1997). Neuropsychological outcome, post concussion symptoms, and forensic considerations in mild closed head trauma. *Seminars in Clinical Neuropsychiatry, 2*, 196–206.

Larrabee, G. J. (2000a). Association between IQ and neuropsychological test performance: Commentary on Tremont, Hoffman, Scott, and Adams (1998). *The Clinical Neuropsychologist, 14*, 139–145.

Larrabee, G. J. (2000b). Forensic neuropsychological assessment. In R. D. Vanderploeg (Ed.), *Clinician's guide to neuropsychological assessment* (2nd ed., pp. 301–335). Mahwah, NJ: Erlbaum.

Larrabee, G. J. (2003). Detection of malingering using atypical performance patterns on standard neuropsychological tests. *The Clinical Neuropsychologist, 17*, 410–425.

Larrabee, G. J., & Crook, T. H. (1988). Assessment of drug effects in age-related memory disorders: Clinical, theoretical, and psychometric considerations. *Psychopharmacology Bulletin, 24*, 515–522.

Larrabee, G. J., Kane, R. L., Schuck, J. R., & Francis, D. E. (1985). The construct validity of various memory testing procedures. *Journal of Clinical and Experimental Neuropsychology, 7*, 239–250.

Larrabee, G. J., Largen, J. W., & Levin, H. S. (1984). Sensitivity of age-decline resistant ("hold") WAIS subtests to Alzheimer's disease. *Journal of Clinical and Experimental Neuropsychology, 7*, 497–504.

Larrabee, G. J., Trahan, D. E., & Levin, H. S. (2000). Normative data for a six-trial administration of the Verbal Selective Reminding Test. *The Clinical Neuropsychologist, 14*, 110–118.

Lees-Haley, P. R., & Brown, R. (1993). Neuropsychological complaint base rates of 170 personal injury claimants. *Archives of Clinical Neuropsychology, 8*, 203–209.

Lees-Haley, P. R., English, L. T., & Glenn, W. J. (1991). A fake bad scale on the MMPI-2 for personal injury claimants. *Psychological Reports, 68*, 203–210.

Lees-Haley, P. R., Smith, H. H., Williams, C. W., & Dunn, J. T. (1996). Forensic neuropsychological test usage: An empirical survey. *Archives of Clinical Neuropsychology, 11*, 45–51.

Leonberger, F. T., Nicks, S. D., Larrabee, G. J., & Goldfader, P. R. (1992). Factor structure of the Wechsler Memory Scale-Revised within a comprehensive neuropsychological battery. *Neuropsychology, 6,* 239–249.

Lezak, M. D., Howieson, D. B., & Loring, D. W. (2004). *Neuropsychological assessment* (4th ed.). New York: Oxford University Press.

Lilienfeld, S. O., Lynn, S. J., & Lohr, J. M. (2003). Science and pseudoscience in clinical psychology. In S. O. Lilienfeld, S. J. Lynn, & J. M. Lohr (Eds.), *Science and pseudoscience in clinical psychology* (pp. 1–14). New York: Guilford Press.

Luria, A. R. (1966). *Higher cortical functions in man.* New York: Basic Books.

McFie, J. (1975). *Assessment of organic intellectual impairment.* New York: Academic Press.

McKinzey, R. K. (2000). A research update: Neuropsychological assessment. *For the Defense, 23,* 62–63.

Meehl, P. E. (1978). Theoretical risks or tabular asterisks: Sir Karl, Sir Ronald, and the slow progress of soft psychology. *Journal of Consulting and Clinical Psychology, 46,* 816–834.

Meehl, P. E., & Rosen, A. (1955). Antecedent probability and the efficiency of psychometric signs, patterns, or cutting scores. *Psychological Bulletin, 52,* 194–216.

Meyer, G. J., Finn, S. E., Eyde, L. D., Moreland, K. L., Dies, R. R., Eisman, E. J., et al. (2001). Psychological testing and psychological assessment. A review of evidence and issues. *American Psychologist, 56,* 128–165.

Milberg, W. P., Hebben, N., & Kaplan, E. (1996). The Boston Process Approach to neuropsychological assessment. In I. Grant & K. M. Adams (Eds.), *Neuropsychological assessment of neuropsychiatric disorders* (2nd ed., pp. 58–80). New York: Oxford University Press.

Miller, E. (1983). A note on the interpretation of data derived from neuropsychological tests. *Cortex, 19,* 131–132.

Miller, L. S., & Rohling, M. L. (2001). A statistical interpretive method for neuropsychological test data. *Neuropsychology Review, 11,* 143–169.

Mittenberg, W., Azrin, R., Millsaps, C., & Heilbronner, R. (1993). Identification of malingered head injury on the Wechsler Memory Scale-Revised. *Psychological Assessment, 5,* 34–40.

Mittenberg, W., Patton, C., Canyock, E. M., & Condit, D. C. (2002). Base rates of malingering and symptom exaggeration. *Journal of Clinical and Experimental Neuropsychology, 24,* 1094–1102.

Popper, K. R. (1959). *The logic of scientific discovery.* New York: Basic Books.

Powell, B. D., Brossart, D. F., & Reynolds, C. R. (2003). Evaluation of the accuracy of two regression-based methods for estimating premorbid IQ. *Archives of Clinical Neuropsychology, 18,* 277–292.

Powell, J. B., Cripe, L. I., & Dodrill, C. B. (1991). Assessment of brain impairment with the Rey Auditory Verbal Learning Test: A comparison with other neuropsychological measures. *Archives of Clinical Neuropsychology, 6,* 241–249.

Psychological Corporation. (2001). *WTAR. Wechsler Test of Adult Reading. Manual.* San Antonio, TX: Author.

Reitan, R. M., & Wolfson, D. (1993). *The Halstead-Reitan Neuropsychological Test Battery. Theory and clinical interpretation* (2nd ed.). South Tucson, AZ: Neuropsychology Press.

Reitan, R. M., & Wolfson, D. (1996). Theoretical, methodological, and validational bases of the Halstead-Reitan Neuropsychological Test Battery. In I. Grant & K. M. Adams (Eds.), *Neuropsychological assessment of neuropsychiatric disorders* (2nd ed., pp. 3–42). New York: Oxford University Press.

Rey, A. (1964). *L'examen clinique en psychologie* [The clinical examination in psychology]. Paris: Presses Universitaires de France.

Reynolds, C. R. (2001). Commentary on the American Academy of Neurology report on neuropsychological assessment. *Archives of Clinical Neuropsychology*, *16*, 199–200.

Rohling, M. L., Meyers, J. E., & Millis, S. R. (2003). Neuropsychological impairment following traumatic brain injury: A dose–response analysis. *The Clinical Neuropsychologist*, *17*, 289–302.

Russell, E. W. (1990, June). Twenty ways of diagnosing brain damage when there is none. Paper presented at the meeting of the Florida Psychological Association, St. Petersburg Beach, FL.

Russell, E. W., and Kolitz-Russell, S. L. (2003). Twenty ways and more of diagnosing brain damage when there is none. *Journal of Controversial Medical Claims*, *10*, 1–14.

Schretlen, D. J., Munro, C. A., Anthony, J. C., & Pearlson, G. D. (2003). Examining the range of normal intraindividual variability in neuropsychological test performance. *Journal of the International Neuropsychological Society*, *9*, 864–870.

Scott, J. G., Krull, K. R., Williamson, D. J. G., Adams, R. L., & Iverson, G. L. (1997). Oklahoma Premorbid Intelligence Estimation (OPIE): Utilization in clinical samples. *The Clinical Neuropsychologist*, *11*, 146–154.

Sherer, M., Scott, J. G., Parsons, O. A., & Adams, R. L. (1994). Relative sensitivity of the WAIS-R subtests and selected HRNB measures to the effects of brain damage. *Archives of Clinical Neuropsychology*, *9*, 427–436.

Slick, D. J., Sherman, E. M. S., & Iverson, G. L. (1999). Diagnostic criteria for malingered neurocognitive dysfunction: Proposed standards for clinical practice and research. *The Clinical Neuropsychologist*, *13*, 545–561.

Spreen, O., & Strauss, E. (1998). *A compendium of neuropsychological tests* (2nd ed.). New York: Oxford University Press.

Stuss, D. T. (1995). A sensible approach to mild traumatic brain injury. *Neurology*, *45*, 1251–1252.

Swets, J. A. (1973). The relative operating characteristic in psychology. *Science*, *182*, 990–1000.

Tranel, D. (1996). The Iowa-Benton School of neuropsychological assessment. In I. Grant & K. M. Adams (Eds.), *Neuropsychological assessment of neuropsychiatric disorders* (2nd ed., pp. 81–101). New York: Oxford University Press.

Tremont, G., Hoffman, R. G., Scott, J. G., & Adams, R. L. (1998). Effect of intellectual level on neuropsychological test performance: A response to Dodrill (1997). *The Clinical Neuropsychologist*, *12*, 560–567.

Trope, Y., Gervey, B., & Liberman, N. (1997). Wishful thinking from a pragmatic hypothesis-testing perspective. In M. S. Myslobodsky (Ed.), *The mythomanias: The nature of deception and self-deception* (pp. 105–131). Mahwah, NJ: Erlbaum.

Volbrecht, M. E., Meyers, J. E., & Kaster-Bundgaard, J. (2000). Neuropsychological outcome of head injury using a short battery. *Archives of Clinical Neuropsychology*, *15*, 251–265.

Wechsler, D. (1945). A standardized memory scale for clinical use. *Journal of Psychology*, *19*, 87–95.

Wechsler, D. (1955). *WAIS manual*. New York: The Psychological Corporation.

Wechsler, D. (1981). *WAIS-R manual*. New York: The Psychological Corporation.

Wechsler, D. (1987). *Wechsler Memory Scale–Revised manual*. San Antonio, TX: The Psychological Corporation.

Wechsler, D. (1997). *WAIS-III. Administration and scoring manual*. San Antonio, TX: The Psychological Corporation.

Wedding, D., & Faust, D. (1989). Clinical judgement and decision making in neuropsychology. *Archives of Clinical Neuropsychology*, *4*, 233–265.

Woods, S. P., Weinborn, M., & Lovejoy, D. W. (2003). Are classification accuracy statistics underused in neuropsychological research? *Journal of Clinical and Experimental Neuropsychology*, *25*, 431–439.

Zakzanis, K. K., Leach, L., & Kaplan, E. (1999). *Neuropsychological differential diagnosis*. Lisse, The Netherlands: Swets and Zeitlinger.

2

Neuropsychology and the Law: Principles of Productive Attorney– Neuropsychologist Relations

MANFRED F. GREIFFENSTEIN
LARRY COHEN

Forensic neuropsychology is defined as the presentation of neuropsychological evidence to answer legal questions. Neuropsychological testing for legal purposes has grown from the occasional referral to a critical component of private practice. There is much evidence for the growth of forensic neuropsychology. As reported by Sweet, Moberg, and Suchy (2000), referral from legal sources is currently the main engine of private practitioner income. Published research addressing empirical questions raised by forensic involvement has also grown steadily. The journal *Forensic Neuropsychology*, edited by Jim Hom and exclusively devoted to forensic issues, first appeared in 1999. Sweet, King, Malina, Bergman, and Simmons (2002) compiled a decade's worth of abstracts from three major neuropsychology journals and reported the number of articles addressing forensic issues more than tripled between 1990 and 2000.

Given the proven growth of legal applications for neuropsychology, it logically follows that neuropsychologists have increased personal interactions with agents of the legal system. These agents include attorneys, claims adjustors, and judges, but attorney contacts account for most these interactions. For this reason, the nature of the attorney–neuropsychologist interaction merits considerable discussion. These interactions can have many positive consequences, including enhanced income, interprofessional understanding, and research opportunities. There can also be negative consequences. These include increased scrutiny in the public eye of cherished methods and beliefs. Attorney coaching is also a risk as this violates a psychologist's crucial assumption of a naïve test taker (Youngjohn, 1995).

The purpose of this chapter is to outline important components of the attorney–neuropsychologist interaction, understand them, and manage them. The reader should be mindful of the terminology used in this chapter. The term *forensic neuropsychologist* (FN) simply means any neuropsychologist who provides opinions in a legal setting irrespective of the frequency of this work. The definition does not denote a practitioner who restricts his or her practice to forensic work. To achieve practice content neutrality, we strive to extract general principles by focusing on elements of professional conduct common to both plaintiff and defense experts, between prosecutor and defendant's experts. For this reason, the terms *retaining* and *opposing*, *examining* and *cross-examining* attorneys are used when possible. These terms are used descriptively and do not connote a value judgment. There are, however, some issues unique to plaintiff's experts and some issues unique to defense experts. In these matters, the terms *plaintiff* and *defense* are used for accuracy's sake, but they are still applied without prejudgment.

We strive for neutrality on assessment orientation (process/flexible approach, fixed battery, flexible battery), legal context (civil, criminal, probate), or practice pattern (mostly plaintiff or defense, full-time versus occasional forensics). If possible, we stress universal aspects of all approaches to neuropsychological testing. The terms *neuropsychological tests*, *neurocognitive methods*, and similar wording are used to denote any procedure relying on quantitative or qualitative scores to arrive at conclusions about impaired or intact cognitive abilities. However, neutrality must be tempered by the existence of mainstream neuropsychology practices.

The test selection examples offered are of the *flexible battery* approach, as opposed to uniform administration of the same tests to all patients (fixed battery) and the pure flexible approach (individualized test selection for every patient). The flexible battery is defined as variable but routine groupings of tests for different types of patients. A core set of tests is given to the same class of patients (e.g., a dementia screening or closed head injury [CHI] battery). Additional measures may be added to answer unique questions raised by a case (Bauer, 1994). The flexible battery approach is a sound approach that combines the best elements of all approaches (Benton, 1992; Doerr, 1991). Even proponents of the so-called fixed battery approach often add measures not recommended by the test's creator (e.g., the addition of memory tests to overcome deficiencies of the Halstead-Reitan Battery [HRB]). Hence, most fixed battery proponents are actually practicing flexible battery administration. Practice pattern surveys show the flexible battery approach not only is the majority preference (Lees-Haley, Smith, Williams, & Dunn, 1996), but also is gaining an increasingly greater number of adherents (Sweet, Moberg, & Westergaard, 1996) and presently enjoys broad sponsorship in the neuropsychology community (Sweet & Moberg, 2000).

Nevertheless, irrespective of which test grouping used, we recognize that even the soundest neuropsychological tests should never be interpreted blindly in isolation from a context or important nonquantifiable data. Matarazzo and Herman (1985), discussing approaches to interpreting Verbal–Performance differences on IQ tests, provided a principle that can also serve as a useful generalization for FNs: They noted: "A (VIQ versus PIQ) difference score is merely the initial datum that should stimulate the clinician to search for corroborating, extra-test evidence from the clinical or social history that such a difference is associated with a potentially significant diagnostic finding" (p. 928).

The useful general principle emerges when one replaces "VIQ–PIQ (Verbal IQ–Performance IQ) difference score" with the term "an abnormal neurocognitive score." This principle of multimethod, converging evidence should be applied to any neuropsychological interpretation proffered in court (see chapter 1 on scientific approaches).

BASIC PRINCIPLES OF NEUROPSYCHOLOGIST–ATTORNEY INTERACTIONS

We promote four basic principles of productive neuropsychologist–attorney interactions. These principles are interwoven with each phase of the attorney–neuropsychologist interaction; for the remainder of this chapter; we apply them to these phases, although some principles have more weight than others in a particular phase:

- Understand legal bases.
- Practice good neuropsychology.
- Adhere to ethical principles.
- Be courtroom familiar.

Understanding legal bases means the FN develops a working knowledge of key law and legal practices. Preparation for forensic neuropsychology does not require an especially deep or broad understanding of legal principles. It does require knowing the most applicable evidentiary law, landmark legal cases relevant to psychology, and the basic civil rights of plaintiffs and criminal defendants. Even the most elementary forensic psychology texts provide a sufficient understanding of the law and courtroom procedures to engage in forensic consulting (Andrew, Benjamin, & Kazniak, 1991; Glass, 1991). However, understanding legal bases also includes understanding legal *culture*. The section on conflicting agendas is devoted exclusively to developing an understanding of legal culture.

One author (L. Cohen) frequently uses the phrase "practicing good neuropsy-chology" in his many legal orientation workshops for neuropsychologists. The principle simply means the FN embraces the scientist/practitioner role by relying on both the body of scientific knowledge and sound clinical judgment while conducting legal work. The scientific component of the FN's work requires placing the legal question and assessment methods in the context of peer-reviewed scientific literature. This principle is very general as it must recognize that there are a number of approaches to neuropsychological testing. But, what is important is the FN's ability to defend the chosen method on empirical grounds. Hence, consideration of the well-established dose–response relation-ship between head injury severity and neuropsychological outcome (Dikmen, Machamer, Winn, & Temkin, 1995; Rohling, Meyers, & Millis, 2003; Vol-brecht, Meyers, & Kaster-Bundgaard, 2000) is used to justify conclusions about causation of current neurocognitive performance.

Although empiricism is important in justifying methodology and conclusions, there will not be a published study for every question that arises in legal dis-putes. Each legal case will have unique aspects that can only be addressed by clinical judgment (i.e., extrapolation and logic). When confronted with a 58-year-old schoolteacher and asked whether she can return to work 1 year after a mild concussion, do not bother to look for studies entitled "Prediction of Return to Work Status in Mildly Injured Teachers" or "Predicting the Elements of Teacher Behavior From Neuropsychological Tests." In this case, the FN must exercise sound judgment in generalizing from the data and literature to a specific claimant's (or defendant's) behavior or disability status. Even that champion of actuarial approaches, Paul Meehl, recognized the need to make sound general-izations from related studies and to use case-specific data to modify conclusions in the absence of the perfect on-point study (Meehl, 1954).

Ethical questions are more likely to be raised by forensic work than in any other setting. It is very important to adhere to ethical principles in all aspects of forensic work. This seems self-explanatory as nobody views himself or herself to practice unethically. Nevertheless, courtroom experience offers constant and often subtle pressures to deviate from sound scientific, clinical, and logical prac-tices. Every phase of legal work raises a different ethical issue. The FN should be aware of the unique ethical issues associated with each phase of attorney-neuropsychologist interactions. The very nature of the adversarial system poses the following unique challenge to the neuropsychologist: Legitimate courtroom practices and ethical attorney behavior would be considered abhorrent and un-ethical if practiced by a neuropsychologist.

The difficulty lies in recognizing ethical dilemmas and the appropriate coping response. Even the most ethically scrupulous neuropsychologist must be pre-pared to cope with unfair ethical charges raised by advocates pretending to be neuropsychology experts and by unsavory attorneys. Recognizing the burden of behaving ethically is made more difficult by weaknesses and ambiguity in published ethical guidelines. In cases of ambiguity, the FN must make an honest attempt to distill the gist or "spirit" of the code in ways that are not self-serving (Shapiro, 2000). Refer to chapter 3 for a broader and in-depth exploration of ethical issues.

The principle of being *courtroom familiar* means the FN is able to recognize courtroom dynamics, trial procedures, interpersonal transactions, and personalities (Brodsky, 1991). There are many indicia of courtroom familiarity (Brodsky & Robey, 1973). These may include knowledge about the presiding judge, knowledge of the opposing attorney, absence of the "star witness" mentality, minimal emotional reactions to aggressive subpoenas, and easy concession of minor points during cross-examination. This principle is similar to the principle of understanding legal bases, but we kept it separate because developing courtroom familiarity requires extensive knowledge, some of it arcane and specific to a locale or jurisdiction. Courtroom familiarity also differs because it represents an outcome of forensic experience; understanding legal bases is a precondition for starting forensic work.

Following the section on clashing worldviews, the remainder of the chapter describes the four main phases of attorney–neuropsychologist interactions: the preassessment, assessment, trial, and posttrial phases. The four basic principles of productive interactions are then applied to each phase as appropriate.

FUNDAMENTAL CONFLICTS BETWEEN SCIENTIST/ PRACTITIONER AND LEGAL MODELS

The first part of understanding legal bases is adjustment to the inevitable conflict between neuropsychological and legal methods. The FN must recognize these basic conflicts to develop a productive relationship with the attorney and the trier of fact. The three basic conflicts encountered by the FN are (a) conflicting agendas, (b) conflicting methods, and (c) conflicting relationships.

Conflicting Agendas

The most basic and pervasive conflict to recognize is *objectivity versus partisanship*. In a typical clinical setting, neuropsychologists pursue a goal of describing a person's sensory, motor, retentive, cognitive, and personality characteristics in an objective and reasonably certain way. All conclusions are at least partially grounded in scientific findings, and logical inferences are tightly linked to facts. In contrast, criminal and civil proceedings in America take place in an *adversarial setting*. Attorneys are advocates. Winning and losing cases are more important than accuracy and objectivity. Justice is more important that truth. The attorney's goal is to present a strong case for his or her client while simultaneously minimizing, even mocking, the opposing attorney's arguments. Although attorneys are not allowed to lie, they have no affirmative obligation to the truth.[1]

Failure to acknowledge the basic conflict will ensure a poor working relationship and quickly sour an interest in forensic work. The novice FN becomes dismayed when the retaining attorney invokes the "work product rule" and insists a report not even be written. The FN concludes that the retaining attorney is dishonest, incompetent, or simply unappreciative of her well-developed diagnostic skills. If asked to write a report and make an appearance at court, the FN becomes annoyed that the cross-examining attorney spends 10 minutes asking about a minor scoring error, but does not affirm the 99.9% accuracy in all other scoring. The FN concludes this attorney is unfair.

These perceptions, although often true, betray the FN's misunderstanding of legal culture. An accurate, comprehensive, and balanced report may be harmful to an attorney's case. Because most FNs would be alarmed at any colleague writing a one-sided report that minimizes inconvenient findings and highlights only a minor finding, the FN should realize that it is considered ethical and fair for an attorney to present a case in just such a partisan form. An attorney's acceptance or rejection of his or her FN's report may make sense in the context of this adversarial system.

In rare circumstances, the court may retain the FN as an expert. Federal Rule of Evidence (FRE; 1975) 706 allows a court to authorize its own expert at the expense of both parties. Having the court for your client mitigates the conflicts to some degree because judges are much more interested in everything a FN has to say, and there is less pressure to tailor findings to an advocate's needs. The court's only role is to protect the process of the adversarial system without taking sides. However, court-appointed expertise is uncommon in civil proceedings and perhaps found only in juvenile law. Even in this more desirable circumstance, the FN is still subject to aggressive cross-examination by an advocate.

Conflicting Methods

Another pervasive conflict is *differing standards of proof* (Blau, 1998). FNs are trained in the scientist/practitioner model, which relies on two prongs: conservative evidentiary standards and replication. A common standard of proof used by FNs to justify selection of measures is a zero-order validity study (Grove & Barden, 1999). This is the demonstration of a statistically significant correlation between a neurocognitive measure and a neurological criterion. The statistical threshold for a significant zero-order correlation is conventionally (but not universally) considered to be at least $p < .05$ and ideally $< .01$. This means the test–criterion association potentially discriminating groups is erroneously caused by chance is only 1 of 20 cases. This error rate of 1–5% in experimental (or quasi-experimental) designs means the neuropsychologist is 95–99% confident that the neurocognitive measure's ability to differentiate groups is not caused by chance.[2]

However, many factors can produce artifactual findings in a single study, such as small sample size (insufficient power), number of variables studied (familywise error), plain serendipity (Type I error), and uncontrolled between-group differences (internal validity threat). Thus, replication, preferably in another laboratory, is added as a second requirement. Scientific standards of proof are uniform across settings and are not altered as a function of socially desired versus potentially unpopular outcomes. In summary, neuropsychological consensus requires conservative statistical evidence and consistent results across different settings.

In contrast, the courts require less-conservative evidentiary standards and desire to resolve cases over shorter time frames (Hess, 1999a). The uniqueness of each case and desire for speedy justice make replication over time a practical impossibility. In addition, legal evidentiary standards themselves float; that is, they depend on the gravity of the legal outcome. Per Kagehiro (1990), these evidentiary thresholds (with proposed confidence levels in parentheses) are preponderance of the evidence (51%), clear and convincing evidence (75%), and reasonable doubt (90%). The preponderance-of-the-evidence standard means the trier of fact favors parties having at least 51% of the evidence in their favor. This is the evidentiary standard in personal injury cases. Criminal courts rely on a beyond-a-reasonable doubt standard, but as observed by Hess (1999a), even this level of legal evidence barely approaches the lower limit of the $p <$ .05 standard common in scientific psychology.

Another methods conflict is *responsivity to social and political forces*. Scientific neuropsychology, in principle at least, is supposed to be resistant to changing fads, laws, popular beliefs, and political forces. However, legal decisions not only are influenced by popular beliefs and political trends, but also are expected to be influenced. The assertion that the Constitution is a "living document" is an example of political forces affecting legal interpretation. This leads to the anomalous situation of different evidentiary requirements for the same neuropsychological methodology dependent on the legal question (Tenopyr, 1999). For example, the use of IQ tests in employment and school settings is held to very rigorous standards following the *Griggs et al. v. Duke Power* (1971) ruling. In contrast, despite the proven insensitivity of IQ tests to remote mild head injuries (Binder, 1997; Binder, Rohling, & Larrabee, 1997; Dikmen, Temkin, Machamer, & Holubkov, 1994; Dikmen et al., 1995), neuropsychologists are typically not barred from using "subtle" intelligence subtest differences as evidence for "brain damage" (Faust, Ziskin, & Hiers, 1991). These variable practices make no scientific sense, but they perfectly mirror legal values, which consider most scientific data probative.

Conflicting Roles

Conflicts in the forensic arena are not necessarily between the law and neuropsychology. Role conflicts arise *within* the FN as the FN moves from a clinical to a legal setting and are often termed *dual roles*. One such conflict is *treater versus expert*. In clinical settings, even the most objective neuropsychologist treats the patient with empathy. The treater advocates for the patient's best interests, including support for disability payments even if the objective evidence does not support it. Supporting a patient's demands for compensation has a long tradition in clinical psychology because the legal requirement of proving damages may interfere with the therapeutic goal of improving psychological well-being. Fenichel (1945), discussing how secondary gain prolonged recovery from traumatic neuroses, advised: "Perhaps the idea of giving one single compensation at the right time may be the best way out" (p. 126). In contrast, the expert is supposed to be objective at all times and to assert truths the plaintiff does not want to hear or that may be damaging to his or her case. The magnitude of the conflict further depends on the treatment model. Treaters who are aggressive advocates are especially vulnerable to this dual-role conflict and perhaps should not be allowed to testify as experts at all except to the contents of their report.

Collegiality versus opposition is another conflict that requires some adjustment. In nonforensic settings, neuropsychologists operate in a collegial fashion with their colleagues. They share data with each other, strive for points of agreement in conceptualization of a patient's cognitive problems, and collaborate on research. In a forensic setting, FNs are often asked to critique the work of another neuropsychologist who has been hired by the other side.

Specific Contemporary Conflicts

The core conflicts discussed to this point are structural and endemic to every case in which FNs become. They can only be adjusted to not changed in any substantial manner. However, there are also situations the FN will confront on an episodic basis for which the law and neuropsychology clash. The FN may exercise some control or have considerable input how these conflicts are resolved. The response to each of these conflicts is a matter of controversy, and a variety of solutions is available.

Access to raw data

Legal decisions, like scientific ones, are based on evidence. The rules of evidence in every jurisdiction allow attorneys to obtain the data on which the opposing expert bases his or her opinions. This process is termed *discovery*. In civil and criminal settings, discovery rights are absolute, and no expert witness is immune from the discovery process. Cardiologists must provide electrocardiogram tracings, and blood spatter experts must provide bloody clothes. The evidentiary base on which neuropsychologists rely typically includes test scores, records, interview notes, and mental status observations. It is inevitable that most FNs are eventually asked to provide a copy of their case file, hereinafter referred to as "raw data," to either retaining or opposing counsel.

In developing responses to requests for data disclosure, it is important to define terms. What exactly is meant by raw data? Matarazzo (1990) defined the several different types of raw data subject to discovery. Such data includes (a) written reports, (b) handwritten interview notes, (c) numerical scores (e.g., raw counts of number correct or standardized scores), (d) test stimuli, (e) the participant's actual responses to test stimuli, and (f) test manuals. As a practical matter, most forensic case files will not contain stand-alone test stimuli and actual manuals. Even aggressive attorneys rarely demand test manuals. The clash between the law and neuropsychology usually results from demands to discover raw data in categories (c) and (e): test forms containing verbatim responses and scoring sheets/formulas. A conflict arises because the law recognizes an absolute right to discover raw data, but the ethics code under which most neuropsychologists operate has been interpreted by some as placing strong prohibitions against data sharing. The term *interpreted* is chosen because of the ambiguous and contradictory nature of ethical guidelines.

Historically, the 1992 edition of the "Ethical Principles of Psychologists and Code of Conduct" (American Psychological Association [APA], 1992; hereinafter referred to as the 1992 code) has typically been cited as the authority controlling the treatment of raw data requests from nonpsychologists. A number of the 1992 code's principles bear directly on either forensic activities or the disclosure of raw test data to nonpsychologists. Unfortunately, there has been no consensus in responding to subpoenas, and a wide range of views on handling raw data is reflected in actual practice.

Essig, Mittenberg, Peterson, Strauman, and Cooper (2001) surveyed FNs about their raw data practices. They reported 61% of FNs did not share data in half or more of their forensic cases, and 39% reported honoring the request in the majority of cases. Looking at the extremes only, 12% of FNs refused to forward raw test data at any time, and 18% reported sharing data with the opposition regularly. One reasonable interpretation of this data is that 30% take the polarized views reflected in the commentary literature (discussed later in this section), and the middle 70% disclose data on an irregular basis. Essig et al. did not explore the contingencies of the middle group's practices.

Pieniadz and Kelland (2001) sought to explore the contingencies of data disclosure, but restricted their neuropsychologist survey to the issue of including test scores in the report body. They found 35.5% regularly included scores (the "Yes" group), and 64.5% (the "No" group) did not. The main reasons for including scores were "integrity/thoroughness" and "future comparison" (both 100%

of Yes group). The main reasons for excluding specific scores were "data protection" (90% of No group) and to "maintain the process focus" (50%). Adherents of the process approach were more likely to refuse test score inclusion
than flexible battery adherents. Although survey data are limited, it appears
neuropsychologists lack uniformity and offer many different reasons for including, excluding, or variably supplying the data that serve as the basis for their
opinions.

Reasons for this lack of practice standard may lie in the 1992 code's many
ambiguities and frank contradictions. For example, neuropsychologists who refuse to comply with subpoenas for raw test data may rely solely on ethical
standard 2.02(b), which reads:

Psychologists refrain from misuse of assessment techniques, interventions, results and
interpretations and take reasonable steps to prevent others from misusing the information
these techniques provide. This includes refraining from releasing raw test results or raw
data to persons other than to patients or clients as appropriate, who are not qualified to
use such information.

However, this principle appears to be contradicted by another principle, 1.23(b),
to wit:

When psychologists believe that records of their professional services will be used in
legal proceedings involving recipients of or participants in their work, they have a responsibility to create and maintain documentation consistent with reasonable scrutiny in
an adjudicative forum.

Similarly, Section 7.0 of the code deals exclusively with professional behavior
in forensic settings. Standard 7.02 (Forensic Assessments) asks for psychologists to "provide appropriate substantiation for their findings"; Principle 7.04
(Truthfulness and Candor) demands neuropsychologists "describe fairly the
bases for their testimony and conclusions." It is not clear how neuropsychologists can keep data from attorneys but simultaneously provide data for scrutiny
in the courtroom. Some FNs try to resolve the contradictions by treating principles in hierarchical fashion, viewing some principles as subordinate or superior
to others. However, such superordinate/subordinate readings are purely idiosyncratic and even self-serving and have no support in 1992 code text or history.

Review of commentary articles reveals a wide array of opinions, which may
be broadly classified into two camps for didactic purposes: exceptionalism and
legal primacy. The *exceptionalism* posture interprets the 1992 code's standards
as advocating broad nondisclosure of any form of test datum. The *exceptionalism* posture is premised on the view that neuropsychological test scores are
different from any other form of scientific datum and must be treated differently
irrespective of the law. An example of this view is that of Tranel (1994).

In Tranel's view, the 1992 code is "clear" on barring disclosure, and he relies
solely on Standard 2.02(b) as his authority. Tranel's interpretation goes so far

as to bar the reporting of test scores in the report text. In Tranel's view, the latter is necessary to avoid (a) "potential misuse" and (b) dissemination of test items into the public domain. For example, potential misuse in a legal context is an attorney cross-examining a neuropsychologist on individual items rather than aggregate scores. The public dissemination concern is the idea that neuro-psychological tests assume a naïve participant, and exposure to scores in text may influence future test participants with access to court transcripts.

The legal primacy posture is best exemplified by Lees-Haley and Courtney's (2000) commentary in a special issue of *Neuropsychology Review*. They rejected the exceptionality posture of Tranel (1994) and instead viewed the 1992 code in terms of civil rights and due process. They warned that broad nondisclosure creates a special class of experts who are not subject to *legally mandated* court-room practices, a violation of due process. They cited Standard 1.23(b) (Documentation of Professional Work) as their main authority. Lees-Haley and Court-ney described the futility of resolving contradictions in 2.02b, providing a list of absurd outcomes that may result from the 1992 code's contradictory lan-guage. They also noted that the *potential misuse* term is itself misused by neu-ropsychologists who do not like the unpleasant experience of cross-examination. They noted, for example, that the 1992 code allows disclosing raw test data to a patient contingent on the FN's personal definition of "appropriate," yet simultaneously withholding the same data from another psychologist (usually a defense expert) who does not meet the FN's personal definition of a neuropsy-chologist.

Tranel (2000) considered this outcome contrived, but one of us (M. F. Greif-fenstein) has on occasion been refused access to raw data on the grounds that American Board of Clinical Neuropsychology (ABCN) certification was without merit. We would like to point out another absurd outcome: If in-text test scores were disallowed, every school psychologist in this country would be subject to ethical sanctions for reporting IQ subtest profiles. Some may also view this possibility as contrived, but it is no more contrived than the fear that thousands of dishonest jurors will return to court after a verdict to obtain copies of files containing raw test data.

Clashing opinions on data disclosure policy may be moot as this book goes to press. The code has been rewritten, and a final draft was approved during the August 2002 APA Convention (hereinafter referred to as the 2002 code). The 2002 code addresses the ambiguities in the 1992 code and better reflects the evolving relationship between psychology and law (Fisher, 2003). For example, the defi-nition of raw data is subdivided into two classes in the spirit of Matarazzo (1990), making a clear distinction between scored test forms from a case file versus test manuals. Each is given separate treatment: Standard 9.04 deals with scored protocols in the individual case, and Standard 9.11 deals with test manu-als and stimuli. Standard 9.04 appears to allow release of scored protocols in response to a valid subpoena without the ambiguous "reasonable steps" contingency.

Standard 9.04 allows for more uniform treatment of individual raw data than the old Standard 2.02(b): Raw test data can still be disclosed to a patient/participant, but without the language that some have used to justify withholding evidence from attorneys. In contrast, Standard 9.11 appears to place more restrictions on disclosure of manuals/stimuli. This separate treatment of manuals may allay the fears of public dissemination, with the main reason usually given to withhold *any* data (Tranel, 1994; Naugle & McSweeny, 1995). The 2002 code is not perfect, and it does not deal with the situation of neuropsychological measures that contain the test stimuli on the scoring forms (e.g., the Rey-Osterrieth Complex Figure). Nevertheless, the 2002 code is a reasonable advance toward resolving perceived conflicts between ethics and the law.

Although we accept the legal primacy position as more convincing because it fits better with the American system of due process, we are not advocating for uncontrolled release of data or materials. The official position of the National Academy of Neuropsychology (NAN Policy and Planning Committee, 2000) offers some realistic threats to the public good (e.g., a truly impaired pilot who self-coaches to achieve passable scores). We advise a policy of graded disclosure subordinated to the requirements of local law. We argue that the 2002 code supports a range of disclosing responses from minimal to limiting, depending on (a) the type of test data requested and (b) local law. A valid subpoena is sufficient for disclosing a test participant's scored protocols and history notes.[3] Only Illinois-based neuropsychologists are barred by law from disclosing scored protocols to an officer of the court, consistent with that state's law.

We agree with Lees-Haley and Courtney (2000) that vigorous attempts to withhold data from attorneys create a special class of experts. If allowed to withhold the evidentiary base for their opinions, FNs are in essence given the procedural right to dictate the terms of their cross-examination. A neuropsychologist's testimony would boil down to an unassailable *ipse dixit* argument, "Its so because I say it is so."

In contrast, we agree a request for test materials such as freestanding stimuli (e.g., the actual blocks from Block Design) and the test manual (e.g., the Wechsler Abbreviated Scale of Intelligence™ [WASI] manual itself) requires a more restrictive response. There is a more compelling public interest at stake. A test manual with associated test stimuli is unarguably a guide for coaching and cheating. Hence, the dangers of public dissemination in this circumstance are clearer in ways a scored individual protocol is not. In this case, the FN should take extra steps to ensure the manual does not get into the public record. A request for a judge's order to seal records containing test manual copies at the conclusion of the trial would be appropriate. In summary, the 2002 code recognizes the primacy of law over a specific profession's ethics. Although still not ideal, it is an improvement over the 1992 code.

Third-party observation

A number of jurisdictions give attorneys the right to sit in on independent medical examinations (IMEs). The specific wording of these statutes grant the right for a personal "physician" of the plaintiff's choosing to be present during an IME, or they grant the right of an attorney to be present during a "medical" examination. However, it is a matter of controversy within the legal profession itself whether these statutes broadly cover any third-party observation (TPO) or whether they should be narrowly construed. The controversy centers on the terms *physician* and *medical*, whether these terms should be narrowly construed as referring to physical examinations by medical doctors or whether they can refer to any third-party examination. Trial judges have great latitude in defining the scope of these terms. It is inevitable that every FN will be confronted with this demand.

Case law to date appears to favor a narrow construction, limiting TPO to physical examinations conducted by medical practitioners. Many appeals courts appear to recognize that the validity of psychological test responses (and by implication neuropsychological testing) is more likely to be affected by TPO than physical responses in medical examinations. State appeals and federal court rulings barring TPO are too numerous to mention here, but there are three federal rulings worth mentioning that bear directly on neuropsychology.

In *Cline et al. v. Firestone Tire* (1988), the plaintiff moved for a protective order (*Federal Rule of Civil Procedure*, 1975, Rule 26) barring a neuropsychology IME unless strict conditions were met. The U.S. District Court of West Virginia held that plaintiff was not entitled to have an attorney present. In another case, a Minnesota district court denied the plaintiff's motion to record or observe the examination (*Tomlin v. Holecek*, 1993). The court reasoned that TPO would influence the plaintiff to "guard, alter or disguise" test responses during both the history-taking and testing phases. In *Ragge v. MCA/Universal Studios* (1995), the U.S. District Court for California denied the plaintiff's request for a third-party observer during a neuropsychological IME. One factor tying these three and many other related cases together is that the burden rests on the moving party (the one who wants an observer) to show good cause for potentially affecting an evaluation's validity.

If the FN is confronted with a TPO demand, he or she can productively assist the retaining attorney by citing important literature. There is a rich social psychology literature showing TPO affects some cognitive test scores in a direction of worse performance. The impact of observation on perceptual-motor performance has even been given its own name: the "social facilitation effect."

There are many key studies relevant to neuropsychology. Kehrer, Sanchez, Habif, Rosenbaum, and Townes (2000) examined the effects of a TPO on neuro-cognitive test performance. They reported performance decrements on tests of attention, speed of information processing, and verbal fluency, but no effect on motor speed and cognitive flexibility. Constantinou, Ashendorf, and McCaffrey (2002) examined the effects of an audio recorder and found a decrement in memory scores, but not on motor measures. Using a single-case, ABAB experi-mental design, Binder and Johnson-Greene (1995) described a patient perform-ing worse on malingering measures when her mother was present than when she was absent. J. L. Butler and Baumeister (1998) reported that even warm, supportive observers caused decrements on skilled tasks relative to unmonitored performance. The Binder and Johnson-Greene and Butler and Baumeister stud-ies suggested that plaintiff's arguments for having an "agent" or "supportive family member" present during a neuropsychological examination are not scien-tifically supportable. McCaffrey, Fisher, Gold, and Lynch (1996) offered practi-cal guidelines for responding to attorney requests for observation.

Unlike the raw data issue, there does appear to be a strong practice consensus regarding the presence of third-party observers. Essig et al. (2001) reported that 88% of FNs never allow TPO, and 11% allow it on rare occasion. Not a single FN allowed such observation on a regular basis. Major neuropsychology organi-zations have published strongly worded policies discouraging the practice except in very limited circumstances (Axelrod et al., 2000). In our view, TPO is a legal tactic designed to intimidate neuropsychologists, not to protect the rights of the plaintiff. Plaintiff attorneys do have a right to sit in on the interview portion because there is a more compelling interest to protect legal rights. For example, discussion of liability issues (who caused the accident) is outside the purview of neuropsychologists.

PHASES OF THE ATTORNEY–NEUROPSYCHOLOGIST INTERACTION

The FN can expect interactions with attorneys to go through a series of typical steps. Each step requires different preparatory and cognitive activities and has differing ethical issues. The typical phases of attorney–neuropsychologist inter-action include the preassessment, assessment, report-writing, discovery, testi-mony (deposition or trial), and posttrial phases.

Preassessment Phase

Initial meeting

First contact with an attorney contains a number of crucial elements. The first decisions the FN makes are (a) acceptance or rejection of involvement and

(b) the specific role that will be played. The FN engages in preliminary data collection to support this decision-making process. At a bare minimum, the FN should ask the retaining attorney for three pieces of information: (a) a brief case synopsis, (b) a short list of hypothetical questions to be asked of the FN, and (c) availability of the plaintiff. Other requested information may include anticipated court dates, discovery deadlines, and amount and type of records to be reviewed. This conversation need not last more than 5–10 minutes.

The brief case summary is critical for a number of reasons. The fact set will help determine goodness of fit between your expertise and the case, the elements of the assessment approach, and the amount of time you will spend. More important, the case summary represents the first challenge to your objectivity. The attorney's synopsis is from the viewpoint of an advocate, so the FN must be alert to one-sided portrayals of the case. It is here that the process of resisting the "pull of affiliation" should start (Brodsky, 1991).

Attorneys contact FNs in the belief that neuropsychological analysis will support their medical–legal theory. Thus, they may try to prejudice you right from the outset by providing a biased summary that omits or distorts key facts. A plaintiff attorney may state, "I don't believe in trying mild concussion cases, but I have a client who sustained a severe CHI in a horrible accident 2 years ago, and he hasn't worked since." You later find out the injury was only minor orthopedic strain. A defense attorney may say, "The plaintiff has a long history of drug and alcohol abuse, he hasn't worked in 2 years, and I'm sure his brain was fried before the accident." You later receive records showing a trauma neurosurgeon had to remove 10 cc of destroyed prefrontal lobe tissue. Give attorneys latitude by accepting that there will be some attempt to prejudice you; acceptance or rejection of the case depends on the magnitude of the prejudice. Refuse involvement only if the attorney grossly misrepresents the facts or limits your access to key records.

The hypothetical questions of the retaining attorney determine the activities and roles the FN takes on. The hypothetical question is designed to elicit an opinion that summarizes all the psychological and neuropsychological issues in a brief conclusion understandable to the typical juror (Blau, 1998). The attorney may not yet know the specific questions that he or she will ask during trial, but can gave you general questions that summarize the issues relevant to a neuropsychologist, such as "Did the accident (or failed medical treatment) cause brain damage?" Asking for preliminary hypothetical questions allows the FN to determine whether he or she can potentially frame conclusions in a reasonably probable way, or whether the question even falls within his or her expertise.

This is also an opportunity to discuss your views and forensic history candidly as these considerations shape the general thrust of your future opinions. If a plaintiff attorney contacts you and you do not believe that common adult whiplash causes diffuse axonal injury or that minor concussion causes disproportionately severe long-term disability, say so. The plaintiff attorney will appreciate your candor. Alternatively, if contacted by a defense attorney and you believe that 10 years of cannabis is unlikely to predict preaccident brain damage, also say so at the outset. Even if the attorney decides not to use you, you have established credibility and trust.

Access to the plaintiff (or criminal defendant) is the third key issue to clarify. Neuropsychological and psychological testing requires conditions similar to those of the standardization group described in the test's instruction manual. If the case demands a comprehensive neuropsychological assessment, the FN should insist the plaintiff (or defendant) be examined at the FN's offices. Some prisons do contain secure, quiet interview rooms. Otherwise, if the case comes with severe restrictions imposed by a judge or lack of an appropriate testing room, the FN should refuse.

Another potential issue is third-party observers. In some jurisdictions, case law is interpreted as allowing attorneys (or personal physicians) to be present during independent neuropsychological examinations. Unless the FN's office is equipped with closed-circuit TV (e.g., a good baby video monitor with audio) or one-way mirrors, the FN should refuse to have an observer present in the room with the technician and plaintiff. Any psychologist who offers him- or herself as a third-party observer and insists on sitting in the testing room itself is subject to an ethical complaint.

In some cases, attorneys have already stipulated in advance to place severe limitations on neuropsychological testing without contacting the FN first (e.g., signing a court order allowing videotaping of the test administration). The FN should firmly refuse any involvement in situations for which the retaining attorney stipulated to constraints on a neuropsychologist's testing practices without first consulting the FN. You can help that attorney to avoid the same mistake in the future by providing documentation of the problematic nature of TPO in psychological testing.

Some states allow videotaping of any IME. In such cases, it is important to make involvement contingent on a protective court order restricting videotape reviewing rights and returning all copies of the tape to the FN at the conclusion of litigation (NAN Policy and Planning Committee, 2000). If the court mandates no such assurances, the FN should refuse involvement. The retaining attorney can still have the option of an emergency appeal for application of an abuse of discretion standard to the trial judge's behavior.

In summary, acceptance of the case depends on (a) relevance to one's expertise, (b) sufficient access to data on which to base an opinion, and (c) absence of potential conflicts. If the FN has a prior relationship with any party to the suit, this relationship needs to be considered. "Treating" neuropsychologists should proceed especially gingerly because both the plaintiff and the plaintiff attorney become clients. The remainder of this section assumes the FN's acceptance of involvement.

Role selection

The next crucial element during initial contact is role selection. The FN must determine which of the potential roles to choose. The basic choices are (a) fact witness, (b) expert witness, and (c) litigation consultant. The fact ("reporting") and expert witness roles both involve live testimony either in court or by deposition. As a fact witness, the FN can only report facts about the patient. The testifying expert is a FN who reports opinions at trial or during a deposition. Two crucial features distinguish the expert witness from the fact witness: The expert is allowed to report hearsay ("The plaintiff said . . .") and is allowed to offer an opinion ("Smith's memory problems were caused by a penetrating missile wound to the brain"). In contrast, the fact witness reports information gleaned through the senses only, without any interpretation ("I saw Jones shoot the gun at Smith's head" or "I saw the plaintiff for an examination on July 5, 1999").

If an original examiner who saw the patient on referral from a physician prior to involvement (assuming an attorney did not start the referral chain), that neuropsychologist is technically a fact witness. As a practical matter, however, the line between a fact witness who is a doctor and a testifying expert is blurred. A treating doctor, reading from a report, states, "I gave a diagnosis of closed head injury." That is an expert opinion disguised as a factual report. It is rare for judges to impose any testimonial limitation on a treating doctor, so in practice, a treating doctor is treated the same as a testifying expert.

The role of litigation consultant means the FN works "behind the scenes" to educate the attorney about basic neuropsychological terms and principles, examine test data supplied by another neuropsychologist, offer alternative theories of the facts from a neuropsychological perspective, and design cross-examination questions for the opposing neuropsychologist (Derby, 2001). Any documents developed in this role are subject to the attorney work product rule, meaning the FN remains anonymous, and his or her contributions are not discoverable. However, if a treating or testifying neuropsychologist is also hired as a litigation consultant (to examine the other side's raw test data), the work product rule does not apply, and all conversations or documents related to these activities are discoverable. It is advisable to avoid these kinds of dual roles unless you are willing to disclose your conversations with the attorney.[4]

The last facet of role selection is determination of the pertinent issues on which the FN will offer opinions. Neuropsychological evidence is deemed helpful in assisting the trier of fact in a broad range of civil and criminal cases. Table 2-1 summarizes the kinds of legal settings in which FNs find themselves and the specific issues they are asked to address. The experienced FN should

TABLE 2-1. Partial Summary of Legal Settings and Issues Relevant
to Forensic Neuropsychology

COURT SETTING	SPECIFIC LEGAL ISSUE	NEUROPSYCHOLOGICAL ISSUES
Probate	Testamentary competence	• Postmortem analyses of cognitive state on critical legal dates • Recent and remote memory • Social perception and delusional status
	Capacity for contracts, trusts	• Vulnerability to persuasion • Recent memory • Delusional status
	Competency to testify	• Usually an issue with children; determine cognitive developmental stage
	Guardianship	• IQ • Functional abilities • Judgment
Administrative	Worker's compensation	• Old versus acquired cognitive deficits
	Social Security Disability	• Prediction of functional deficits
Civil	Causation	• Neurogenic versus psychosocial factors • Closed head injury • Low-dose exposure to organic solvents • Black mold causing occult central nervous system damage
	Damages	• Acquired versus old cognitive weaknesses • Post-traumatic versus premorbid psychological attributes • Primary and secondary gain, symptom validity
	Disability under Americans With Disabilities Act	• Formal diagnosis of cognition-based disability • Prediction of accommodations to remediated deficit
Criminal	*Mens rea* or Not guilty by reason of insanity	• Transient amnestic disorder • Dysexecutive syndrome
	Competent waiver of *Miranda* rights	• Auditory comprehension • Reading comprehension
	Competence to stand trial	• Attention • Comprehension • Memory

have learned how to map legal terminology into neuropsychological terminology. Communication between attorney and FN is facilitated when there is a good understanding of which neuropsychological issues are associated with which jurisdictional requirement and vice versa (Grisso, 1988).

The retaining attorney (or claims adjustor) may ask the testifying expert to examine the claimant for evidence of impaired brain functions and disturbed personality. There is no doctor–patient relationship, and such an evaluation is termed an IME. IMEs are typically requested by defense attorneys in civil suits, although plaintiff attorneys ask for them as well when treating doctors are unwilling to be involved. Testimony can also be based on records review only, although this places limitations to the scope of opinions. Both the 2002 code and older 1992 code advise a direct examination in legal cases, but testimony based on records review only is permissible if one testifies to the limitations. Case law upholds neuropsychologists' qualifications to testify on the basis of records alone (*Hutchison v. American Family*, 1994).

The preassessment phase is crucial with respect to ethical adherence. It is here that the FN may be offered dual or even triple roles. Ethical Standard 7.03, from the Forensic Activities section (APA, 1992), states: "In most circumstances, psychologists avoid performing multiple and potentially conflicting roles in forensic matters." A good example of a dual-role conflict is a treater not only testifying for the plaintiff, but also asked to prepare the plaintiff attorney for cross-examination of the defense expert. To avoid this, the FN should insist on a single role: Testifying expert, treater, or trial consultant. Some legal journals (e.g., *Lawyer's Weekly*) publish commentary advising the use of the "objective treater to also analyze the defense neuropsychologist's raw test data and advise on proper cross-examination questions."[5] Acting as a treater and testifying and providing background consulting are unambiguous dual roles that turn the treater into an agent of the attorney.

To combat this, the FN needs to keep in mind the pervasive principle running throughout this chapter: What many attorneys consider good practice is questionable or clear unethical practice for a neuropsychologist. The FN does not have to do everything an attorney expects. As pointed out by Brodsky (1991), bias and ethical conflict occur when the psychologist allows the "pull of affiliation" to subtly enmesh the treater or expert into dual advocacy roles.

Trial consulting work has special ethical ramifications that get limited attention. McSweeny (1997) interpreted the 1992 code Standard 1.16(a) (Misuses of Psychologists' Work) to support a conclusion that trial consulting work by its very nature may be unethical. He reasoned that, because FN trial consultants are typically anonymous, there is no "corrective mechanism" present as required by 1.16(a). Although we believe that trial consulting is not an inherently unethical activity, we agree with McSweeny (1997) that such "behind-the-scenes" work places a special burden on FNs that is found nowhere else in legal work.

Anonymity creates a psychological state with reduced likelihood of negative consequences for behavior. This absence of "moral hazard" may uninhibit aggressive tendencies. Examples of aggressive behavior include designing cross-examination questions that misuse neuropsychological test data, providing irrelevant personal anecdotes attacking the opposing neuropsychologist, or biasing neuropsychological interpretation away from the best-fitting, but inconvenient, diagnosis. A good example of questionable ethical behavior is for the FN consultant to tell the retaining attorney that "fixed batteries such as the Halstead-Reitan are the only measures accepted in the neuropsychology community," "process neuropsychology is the only method for detecting deficits," or "age and education corrections do not need to be used."

In other words, anytime a consulting FN replaces accepted practice parameters with a polarizing polemic, a potential ethical violation may be taking place. An FN who regularly performs such work should note that anonymity is not guaranteed. In federal law, there are exceptions to the anonymous trial consultant rule, and under certain circumstances, an attorney must provide the name of the previously secret consultant.

The trial consultant's work product should be shaped by two parameters: (a) offer advice based on honestly debatable issues of fact and (b) provide consultation as if your identity will eventually be revealed. For example, reliance on age-based corrections or comparisons is not an honestly debatable issue. This is a well-established and sound practice parameter. It would be ludicrous for an FN to argue that age corrections are not needed for neuropsychological tests while simultaneously relying on instruments with age-specific deviation metrics (e.g., Wechsler intelligence scales). What is honestly debatable, however, is the particular choice of age-based normative tables to use with any given neuropsychological measure because there are competing normative databases for the same measure (Mitrushina, Boone, & D'Elia, 1999).

The conflict between treater and attorney's agent is the most common form dual-role conflict takes. Greenberg and Shuman (1997) provided an exhaustive analysis of all the problems inherent in treaters asked to be expert witnesses and trial consultants. The number of potentially conflicting roles is dizzying. As one example, Greenberg and Shuman pointed out that if the treater accepts the role of consultant, then the patient is no longer the client, but the plaintiff attorney is. There may also be circumstances for which the civil defense attorney or prosecutor asks a treater to testify. This is also problematic. In such cases, the treater should insist on being a reporting (fact) witness only and answer questions by reading from their reports. Shuman, Greenberg, Heilbrun, and Foote (1998) went even further; they made the provocative argument that treaters should not be allowed to testify, and attorneys from both sides should be forced to retain independent examiners.

Compensation for services

The last step is determining compensation for services. This is usually handled in the initial meeting. The fees should be reasonable, that is, no different from the fees charged for clinical examinations, assuming similarities in battery composition and testing duration. There is no clinical equivalent to deposition or trial testimony, so it is customary for experts to charge a much higher hourly rate or to charge a minimum fee irrespective of the deposition's length. This is justifiable because the FN has no way of predicting how long a deposition will take or how long he or she will sit in a court corridor. The higher rate for testimony is justified by loss of a day's income from regular activity. Avoid the temptation to charge more for a forensic assessment than a clinical test battery of the same size and content. Nothing shows bias more than a differential fee schedule for the same underlying activity.

The FN should maintain a detailed, annually updated fee schedule that describes the hourly, bundled, or per diem charges. This list can easily be faxed or electronically mailed. The list should include a basic hourly rate for records review or conferences, an hourly rate or bundled fee for neuropsychological testing, fees for briefer forms of testing (e.g., ordinary psychological evaluation or chronic pain behavior evaluation), and deposition or trial testimony and fee policies regarding travel time. Some FNs use staff such as paralegals or graduate students to perform literature searches, review records, write case synopses, or conduct statistical analyses. Supporting staff's time for nontesting activity should be billed at a lower rate. If you rely on such staff, do not pretend you did the work yourself.

The fee schedule should also include an explicit billing policy for live testimony. Some experts bill for trial testimony on a "portal-to-portal" basis (the time you leave home until the time you walk back into your home after testifying); others charge less for commuting time, but start the meter on seating themselves on a bench outside the courtroom. Irrespective of your preferences, the policy should be written clearly on your fee schedule. Also, consider creating a per diem charge if testimony involves traveling to a different city or sitting in court all day. This is reasonable and fair. If you insist on an hourly rate for extensive travel and include the time you slept on the plane or watched a movie in the hotel room the night before trial, you will open yourself to very embarrassing questions, such as, "So doctor, you are billing $500 for every hour you slept?" A per diem charge is easily defensible for the same reasons as a minimum deposition charge: You have to keep a large time slot open during which you would normally perform other billable work.

The FN may wish to ask the attorney to initial and date the fee schedule or sign a brief agreement to pay for services rendered. Per the advice of Blau

(1998), do not fall for vague promises such as "Don't worry, you'll get paid" or "I'll protect your fee." Some NPs demand retainer fees before initiating any work, and this practice dissolves the issue of having a personal financial interest in the outcome. Some plaintiff attorneys will insist you accept a lien on any settlement or jury verdict. Avoid this arrangement at all costs. Accepting this arrangement introduces bias. You have created a financial interest in the outcome of a trial, increasing the pull of affiliation to the retaining side and creating a dual-role conflict (e.g., moneylender vs. treater). Contingent fee arrangements are specifically barred by memberships in some forensic psychology organizations. For example, the American Academy of Forensic Psychology requires adherence to specialty ethical guidelines (Committee on Ethical Guidelines, 1991), which are required in addition to general APA guidelines (APA, 1992, 2002).

Assessment Phase

This section describes the data collection process to gather evidence on which future opinions will be based. This is the point at which the principle of "practicing good neuropsychology" most applies. An important first step in good practice is relying on multimethod, convergent means of data gathering. A convergent evidentiary model allows greater confidence in one's opinions and makes rejection of hypotheses more credible. Diagnoses of posttraumatic brain damage, malingering, or cognitive recovery to baseline are more easily supportable with multiple methods.

Some FNs believe in blind interpretation of test scores without any reliance on demographics or history. This is not advisable because context is undeniably crucial in neuropsychological interpretation. For example, Heaton, Smith, Lehman, and Vogt (1978) found that even expert neuropsychologists could not distinguish the Halstead-Reitan protocols of severe head injury from volunteer fakers when only given score summary sheets.

Some FNs heavily weight interview data and symptom report alone as evidence for cerebral dysfunction. This is termed *diagnosis by clinical history*. But, reliance on such an impressionistic approach alone is not empirically or logically supportable because subjective cognitive complaints are nonspecific, have no proven ability to predict cerebral status, and do not correlate with neurocognitive test scores (Chelune & Heaton, 1986; Satz et al., 1998).

Three recommended basic convergent evidence methods of the assessment phase are review of outside records, direct and collateral interview, and neurocognitive and psychological test administration. Lally (2003) referred to these three evidentiary sources as the "tripod" on which psychological testimony rests and argued that this approach places psychologists at an advantage over other mental health professionals. Also see chapter 1, this volume, on scientific approaches. Each method by itself is fallible.

Records review

Self-report, especially by interested parties in a lawsuit, simply cannot be relied on as the only basis for establishing preinjury functioning. Considerable research has shown a substantial number of litigants with brain damage claims may give biased histories, in some cases biasing history to the point of outright distortion (Faust, 1995). One form of reporting bias takes positive inflation of preinjury cognitive and mental health status (Greiffenstein & Baker, 2001; Johnson-Greene et al., 1997).

Mittenberg, DiGiulio, Perrin, and Bass (1992) asked late postconcussion claimants and uninjured matched controls to retrospectively rate past memory skills. The late postconcussion group grossly underreported premorbid memory slips relative to the controls. Greiffenstein, Baker, and Johnson-Greene (2002) asked litigating postconcussion patients and nonlitigating neuropsychiatric patients to estimate their scholastic preinjury grade point average. The postconcussion claimants grossly overestimated their grade point average. Even schizophrenics and patients with dementia were more accurate than postconcussion litigants were. Nelson, Drebing, Satz, and Uchiyama (1998) asked patients with CHI and college students to self-report differences before and following a "brain event." They found that the patients with CHI reported many fewer emotional problems in the past than the college students did.

Review of relevant records provides a means of overcoming bias in self-report. Records review also achieves many other goals, including (a) establishing the severity of the original neurological injury, (b) estimating cognitive and functional baseline, (c) finding or ruling out medical conditions with neurological implications, and (d) variability versus stability of neuropsychological test scores if claimant was previously tested. Records also supply the context in which to determine whether abnormal test scores represent an acquired versus an old weakness. Performance on the Speech Sounds Perception Test, with its requirement of phonetic attack skills, would be viewed differently in a person whose school records show completion of the sixth grade than a person with a college degree. Finally, records allow assessment of biased reporting. If a person claims 3 days of anterograde amnesia, but emergency room records show the person reported being only "stunned," this is important evidence to establish whether a brain injury claim is genuine. On the other hand, claimant self-report that correlates with medical findings in the earliest records improves credibility.

The weaknesses of relying on records alone need to be emphasized. Records are fallible and are possibly the weakest portion of the evidentiary tripod. Unlike the interview and testing data collection phases, the records review phase is impossible to standardize. Unlike other countries with strong centralized record keeping and universal standards, Americans vary greatly in the school systems they attend, the tests they are given, and the medical practices to which they are exposed. Some legal cases contain volumes of detailed records; others contain a few illegible progress notes. Records also vary greatly along the dimension of subjectivity and objectivity. A computerized tomographic scan is more objective than psychiatric diagnoses given by a primary care physician. The FN should ask the retaining attorney to obtain records most likely to contain relatively objective data: school records that include results of standardized testing, date-of-incident records that contain neurological and mental status testing, neuro-imaging studies, routine and 24-hour electroencephalographic studies, and phar-macy records.

Cripe (2002) listed the many pitfalls of relying exclusively on records and advised of the need to correlate records with other evidence. The main problem is logical, namely, the assumption of veridicality: Do the words used accurately describe what transpired in the past? However, this is exactly the assumption made in the law, memorialized in the doctrine of *res ipsa loquitor*, "the thing speaks for itself." This means that certain matters do not have to be explained or supported any further than what is already obvious.

This is another example of the conflict between methods of the law and psy-chological decision making. Just because a plaintiff's preinjury medical record contains diagnoses of "anxiety" and "depression" does not necessarily mean the diagnoses are accurate. Conversely, the absence of preinjury anxiety and depres-sion diagnoses does not mean a plaintiff was free of psychological problems. The accuracy of past diagnoses needs to be confirmed using a convergent, multi-method approach every bit as much as characterizations of present functioning.

Other problems include limited sampling or lack of standardization, different report-writing styles, narrow focus, subjective or biased interpretations, and lack of validation. As an example of limited sampling and lack of standardization, one emergency department may require interval applications of the Glasgow Coma Scale; others may require "attention and orientation" testing only. This can make staging of the original neurological insult problematic. As an example of narrow focus, some psychiatrists explore only Axis I diagnoses and never explore pervasive personality patterns for Axis II diagnoses. They usually write "deferred" or "none" for Axis II diagnoses. The absence of psychiatric records also does not mean the absence of psychopathology in the past. For example, persons with antisocial traits, poor insight, or personality disorders are unlikely to seek mental health counseling.

Interview

Neuropsychological assessment consists of much more than just administering and scoring tests. Collection of interview material during a face-to-face inter-view is a critical component of the assessment phase (Sweet, 1991). The inter-view of the plaintiff (or defendant) is used to gather two forms of impressionis-tic data: history and mental status examination (MSE). The history collected from the claimant includes the precipitating event(s); evolution of cognitive and psychological complaints; treatment efforts, including referral patterns; present complaints, present and past social status; and developmental, educational, and past medical histories. The present complaints may be divided into cognitive, emotional, somatic, and behavioral components.

The history is crucial because it provides the context in which to interpret the subsequent test scores. The context for interpretation is developed by distilling historical information into a few areas, such as (a) the severity of the initial neurological injury, (b) background variables that help establish preinjury aptitude and achievement levels, and (c) establishment of the symptom time line. A typical approach to interviewing is to develop a structured interview form. This confers standardization on the interview process (see Test Administration section).

The MSE component is a systematic monitoring of behavioral cues during the interview, cues that will be integrated into the total impression and final opinions (Cronbach, 1984; Strub & Black, 1988). The MSE includes a description of the claimant's speech and language, verbal content and discourse organization, logic and reasoning, affect, mental trends, nonverbal behavior, and social relatedness. The MSE is another form of convergent evidence that should be correlated with history, records, and test scores to prove or disprove brain injury claims. This process of correlating and weighing data sources is impressionistic, assumes a sensitive and adequately trained observer (Sweet, 1991), and should be described as such during testimony.

There are some important differences between forensic and clinical neuropsychological interviewing. One difference is the in-depth exploration of the symptom time line and cognitive–attitudinal factors. Brain disease such as CHI is not only determined by a set of complaints and findings, but also its clinical course is a part of the definition. Cognitive symptoms that suddenly erupt or evolve long after a head injury are not consistent with the disease of CHI; rather, true CHI symptoms appear in maximum intensity immediately following head trauma. For this reason, it is important to inquire when the symptoms started. This of course should be correlated with the records.

Cognitive–attitudinal factors are also important. Clinicians are less concerned about why patients believe what they do. FNs, however, should devote some time to exploring the claimant's beliefs regarding the nature of their cognitive problems, their expectancies of outcome, and the sources for their beliefs. That is because the process of litigation exposes claimants to influences and experiences not present in straightforward clinical situations. This exploration can provide insights into prognosis and separation of neurogenic from psychogenic, situational, and secondary gain factors.

One source of nonneurogenic influence is suggestion by authority figures. Direct coaching by attorneys is a documented occurrence (Youngjohn, 1995).

In a survey, a majority of trial lawyers viewed it as their duty to expose plaintiffs to psychological test content in preparation for defense-requested evaluations (Essig et al., 2001). Even well-meaning neuropsychologists may further spoil data by giving inappropriate warnings about symptom validity detection (Youngjohn, Lees-Haley, & Binder, 1999).

Other influences include the plaintiff's participation in protracted litigation, education in head injury symptoms through a "traumatic brain injury [TBI] education group," and Internet research; symptom suggestion by doctors may lead some claimants to monitor their every memory act with intense diligence. This can result in the plaintiff innocently misinterpreting normal forgetting episodes as evidence for a CHI. In this case, causation of memory complaints may lie in misdiagnosis of brain damage by aggressive treaters. In contrast, a person who reports memory problems starting immediately following head trauma with at least some improvement over time is more likely to have a neurogenic cause.

Test administration

Test selection in a forensic arena is guided by the same general principles as during a regular clinical neuropsychological examination. The courtroom experience is more relaxing, and the answers to aggressive questions suggest themselves more readily a good neuropsychological examination was conducted at the beginning. Despite myths and beliefs to the contrary, there is no legal requirement that only commercially available, so-called fixed batteries are admissible (Reed, 1996). Test selection should be based what we term a "sound assessment doctrine." The proposed elements of a sound forensic neuropsychological assessment are as follows:

• Use a standardized approach.
• Never rely on single tests.
• Use tests in common use that have a sound scientific basis.
• Always assess effort and symptom validity.
• Use tests with a sound normative basis.
• Use logical and relevant test selection.
• Avoid "homemade" and novel approaches.
• Avoid blind interpretation of commercial fixed batteries.

An assessment method is *standardized* when a procedure is described with sufficient clarity to allow different examiners to collect data in the same manner with minimum error (Anastasi & Urbina, 1997; Grisso, 1988). Practically speaking, standardized measures typically refer to commercially available published tests and measures, although such a definition is too restrictive. Nevertheless, even a self-report history form is considered standardized if the same questions, response formats, items, and printed form are used with every examinee. Parenthetically, the terms "standardized" and "reliability/validity" are mistakenly used interchangeably by laypeople and even by testifying neuropsychologists.

Avoidance of single tests is the corollary of relying on a group of routine tests (Bigler & Ehrfurth, 1981). Single tests, although they may show modest sensitivity to some forms of cerebral dysfunction (Frankle, 1995; Lacks, 1982), are not likely to answer questions before the court or may even miss severe neuropathology (Bigler & Ehrfurth, 1980). From a legal standpoint, most personal injury suits and criminal cases raise complex issues that cannot be answered by a single neurocognitive measure (or a single fixed battery). A person who sustains a moderate brain injury but reports a premorbid history of learning disability and attention deficits cannot be satisfactorily evaluated with a single measure. Single neurocognitive measures come from an era during which the only diagnostic question was one of "organicity," that is, whether there was brain damage or not. Most neuroimaging technologies allow this question to be answered satisfactorily, and the value of neuropsychological tests is to correlate cognitive and behavior changes with the neuroimaging results.

Neuropsychological measures with a sound scientific basis in common use are those with proven validity as shown in peer-reviewed scientific journals. Measures and techniques that are commonly practiced and at least meet minimum scientific and empirical foundations are the only ones that should be used. Strong evidence for the validity of a neuropsychological measure is proven ability to detect cognitive deficits in persons known to have such defects (sensitivity) or ability to determine the absence of deficit in persons known to be deficit free (specificity).

There is no neuropsychological measure (or battery) that demonstrates both excellent sensitivity and specificity in all imaginable clinical situations. Single studies demonstrating both excellent sensitivity and specificity for a measure can be used for admissibility purposes, but they do not apply to the weight of evidence. It is often the case that many other studies will also show that same measure to be abnormal in persons with putatively normal brains. Sensitivity and specificity are usually tradeoffs and depend on many factors, including the base rate of the target symptom measured and task difficulty. Most common neuropsychological measures should have at least good sensitivity (poorer scores in brain-damaged persons) and modest specificity, or they should demonstrate excellent specificity (better scores in normal people) and modest sensitivity. Specificity tends to be variable because nonneurological conditions can affect test scores (e.g., abnormal scores in depressed, older, or intellectually marginal persons).

Neuropsychological performance tests, which measure how good somebody typically is at a cognitive skill, demonstrate good sensitivity (sensitive to brain damage), but variable specificity (affected by factors other than brain damage). In contrast, neuropsychological symptom scales measure abnormal behaviors, not normal ones. A good example of such a scale is the Aphasia Screening Test. This measure has excellent specificity (few false positives), but low sensitivity (the majority of brain-damaged persons are not classically aphasic). A defensible forensic test battery should include both sensitive measures (cognitive performance) and specific measures (e.g., aphasia testing when appropriate). The important concluding maxim is this: The nonspecificty of most neuropsychological tests is the main reason for never interpreting scores in isolation from collateral records and history.

The FN should always give neurocognitive symptom validity tests (NSVTs). Forensic settings contain strong incentives for distorting test scores or interview data (positive reinforcement) while simultaneously providing disincentives for returning to a productive lifestyle (negative reinforcement). There is no legitimate reason for avoiding these measures in a forensic context. The base rate for invalid response styles in litigated brain damage claims is high, even when stringent criteria for malingering are applied.

For example, Binder and Willis (1991), using the Portland Digit Recognition Test, gave a malingering diagnosis if a minor injury litigant scored worse than the poorest performing patient with severe brain injury did. They still found roughly a third of litigating remote concussion patients met their criteria for malingering. When less-stringent but still rigorous criteria are applied, an elevated base rate of malingering in litigated postconcussion syndrome is the rule and not the exception (Greiffenstein, 2003; Mathias, Greve, Bianchini, Houston, & Crouch, 2002).

Modestly high base rates for malingering, defined as from one third to two thirds of a population, provide maximal diagnostic efficiency and incremental hit rates for validated symptom validity tests (Mossman, 2000a, 2000b). There is also good evidence for an inverse dose–response effect in litigated neurological injury: The more minor the neurological injury is, the greater is the likelihood of response distortion (Albers, Wald, Garabrant, Trask, & Berent, 2000; Green, Iverson, & Allen, 1999; Greiffenstein, 2003; Miller & Cartlidge, 1972).

Finally, a multistrategy approach to examining response distortion should be taken (Sweet, 1999b). Poor effort and malingering are not only seen on memory tests. There are other documented forms of noncompliance, such as exaggeration of motor deficits (Greiffenstein, Baker, & Gola, 1996), overidealized premorbid baseline (Greiffenstein, Baker, & Johnson-Greene, 2002), amplification of somatic problems (Larrabee, 1998), and excessive subjective complaining (Greiffenstein, Baker, Gola, Donders, & Miller, 2002). A review of particular NSVTs is beyond the scope of this chapter and is covered in more detail in chapter 4 of this volume.

Neuropsychological measures with a *sound normative base* mean that you have an objective basis for classifying cognitive scores as normal, abnormal, deficient, weak, or superior. Without a normative basis, characterization of test scores as normal or abnormal is prone to guesswork. A normative basis for a measure is established when it is given in standardized fashion to many community-residing, neurologically normal persons. This process provides normative tables, which are grouped data showing the range of performances typical for the majority of normal persons. Good normative tables allow the FN to classify a person's cognitive functions comfortably in terms of distance from the normal range.

Normative tables are typically organized by age, but can also be organized by education, gender, and intelligence. Many validated neuropsychological measures also come with normative tables. Experts who completely eschew use of normative tables, who rely on "one-size-fits-all" cutting scores, or who base their score classifications on "experience" or "internal norms" will not only fail a *Daubert v. Merrell Dow* (1993) challenge, they will fail even a tepid cross-examination. Most normative tables offer age-specific performance breakdowns, but the FN is wise to use multiple types of normative tables to promote convergence of methods. For example, there has been considerable research into the impact of IQ levels of neuropsychological performance (Tremont, Hoffman, Scott, & Adams, 1998) separate from the influence of age.

Relying on measures with logical basis means using tests that have lucid links and clear relevance to the legal issues at hand. The *Joiner v. General Electric* (1997) legal decision, discussed in the section on admissibility, allows a trial judge to disqualify even sound methods if they have no lucid link to the case at hand. A neuropsychological measure that is valid, standardized, and well normed is not necessarily a logical choice in a given legal issue. There would be no reason to give the Mattis Dementia Rating Scale to a person exposed to low levels of organic solvents because dementia is not suspected and has not been documented.

Another example is the General Neuropsychological Deficit Scale (GNDS) version of the HRB (Reitan & Wolfson, 1985). The GNDS was validated against persons with terminal brain cancer and other severe cerebral dysfunction (Wolfson & Reitan, 1995). The GNDS is certainly acceptable in severe brain damage cases before the court, but it has not been shown to prove the existence of permanent deficits in patients with minor brain injury (Dikmen et al., 1995). Thus, there is no logical link with remote minor head injury claims. Interestingly, the GNDS may be better at proving the existence of preinjury learning disability than at proving permanent mild cognitive problems in persons with minor head injury (Oestreicher & O'Donnell, 1995).

In summary, the general principle is forensic neuropsychological assessment relies on multiple standardized measures of both effort and function that have sound scientific, normative, and logical bases. A flexible battery relying on a routinely administered core of tests with each test in the battery showing at minimum modest correlation with the neurological condition at issue is the preferred approach. Some may hold a contrary view. Russell (1998) opined it was necessary to validate every grouping of tests *as a group* to enter the legal arena (e.g., Russell's version of the HRB would be acceptable in court). However, there is no logical, scientific, or legal basis to this opinion. Logically, it is no more necessary for neuropsychologists to prove the validity of any grouping of tests than it is necessary for medical doctors to validate a fixed set of diagnostic procedures to apply to every patient.

Empirically, Volbrecht, Meyers, and Kaster-Bungaard (2000) constructed a semiflexible test battery made up of *individually* validated neurocognitive measures from different conceptual domains (memory, learning, sustained attention, etc.). Volbrecht et al. demonstrated this semiflexible battery's predictive validity by showing a dose–response relationship with brain injury severity and showed discriminant validity in the differentiation of various clinical groups.

Legally speaking, Russell (1998) and similar Halstead-Reitan proponents failed to understand the general contours of *Daubert*: It has a liberal thrust. *Daubert* only requires some peer-reviewed evidence that a methodology is valid. Hence, the term *methodology* cannot be narrowly constructed to mean a "group of simultaneously validated procedures." A logical implication of Russell's (1998) beliefs would be that under *Daubert*, testifying geologists would have to use the same finite set of measures irrespective of which issue they are testifying regarding. This of course is absurd.

The ethics of the assessment phase are guided by multiple standards. The use of obsolete tests should generally be avoided (Standard 9.08 in the 2002 code). Obsolete does not mean measures that are simply old, but it definitely means old measures without any contemporary normative tables (e.g., use of the Wechsler-Bellevue or Wechsler Adult Intelligence Scale). However, the Wechsler Memory Scale, despite being 60 years old, has relatively contemporary normative tables (Spreen & Strauss, 1991, 1998). All measures should have some reliability and validity data from published peer-reviewed studies. A technique supported only by a single poster presentation may not be supportable. "Homemade" tests without any supporting data should be avoided at all costs. If not, the face valid reasoning should be stated in the report and the unknown reliability and validity acknowledged during testimony.

Report-Writing Phase

Neuropsychologists entering the forensic area for the first time treat written reports like clinical reports. However, there are numerous differences between the two, including differences in audience, objectives, vocabulary, level of detail, and treatment of the unspoken (Derby, 2001). The differing matters of style and report content are summarized in Table 2-2 and discussed in more detail next.

TABLE 2-2. Differences Between Clinical and Forensic Neuropsychology Reports

REPORT CHARACTERISTICS	CLINICAL SETTING	FORENSIC SETTING
Audience	Physicians, mental health professionals	Attorneys, judges, hearing officers, claims adjustors
Audience's main interest	Medical issues: neurocognitive diagnosis, prognosis, treatment	Narrow legal issues: causation, damages, competency
Level of detail	Report all meaningful cognitive and personal characteristics to better understand patient	Report details to establish important facts and support main inferences; avoid prejudicial details if not at issue
Vocabulary	Freely use trait labels ("egocentric"), cognitive deficit terms ("perseveration"), diagnostic terms ("dementia"), acronyms ("TIA")	Use understandable terms, avoid technical jargon in narrative, although may be unavoidable when reporting scores
Controlling mental set	Write as if the patient's general welfare depends on your opinion	Both consider general welfare and write as if you are under oath; be careful and definitive
Causation	Rarely considered, unknown for most mental disorders	State whether cause of action is a contributing factor to abnormal cognitive findings
Fact reporting	Treat history as fact unless proven otherwise (e.g., "The patient was on disability before the accident")	Stress the attribution of facts (e.g., "The claimant described himself as disabled before the accident")
Functional patterns	Predict activities of daily living	Provide a nexus, that is, explain the reasoning linking test scores to predictions of altered living skills
Diagnosis	Fit the person to the diagnostic category (i.e., formal *Diagnostic and Statistical Manual of Mental Disorders*, 4th ed., diagnosis)	Fit the category to the person; describe in concrete terms (see text for examples)
Behavior observations	Typically brief, limited to factors relevant to administration and scoring of tests	Longer and more detailed; correlate mental status with test scores and legal claims

The most obvious difference in report styles is audience and the related difference of report function. The clinician writes for physicians and mental health professionals, but the FN writes for a lay audience with administrative or legal backgrounds. The main report function for a clinician is neurocognitive diagnosis, psychological diagnosis, prognosis, and treatment. This report function is invariant across medical referral sources. In contrast, attorneys, judges, claim adjustors, and juries are concerned with narrow issues of law. Thus, report functions can vary widely (cf. Table 2-1).

In general, the primary function of the FN report is to offer opinions on the link between neuropsychological findings and the issue before the court. In personal injury cases, FNs address the issue of causation and damages, but causation may not be an issue in probate or criminal cases. In criminal cases, there are six different types of competence, including competence to plead guilty, waive right to counsel, and stand trial (Grisso, 1988, p. 3). Refer to chapter 12 on criminal contexts in this volume for further information. In essence, the FN report writer needs greater mental flexibility in tailoring the report to the specific legal issues.

The most important difference between clinical and forensic reports is the question of causality. Did the event in question (termed the "cause of action") cause any alterations in brain function? Many jurisdictions rely on a "proximate cause" criterion, meaning an act, event, or omission that results in the damage claims made, although it may not necessarily be the nearest or last cause. There is much legal controversy about what qualities an agency must possess in relation to an outcome to deserve the title cause, and we are not concerned with that discussion here.

What the FN should recognize is that courts are very concerned with *simple* causal ideas such as, "Did this car accident cause any cognitive or brain problems"? Most neuropsychologists recognize there is rarely a single cause for any psychological or neuropsychological disorder, barring rare neurobehavioral syndromes such as alexia or reduplicative paramnesia. Neuropsychologists are taught to think in multifactorial terms, and clinicians rarely address single causes in their reports, if they address cause at all. But, a forensic setting requires an answer to the question in a reasonably certain way. Remember, the standard of proof in personal injury cases is 51% or better, meaning the FN needs only reasonable certainty. A FN's statement that "the accident/mold exposure/toxic substances (is/is not) a factor in the claimant's neuropsychological presentation" represents a nice balance between the need for a simple causation statement and the need to consider multiple factors.

Another important difference between clinical and forensic reports is characterization of fact status. Clinical report writing requires economy and an assumption of accuracy. Hence, the reporting style may treat unsupported statements as statements of fact. A common statement in clinical reports is the following: "The patient comes for neuropsychological testing 8 months after a closed head injury." This sentence assumes "closed head injury" is a valid diagnosis, which may or may not be accurate. In a forensic report, the FN must attribute unsupported "factual sounding" statements to the source to make it more factual. A more factual restatement of the lead-in sentence in a forensic context would be, "The claimant comes for neuropsychological testing, believing she suffered a closed head injury." This protects you (especially plaintiff witnesses) from the accusation in court that you prejudged brain damage before you even laid eyes on the patient. Beginning all alleged statements of fact with "The claimant states" or "reports" is more factual and objective.

Another important difference between a clinical and a forensic report is the type and range of detail. In a clinical report, the focus is on describing *all* the meaningful psychological and cognitive characteristics of the person. The forensic report should focus only on the *most relevant* factors that contribute to a neuropsychological or psychological opinion. Grisso (1988) discussed the different philosophies of forensic report writing and recommended "striking a balance on detail." This means the report should include enough detail to establish important facts or track essential inferences; it should not include all of the neurocognitive or psychological observations that could be made, irrespective of how crucial such factors may be in clinical settings. The mention of a psychologically meaningful, but legally irrelevant, characteristic may introduce bias into the report that is more prejudicial than probative.

A good example of this is the issue of sexual orientation. In a personal injury context, a plaintiff's homosexuality may or may not be relevant. Drawing from one of our (M. F. Greiffenstein) personal files, mention of a plaintiff's lesbian status was omitted in one case because she was claiming only memory difficulties, not any psychological damages. She was committed to her lifestyle and reported no disruption of daily function related to her orientation. Thus, there was no relevance to the legal issue of damages. However, homosexuality was mentioned as a key factor in another case. The plaintiff had been absurdly diagnosed with "organic anxiety disorder" blamed on a 2-year-old minor injury. Preinjury records indicated the plaintiff voiced conflict between his desire for men and his father's demand he get married and produce grandchildren. The plaintiff gave up his male companion and married shortly after the accident. In this case, the report details established an important fact (preinjury voicing of sexual orientation conflict) and tracked an essential inference (the pressure of deception was a reasonable alternative cause of present anxiety symptoms) relevant to the damages issue. In summary, it is important to add emotionally charged details only if they contribute to understanding the plaintiff's (or criminal defendant's) legal claims.

Forensic neuropsychologists must strive to communicate in plain language and limit use of technical terms. This is very difficult to do in practice because most FNs are trained to use concise vocabulary that conveys rich meaning to similar-minded professionals. One mental exercise that may be useful to testifying experts is to develop a "dictionary" of commonly used jargon that supplies "definitions" that laypeople can understand. This is especially useful prior to trial. Table 2-3 contains a list of common neuropsychological terms. For example, the phrase "the protocol was characterized by strong perseverative tendencies in response to feedback" can be translated as "Mr. K showed a tendency to repeat the same mistake over and over, even when given clues about the correct answer."

The clinical and FN reports also differ on the importance of behavior observations. The clinical writer briefly comments on the gross neurological or cognitive functions necessary to support standard test administration (e.g., they are

TABLE 2-3. Proposed List of Neuropsychological Terminology Translated into Layperson's Terms

TECHNICAL DEFINITION[a]	CONCEPT	LAYMAN DEFINITION
The superiority of one cerebral hemisphere for processing specific tasks	Cerebral dominance	The right or left brain is better at one form of mental processing than another
Persistence of the same response despite its inappropriateness	Perseveration	Repeating the same mistake over and over despite feedback it is wrong
Cognitive abilities necessary for goal-directed action and adaptation to a range of environmental conditions and demands	Executive functions	A group of mental abilities concerned with planning and achieving goals
A disturbance in visually guided constructional activity	Constructional dyspraxia	A special difficulty often seen with right brain problems in drawing, copying, or building things
A generalized loss of cognitive functions resulting from cerebral disease occurring in clear consciousness (i.e., absence of confusional state)	Dementia	A brain disease in which many mental abilities are lost at the same time even though the patient remains alert and attentive

[a]Technical definition obtained from Loring (1999).

adequately oriented and attentive, have functional vision and hearing, etc.). In forensic settings, behavior observations are more comprehensive and detailed to promote convergent reasoning. Convergent reasoning is promoted through the correlation of mental status observations with other data, such as test scores and objective injury characteristics. The allegation of neuropsychological damages always includes claims of functional deficits (i.e., disruption of daily activities or attitudes deemed important by society). Examples of functional impairments include capacity for forming criminal intent, permanent work disability, or marital problems.

For this reason, it is important to correlate detailed mental status observations with test scores and relate these findings to the legal issue. A patient's conduct in the waiting room would not be mentioned in a routine clinical report, but an observation of a criminal defendant reading a magazine in the waiting room, but scoring at chance levels on the Peabody Individual Achievement Test (PIAT) Reading Comprehension Test would be relevant in a competent waiver of *Miranda* rights issue. There would also be lack of correlation between a plaintiff who claims severe memory loss but serves as sole historian during the interview, even correcting her spouse on dates and times. On the other hand, a plaintiff who repeats the same topic throughout the interview and makes many perseverative errors on the Wisconsin Card Sorting Test (WCST) shows better correlation.

The approach to formal diagnosis also differs. In forensic settings, the FN should avoid strict categorization in the narrative (exclusive of the formal axial diagnosis) and use more descriptive, probabilistic-sounding statements in describing neuropsychological characteristics. Fit the category to the person, not the person to the category (Weiner, 1999). For example, in the case of findings favoring the plaintiff's position, a conclusory statement such as "The accident caused closed head injury syndrome of 5 years' duration" is not advisable. Instead, consider a statement such as "Mrs. Jones's present difficulties in recalling new information and subjective complaints resemble those seen in persons with proven brain tissue loss after blunt head trauma. The accident is a factor in the present results."

If you discover findings that favor the defense, consider the following: Make the negative diagnosis conditional and then add a positive descriptive statement. For example, "Although it is not possible for any one-time examination to rule out closed head injury symptoms in the past, the present examination does not contain any evidence for present neuropsychological impairment. Mrs. Jones presently closely resembles persons who are neurologically normal and enjoy a wide range of intact cognitive, perceptual, and motor abilities." In this way, the neuropsychologist provides differential certainty depending on time, that is, higher certainty about the present and lower certainty about the past. Weiner

(1999) described this language as promoting interprofessional convergence of psychologists' style of probabilistic statements and attorney's preponderance-of-the-evidence standards.

A simple diagnosis and formal axial diagnosis may be sufficient for clinical reports. However, in a forensic report, providing a diagnosis to address the causation issue is considered a "mere conclusory comment." In the example given above of "closed head injury of 5 years' duration," there is no stated nexus between the event 5 years earlier and the conclusion. A *nexus* refers to a network of lucid links between the cause of action, diagnostic methods, and the conclusion. In simplest terms, the FN must explain the reasons the plaintiff still suffers cognitive impairments so many years later. Simply diagnosing CHI on the sole basis of obtaining abnormal results *after* the incident is not logically supportable. This is the logical error of *post hoc, ergo proptor hoc* (Larrabee, 1990).

In addition, in the case of negative findings with respect to behavioral sequelae of head injury, it is useful also to provide a positive theory of the plaintiff's behavior. What is a reasonable basis for the memory complaints if not impaired brain function? Statements about the impact of mood, age, psychological syndromes, attribution style, physical status, medication status, and social demand features can be made if such opinions are grounded in actual findings. The following opinion is an example of an alternative theory of complaints that is grounded in differential diagnosis: "Mr. Doe's memory complaints are shaped by his sad mood, significant others' tendency to overfocus on any mistake, and the resulting mistrust of his own thought processes." In this case, the FN's evidence for this opinion was a history of remitting/relapsing depression predating an accident, a current spike-2 Minnesota Multiphasic Personality Inventory (MMPI) profile (a profile dominated by a deviant elevation on the Depression scale), an overly solicitous family, and a speech pathologist who treated any forgetting episode as "evidence for TBI."

The ethical aspects of the report-writing phase are controlled by all standards in Section 2.0 of the 1992 code (Evaluation, Assessment, or Intervention) and Section 9.0 (Assessment) of the 2002 code (APA, 2002). Ethical Standard 9.06 (APA, 2002) implies an ethical reason for relying on convergent evidence to interpret test scores. Please refer to this volume's chapter 3 on ethics for a more detailed discussion.

The Trial Phase

Discovery phase

Discovery is a preliminary process for compiling facts relevant to the case. All parties to a suit have the statutory right to ask for all documents that form the basis of an opinion. Most states' discovery rules are based on the FRE (1975), although there are some jurisdictional differences of which the FN should be aware. Discovery is designed not only to collect information; but also to narrow the dispute into main issues. In the case of the FN, the opposing side wants an early look at the FN's opinions, bases for that opinion, and pertinent personal information about the FN. Typically, attorneys demand key information from the opposing side, with demands taking the form of an interrogatory or a discovery deposition. An interrogatory is a typed list of questions. Discovery depositions are also attempts to (a) determine what the FN knows and does not know, (b) pin the expert down to a final opinion, and (c) sample the witness's testifying behavior. A discovery deposition can only be used for impeachment purposes at trial, meaning it can be used to develop inconsistencies at trial.

It does not matter if you are a treating doctor or an independent examiner; your complete case file is discoverable. If you have offered trial consulting services in addition to testimony, all notes and documents prepared for the retaining attorney are also discoverable. Although practices vary, most states have broad discovery rules. Neuropsychologists should expect the entire file to be subpoenaed. This includes interview notes, test forms, computerized scoring reports, correspondence, records reviewed, notes, and billing statements.

Admissibility

An important element of neuropsychologists' legal involvement is the admissibility of their data and opinions. Federal, state, and case laws provide criteria, or "legal tests," that determine which evidence is admitted into trial. Rules governing admission of expert testimony are codified in the FRE, particularly FRE Rules 702–706. Key case law governing admission includes the "Daubert trilogy" discussed below.

Understanding legal bases of admissibility includes knowledge of the applicable FRE. The most applicable one is FRE 702, which states:

If scientific, technical, or other specialized knowledge will assist the trier of fact to understand the evidence or to determine a fact in issue, a witness qualified as an expert by knowledge, skill, experience, training, or education, may testify thereto in the form of an opinion or otherwise.

This means an expert has training in areas that the average juror or judge is not expected to understand. The FN assists the juror (or judge) in either understanding the evidence (e.g., explaining CHI) or determining a fact in issue (e.g., whether the car accident caused a brain injury in the plaintiff). FRE represents a broad liberalization of the term "expert," and most neuropsychologists would have no difficulty qualifying under this rule.

The judge is given broad discretion in applying admissibility rules. Understanding admissibility guidelines is crucial to a productive attorney–neuropsychologist interaction because you must convince the attorney that your methodology and opinions will survive a legal challenge. Challenges to neuropsychological testimony may take three forms: (a) general competence of psychologists to testify, (b) scope of neuropsychological testimony, and (c) challenges to particular neuropsychological methods or tests.

Challenges to general competence to testify are rare. Courts have officially recognized psychologists as competent experts since the *Jenkins v. United States* (1962) appellate court decision. Jenkins was a felon who mounted an insanity defense against sexual assault charges, but the trial judge threw out testimony from all psychologists and one psychiatrist who relied on IQ scores. The trial judge ruled psychologists lacked medical training, a prerequisite for testifying about "mental disease." The trial judge was reversed on appeal.

The majority opinion was that two factors should guide admission of psychological evidence: the actual experience of the witness and the probative value of the testimony. As neuropsychological tests may sometimes be the only evidence of cognitive dysfunction in brain injury claims, neuropsychological testimony easily meets the probative prong. Proving "actual experience" means documentation of coursework, training, and work experience relevant to neuropsychology (Greiffenstein, 2002). The general competence of neuropsychologists to testify was challenged at the trial and appellate court levels in *Simmons v. Mullins* (1975). Relying on both *Jenkins v. United States* (1962) and the newly published FRE, this Pennsylvania appeals court ruled that neuropsychologists could testify because they were nonmedical professionals with specialized knowledge about measuring cognitive change.

Challenges to scope of neuropsychological testimony are more common, but typically involve only one issue: causation. There have been many published appeals challenging the ability of FNs to make inferences about physical changes in the brain blamed on the cause of action. In other words, can the neuropsychologist infer brain changes from test score or observational evidence? This body of case law contains mixed rulings both adverse to and supportive of neuropsychological testimony, depending on geographic location and type of brain damage claim.

A supportive ruling was made by the Iowa Supreme Court in *Hutchison v. American Family Mutual Insurance* (1994). This court ruled that neuropsychologists are qualified both to diagnose the general state of the brain and whether the cause of action (e.g., car accident) was a factor in altered brain status. In the CHI claim of *Valiulis v. Scheffeos* (1989), an Illinois appellate court also supported neuropsychological causation testimony, noting that medical doctors themselves rely on neuropsychologists to answer this question.

However, testimonial scope rulings appear to be unfavorable to neuropsychologists in a different context: claims of neurotoxic brain injury. In this body of law, the ability of neuropsychologists to infer subtle (i.e., unobservable) brain changes is challenged, typically by defense attorneys. A few critical cases bear mentioning. In *Schudel v. General Electric* (1995), plaintiffs proffered neuropsychological evidence for brain damage caused by organic solvents and poly-chlorinated biphenyls (PCBs). The federal appeals court for the Ninth Circuit ruled neuropsychological testimony is limited to damages, but cannot address physical causation. It was up to medical doctors or the jury to draw any connection between claimed neurocognitive deficits and toxic exposure. *Chandler Exterminators v. Morris* (1992) is another neurotoxic tort case. The Georgia Supreme Court affirmed the trial court's decision to bar a neuropsychologist's testimony that linked neurotoxicants with abnormal test scores. Under pressure from advocacy groups, the Georgia legislature wrote new law specifically allowing neuropsychologists to offer brain injury testimony in that state.

Challenges to specific neuropsychological tests and measures are also common and should be taken very seriously. In this case, the FN is recognized as an expert and competent to testify by both sides. However, this type of challenge questions the scientific basis of one or more of the expert's specific methods, measures, or conclusions. For example, a plaintiff attorney may challenge the use of a particular malingering detection method, or a defense attorney may challenge reliance on a list of "brain damage signs." Challenges to specific methods are brought under the *Frye v. United States* (1923) and *Daubert* rulings. These are famous rulings that lay out concrete criteria for admission of specific methodologies.

The *Frye v. United States* (1923) ruling originated with a felon arguing the trial judge should not have barred scientifically based exculpatory evidence. The defendant's experts were prepared to testify Frye was innocent because of results from an early form of the polygraph. This federal appeals court affirmed the trial judge's disqualification of the polygraph based on what is termed the *Frye* standard: Only those scientific methods and concepts that have gained *general acceptance* in a particular field are admissible. In this light, the polygraph was considered too experimental.

This general acceptance standard held sway for 70 years until challenged in the famous *Daubert v. Merrell Dow* (1993) Supreme Court decision. The *Daubert* court agreed with plaintiffs that the FRE supplanted *Frye*. To be admissible, scientific testimony must meet two very broad criteria: They must be (a) scientifically valid and (b) relevant to the case at hand. The *Daubert* court offered trial judges a partial list of specific guidelines to determine the scientific validity prong. This nonexhaustive list includes

1. Falsifiability, that is, has the methodology been tested, or is it even testable?
2. Peer review, that is, has the methodology been published or subjected to peer review?
3. Does the method show an acceptable error rate, or is there potential for testing the error rate? (The word *potential* implies this is a restatement of the falsifiability test.)

4. Have the principles or methodology gained general acceptance? (*Frye* again.)

5. Is there a technical manual or other guide to control use of the instrument?

The Supreme Court further refined the *Daubert* "criteria" in two other major decisions. In *General Electric v. Joiner* (1997), the court ruled the *Daubert* standard applied to an expert's deductive processes even in the presence of sound and accepted methods. In this case, a trial judge threw out an expert's testimony that the plaintiff's lung cancer was caused by PCB exposure because this deduction was based on inapplicable epidemiological and animal studies. The *Joiner* court agreed the plaintiff was not exposed to the same circumstances reported in the epidemiological studies and was not injected with extreme PCB levels like a laboratory animal. Hence, the expert could not explain why these studies applied to the instant case, signaling irrelevance. In short, *Joiner* requires judges to examine the reasoning processes experts use to bridge the gap between data and conclusions. In *Kumho Tire v. Carmichael* (1999), the court recognized the *Daubert* opinion was too narrowly linked to the term *scientific* in FRE 702. The *Kumho* decision extended *Daubert* standards to cover all forms of expertise, including but not limited to technical and experiential testimony.

The psychology and neuropsychology community's reception of the "*Daubert* trilogy" has been one of mixed feelings tinged with foreboding. A field-restricted search of PsycInfo we conducted in December 2003 retrieved 80 published psychology articles containing the term "Daubert" in the title or abstract. Most were commentary articles about *Daubert*'s imagined impact on psychological practice. For example, Grove and Barden (1999) warned that a number of diagnoses, such as posttraumatic stress disorder and multiple personality disorder would not survive scrutiny under the new standards. Of these 80 references, 10 included the term "neuropsychological" in the title or abstract. These commentary articles offered either dire predictions of neuropsychology's future in the courtroom or argued for narrow inclusion of favored methods.

Posthuma, Podrouzek, and Crisp (2002) warned that *Daubert* poses a serious challenge to neuropsychological testimony in mild head injury cases. As remote minor head trauma cases make up the bulk of forensic neuropsychological referrals, an implication is that much of our forensic work will disappear.

Reed (1996) interpreted *Daubert* to mean that only the commercially available fixed batteries (e.g., the HRB) would survive a *Daubert* challenge, and that flexible test batteries would not be admissible. Insofar as most neuropsychologists adhere to a flexible battery approach and only a small minority advocate fixed batteries, Reed's implication is that most neuropsychologists would not receive court work.

Reitan and Wolfson (2002) opined that most neuropsychological measures are "lacking" in conformity to *Daubert* criteria, except Reitan's own test battery.

Lees-Haley, Iverson, Lange, Fox, and Allen (2002) expected "many inadmissibilities" of MMPI-2 validity scales, but acknowledged it meets the general acceptance prong of *Daubert*.

Our view is that *Daubert* has had minimal to no impact on neuropsychological practices and is unlikely to have a negative impact in the future. In fact, we view neuropsychologists as uniquely suited to meet the challenges of *Daubert*. We agree with Lally (2003) that psychologists are better positioned to respond to *Daubert* challenges than mental health professionals who rely on interview and self-reported history, such as social workers and psychiatrists. Our optimism is based on multiple grounds. Our optimism is also based on textual analysis of *Daubert* combined with empirical and anecdotal evidence.

An integrated reading of the *Daubert* trilogy and the FRE (1975) indicates the judge's gatekeeping role is a liberal mandate, which encourages acceptance of even novel and recent methodologies. The *Daubert* elements are also unweighted and polythetic criteria. This means no single element is necessary, and any single element or combination of elements is sufficient to admit evidence. Practically, this means the trial judge can rely on only a single element if he or she chooses (e.g., the *Frye* general acceptance criteria alone).[6] There is case law and anecdotal evidence for this view. In a brutally candid single case report, McKinzey and Ziegler (1999) acknowledged their failure to mount a convincing *Daubert* challenge to a "flexible test battery." In their case, the judge ruled that a flexible test battery was valid because of the general acceptance doctrine alone.

There is much empirical evidence for the nonthreat of *Daubert* to forensic neuropsychology. Neurocognitive symptom validity tests have survived many *Daubert* challenges. Mossman (2003) conducted a Lexis[TM] search in December 2002 and retrieved 18 published federal and state cases referring by name to NSVTs. Five of these cases involved application of *Daubert* reliability factors to use of NSVTs, and the courts found such tests admissible in all cases.

Why the failure of dire predictions to come true? The method skeptics or narrow-practice advocates (those who warn that *Daubert* will only favor a narrow range of instruments) seem to confuse the important legal distinctions between *admissibility* and *weight*. Admissibility is a judge's decision that evidence has probative value, that is, is it relevant, can it determine the outcome of the case, and should the jury see it? The judge only analyzes the relevance of the evidence and does not make value judgments about relative importance. Hence, a test of modest validity has equal footing with a test of great validity during an admissibility hearing. Both are probative. In contrast, weight is a jury decision and refers to perception of the evidence's importance and believability *after* it is admitted.

Reed's (1996) and Reitan and Wolfson's (2002) conclusion that only fixed test batteries will pass *Daubert* analysis is incorrect because it is based on such confusion. They seem to believe that perceived superiority is relevant to admissibility, but their arguments for superiority only go to weight. Reed cited the case of *Chapelle v. Ganger* as proof of his conclusion, but even cursory study of the judge's written decision revealed *all* neuropsychological testimony was admitted.[7] The judge only put greater weight on testimony from a fixed battery advocate for reasons that had nothing to do with battery composition. There was no *Daubert* challenge to a flexible test battery at all. There was only a *Daubert* challenge to a vocational counselor offering intuitive testimony.

The FN must still be prepared to cope with occasional challenges to portions of the test battery. Challenges to specific neuropsychological tests take the form of *Daubert* or *Frye* hearings held *in limine*. This means the court hears evidence pro and con away from the jury. The opposing attorney files a motion asking the court to exclude a particular test measure or a particular conclusion from admission. Most states have adopted the *Daubert* standards into their own rules of evidence, but many states still rely on *Frye* or *Frye* hybrids (e.g., *Frye-Davis* in Michigan).

The FN helps the retaining attorney prepare the response (or even the motion itself) by applying the *Daubert* criteria to a particular test's (or inference's) knowledge base. For example, if there is a challenge to use of the WCST to determine frontal lobe damage in a head injury claim, the FN could supply the retaining attorney with the test manual (meeting Element 5 above). The validity and falsifiability of the WCST can be shown by citing studies that correlate WCST performance with frontal activity or damage (e.g., Boone et al., 1999; Pendleton and Heaton, 1982; Robinson, Heaton, Lehman, & Stilson, 1980; Steinberg, Devous, & Paulman, 1996), and the sensitivity and error rate can be shown with Robinson et al. (1980). The general acceptance of the WCST can be shown through its mention in commonly used test compendiums (Spreen & Strauss, 1991) or by citing test user surveys. For example, Butler, Retzlaff, and Vanderploeg (1991) reported 73% of respondents use the WCST routinely. Of course, the large number of articles published on the WCST easily meet the peer review and publication element of the *Daubert* standards.

Deposition or testimony phase

Once the admissibility of neuropsychological methods is established, the neuropsychologist–attorney interaction moves to the next step: The FN offers oral or written opinions under oath for scrutiny by opposing counsel and the trier of fact (judge or jury). Sworn testimony can be offered in written form (interrogatory or affidavit) or in oral form through a deposition or in the courtroom. A deposition is a form of legal discovery in which litigants question witnesses to determine what testimony they will offer at trial.

A deposition is a very formal process in which a court reporter transcribes questions and answers into a typed record. A discovery deposition is conducted solely by the opposing counsel and represents a preliminary effort to obtain information about opinions, narrow the dispute into the most pertinent issues, and evaluate potential courtroom demeanor of the FN. A discovery deposition cannot be introduced at trial except to impeach the witness. A *de bene esse* deposition is more commonly referred to as a "trial deposition," and it is intended to preserve a FN's testimony if he or she is not available to appear live at trial. Alternatively, but more rarely, the FN's live testimony can also be offered at trial in front of the judge and jury.

A trial deposition or live trial testimony is broken into two phases: direct examination and cross-examination. Direct examination occurs first and is defined as testimony elicited by the retaining attorney. The direct examiner first tries to establish qualifications to testify as an expert with questions about academic degrees, neuropsychology coursework at the graduate school level, predoctoral and postdoctoral training in psychology and neuropsychology, employment history, relevant experience, and publications. Opposing counsel may on occasion challenge credentials during direct examination by asking the court to *voir dire* the FN. *Voir dire* means "to tell the truth" and is a preliminary examination of competence to testify through additional questions about credentials. The trial judge then decides whether your testimony is allowed. Qualification as a witness is rarely a problem for FNs. In addition, the FRE (1975) 702–705 (and the related state evidentiary rules) give broad latitude to trial judges to consider many factors, including experience in the absence of publication or board certification. In summary, the *voir dire* does not pose a major threat in most cases. However, opposing attorneys can continue to emphasize questionable or insufficient credentials during cross-examination.

The direct examination continues after the FN has been qualified. The questions are open ended but designed to elicit brief and simple opinions favorable to the retaining attorney. Most retaining attorneys use the FN's report outline and headings to organize questions, which mirror the same temporal sequence of steps taken by the FN before issuing a final report (e.g., taking history, administering and scoring tests, integrating multiple data sources, formulating a diagnosis). Cross-examination begins immediately following the conclusion of direct examination. The opposing counsel asks questions from two general categories: questions designed to elicit weaknesses or flaws in the FN data gathering or logic and questions designed to prove bias or lack of independence.

Productive attorney–neuropsychologist interactions during the trial phase cannot be managed or controlled in the same way as during any pretrial stage. The FN's interactions with retaining and opposing attorneys are now public. The attorneys and court rules govern behavior. Hence, the FN should focus on his or her style of interacting with the jury. The cross-examining attorney has the right to ask questions and receive responsive answers. *Responsive* means the answer is relevant; it does not mean you have to give the answer desired.

There is no legal requirement that an FN must answer "yes" or "no," despite the desire of some attorneys to have you believe this. Brief narrative answers are allowable.

Productive attorney–neuropsychologist interactions now depend on the elements of expert witness control. These are behaviors and attitudes you have wide latitude in determining. The FN has control over nonverbal behaviors (demeanor and gaze), agency (active vs. passive answering), speech characteristics (pace and volume), and speech content (scope of answers, definitions offered) and manifest attitude (deliberate, unbiased) and general style of communication (objective, advocative, educating).

The general elements of expert witness control refer to a consistent style of communication across your entire testimony. The best general style is defining your role as one of educating the jury. The corollary of this is never be an advocate. You are not there to persuade, entertain, advocate, crusade for justice, pursue quixotic ideals, or validate your own sense of self-importance. Your objectivity will be measured by how you educate the jury in principles of neuropsychology and how you applied those principles to the issue at hand. You advance this style by responding deliberately without excessive qualification, patiently explaining definitions in simple terms without using technical words or making gratuitous assumptions about the fact finder's technical knowledge. Be honest about your experience, knowledge, and the neuropsychological literature. Jurors are likely to come from more modest backgrounds than the expert, but they do not need a high degree to recognize puffery, manipulation, and gross violations of common sense when they hear it.

Another stylistic element is maintaining objectivity. This does not mean you cannot have a point of view or philosophy or that you should never be passionate. Despite cherished myths to the contrary, do not brag that your objectivity is proven by statements such as "I do 50% of work for plaintiffs and 50% for defense." A 50/50 split can easily be evidence for the opposite: You give a favorable opinion to the side that reaches the telephone first. If you commonly give opinions favoring certain positions over others, this could actually be more objective if your opinion percentages approximate the base rate for a given condition, diagnosis, or phenomenon.

For example, if you happen to find that 40% of minor head injury litigants show positive malingering signs on memory tests, this would be more objective given the high prevalence of malingering in late postconcussive claimants (Binder & Willis, 1991; Gianoli, McWilliams, Soileau, & Belafsky, 2000; Greif-fenstein, Baker, & Gola, 1994). For example, Mittenberg, Patton, Canyock, and Condit (2002) surveyed forensic neuropsychologists representing a pool of more than 33,000 forensic cases and reported a 40% base rate of invalid effort. Given the high prevalence of invalid effort, the FN who never diagnoses or even suspects invalid effort should be considered biased. If you find permanent brain dysfunction in 95% of the mild TBI litigants you examine, these conclusions may be biased because they go against the base rate for residual deficits in mild head trauma (Binder et al., 1997). Conversely, if you only find evidence of permanent brain dysfunction in persons who have taken over 30 days to follow commands, you may also show bias because persisting deficits are common in persons with shorter periods of coma (Dikmen et al., 1995). The point is that witness bias is not measured by simply calculating the number of plaintiff versus defense (or prosecution versus defense) referrals.

Nonverbal behaviors are also important for attorney–neuropsychologist interactions during the trial phase. Maintain consistency of demeanor across both the direct and cross-examination phases. It is helpful to consider the familiar psychological concept of "examiner characteristics," in which the tester's personality, biological traits, and nonverbal behavior influence responses to psychological tests. This applies equally to the courtroom and entails the characteristics of the questioning attorney influencing your responses.

Direct and cross-examinations contain entirely different questions, methods, and aims associated with different personalities. The direct examination elicits evidence to support an opinion, and the cross elicits testimony that disproves it. The direct examiner is friendlier and less controlling; the cross-examiner is less friendly and more controlling. The retaining attorney encourages discourse with more open-ended questions, and the opposing attorney limits you with closed-end questions. The FN has no procedural right to dictate the content of direct or cross-examination. The FN does have control of demeanor. This means consistency in tone, posture, gaze, prosody, and movement. For example, when the retaining attorney's direct examination is done, turn in the witness chair and squarely face the opposing attorney. This signals you are giving as much attention to the opposing side as you did the retaining side. Continuing to stare in the old direction appears dismissive and inattentive.

The FN may also control the timing and scope of answers. You do not have to answer quickly or match the pace of the questioner. As a general maxim, effective answers to questions concisely address more than one issue. A reasonably brief answer simultaneously (a) shows honesty and integrity, (b) shows responsivity to the question, (c) educates the jury, (d) defines the issue in your terms, and (e) reiterates the bases for your opinion. It is not possible to achieve all goals with any one answer, unless one launches into a numbing discourse before being cut off by the judge. But, effective answers (other than genuine Yes–No questions) should cover at least two issues.

However, the most difficult aspect of expert witness control during testimony is speech content. This takes much experience and an adequate knowledge base. Passive answering means responding only to the overt, literal meaning of the question. The effective FN engages in active answering whenever possible. An active answer is responsive not only to the overt question, but also to the latent content. It is responding to the latent content that differentiates the knowledge-able and effective witness from the less-effective witness. This interchange be-tween a defense attorney and plaintiff's neuropsychologist shows an active an-swer in response to a general question:

Q: So neuropsychological test scores can be abnormal, but a person's brain can still be functioning normally?

A: It is true that one or a few abnormal test scores are common in the general population. However, it is Ms. Jones's high number and pattern of abnormal scores that led to my diagnosis of brain problems.

In this case, the active answer addressed the imprecision of the question, namely, ambiguity of number (How many abnormalities can a normal person produce?). The latent issue raised by the question was which criteria differenti-ate abnormal brain states from nonneurological explanations. "Yes" may some-times be an adequate answer in the right context, but may have left misimpres-sions with the trier of fact, such as (a) this plaintiff scored abnormally on only a few measures, (b) the expert never considered alternative explanations, or (c) the witness was biased toward finding brain damage. The point is that active answers are allowable, control misimpressions, educate the trier of fact, and provide a lucid link between general questions and the specific matter at hand.

Another element of attorney–neuropsychologist interactions during trial is anticipation of difficult questions designed to trap, embarrass, or impeach you. There are many such questions, termed *gambits*, designed to make you look ill-informed, stupid, biased, or out of touch with mainstream neuropsychology. Although such questions can be legitimate and such characteristics could accu-rately apply to you, this chapter assumes a conscientious and knowledgeable NP. The following represents a small list of the most common gambits for which you should always be prepared: false alternatives, upsetting the witness, learned treatise (LT), and credentials challenge.

The gambit of *offering false alternatives* is one of the most commonly used methods of confusing the witness. The question asks the FN to choose between two competing explanations, usually phrased in an either/or manner. For exam-ple, after establishing that malingering measures were consistently negative in a plaintiff, the attorney asks, "Now doctor, either my client is malingering or is brain damaged, correct?" This statement assumes (note: latent content) that malingering and cerebral dysfunction are mutually exclusive and further as-sumes that no other diagnoses exist. The courtroom-unfamiliar neuropsycholo-gist may think that courtroom procedure dictates choosing only the alternatives provided by the attorney. The best response is one that rejects the underlying premise while simultaneously educating the trier of fact. A defensible answer would be "The absence of faking does not prove brain damage. Good effort only means the test scores are valid. In this case, Mr. Smith's good efforts produced test scores indicating normal memory for recent events." Here, in concise and plain fashion, the witness rejected the false alternative gambit, educated the jury (validity scales measure effort, not brain damage), proved his or her basic fairness ("Mr. Smith's good efforts"), and took the opportunity to restate the basic opinion ("test scores indicating normal memory").

Upsetting the witness is an attempt to raise the frustration level of the witness. There is a popular maxim that governs attorney behavior: "If you have the facts on your side, argue the facts. If you have the law on your side, argue the law. If you have neither facts nor law on your aside, attack!" Largely, most attorneys conduct themselves civilly. Great attorneys can conduct aggressive cross-examinations tempered by respect for the doctor's standing and credentials. Nevertheless, some attorneys try to provoke expert witnesses with inappropriate assaults in an attempt to elicit an overly emotional response. The hope is the expert witness explodes, lessening the witness's objective stance.

The best approach is to strip the emotion from the hostile question and uncover and respond to the (presumably rational) latent issue. More concretely, the expert answers with a two-part response: (a) The first clause restates the question in objective terms, and (b) the second clause answers the restated question in professional terms. Note this is a variation of the admit–deny tactic recommended by Brodsky (1991). For example, consider the following interchange:

Q: Doctor, isn't it true that some neuropsychologists have questioned your ethics in similar legal cases?

A: If you are asking whether I have been the subject of an ethics investigation, the answer is no." (A variation that is useful when an opposing neuropsychologist attacks you: "If you are asking if other neuropsychologists were upset that I disagreed with them on an some issue, the answer is yes.")

In this example, the expert stripped away the hostile insinuation and extracted a legitimate issue. Note that the question itself is legally improper because the attorney is testifying, not developing facts. Attorneys are not allowed to ask questions that assume facts not in evidence. The question is an obvious attempt to smear the witness with hearsay insinuation. Nevertheless, a common problem for experts is that not all retaining attorneys will know to object, and not all trial judges will sustain an objection to unfair questions. The FN must be prepared to cope with situations in which attorneys are given unusual latitude. You cannot offer legal objections yourself.

The FN must recognize the *LT gambit* and its variants. Under such a line of questioning, the FN is confronted with neuropsychology texts, journal articles, published commentary, and even interview transcripts with well-known neuro-psychologists. The attorney tries to get the expert to acknowledge a book/article/author/sentence/paragraph as "authoritative." A common question is "Don't you agree that Dr. Schmendrik's book *Neuropsychological Testing* is authoritative?" or "You have to agree that Dr. Legend Owen Mind is one of the great authorities in neuropsychology." The courtroom-unfamiliar expert does not know the legal ramifications of agreeing that a treatise is authoritative: Accepting a learned treatise means you must agree with every statement in the document. The eager-to-please witness who answers "Yes" will next be treated to a list of inconsistencies between his or her opinion and those of the alleged authoritative text.

The general principle is to refuse the gambit in every single case. This is both honest and scientifically defensible, but often difficult to do. Unless the expert is a polymath and absolute master of all neuropsychology writings, you should always refuse to agree. To maintain consistency, you must even refuse to acknowledge your own publications as authoritative in the legal sense, even if some expert witness guides advise you against this.[8]

There are a number of approaches to deal with the persistent LT gambit. A general approach is to acknowledge a book's relative importance or personal usefulness ("Its an important text that I sometimes rely on") while simultaneously denying overarching authority ("but nothing in neuropsychology is authoritative"). Another way is to provide answers that inform the jury that sound scientific and clinical practices never rest in any single individual or book. This is particularly true in neuropsychology. Hence, in response to questions about a book or specific journal, the FN witness might respond "With over 100 journals in neuropsychology and neurology coming out every month and thousands of articles in general psychology, no one article is that important." In response to the authoritative person variant, reasonable answers may be as follows: "Thousands of men and women have contributed to the field of neuropsychology, and I recognize Dr. Costas as one of those contributors" or "Dr. Legend Owen Mind is an important contributor to neuropsychology, but I don't necessarily agree with everything he has written."

When the opposing attorney wants you to agree or disagree with a statement he or she has read, another tactic is to ask for the book/article/document that the attorney is holding. The opposing counsel usually offers you a document containing a highlighted paragraph, sentence, or in some cases just half a sentence. Politely demur and state that although you are able to read, it would have no meaning unless you could read the whole chapter. It is very common for an attorney to read a sentence out of context, even though the entire paragraph or chapter may make clear the sentence has a meaning other than the one intended. Could you get a 60-minute break to read the whole chapter? In the appropriate context, more courtroom-familiar witnesses can fine-tune the answer to demonstrate powerfully to the jury that even alleged "authorities" frequently change their opinion. Going back to the first question, an answer might be, "Given that Dr. Lezak has published many different editions of her book and updated her opinions, it can't be authoritative. Which of the updated editions of Lezak did you have in mind?" However, this is a gambit for which assertiveness does not cause the attorney to beat a hasty retreat. The attorney may persist in an effort to make the witness look evasive, pompous, or out of touch with scholarship. Unlike other gambits, the FN should be prepared for persistent questions designed to make you look out of touch.

Even the most courtroom familiar and knowledgeable should expect a credentials challenge during the cross-examination. The title of *neuropsychologist* is a designation especially vulnerable to this attack because there is no controlling authority for determining this status. The majority of states only regulate use of the term *psychologist*.[9] Once recognized by the state as a psychologist, specialties' designations depend on the individual's subjective self-appraisal. FNs should prepare themselves for this approach by briefly outlining the features of their background that support their self-designation.

Greiffenstein (2002) offered an objective checklist approach for attorneys to select neuropsychologists, but FNs can adopt this same approach to prepare a list of qualifying attributes for the retaining attorney to use during direct examination. This helps to establish a foundation for qualifying you as an expert. The FN should divide the list into four broad areas: education (university, degree, major, minor, supervised training, relevant workshops); experience (employment, consultantships, diversity of neurological conditions); certification (board type and rigor of board); and publications (dissertation, publications, abstracts, commentary articles, book chapters).

This list is not exhaustive, and FNs may wish to emphasize other attributes, such as number of workshops, teaching experience, or diversity of experience. Make sure the list is up to date and provide sufficient detail to avoid leaving a misimpression. For example, an expert once listed "University of Michigan 1980–1982" under the heading "Postdoctoral Experience," leading the retaining attorney to believe the expert was a full-time postdoctoral fellow at a prestigious institution. However, the expert left out the crucial fact he only attended irregular group supervision sessions offered by a retired professor in the Ann Arbor area.

If the attack on the neuropsychology title fails (it usually does), the focus becomes the particulars of the case at hand. If the case is one of permanent brain damage following low-dose exposure to organic solvents, for example, the questioning will focus on the FN's lack of publications in this area or lack of experience with the particular diagnosis. If this issue has already been discussed with the retaining attorney, the FN's strategy is to answer these questions by presenting the bases for generalizing neuropsychological techniques to diverse populations (a restatement of Brodsky, 1991). You do this by stressing the basic commonalities among all patients from a neurological standpoint. For example, in the case of memory disorder, you would stress that all patients irrespective of social class, race, or illness share basic commonalities, including the fact they have brains with right and left halves, and the parts of the brain that control memory formation are basically invariant from one person to the next with rare exception. Witness this interchange:

Q: Isn't it true that you have never performed neuropsychological testing on railroad workers exposed to organic solvents or published anything about it?

A: Neuropsychological tests are designed for use with a wide variety of patients with suspected brain disorders, including railroad workers, but I agree this is the first time I have seen a railroad worker in litigated circumstances.

Or, the answer could be as follows:

A: We use memory measures to examine memory complaints in thousands of different people, including railroad workers, but this is the first time I personally have looked at memory complaints blamed on solvents by a railroad worker.

The expert in this case has accomplished multiple things: He or she has answered honestly about lack of experience with railroad workers claiming solvent exposure (responsive to the surface question). The expert also educated the jury on latent issues such as (a) stressing long and deep experience with many different kinds of patients, (b) the generalizability of neurocognitive measures to different communities, and (c) deflation of the question's false conceit of the "special plaintiff understood only by my expert." If the attorney presses now, he or she will appear to give the message that railroad workers from his or her state (or county or town) have peculiar brains that are different from any other jurisdiction in the country. This will not go over well with the folks in the attorney's community.

The trial phase challenges the neuropsychologist to present well-founded opinions that do not misstate or distort principles of neuropsychology. Ethical treatment of this is covered in Standards 1.06 of the 1992 code and Section 2.04 of the 2002 code (Basis for Scientific and Professional Judgments). It is inevitable that some neuropsychologists will voice opinions that are outliers relative to the mainstream of common practices. This is not necessarily unethical. The mainstream or consensus opinion is not automatically the best or most valid one. The FRE 702–705 combined with the *Daubert* (1993), *Kumho* (1999), and *Joiner* (1997) court decisions were designed to allow novel but potentially provable ("falsifiable") approaches into the courtroom.

Sometimes, outlying opinions are so unfounded that appellate courts limit neuropsychologist's scope of testimony. In the case of *Grenitz v. Tomlain* (2003), the Florida Supreme Court withdrew from earlier legal precedent that had given neuropsychologist's broad scope because of a witness's testimony. The witness claimed that the Object Assembly subtest of a Wechsler IQ test was able to differentiate *in utero* from *intrapartum* brain damage. Some medical organizations have started to take action against unfounded testimony on the grounds that legal testimony is an extension of practicing medicine and thus subject to oversight. Two neurosurgeons (in separate jurisdictions) were sanctioned for purportedly misstating practice standards (Albert, 2002). One neurosurgeon responded by suing a national neurosurgery organization, lost at the trial level, then appealed. The U.S. Supreme Court upheld the lower courts, ruling that professional societies must discipline members concerning improper courtroom testimony (*Austin v. AANS*, 2002; see Adams, 2002).

Posttrial Phase

An issue that receives little attention in expert witness guidebooks is posttrial considerations. Your involvement should not end after the verdict. This should be a time of reflection. First, never call the retaining attorney to find out the verdict. Strong interest in the outcome of a trial means you have an emotional stake in winning and losing.

Second, engage in an honest self-appraisal of your methods and testimony. This requires painful recollection of the cross-examination. Was the cross-examination skillful? Did the aggressive questions uncover *genuine* weaknesses in your reasoning, or were they merely designed to assassinate your character? An honest self-appraisal not only improves future testimony, but also can inform your routine clinical work. For example, one of us (M. F. Greiffenstein) used to rely heavily on qualitative signs as evidence for brain impairments. After a few unpleasant depositions, it became evident that these "signs" were sometimes seen in the context of *normal* aggregate scores. The base rate for this kind of error was actually quite high in the normal population. Another area for self-appraisal is reliance on Verbal–Performance IQ differences. A typical overinterpretation is "Mr. Doe's PIQ is 15 points lower than his VIQ, proving traumatic damage to the right brain." Actually, VIQ–PIQ splits are the rule and not the exception in the IQ protocols of persons with intact brains (Kaufman, 1990; Matarazzo, 1972; Matarazzo, Bornstein, McDermott, & Noonan, 1986). After that point, I relied more on a quantitative approach, using process neuropsychology methods as an additional tool, not a complete approach.

The posttrial phase is the best time for an "integrity check" (Brodsky, 1999). This is a self-appraisal of objectivity and fairness. Maintaining objectivity requires a number of steps, including awareness of the pull to affiliate with the retaining side. For example, if you catch yourself making multiple telephone calls to the retaining attorney to breathlessly announce a new insight, you may have succumbed to the pull of affiliation.

Second, you may assess the degree of emotional and financial involvement in the outcome. Do you eagerly await a phone call from the defense attorney telling of the jury's "no cause" verdict, or are you planning to spend the money you will be paid if the jury gives the plaintiff a favorable verdict? As mentioned, a simple ratio of plaintiff-to-defense cases is not compelling evidence for objectivity versus partisanship. It is a reality that most experts tend to be retained by one side more than another. There are many reasons for this, including word of mouth, aggressive versus conservative neurodiagnostic approaches, and scientist–practitioner ethos versus pure clinical orientation. In criminal contexts, psychologists testify for the defense more than the state, probably because psychologists' sympathies lie with mentally disturbed offenders. Many forensic psychologists proudly list "Death Penalty Mitigation" on their business cards, but few list "Death Penalty Aggravation" as a selling point. This is not to say that every bias is bad. All experts have biases toward a type of conclusion or method of analysis, and these should be readily acknowledged.

As discussed by Brodsky (1999), forensic neuropsychologist Edward Colbach (Colbach, 1981) recommended calculating a Validity Quotient (VQ). This is calculated by dividing the total number of court decisions into the number of court decisions for which opinion and verdict matched. Hence, if your opinion and the jury's have matched every time, the VQ would be 100%. However, like Brodsky (1999), we strongly advise against using this method. The VQ requires calling the retaining attorney to get the verdict. This is nothing more than the pull of affiliation, a wish to be "on the winning side." Second, the VQ assumes that a legal verdict validates or invalidates a psychologist's opinion. However, this thinking betrays certain grandiosity, that somehow the FN's opinion is the most critical in determining a fact at issue. Many factors go into trier-of-facts decision-making processes, including the competency of attorneys, the likability of litigants, other expert witness testimony, liability issues, and other legal issues having nothing to do with a FN's work. If you strongly believe in the VQ, you may be prone to the "star witness" mentality.

The best method for estimating objectivity is to correlate personal opinions with known base rates for certain conditions. Of course, estimating base rates is art as well as science. The idea is to determine whether you find cognitive dysfunction related to the cause of action much more often than the base rates allow or less cognitive dysfunction (or psychopathology) than expected. This issue could be thought about in the same way attorneys do: A judge's basic fairness is not determined if the judge sustains plaintiff's or defense's objections in a 1:1 ratio. That is not fairness; that is just scorekeeping. Instead, fairness is determined by how close the judge's rulings adhere to the letter of law. Hence, a fair judge could still easily rule 90% in favor of plaintiff and 10% in favor of defense in a particular case.

SUMMARY

Practicing principled forensic neuropsychology requires two integrated approaches: aspirational behavior and avoidance of committing wrongful acts (Hess, 1999b). Avoidance of wrongful acts means the FN behaves legally, morally, and ethically. This may include recognition of the seven deadly sins (e.g., avoiding sloth by writing timely neuropsychology reports). Aspirational behavior means constant examination of each act or report concerning its implications for personal development and society. The aspirational approach encourages excellence in our profession and science. Attorneys do FNs a great service by sometimes attacking assessment methods. A good cross-examination can reveal inadequacies in assessment techniques, such as an inadequate normative base and classification hit rates no better than base rate guessing. This can only improve our pursuit of good test instruments.

Aspirational goals include prevention of misuse of the FN's work. Newspapers have been filled with bizarre legal defense theories in sensational crimes, and some neuropsychology experts have contributed to such defenses. For example, one FN opined that a mass killer was legally insane because of "subtle frontal lobe damage," while simultaneously ignoring the defendant's well-organized efforts to cover up the crime and evade detection for over a year. Most states' insanity statutes require evidence of *severe* cognitive dysfunction or severe emotional dysregulation to support a conclusion of legal insanity. The responsible FN must not only weigh the body of scientific knowledge, but also must apply this knowledge to all relevant behaviors displayed by a defendant before agreeing to support an unusual medicolegal theory.

Table 2-4 represents a distillation of the ideas in this chapter. It is similar to the "Rules of Road" tables that the late Ted Blau created for forensic psychologists (Blau, 1998). It is hoped that Table 2-4 contains both the aspirational and moral underpinnings mentioned by Hess (1999b). The reader may wish to add personal ideas.

Both budding and experienced FNs may wish to maintain a basic resource library. We wish to emphasize that an encyclopedic knowledge of the law is not necessary to engage in productive and effective expert witness work. There are, however, key texts and articles that are indispensable. Hess and Weiner's (1999) *Handbook of Forensic Psychology* provides a thorough database in the application of psychological methods to legal questions. There is no chapter on neuropsychology, and the book's limitation is its emphasis on criminal issues. Melton, Petrila, Poythress, and Slobogin's second edition of *Psychological Evaluations for the Courts* (1997) is a veritable encyclopedia of forensic knowledge that

TABLE 2-4. Summary of Four Principles of Productive Attorney–Neuropsychologist Relations With Examples

Knowledge of legal bases
* Understand, accept, and adjust to structural conflicts between legal and scientific outlooks
* Recognize manageable specific conflicts that arise from time to time and develop specific response strategies (e.g., third-party observation request or orders)
* Be familiar with the essentials of the Federal Rules of Evidence, the *Daubert* trilogy, the *Frye* decision, and case law applicable to neuropsychological testing

Practice good neuropsychology
* Adhere to scientist/practitioner model
* Data collection is ideally a tripod consisting of outside records, history and behavioral observations, and test scores; each method by itself is fallible
* Justify selection of all measures on basis of peer-reviewed studies; admissibility law does not require relying on a fixed, commercial test battery
* Design test battery to both legal and clinical issues raised by a particular case
* Avoid use of single or homemade tests, diagnosis of brain damage on symptoms alone

Adhere to ethical principles
* Understand 2002 ethics code both generally and in terms of the specific principles relevant to forensic applications
* Recognize the ethical traps associated with each phase of the attorney–neuropsychologist interaction
* Avoid "pull of affiliation" by recognizing that you do not have to do everything an attorney asks you to do (e.g., avoid not only testifying as a "treating doctor," but also providing anonymous litigation consultation)

Be courtroom familiar
* Rigorously maintain mental set of "educator of trier of fact" when testifying
* Maintain consistency of gaze, demeanor, volume, and prosody during both direct and cross-examination
* Practice "active answering" to questions to educate the jury and avoid misimpressions; there is no legal authority requiring you to answer in "Yes" and "No" fashion
* Recognize common legal gambits and develop acceptable means of responding (e.g., avoid the learned treatise gambit)
* Respond with tactics only when they are genuinely called for; if "Yes" is a complete answer, then answer "Yes"

contains a more detailed discussion of key legal decisions than Hess and Weiner's *Handbook*. Again, there is no chapter on neuropsychology, but the intelligent reader can use this book to make intelligent extrapolations to his or her work.

Sweet's (1999a) edited volume *Forensic Neuropsychology* serves as a good review of foundational knowledge (e.g., essential psychometrics) and the application of neuropsychological methods to specific legal populations (head injury, toxic torts, educational disability). Even though it is now out of print, Doerr and Carlin's (1991) *Forensic Neuropsychology* provides simple explanations of basic legal concepts that are perfect for the novice FN. The book's weaknesses are that it was written before the *Daubert* decision and the scientific references are dated.

Every neuropsychologist should have copies of the *Daubert* trilogy. The *Daubert*, *Joiner*, and *Kumho* cases can be downloaded from Cornell Law School's Web site: http://supct.law.cornell.edu/supct/index.html. If you are interested in researching federal and state appellate cases relevant to neuropsychology, the Lexis-Nexis™ service allows relatively inexpensive downloading of individual opinions at http://www.lexisnexis.com/. The 2003 *Federal Rules of Evidence* and *Federal Rules of Civil Procedure* are available through West Publishing at http://west.thomson.com, although there has been little modification over their first publication in 1975.

Neuropsychologists frequently ask us about specific responses to especially difficult direct and cross-examination questions. Coping with cross-examination is partly science, but mostly art. Stanley Brodsky's 1991 and 1999 books on psychological testimony are essential reads: *Testifying in Court: Guidelines and Maxims for the Expert Witness* and *The Expert Expert Witness*, respectively. These books offer powerful tools for providing genuine, responsive, and respectful answers to the most difficult questions. The Faust, Ziskin, and Hiers (1991) volume *Brain Damage Claims: Coping With Neuropsychological Evidence* is a good resource for self-examination of weaknesses in one's assessment approach. In our view, Faust et al. have received much unfair criticism for their "method skepticism" of psychological techniques in the courtroom. Their critique has actually been an impetus to much research that has strengthened neuropsychology's position in the courtroom. Witness the explosion of research into developing symptom validity tests in the 1990s that started shortly after publication of Faust et al.'s critiques. Their approach is a good example of the aspirational arm of principled forensic neuropsychology.

NOTES

1. The adversarial system arises out of a medieval religious context, the trial by ordeal. However, not all legal systems operate with an adversarial ethos. Continental Europe is subject to the Napoleonic Code, in which attorneys have an affirmative obligation to the truth.
2. Error rate is used here in its experimental sense; that is, error rate is the probability that a group difference in test score may be caused by chance rather than a brain lesion. The other sense of error rate is in an actuarial context (i.e., the number of false positives and false negatives in predicting group membership). However, there is no consensus as to a minimum accepted error rate except the broad standard of improving over base rate prediction.

3. A commonly held myth is that only subpoenas signed by a judge need be honored. The reality is that, in most jurisdictions, judges have delegated much of their subpoena authority to attorneys. In Michigan, for example, the typed signature of a court clerk is sufficient to render a subpoena valid. That is not to say that the FN has no rights in response to a subpoena.

4. The attorney–work product doctrine adds another complication to the opinion that psychologists only send raw data to the opposing side's psychologist. An attorney who hires an FN background consultant does not wish to let this arrangement be known. Being forced to reveal the identity of the neuropsychologist to receive raw test data is another violation of an attorney's prerogatives, again giving some neuropsychologists the de facto procedural right to dictate legal practices.

5. Attorneys' perceptions of experts provide good examples of how advocacy affects attitudes. Plaintiff attorneys uniformly term the so-called treating doctors they retain "objective," but doctors hired by the defense are "all biased." Defense attorneys, on the other hand, view treaters as biased because treaters by their very nature are advocates. Treaters may also have a strong financial interest in the outcome of the trial (e.g., the insurer is forced to pay their bills after verdict). Defense attorneys consider their own experts to be more objective because they are paid irrespective of who wins or loses.

6. After hearing *Daubert*, the Supreme Court remanded the case back to the trial judge to apply the new standard to the facts. The trial judge again rejected plaintiff's expert testimony on the same grounds he did at trial: The testimony was not valid or relevant for lack of any general acceptance. Note that the *Frye* rule is one of the *Daubert* elements.

7. *Chappelle v. Ganger* was a bench trial of a brain injury claim. The judge's written decision indicated that even *partial* HRB protocols from two other neuropsychologists were admitted into evidence. This fact alone refutes Reed and Reitan's conclusions. Defense counsel moved for a *Daubert* hearing only to bar the testimony of a vocational specialist who had performed no testing and offered no peer-reviewed study to back up his opinion that the plaintiff would never work.

8. Expert witness guides written solely by attorneys need to be viewed critically. The attorneys who write these texts still have a stake in controlling experts' responses and channeling them in favorable directions. For example, Babitsky and Mangravitis's (1997) book, an otherwise excellent resource, implies the learned treatise approach is irresistible and warns the reader that refusing the gambit makes the witness look foolish. Of course, only attorneys will benefit if most experts come to believe this. Consider this: If you go to Las Vegas and the casino provides you with a complimentary copy of *How to Beat the House Every Time*, wouldn't you be skeptical?

9. As of this writing, only Louisiana and Virginia offer specialty licensing for neuropsychology.

REFERENCES

Adams, D. (2002, February 4). U.S. Supreme Court denies appeal of physician discipline case. *American Medical News*. Retrieved September 2002 from http://www.ama-assn. org/sci-pubs/amnews/pick_02/prse0204.htm

Albers, J. W., Wald, J. J., Garabrant, D. H., Trask, C. L., & Berent, S. (2000). Neurologic evaluation of workers previously diagnosed with solvent-induced toxic encephalopathy. *Journal of Occupational and Environmental Medicine, 42*, 410–423.

Albert, T. (2002, April 8). *American Medical News*. On the hot seat: Physician expert witnesses. Retrieved September 2002 from http://www.ama-assn.org/sci-pubs/amnews/pick_02/prsa0408.htm#rbar_add

American Psychiatric Association. (1994). *Diagnostic and statistical manual of mental disorders* (4th ed.). Washington, DC: Author.

American Psychological Association. (1992). Ethical principles of psychologists and code of conduct. *American Psychologist, 47,* 1597–1611.

American Psychological Association. (2002). Ethical principles of psychologists and code of conduct. *American Psychologist, 57,* 1060–1073.

Anastasi, A., & Urbina, S. (1997). *Psychological testing* (7th ed.). Upper Saddle River, NJ: Prentice-Hall.

Andrew, G., Benjamin, H., & Kazniak, A. (1991). The discovery process: Deposition, trial testimony and hearing testimony. In H. O. Doerr & A. S. Carlin, (Eds.), *Forensic neuropsychology* (pp. 17–32). New York: Guilford Press.

Axelrod, B., Barth, J., Faust, D., Fisher, J., Heilbronner, R., Larrabee, G., et al. (2000). Presence of third party observers during neuropsychological testing: Official statement of the National Academy of Neuropsychology. *Archives of Clinical Neuropsychology, 15,* 379–380.

Babitsky, S., & Mangraviti, J. J. (1997). *How to excel during cross-examination. Techniques for experts that work.* Falmouth, MA: SEAK Press.

Bauer, R. (1994). The flexible battery approach to neuropsychological assessment. In R. D. Vanderploeg (Ed.), *Clinician's guide to neuropsychological assessment* (pp. 259–290). Hillsdale, NJ: Lawrence Erlbaum.

Benton, A. L. (1992). Clinical neuropsychology: 1960–1990. *Journal of Clinical and Experimental Neuropsychology, 14,* 407–417.

Bigler, E. D., & Ehrfurth, J. W. (1980). Critical limitations of the Bender Gestalt Test in clinical neuropsychology: Response to Lacks. *International Journal of Clinical Neuropsychology, 2,* 88–90.

Bigler, E. D., & Ehrfurth, J. W. (1981). The continued inappropriate singular use of the Bender Visual Motor Gestalt Test. *Professional Psychology: Research and Practice, 12,* 562–569.

Binder, L. M. (1997). A review of mild head trauma: II. Clinical implications. *Journal of Clinical and Experimental Neuropsychology, 19,* 421–431.

Binder, L. M., & Johnson-Greene, D. (1995). Observer effects on neuropsychological performance: A case report. *Clinical Neuropsychologist, 9,* 74–78.

Binder, L. M., Rohling, M. L., & Larrabee, G. J. (1997). A review of mild head trauma: I. Meta-analytic review of neuropsychological studies. *Journal of Clinical and Experimental Neuropsychology, 19,* 432–457.

Binder, L. M., & Willis, S. C. (1991). Assessment of motivation after financially compensable minor head trauma. *Psychological Assessment, 3,* 175–181.

Blau, T. H. (1998). *The psychologist as expert witness* (2nd ed.). New York: Wiley.

Boone, K. B., Miller, B. L., Lee, A., Berman, N., Sherman, D., & Stuss, D. T. (1999). Neuropsychological patterns in right versus left frontotemporal dementia. *Journal of the International Neuropsychological Society, 5,* 616–622.

Brodsky, S. L. (1991). *Testifying in court. Guidelines and maxims for the expert witness.* Washington, DC: American Psychological Association Press.

Brodsky, S. L. (1999). *The expert expert witness.* Washington, DC: American Psychological Association Press.

Brodsky, S. L., & Robey, A. (1973). On becoming and expert witness: Issues of orientation and effectiveness. *Professional Psychology, 3,* 173–176.

Butler, J. L., & Baumeister, R. F. (1998). The trouble with friendly faces: Skilled performance with a supportive audience. *Journal of Personality and Social Psychology, 75,* 1213–1230.

Butler, M., Retzlaff, P. D., & Vanderploeg, R. (1991). Neuropsychological test usage. *Professional Psychology: Research and Practice, 22,* 510–512.

Chandler Exterminators Inc. v. Morris, 200 Ga. App. 816 (1992).

Chelune, G., & Heaton, R. (1986). Neuropsychology and personality tests and their relation to patient's complaints of disability. In G. Goldstein and R. Tarter (Eds.), *Advances in clinical neuropsychology* (Vol. 3). New York: Plenum Press.

Cline et al. v. Firestone Tire, 118 FRD 588 (1988).

Colbach, E. M. (1981). Integrity checks on the witness stand. *Bulletin of the American Academy of Psychiatry and Law, 9,* 285–288.

Committee on Ethical Guidelines for Forensic Psychologists. (1991). Specialty guidelines for forensic psychologists. *Law and Human Behavior, 15,* 655–665.

Constantinou, M., Ashendorf, L., & McCaffrey, R. J. (2002). When the third party observer of a neuropsychological evaluation is an audio-recorder. *Clinical Neuropsychologist, 16,* 407–412.

Cripe, L. (2002). Limitations of records reviews. *Division of Clinical Neuropsychology Newsletter 40, 20,* 7–8.

Cronbach, L. (1984). *Essentials of psychological testing* (4th ed.). New York: Harper and Row.

Daubert v. Merrell Dow, 509 U.S. 579 (1993).

Derby, W. N. (2001). Writing the forensic neuropsychological report. In C. G. Armengol, E. Kaplan, & E. J. Moes (Eds.), *The consumer oriented neuropsychological report* (pp. 203–224). Lutz, FL: PAR.

Dikmen, S. S., Machamer, J. E., Winn, H. R., & Temkin, N. R. (1995). Neuropsychological outcome at 1-year post head injury. *Neuropsychology, 9,* 80–90.

Dikmen, S. S., Temkin, N. R., Machamer, J. E., & Holubkov, A. L. (1994). Employment following traumatic head injuries. *Archives of Neurology, 51,* 177–186.

Doerr, H. O. (1991). Issues in initial contact: Neuropsychologist–attorney–patient. In H. O. Doerr & A. S. Carlin (Eds.), *Forensic neuropsychology* (p. 40). New York: Guilford Press.

Doerr, H. O., & Carlin, A. S. (1991). *Forensic neuropsychology* (p. 242). New York: Guilford Press.

Essig, S. M., Mittenberg, W., Peterson, R. S., Strauman, S., & Cooper, J. T. (2001). Practices in forensic neuropsychology: Perspectives of neuropsychologists and trial attorneys. *Archives of Clinical Neuropsychology, 16,* 271–291.

Faust, D. (1995). The detection of deception. *Neurologic Clinics, 13,* 255–265.

Faust, D., Ziskin, J., & Hiers, J. B. (1991). *Brain damage claims: Coping with neuropsychological evidence.* Los Angeles: Law and Psychology Press.

Federal rule of civil procedure. (1975). St. Paul, MN: West.

Federal rules of evidence for United States courts and magistrates. (1975). St. Paul, MN: West.

Fenichel, O. (1945). *The psychoanalytic theory of neurosis.* New York: Norton.

Fisher, C. B. (2003). Release of test data and the new APA ethics code. *American Psychology Law Society News, 23,* 1–6.

Frankle, A. H. (1995). A new method for detecting brain disorder by measuring perseveration in personality responses. *Journal of Personality Assessment, 64,* 63–85.

Frye v. United States (D.C. Cir. 1923) 293 F. 1013.

Gianoli, G., McWilliams, S., Soileau, J., & Belafsky, P. (2000). Posturographic performance in patients with the potential for secondary gain. *Otolaryngological, Head and Neck Surgery, 122,* 11–18.

Glass, L. S. (1991). The legal base in forensic neuropsychology. In H. O. Doerr & A. S. Carlin (Eds.), *Forensic neuropsychology* (pp. 3–16). New York: Guilford Press.

Green, P., Iverson, G. L., & Allen, L. (1999). Detecting malingering in head injury litigation with the Word Memory Test. *Brain Injury, 13,* 813–819.

Greenberg, S. A., & Shuman, D. W. (1997). Irreconcilable conflict between therapeutic and forensic roles. *Professional Psychology: Research and Practice, 28,* 50–57.

Greiffenstein, M. F. (2002). Selecting a neuropsychologist as an expert witness. *Michigan Bar Journal, 81,* 45–46.

Greiffenstein, M. F. (2003). Neuropsychology research out of a private practice setting. In G. L. Lamberty (Ed.), *The practice of clinical neuropsychology* (pp. 125–142). New York: Swets and Zeitlinger.

Greiffenstein, M. F., & Baker, W. J. (2001). Comparison of premorbid and postinjury MMPI-2 profiles in late postconcussion claimants. *Clinical Neuropsychologist, 15,* 162–170.

Greiffenstein, M. F., Baker, W. J., & Gola, T. (1994). Validation of malingered amnesia measures in a large clinical samples. *Psychological Assessment, 6,* 218–224.

Greiffenstein, M. F., Baker, W. J., & Gola, T. (1996). Motor dysfunction profiles in traumatic brain injury and postconcussion syndrome. *Journal of the International Neuropsychological Society, 2,* 477–485.

Greiffenstein, M. F., Baker, W. J., Gola, T., Donders, J., & Miller, L. (2002). The fake bad scale in atypical and severe closed head injury litigants. *Journal of Clinical Psychology, 58,* 1591–1600.

Greiffenstein, M. F., Baker, W. J., & Johnson-Greene, D. (2002). Actual versus self-reported scholastic achievement of litigating postconcussion and severe closed head injury claimants. *Psychological Assessment, 14,* 202–208.

Grenitz v. Tomlian, 858 So. 2d 999 (2003 Fla.)

Griggs et al. v. Duke Power Co., 401 U.S. 424 (1971).

Grisso, T. (1988). *Competency to stand trial. A manual for practice.* Sarasota, FL: Professional Resources Exchange.

Grove, W. M., & Barden, R. C. (1999). Protecting the integrity of the legal system: The admissibility of testimony from mental health experts under *Daubert/Kumho* analyses. *Psychology, Public Policy, and Law, 5,* 224–242.

Heaton, R., Smith, H. H., Lehman, R. A., & Vogt, A. T. (1978). Prospects for faking believable deficits on neuropsychological testing. *Journal of Clinical and Consulting Psychology, 5,* 892–900.

Hess, A. K. (1999a). Defining forensic psychology. In A. K. Hess & I. B. Weiner (Eds.), *The handbook of forensic psychology* (2nd ed., pp. 24–47). New York: Wiley.

Hess, A. K. (1999b). Practicing principled forensic psychology: Legal, ethical and moral considerations. In A. K. Hess & I. B. Weiner (Eds.), *The handbook of forensic psychology* (2nd ed., pp. 673–699). New York: Wiley.

Hess, A. K., & Weiner, I. B. (1999). *The handbook of forensic psychology* (2nd ed., p. 756). New York: Wiley.

Hutchison v. American Family Mutual Insurance, 514 N.W., 2d 882 (Iowa 1994).

Jenkins v. US, 307 F.2d 637 (1962).

Johnson-Greene, D., Dehring, M., Adams, K. M., Miller, T., Arora, S., Beylin, A., et al.. (1997). Accuracy of self-reported educational attainment among diverse patient populations: A preliminary investigation. *Archives of Clinical Neuropsychology*, *12*, 635–643.

Joiner v. General Electric, 522 U.S. 136 (1997).

Kagehiro, D. (1990). Defining the standard of proof in jury instructions. *Psychological Science*, *1*, 194–200.

Kaufman, A. S. (1990). *Assessing adult and adolescent intelligence*. New York: Allyn and Bacon.

Kehrer, C. A., Sanchez, P. N., Habif, U., Rosenbaum, J. G., & Townes, B. D. (2000). Effects of a significant-other observer on neuropsychological test performance. *Clinical Neuropsychologist*, *14*, 67–71.

Kumho Tire v. Carmichael, 526 U.S. 137 (1999).

Lacks, P. (1982). Continued clinical popularity of the Bender-Gestalt Test: Response to Bigler and Ehrfurth. *Professional Psychology: Research and Practice*, *13*, 677–680.

Lally, S. J. (2003). What tests are acceptable for use in forensic evaluations? A survey of experts. *Professional Psychology: Research and Practice*, *34*, 491–498.

Larrabee, G. J. (1990). Cautions in the use of neuropsychological evaluation in legal settings. *Neuropsychology*, *4*, 239–247.

Larrabee, G. J. (1998). Somatic malingering on the MMPI and MMPI-2 in personal injury litigants. *Clinical Neuropsychologist*, *12*, 179–188.

Lees-Haley, P. R., & Courtney, J. C. (2000). Reply to the commentary on "Disclosure of tests and raw test data to the courts." *Neuropsychology Review*, *10*, 181–182.

Lees-Haley, P. R., Iverson, G. L., Lange, R. T., Fox, D. D., & Allen, L. M., III. (2002). Malingering in forensic neuropsychology: *Daubert* and the MMPI-2. *Journal of Forensic Neuropsychology*, *3*, 167–203.

Lees-Haley, P. R., Smith, H. H., Williams, C. W., & Dunn, J. T. (1996). Forensic neuropsychological test usage: An empirical survey. *Archives of Clinical Neuropsychology*, *11*, 45–51.

Loring, D. (1999). *International Neuropsychology Society (INS) dictionary of neuropsychology*. New York: Oxford University Press.

Matarazzo, J. D. (1972). *Wechsler's measurement and appraisal of adult intelligence* (5th ed.). New York: Oxford University Press.

Matarazzo, J. D. (1990). Psychological assessment versus psychological testing: Validation from Binet to the school, clinic, and courtroom. *American Psychologist*, *45*, 999–1017.

Matarazzo, J. D., Bornstein, R. A., McDermott, P. A., & Noonan, J. V. (1986). Verbal IQ versus Performance IQ difference scores in males and females from the WAIS-R standardization sample. *Journal of Clinical Psychology*, *42*, 965–974.

Matarazzo, J. D., & Herman, D. O. (1985). Clinical uses of the WAIS-R: Base rates of differences between VIQ and PIQ in the WAIS-R standardization sample. In B. B. Wolfman (Ed.), *Handbook of intelligence* (pp. 899–932). New York: Wiley.

Mathias, C. W., Greve, K. W., Bianchini, K. J., Houston, R. J., & Crouch, J. A. (2002). Detecting malingered neurocognitive dysfunction using the Reliable Digit Span in traumatic brain injury. *Assessment*, *9*, 301–308.

McCaffrey, R. J., Fisher, J. M., Gold, B. A., & Lynch, J. K. (1996). Presence of third parties during neuropsychological evaluations: Who is evaluating whom? *Clinical Neuropsychologist*, *10*, 435–449.

McKinzey, R. K., & Ziegler, T. G. (1999). Challenging a flexible neuropsychological battery under *Kelly/Frye*: A case study. *Behavioral Sciences and the Law*, *17*, 543–551.

McSweeny, A. J. (1997). Regarding ethics in forensic neuropsychological consultation: A comment on Guilmette and Hagan. *Clinical Neuropsychologist, 11*, 291–293.

Meehl, P. E. (1954). *Clinical versus statistical prediction: A theoretical analysis and a review of the evidence.* Minneapolis: University of Minnesota Press.

Melton, G. B., Petrila, J., Poythress, N. G., & Slobogin, C. (1997). *Psychological evaluations for the courts. A handbook for mental health professionals and lawyers* (2nd ed., p. 794). New York: Guilford Press.

Miller, H., & Cartlidge, N. (1972). Simulation and malingering after injuries to the brain and spinal cord. *Lancet, 1*, 445–452.

Mitrushina, M. N., Boone, K. B., & D'Elia, L. F. (1999). *Handbook of normative data for neuropsychological assessment.* New York: Oxford University Press.

Mittenberg, W., DiGiulio, D. V., Perrin, S., & Bass, A. E. (1992). Symptoms following mild head injury: Expectation as aetiology. *Journal of Neurology, Neurosurgery and Psychiatry, 55*, 200–204.

Mittenberg, W., Patton, C., Canyock, E. M., & Condit, D. C. (2002). Base rates of malingering and symptom exaggeration. *Journal of Clinical and Experimental Neuropsychology, 24*, 1094–1102.

Mossman, D. (2000a). Interpreting clinical evidence of malingering: A Bayesian perspective. *Journal of the American Academy of Psychiatry and Law, 28*, 293–302.

Mossman, D. (2000b). The meaning of malingering data: further applications of Bayes' theorem. *Behavioral Sciences and Law, 18*, 761–779.

Mossman, D. (2003). Daubert, cognitive malingering, and test accuracy. *Law and Human Behavior, 27*, 229–249.

NAN Policy and Planning Committee. (2000). Test security: Official position statement of the National Academy of Neuropsychology. *Archives of Clinical Neuropsychology, 15*, 383–386.

Naugle, R., & McSweeny, A. J. (1995). On the practice of routinely appending neuropsychological data to reports. *Clinical Neuropsychologist, 9*, 245–247.

Nelson, L. D., Drebing, C., Satz, P., & Uchiyama, C. (1998). Personality change in head trauma: A validity study of the Neuropsychology Behavior and Affect Profile. *Archives of Clinical Neuropsychology, 13*, 549–560.

Oestreicher, J. M., & O'Donnell, J. P. (1995). Validation of the General Neuropsychological Deficit Scale with nondisabled, learning-disabled, and head-injured young adults. *Archives of Clinical Neuropsychology, 10*, 185–191.

Pendleton, M. G., & Heaton, R. K. (1982). A comparison of the Wisconsin Card Sorting Test and the Category Test. *Journal of Clinical Psychology, 38*, 392–396.

Pieniadz, J., & Kelland, D. Z. (2001). Reporting scores in neuropsychological assessments: Ethicality, validity, practicality and more. In C. G. Armengol, E. Kaplan, & E. J. Moes (Eds.), *The consumer-oriented neuropsychology report* (pp. 123–140). Odessa, FL: Psychological Assessment Resources.

Posthuma, A., Podrouzek, W., & Crisp, D. (2002). The implications of *Daubert* on neuropsychological evidence in the assessment of remote mild traumatic brain injury. *American Journal of Forensic Psychology, 20*(4), 21–38.

Ragge v. MCA/Universal Studios, 165 FRD 605 (1995).

Reed, J. E. (1996). Fixed versus flexible neuropsychological test batteries under the *Daubert* standard for the admissibility of scientific evidence. *Behavioral Sciences and the Law, 14*, 315–322.

Reitan, R. M., & Wolfson, D. (1985). *The Halstead-Reitan neuropsychological test battery. Theory and clinical Interpretation.* Tucson, AZ: Neuropsychology Press.

Reitan, R. M., & Wolfson, D. (2002). Detection of malingering and invalid test results using the Halstead-Reitan Battery. *Journal of Forensic Neuropsychology, 3,* 275–314.

Robinson, A. L., Heaton, R. K., Lehman, R. A., & Stilson, D. W. (1980). The utility of the Wisconsin Card Sorting Test in detecting and localizing frontal lobe lesions. *Journal of Consulting and Clinical Psychology, 48,* 605–614.

Rohling, M. L., Meyers, J. E., & Millis, S. R. (2003). Neuropsychological impairment following traumatic brain injury: A dose–response analysis. *The Clinical Neuropsychologist, 17,* 289–302.

Russell, E. W. (1998). In defense of the Halstead Reitan Battery: A critique of Lezak's review. *Archives of Clinical Neuropsychology, 13,* 365–381.

Satz, P., Forney, D. L., Zaucha, K., Asarnow, R. R., Light, R., McCleary, C., et al. (1998). Depression, cognition, and functional correlates of recovery outcome after traumatic brain injury. *Brain Injury, 12,* 537–553.

Schudel v. General Electric, 120 F.3d 991 (1995).

Shapiro, D. L. (2000). Commentary: Disclosure of tests and raw test data to the courts. *Neuropsychology Review, 10,* 175–176.

Shuman, D. W., Greenberg, S., Heilbrun, K., & Foote, W. E. (1998). An immodest proposal: Should treating mental health professionals be barred from testifying about their patients? *Behavioral Sciences and the Law, 16,* 509–523.

Simmons v. Mullins, 231 Pa. Super. 199, 331 A.2d 892 (Pa. Super. 1975).

Spreen, O., & Strauss, E. (1991). *A compendium of neuropsychological tests.* New York: Oxford University Press.

Spreen, O., & Strauss, E. (1998). *A compendium of neuropsychological tests* (2nd ed., p. 736). New York: Oxford University Press.

Steinberg, J. L., Devous, M. D., Sr., & Paulman, R. G. (1996). Wisconsin Card Sorting activated regional cerebral blood flow in first break and chronic schizophrenic patients and normal controls. *Schizophrenia Research, 19,* 177–187.

Strub, R., & Black, F. W. (1988). *Neurobehavioral disorders: A clinical approach.* Philadelphia: Davis.

Sweet, J. J. (1991). Psychological evaluation and testing services in medical settings. In J. J. Sweet, R. H. Rozensky, & S. M. Tovian (Eds.), *Handbook of clinical psychology in medical settings* (pp. 291–313). New York: Plenum Press.

Sweet, J. J. (1999a). *Forensic neuropsychology. Fundamentals and practice.* Lisse, The Netherlands: Swets and Zeitlinger, p. 535.

Sweet, J. J. (1999b). Malingering: Differential diagnosis. In J. J. Sweet (Ed.), *Forensic neuropsychology. Fundamentals and practice* (pp. 255–285). Lisse, The Netherlands: Swets and Zeitlinger.

Sweet, J. J., King, J. H., Malina, A. C., Bergman, M. A., & Simmons, A. (2002). Documenting the prominence of forensic neuropsychology at national meetings and in relevant professional journals from 1990 to 2000. *Clinical Neuropsychologist, 16,* 481–494.

Sweet, J. J., & Moberg, P. J. (2000). A survey of practices and beliefs among ABPP and non-ABPP clinical neuropsychologists. *Clinical Neuropsychologist, 4,* 101–120.

Sweet, J. J., Moberg, P. J., & Suchy, Y. (2000). Ten-year follow-up survey of clinical neuropsychologists: Part II. Private practice and economics. *Clinical Neuropsychologist, 14,* 479–495.

Sweet, J. J., Moberg, P. J., & Westergaard, C. K. (1996). Five-year follow-up survey of practices and beliefs of clinical neuropsychologists. *Clinical Neuropsychologist, 10,* 202–221.

Tenopyr, M. L. (1999). A scientist-practitioner's viewpoint on the admissibility of behavioral and social scientific information. *Psychology, Public Policy and Law, 5*, 194–202.

Tomlin v. Holecek, 150 FRD 628 (1993).

Tranel, D. (1994). The release of psychological data to nonexperts: Ethical and legal considerations. *Professional Psychology: Research and Practice, 25*, 33–38.

Tranel, D. (2000). Commentary on Lees-Haley and Courtney: There is a need for reform. *Neuropsychology Review, 10*, 177–178.

Tremont, G., Hoffman, R. G., Scott, J. G., & Adams, R. L. (1998). Effect of intellectual level on neuropsychological test performance: A response to Dodrill (1997). *The Clinical Neuropsychologist. 12*, 560–567.

Valiulis v. Scheffeos, 191 Ill. App. 3d 775, 547 N.E. 2d 1290 (Ill. App. 2 Dist. 1989).

Volbrecht, M. E., Meyers, J. E., & Kaster-Bundgaard, J. (2000). Neuropsychological outcome of head injury using a short battery. *Archives of Clinical Neuropsychology, 15*, 251–265.

Weiner, I. B. (1999). Writing forensic reports. In A. K. Hess & I. B. Weiner (Eds.), *The handbook of forensic psychology* (pp. 501–520). New York: Wiley.

Wolfson, D., & Reitan, R. M. (1995). Cross-validation of the General Neuropsychological Deficit Scale (GNDS). *Archives of Clinical Neuropsychology, 10*, 125–131.

Youngjohn, J. R. (1995). Confirmed attorney coaching prior to neuropsychological evaluation. *Assessment, 2*, 279–283.

Youngjohn, J. R., Lees-Haley, P. R., & Binder, L. M. (1999). Comment: Warning malingerers produces more sophisticated malingering. *Archives of Clinical Neuropsychology, 14*, 511–515.

3

Ethical Practice of Forensic Neuropsychology

CHRISTOPHER GROTE

Surveys have demonstrated that neuropsychologists are asked to consult with greater frequency in forensic cases, and that an increased percentage of neuropsychology conference presentations and journal publications have been devoted to related topics such as malingering (Sweet, King, Malina, Bergman, & Simmons, 2002; Sweet, Moberg, & Suchy, 2000). This increase has been accompanied by a flurry of articles, books, and conference presentations related to ethics in forensic neuropsychology (Bush, in press; Bush & Drexler, 2002). This is both appropriate and necessary for at least two reasons.

First, neuropsychologists have to be constantly vigilant of the need to produce unbiased and appropriately informed opinions if courts can be expected to rely on their opinions. Failure to maintain this neutrality could instead lead others to view us as mercenaries whose opinions might be influenced by the needs of those who retain us in adversarial cases. Second, neuropsychologists may not be fully aware of all the potential ethical and legal implications that arise when their reports are used in forensic settings. Their graduate education and training may have focused only on more general ethical issues, such not having sexual relationships with patients (note the term *patient* is used throughout this chapter instead of client, claimant, or litigant; of course, use of this term is not meant to imply that a treating or doctor–patient relationship exists during a forensic neuropsychological examination). Previous training in ethics may not have specifically focused on those issues related to forensic neuropsychological practice, such as informed consent for assessment, release of raw data, or obstacles to presenting unbiased and fully informed opinions in forensic cases.

Although the older literature contains some guidelines on the ethical provision of specialty forensic services (Committee on Ethical Guidelines, 1991), these often did not make specific reference to topics of greatest interest to neuropsychologists. More recent publications are much more helpful to the forensic neuropsychologist. Among these is a recently published official statement from the National Academy of Neuropsychology concerning independent and court-ordered forensic neuropsychological examinations (National Academy of Neuropsychology, 2003b). This document outlines many important topics, including basic ethical precepts, examination procedures, and scope of interpretation of neuropsychological results.

This chapter covers three topics. The first section reviews the "Ethical Principles of Psychologists and Code of Conduct" (American Psychological Association [APA], 2002) and the changes that are of greatest relevance to the practice of forensic neuropsychology. The second section reviews the implications of the recently enacted Health Insurance Portability and Accountability Act (HIPAA). Although this is a very complex set of rules, an attempt is made to determine what effect it will have on the practice of clinical and forensic neuropsychology. The final section of this chapter is an overview of ethical obstacles sometimes encountered in the practice of forensic neuropsychology.

CHANGES FROM THE 1992 TO 2002 "ETHICAL PRINCIPLES OF PSYCHOLOGISTS AND CODE OF CONDUCT"

The APA first published its code in 1953 (APA, 1953). The 2002 version represents the ninth iteration of this document. The 2002 code was published in the December 2002 *American Psychologist* (APA, 2002), but did not take effect until June 1, 2003. The 2002 code was produced after seven drafts in response to over 1,300 comments from APA members and others (Fisher, 2003).

Comparison of "redline" versions of the 1992 and 2002 code, as listed on the APA Web site (APA, 2003), showed what initially appeared to be a significant reorganization and rewording of the principles. Closer inspection suggests that many of the changes are stylistic and not clearly substantive. Binder and Thompson (1995) similarly attempted to describe the changes of greatest importance to the practice of neuropsychology in the 1992 revision of the ethics code and took pains to make the distinction between aspirational goals and enforceable rules. A similar distinction is present in the most recent revision because Principles A through E, which outline pathways to integrity, justice, and so on, are nonenforceable ethical ideals.

An article published in the January 2003 *Monitor on Psychology* (Smith, 2003) and further reviews indicate at least three changes of which forensic neuropsychologists should be aware. These concern the release of raw data, the need to obtain informed consent for assessment, and the use of interpreters for evaluations. Some other changes in the code are also briefly reviewed.

Release of Raw Data

No doubt the reader of this chapter has already been alerted to the fact that the new ethics code has altered policy regarding release of raw data. What may be less clear is how these changes will interface with both HIPAA and state law. The ethics code change probably most relevant to the practice of forensic neuropsychology is found in Standards 9.04 (Release of Raw Data) and 9.11 (Maintaining Test Security). These standards were long debated by the Ethics Code Task Force and received more public comment during the revision period than any other standard (Fisher, 2003).

The end product is a more liberal interpretation than the 1992 code in determining to whom, and when, a psychologist must release "raw data." The 1992 code prevented release to others who were "not qualified" to use the raw data. This was a vague description that led to frequent debate about who was or was not qualified to examine raw data. There was also dissension regarding the 1992 interpretation of raw data and whether this referred to test forms, test materials, test scores, or some combination of these elements. As a result, some neuropsychologists reportedly refused to release copies of patient's test results/forms to other licensed psychologists because they were not board certified by a particular organization or perhaps even because of some personal enmity between the two psychologists.

The 2002 code makes it a bit more clear as to what psychologists should do when asked for their files, although these requests will have to be balanced against one's interpretation of HIPAA and applicable laws in the state of practice. Further, the 2002 code draws a distinction between raw data and test materials. The 2002 Standard 9.11 (Maintaining Test Security) states that "psychologists make reasonable efforts to maintain the integrity and security of test materials"; these are defined as "manuals, instruments, protocols and test questions or stimuli and does not include *test data* as defined in Standard 9.04." This seems to suggest that psychologists should not freely release things such as the Wechsler Adult Intelligence Scale, Third Edition (WAIS-III; Wechsler, 1997) Block Design drawings and blocks or the Wechsler Memory Scale, Third Edition (WMS-III; Wechsler, 1997) Spatial Span blocks, but there are at least two limits to the significance of Standard 9.11.

The differentiation of test data and materials is discussed at length in a position paper from the National Academy of Neuropsychology (www.nanonline.

org), which is a follow-up to the academy's first paper on test security (National Academy of Neuropsychology, 2000). The update reveals the complexity of these issues and makes it clear that there is little obvious consensus among different organizations and individuals in defining and judging these issues. However, it does seem to be the case that test materials are rarely, or never, requested by nonpsychologists. Second, the standard only requires "reasonable efforts" not to release these materials and does not make it clear what this means. Some psychologists may interpret this to mean they only have to explain their potential concerns about misuse of the materials to a nonpsychologist before then releasing them; other psychologists might instead insist on a court order.

Regardless of these quibbles, it is clear that Standard 9.04 has greater relevance concerning the release of test materials or raw data. It states:

(a) The term *test data* refers to raw and scaled scores, client/patient responses to test questions or stimuli, and psychologists' notes and recordings concerning client/patient statements and behavior during an examination. Those portions of test materials that include client/patient responses are included in the definition of *test data*. Pursuant to a client/patient release, psychologists provide test data to the client/patient or other persons identified in the release. Psychologists may refrain from releasing test data to protect a client/patient or others from substantial harm or misuse or misrepresentation of the data or the test, recognizing that in many instances release of confidential information under these circumstances is regulated by law.

(b) In the absence of a client/patient release, psychologists provide test data only as required by law or court order.

Standard 9.04 is more liberal than what was in the 1992 code in that it is fairly clear in telling psychologists to release copies of test forms when directed to by patients or their attorneys. One might attempt to argue that "substantial harm" might result because of this release, but this might be a stretch, especially in light of the new HIPAA regulations. Of course, psychologists who practice in states such as Illinois and Iowa that have laws restricting the release of raw data to nonpsychologists will not be affected by either the new APA ethics code or by HIPAA.

An article in the January 2003 APA *Monitor* (Daw Holloway, 2003b) stated that state law supercedes HIPAA, and of course both of these would trump the APA ethics code when the code conflicts state or federal law. It is also important to know that HIPAA is not applicable when raw data were collected in the process of legal or administrative proceeding (Fisher, 2003). Federal Law 45 C.F.R. 45 164.508 and 164.524[(a)(1)] is part of the HIPAA legislation and states that "Patients do not have the right of access to information compiled in reasonable anticipation of, or for use in, a civil, criminal, or administrative action or procedure."

In terms of release of raw data, it has been written that state law takes precedence over HIPAA, and that HIPAA in turn supercedes any ethical codes (Daw

Holloway, 2003b). Figure 3-1 provides an overview of steps that clinicians may want to consider in determining if or when to release copies of their raw data. It illustrates that a patient, the patient's attorney, or a court must request or order this release; it is difficult to imagine circumstances under which this release could otherwise occur. However, if a patient has requested this release and a court has not ordered the release, the clinician must then determine

When Should Raw Data Be Released?

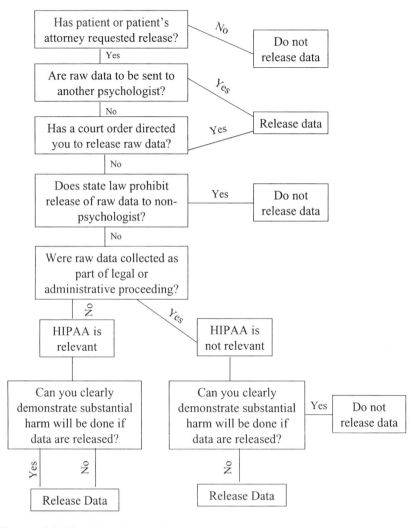

FIGURE 3-1. Flowchart of data release. HIPAA, Health Insurance Portability and Accountability Act.

whether the state in which he or she is practicing has any legislation regarding this issue.

An informal survey of colleagues indicated that at least four of the United States and one Canadian Province each prohibit the release of raw data to nonpsychologists. The cited legislation for each jurisdiction is as follows: Illinois (Section 3 c) of (740 ILCS 110) of the Mental Health and Developmental Disabilities Act of the State of Illinois; Florida [Chapter 490; 64 B19-18.004(3)]; Iowa (Section 1 228.9); Texas (Title 22, Part 21, Rule 465.22); Alberta [Health Information Act Section 11(1)(e)]. Colleagues from other states, including Utah, Hawaii, Arizona, and Oregon, responded that their states had no such restrictions on the release of raw data to nonpsychologists. This obviously is not a comprehensive listing, so it is incumbent on a practicing psychologist to check with the state psychological association or otherwise be aware of state legislation regarding this issue.

Assuming that a psychologist is not prohibited from releasing raw data to nonpsychologists, the next step in this process would be to determine if the request is related to a court or administrative proceeding. If it is *not* related, then HIPAA *does* apply. This is important because HIPAA does not appear to allow for the concept of substantial harm or misuse of the data as an excuse not to send the data (Fisher, 2003). That is, a psychologist's concern that the data will somehow be misused cannot serve as a reason not to send it in nonlegal cases. However, if the request for raw data *is* related to a court or administrative proceeding, then HIPAA *does not* apply. Should there be a substantial reason to believe the data would be misused in such a scenario, the psychologist would be justified in attempting to withhold it. Of course, this refusal may not be the last word as an attorney might be successful in obtaining a court order, which of course would trump any of the psychologist's reasons for not sending the data along. Obviously, this is a complicated situation, and clinicians should proceed cautiously, consult with colleagues, and document their reasons for responding or failing to respond to requests for copies of their raw data.

Informed Consent for Assessment

There now is a requirement for informed consent for assessment. This was not in the 1992 version. Standard 9.03(a) of the 2002 code states:

Psychologists obtain informed consent for assessments, evaluations or diagnostic services, as described in Standard 3.10, Informed Consent, except when (1) testing is mandated by law or governmental regulations; (2) informed consent is implied because testing is conducted as a routine educational, institutional or organizational activity (e.g. when participants voluntarily agree to assessment when applying for a job); or (3) one purpose of the testing is to evaluate decisional capacity. Informed consent includes an explanation of the nature and purpose of the assessment, fees, involvement of third parties, and limits of confidentiality and sufficient opportunity for the client/patient to ask questions and answers.

Standard 9.03(b) states:

Psychologists inform persons with questionable capacity to consent or for whom testing is mandated by law or governmental regulations about the nature and purpose of the proposed assessment services, using language that is reasonably understandable to the person assessed.

Finally, Section 3.10(d) (Informed Consent) needs to be included here:

Psychologists appropriately document written or oral consent, permission and assent.

The 2002 code requires much more of psychologists in explaining and documenting consent for assessment. First, it seems to require making an immediate determination of whether a patient is competent. If there is some reason to doubt this (and the basis for this doubt will probably have to be documented somewhere), then the patient may need to only give *assent*. This seems to be a less-stringent criterion than of *consent*. The former may be generally interpreted as primarily presenting information to a patient and allowing the patient to ask questions or have the opportunity to make objections known. However, it may not always be required that the patient make some sort of indication that he or she understands and agrees to proceed with the assessment if it appears that the patient lacks the ability to do so. In contrast, patients who initially are presumed or known to be competent would be required to give consent, meaning that there is some indication both that they understand what is proposed and that they have agreed to this.

How much detail should neuropsychologists provide in explaining what will happen if a patient is assessed, and how should this be documented? This is not spelled out by the 2002 code and could not be given the inevitable problems that would occur if a "one-size-fits-all" solution had been attempted on what will obviously be a complicated and diverse range of situations.

One possible solution has been proposed by the Board of Directors of the National Academy of Neuropsychology. Their official statement (National Academy of Neuropsychology, 2003c), approved in October 2003, on informed consent in clinical neuropsychology practice includes both a flowchart indicating for which situations either assent or consent should be obtained, as well as a sample template for informed consent. The last document explains some of what the patient should expect during the evaluation (e.g., interview, memory testing), foreseeable risks such as frustration or fatigue, estimated fees and length of evaluation (including that patients are ultimately responsible for the fee), and limits of confidentiality. Presenting such a document to a patient, and the patient eventually signing it, has some obvious merits, particularly in that it provides a strong counterclaim to any later possible patient claims that he or she did not know what to expect.

On the other hand, two potential limits to this approach are foreseen. First, when presenting a written list of foreseeable activities that will occur during an evaluation, such as memory and personality assessment, when does the duty end? Should it go on to alert patients to the possibility that tests of effort (e.g., malingering tests) will be given, or that tests such as the Minnesota Multiphasic Personality Inventory 2 (MMPI-2; Butcher, Dahlstrom, Graham, Tellegen, & Kaemmer, 1984) will include "validity scales"? If intending to confront a patient with a written list of all foreseeable risks inherent in an evaluation, it could easily be argued that this should include issues such as tests of malingering (even though research has demonstrated that "forewarning" malingerers only leads to more sophisticated malingering; Youngjohn, Lees-Haley, & Binder, 1999).

A second potential problem with routinely attempting a written debriefing of informed consent is that it could sometimes lead to a chilling effect on any subsequent relationship the treating or expert neuropsychologist hopes to build with the patient. Some have commented that such advisory efforts may be "overkill" and pointed out that patients are not routinely confronted with such documents when they are referred for blood tests or other medical procedures, and that our attempts to obtain written informed consent may unnecessarily alarm patients when they read disclaimers about "foreseeable risks and discomforts."

Indeed, despite not having previously attempted to obtain written consent routinely, I am unaware of any postevaluation complaints from patients that information had been inappropriately released, that charges had been inappropriately made, or that inappropriate testing had occurred. However, a claim that "nothing bad has ever happened before" will probably not be viewed as a good reason not to pay attention to Standard 9.03.

Perhaps a reasonable solution would be for clinicians to give a verbal explanation of the nature, content, and cost of an intended neuropsychological evaluation and then (presuming the patient has given a verbal assent or consent) proceed to document all this. The neuropsychologist might include in the subsequent report some boilerplate language that consent had been achieved. However, referring parties may not wish for such potentially extraneous information always to be included in reports. Therefore, another solution may be for the neuropsychologist to include some type of form in a patient's chart that might be checked off to indicate that verbal consent had been obtained. It appears that neuropsychologists who do not in any way attempt to document informed consent will put themselves at risk for violation of Standard 9.03 should a patient later dispute an issue concerning the parameters of the evaluation.

Informed Consent for Services of an Interpreter

Informed consent for services of an interpreter is actually Section (c) of Standard 9.03, but has been separated out here because this seems to be an issue different from what is usually considered a routine part of obtaining informed consent for assessment. Ethical Standard 9.03 states that "Psychologists using the services of an interpreter obtain informed consent from the client/patient to use that interpreter, ensure that confidentiality of test results and test security are maintained, and include in their recommendations, reports and diagnostic or evaluative statements, including forensic testimony, discussion of any limitations on the data obtained." Also relevant is Section 9.02(c): "Psychologists use assessment methods that are appropriate to an individual's language preference and competence, unless the use of an alternative language is relevant to the assessment issues."

These standards bring to mind issues raised by Artiola and Mullaney (1998) and others (LaCalle, 1987) that discuss the evaluation of patients who come from a different culture or who speak a different language than the evaluator. There is no doubt that such patients should, when possible, be referred to clinicians who speak the same first language as the patient. Also, the clinician should attempt to use assessment instruments developed and normed for the appropriate ethnic group. Ponton and Leon-Carrion (2001), for example, have written extensively on how to evaluate Hispanic patients appropriately.

It is less clear, however, what to do if a clinician cannot find an appropriate colleague for referral. This problem is especially acute in large cities such as Chicago or New York, where the clinician is likely to encounter patients who speak Urdu, Mandarin, or other myriad languages. It is unlikely that these clinicians will have access to colleagues who either speak these languages or have appropriately normed testing materials available.

What should be done in such circumstances? Although it may be tempting simply to tell a referent that "It can't be done," this runs the risk of denying clients appropriate services. Obviously, responses at the other end of the spectrum may be equally inappropriate. That is, proceeding as if the patient is fluent in English and is familiar with "majority" American culture and not describing the limits of the evaluation in one's report is just as likely to lead to an inappropriate outcome. Instead, each referral of this type will dictate various ways of proceeding, which might range from referral to a colleague, to judicious and limited evaluation, to refusal to accept the referral even in the absence of referring elsewhere.

If a clinician elects to proceed with the use of an interpreter, the new ethical standard does serve as a warning that patients must agree to this, and the interpreter must be cautioned against the inappropriate release of information to nonauthorized others concerning either information about the patient or even the specifics of a test's items or content. Clinicians should also be cautious about asking friends or relatives of the friend to stand in as interpreters because their lack of objectivity may interfere with accuracy. Patients might also be reluctant to disclose personal information fully in interviews if a friend or relative is serving as an interpreter.

Other Changes in the Code

Of course, there are other changes in the 2002 code that conceivably could have an impact on the practice of forensic neuropsychology, but they do not seem to have as obvious implications as the three examples cited above. Here are a few other changes of interest.

Section 9.01(b) and (c) (Bases for Assessment) makes it more clear that psychologists can provide testimony regarding patients even when they have not had the opportunity to do their own evaluation. For example, it now states that when "an individual examination is not warranted or necessary for the opinion, psychologists explain this and the sources of information on which they based their conclusions and recommendations."

Another change of interest is that the old Section 7, Forensic Activities, has been eliminated. This seems just as well because its previously separation might have suggested that a different set of ethical rules applied to forensic cases. Obviously enough, the elimination of the forensics section does not imply that psychologists are now allowed to be as unethical as they please if they are retained by an attorney. It is reassuring to know that the ethically relevant sections of the old standard have been transferred to other sections of the new code.

Finally, a new subsection (9.02[b]) specifies that psychologists use assessment instruments with validity and reliability that have been established for use with members of the population tested. Otherwise, psychologists weigh the strengths and limitations of using such tests.

IMPACT OF THE HEALTH INSURANCE PORTABILITY AND ACCOUNTABILITY ACT ON THE PRACTICE OF FORENSIC NEUROPSYCHOLOGY

At the time of this writing, HIPAA appears to be the 800-pound gorilla about to tear down clinical and research practice as we have always known them. Or will it? Repeated attempts to "nail down" what is changed by this law, which took effect in April 2003, inevitably led to "legalese" and contradictions. There is no doubt, however, that interpretation of HIPAA is state, hospital, or perhaps even clinician specific, but it is still difficult to understand at this juncture whether any related changes will eventually be worth all the fuss and worry that have accompanied the products and services now marketed to the HIPAA anxious.

This review discusses, in three sections, what little seems to be understood about HIPAA at this point. The first section is a brief overview of HIPAA, including its impact on what might be termed some "technical" issues. The second section discusses what appears to be the two most relevant "conceptual" issues for the treating neuropsychologist: accounting of disclosures and a patient's right to limit information contained in a report or chart. These first two sets of issues are meant to apply to "treating" (e.g., nonforensic, non- independent medical examination [IME]) cases. These are briefly reviewed in this text of forensic neuropsychology as they still should be of interest to the practicing neuropsychologist and because some "forensic" cases may initially present as "nonforensic." The third and final HIPAA section reviews implications for forensic neuropsychology cases.

Health Insurance Portability and Accountability Act Overview

Again, HIPAA is an acronym for the Health Insurance Portability and Accountability Act. It was signed into law in 1996, but its provisions did not take effect until April 2003. The law was originally designed to allow people to transport their health insurance from one employer to the next, but of course has morphed into something akin to the beast that ate Cincinnati. HIPAA now pertains to just about everyone who participates in the health care system, including health care providers, health care clearinghouses, and health insurers.

Some requirements of HIPAA might be considered technical. It appears that computers must be sufficiently encrypted when transmitting data about patients, that fax machines and computer screens must be placed in ways that passersby cannot see information about patients, files must be sufficiently protected and locked, and so on. Patients must also be presented with HIPAA disclosure notifications, which will detail how their information is safeguarded and how the patient may access it. Review of the specifics of these issues is beyond the scope of this chapter. The APA and various state organizations have compiled HIPAA kits that might be of use to those who need such assistance.

The Health Insurance Portability and Accountability Act and the Treating Psychologist

Review of HIPAA legislation and related articles raises two issues that seem most likely to have an impact on nontechnical aspects of neuropsychological practice. The first of these concerns the right to obtain an accounting of disclosures of protected health information unless the "disclosure was made to carry out treatment, payment and health care operations as defined under HIPAA" (Office of Legal Affairs, 2001). In other words, patients have the right to know if the neuropsychologist has passed along their information to marketers or other nonhealth professionals. Because most treating psychologists will have been careful not to disclose patient information in ways other than to carry out treatment or to process insurance claims, it is difficult to anticipate how the accounting of disclosures will apply to psychologists in most circumstances. Indeed, psychologists have traditionally been very mindful of patient confidentiality, perhaps more so than colleagues in other professions. The legal counsel to the Massachusetts Psychological Association (Millard, 2002) opined that:

In many ways, psychologists have always had great provisions for privacy, so they will probably be less affected than other health care providers. I don't think the changes will be hugely substantive in the way one practices, but it will bureaucratize the relationship between the psychologist and the patient, because there will definitely be more forms to fill out.

The other area of HIPAA probably most pertinent to the treating neuropsychologist is that of the need to transmit the minimum necessary amount of information. Under this requirement, covered entities—such as managed care companies—are barred from requesting information beyond what is minimally necessary to accomplish payment or other administrative tasks (Daw Holloway, 2003a). This is meant to safeguard confidential information in a patient's file, and it may result in conflicts between psychologists and payers that eventually would have to be resolved by a court.

However, some have questioned whether the minimum necessary provision might be interpreted to permit patients to restrict or amend information in their report or chart, and whether this might mean that a patient could dictate the way in which a report might be written. For instance, a patient might request that a psychologist not include results from effort testing or might state his or her wish that the psychologist not refer to aspects of the patient's background (such as ongoing substance abuse) when interpreting current test results. However, although "covered entities" (those to whom HIPAA applies) have a duty to consider such requests, they also have the right to deny them.

Consultation with a hospital privacy officer indicated that a "clinician's judgment" is paramount in determining what type of information should go into a patient's report. Of course, the patient always retains the right to revoke disclosure of said report and may direct the psychologist not to release the report to anyone. Some patients, even in the time before HIPAA, not only revoked authorization, but also directed that the psychologist destroy all records of contact with that patient. Of course medical records cannot be destroyed because of both state law and APA ethical principles.

So far, this review has failed to demonstrate any definite HIPAA-related changes for the practice of a treating neuropsychologist other than what might be considered technical (such as HIPAA forms), and for the most part many of these may not be substantially different from what was done before HIPAA was enacted. Of course, this does not imply that there are no significant changes in store for the treating neuropsychologist—only that relatively little has been clearly identified as the time of this writing.

The Health Insurance Portability and Accountability Act and Forensic Neuropsychology

The one thing about HIPAA that seems to be spelled out clearly is that it does not specifically apply to the practice of forensic neuropsychology. According to an article written by Celia Fisher, the chair of the APA Ethics Code Task Force, "There are instances, however, when HIPAA constraints are not at issue" (Fisher, 2003). More specifically, the relevant section of HIPAA legislation [45 C.F.R. 45 164.508 and 164.524[a](1)] states that "Patients do not have the right of access to information compiled in reasonable anticipation of, or for use in, in a civil, criminal or administrative procedure." As reviewed, this information has been incorporated into Figure 3-1, which shows the interaction of HIPAA, state law, and APA ethics in determining when and if raw data can be released to others.

To conclude, at this early point in HIPAA time, it appears that this new legislation will have minimal impact on the practice of forensic neuropsychology. For nonforensic cases, it should be kept in mind that the new APA ethical code pertaining to release of raw data was written with HIPAA in mind, and practitioners should be prepared to release copies of requested raw data if their state does not prohibit this.

OBSTACLES TO THE ETHICAL PRACTICE OF FORENSIC NEUROPSYCHOLOGY

It is not enough to be well intentioned or to view oneself as "ethical" to avoid ethical dilemmas and inappropriate outcomes in forensic neuropsychology. Forensic neuropsychologists cannot necessarily rely on common sense, or the opinion of a referring party, as to the correct course of action in ethically questionable situations. Another problem is that many questions or problems cannot be anticipated in advance of occurrence, and there may be little time to seek consultation from colleagues or to think the way through the problem.

Therefore, the rest of this chapter serves as a reference guide for ethical dilemmas that might reasonably be expected to encounter in forensic neuropsychology cases. These are based on situations, and actual questions and comments, encountered by colleagues and myself. These are presented in roughly the same order that they would occur in the evolution of a forensic neuropsychological evaluation. That is, this discussion initiates with dilemmas likely encountered with the first contact with a referring party and concludes with issues related to deposition or trial testimony. References to the relevant sections of the 2002 ethical principles are made for each section.

Competence

Regarding competence (Ethical Standard [ES] 2 Competence; 2.01 Boundaries of Competence), the dilemma has involved the following question: "Will you provide opinions on this child custody case?" Psychologists should agree to be retained only on cases for which their education, training, and knowledge are sufficient for them to offer expert opinions on the issues at hand. At a minimum, this would require them to have knowledge of the relevant literature and sufficient supervised or recent clinical experience with the type of patient/problem referred. Neuropsychologists typically have a doctorate in clinical psychology and as such usually have had experience in other areas besides neuropsychology. This might allow them to serve as experts in cases involving chronic pain, psychopathology, child custody, or a host of other issues, but they should make sure of their ongoing competence before agreeing to be retained.

Psychologists and nonpsychologists alike might refer to the "definition of a neuropsychologist" papers promulgated either by Division 40 (Clinical Neuropsychology) of the APA (1989) or by the National Academy of Neuropsychology (2001) to help determine who might have the necessary credentials to offer a neuropsychological opinion. Both definitions seem to agree that board certification may be or is the best evidence of specialized training and knowledge in neuropsychology.

Method of Retainer

The dilemma concerning the method of retainer (ES 3.06 Conflict of Interest; 6.04 Fees and Financial Arrangements; 6.07 Referrals and Fees) has involved the questions: "Will you work on lien?" and "Will you work for a reduced fee?" Because plaintiff lawyers typically do not collect a fee from a client until a settlement or jury verdict has been awarded, they sometimes will ask experts to wait to get paid. Besides not knowing when this will occur, the psychologist may not even know *if* they will get paid. It is difficult to imagine how an expert can maintain neutrality, say in front of a jury, if he or she knows that none of the fees will be paid unless the plaintiff receives a favorable verdict.

Similarly, disability insurance companies, or defense litigators, may sometimes ask an expert to "cap" their bill for a less-than-usual amount. Although this may not be as problematic as working on lien, it is not without its own set of problems. Working for less than your usual fee may tempt you to cut corners and not do as thorough a job as is necessary or typical.

On the other hand, psychologists should also consider doing *pro bono* work for impoverished clients, which does suggest some reason not to automatically refuse to take some cases either on lien or for reduced fees. Such things should be carefully though through, and you should try to ensure that the work will remain of the highest quality and not be tainted by the manner of retainer before agreeing to one of these alternative financial arraigments.

Suggestions of Bias or Collusion

Suggestions of bias or collusion (ES 2.04 Bases for Scientific and Professional Judgments) has involved the question: "Will you be able to hit a home run on this case?" It is the rare attorney who is so psychopathic or aggressive as to make an up-front suggestion to a potential expert that only a certain opinion is sought, but it happens. It is more common for an attorney or insurance company representative to inquire about a professional's training and experience. Questions about board certification, work setting and experience, and familiarity with a particular clinical issue are entirely appropriate and should be welcomed. However, in some cases the attorney may drop subtle or not-so-subtle hints that certain opinions are sought. It may be the case that an attorney is naïve and inexperienced, and that he or she can be quickly disabused of your willingness to go along for the ride. Of course, some attorneys are not naïve about such issues, and these might be refused one's services.

Attorneys are not the only possible source of bias in a forensic neuropsychological examination. As reviewed in a chapter by Sweet, Grote, and van Gorp (2002), both the neuropsychological expert and the patient may also introduce elements of unfairness or preconceived notions of outcome of an evaluation. Those interested might review Sweet and Moulthrop's (1999b) article on ways to attempt to identify bias in personal work. The subsequent commentary and critique of this article by Lees-Haley (1999), as well as Sweet and Moulthrop's response to Lees-Haley, provide a range of complementary and contradictory views.

Review of Records/Examination of Patient

For the review of records/examination of patient dilemma (ES 9.01 Bases for Assessment), "Don't worry, Doctor, we'll tell you what you need to know about this case" is another question that has been asked. Neuropsychologists unfamiliar with their role may not fully appreciate their duty to exhaust all reasonable means to understand a case before they reach an opinion. They need to be proactive in asking for and receiving appropriate background information. This might include school and work records to estimate premorbid functioning or deposition transcripts of the patient's collaterals to determine their views of how a person's daily life has been affected by an accident or illness.

Medical records can be voluminous in these cases, but the forensic neuropsychologist should routinely attempt to review things such as ambulance and police records, the statements of witnesses, as well as emergency room, hospital, and imaging records. Psychologists should not passively rely on the judgment of the retaining party to determine which records will be sent. Attorneys or insurance companies might send only a subset of a voluminous group of records to a psychologist for review, and it may be the case that these are sufficient for the psychologist to understand the situation. If they are not sufficient, it is the psychologist's duty to ask for additional records, which may or may not be available. If they are not available or not sent for some other reason, the psychologist should document this in his or her records and report and note the effect that this lack of information had on their opinion.

In most cases, a decision needs to be made whether the psychologist is going to request to do his or her own examination of a patient. This request for examination will be often be agreed to by a retaining party, but in some cases, this request may not be granted. This could be because certain deadlines have passed, or the patient's attorney is somehow successful in refusing to accede to such a request.

It should be noted that failure to examine a patient personally does not mean that a psychologist cannot produce opinions. Ethical Standard 9.01(c) addresses this in acknowledging that, in some situations, an individual examination is not warranted or necessary for opinions. Obviously, psychologists will typically have to offer a more limited range of opinions when they only review records and have not seen a patient, but again they are not precluded from offering *any* opinions.

The primary point is that psychologists need to determine what must be reviewed or done for them to arrive at their opinions. They should not rely on the opinions of retaining or opposing parties to determine this. Obstacles should be fought against, and if the result is unsuccessful (records or patient not examined), the effect of this needs to be incorporated into the report.

Safeguarding Psychological Tests

The dilemma of safeguarding of psychological tests (9.04 Release of Raw Data) has involved the following two questions: "We'll let you test our patient only if we tape your evaluation" and "Send your complete file to us." Attorneys have a duty to represent their client's interests, and they do not have to be objective or even "friendly" in how they do this. They often will voice active suspicion of opposing experts and imply that only a biased incompetent could have arrived at certain opinions. Sometimes, they may feel this way even before the patient is evaluated and go to great lengths to ensure that an evaluation will be done "fairly."

Therefore, they may attempt to obtain court orders that allow the examination to be videotaped or audiotaped. Demands might be made to allow an attorney or the attorney's representative (such as another psychologist or a court reporter) to sit in on the evaluation. At the end of the evaluation, attorneys might insist that copies of all test materials be sent to them.

Any of these scenarios should cause the psychologist to invoke Ethical Standard 9.04. Test data should not be released to nonpsychologists unless there is good reason to (see Figure 3-1). In the case of a postevaluation request for raw data, it is nearly inevitable now that requested raw data will have to be copied and sent to someone else. However, this does not mean that psychologists need to agree to infringements on the evaluation itself. Although it may be that attorneys are sincerely interested in ensuring that only appropriate interviewing and testing is conducted, it seems equally, if not more, likely that such requests are meant to intimidate the evaluating psychologist, perhaps even to the point of withdrawing from the case for ethical concerns or because of the unpleasantness of monitoring by an adversarial party.

Psychologists should attempt to educate others about the negative impact that this third-party observation may have on the obtained results. Position papers from the National Academy of Neuropsychology (Axelrod et al., 2000) and the American Academy of Clinical Neuropsychology (2001), as well as other sources (Constantinou, Ashendorf, & McCaffrey, 2002) can be cited in such instances and previously have caused judges to disallow an invasion of the evaluation process. However, because some states may allow an attorney to be present during any IME, the psychologist must be prepared for this and to have ready a series of responses for different scenarios.

It may be that, if forced, a neuropsychologist would agree to allow an attorney to sit quietly behind a client during the interview or testing. Such a stance may be the best that can be hoped in certain cases. However, it is difficult to imagine how a psychologist would allow this observer to interfere with the evaluation process, such as by interrupting with questions, comments, or derisive sneers and snorts. It is also difficult to imagine situations in which a psychologist might allow recording equipment during the administration of psychological tests unless there was some sort of agreement or protective order that prohibited release or further use of these recordings. Additional details on ways to handle requests for release of raw data or test materials can be found in another position paper by the National Academy of Neuropsychology (2003a).

Range and Detail of Interview

The dilemma of range and detail of interview (ES 9.01 Bases for Assessment) has involved the statement "I'm only answering the interview questions that I think are relevant." It may not be unusual for patients to come to an IME with the feeling that the evaluating psychologist is there to help them no matter what (if referred through their attorney) or is there to hurt them no matter what (if referred by their insurer or an opposing attorney). Attempts to convince them of the evaluator's neutrality might be made, but still might be answered by the patient with scorn or disbelief. In any event, a patient's attitude should not determine the number, range, or type of questions asked of him or her.

Despite attempts to build some rapport, some patients may go on to refuse to answer interview questions. This could range from an isolated question or two, to a steadfast refusal to answer any and all forthcoming questions. In such situations, the neuropsychologist must determine if the information is needed to arrive at opinions asked of them. If the information indeed is needed (as will probably be the case because the question was asked in the first place), the clinician then has the dilemma of determining how to proceed. It might be possible to persuade the patient to continue with the interview by pointing out the relevance of the questions. Alternatively, the question might either be asked later in the interview or be rephrased in another way that the patient does not find objectionable. However, the neuropsychologist should not refrain from terminating an evaluation if it appears that the client's resistance is so high as to keep the neuropsychologist from obtaining the needed background information.

Relationships With Litigants and Claimants

Regarding relationships with litigants and claimants (ES 9.03 Informed Consent in Assessments), the dilemma has involved the question, "Doctor, will you send me a copy of my report?" It might seem self-evident that litigants and claimants understand the reason they are referred for a forensic neuropsychological assessment because it could be presumed they have been informed by their attorney or insurance company about this. Because such an assumption cannot be made, it is incumbent on a neuropsychologist to explain the circumstances of the assessment. This debriefing minimally should include an explanation that the patient is referred for an IME and not for treatment. They need to understand that there are limits to confidentiality, and that a report detailing the results will be written. They also need to understand that feedback will not be offered to them unless the neuropsychologist is authorized to do so. Litigants should have an opportunity to ask questions. The patient's understanding of the evaluation might be memorialized by having them sign some sort of IME waiver or disclaimer. However, because some litigants have been forewarned "not to sign anything," it is also acceptable to have a verbal explanation and consent, which is then documented by the psychologist.

Performing a Competent Evaluation

There can be a dilemma of performing a competent evaluation (ES 9.01 Bases for Assessment, 2.03 Maintaining Competence): "You don't need to give my client a malingering test. I can tell you he's honest." As reviewed, neuropsychologists should not enter into cases in which they do not have proper expertise. This would include awareness of recent developments in the field and knowledge of some of the seminal articles about issues discussed. For instance, the articles by Dikmen, Machamer, Winn, and Temkin (1995) and Binder and colleagues (Binder, 1997; Binder, Rohling, & Larrabee, 1997) are extremely important contributions in how to diagnose and understand mild traumatic brain injury, but it is evident that many neuropsychologists are unfamiliar with these articles and seem to have no greater understanding of this topic than what they might have learned in graduate school years or decades ago.

Similarly, some clinicians have argued that tests of effort, or "malingering tests," do not need to be given because they can assess this by virtue of their observation of the patient or because that area of research is not well developed in their opinion. Such comments, of course, run counter to empirical research (Grote, Kooker, et al., 2000; Sweet, 1999; Youngjohn, Spector, & Mapou, 1998). Some of these same clinicians also have argued that it is appropriate to give tests that have not been renormed in over 50 years. The basis for such claims seems quite thin.

The point is that our clinical work is based on scientific investigations, and these are ongoing. Clinicians have a responsibility to keep up with developments in their field. Failure to make reasonable efforts to do so may well justify charges of failure to adhere to the standards of the field and to maintain competence.

Accurate and Full Reporting of Findings

The dilemma of accurate and full reporting of findings (ES 9.01 Bases for Assessment; 9.10 Explaining Assessment Results) could involve the statements: "Doctor, please don't mention that my client was once arrested. It has nothing to do with this case" and "Doctor, don't include my wife's IQ scores in your report. Her employer has no need to know them." A neuropsychological interview is just as important, if not more important, than any test that might be administered (Lezak, 1995). These interviews need to assess a broad range of factors that will assist the neuropsychologist in placing the test data in proper context. Both clinical and forensic patients should routinely be asked questions about their families of origin; educational attainment and achievement; previous medical, psychiatric, and substance abuse histories; and so on.

It is not unusual for such interviews to reveal potentially embarrassing details that a client, or the client's attorney, would prefer not go into a report. Of course, this possibility should have been discussed beforehand during the informed consent for assessment, and these details need not be reported if they do not contribute to an understanding of the patient's neuropsychological status. However, the neuropsychologist should remember that he or she is ultimately responsible for providing a full and correct neuropsychological opinion and may not be able to arrive at such an opinion if he or she agrees to omit relevant biographical details.

Accuracy in Testimony

As to the involvement of accuracy in testimony (ES 9.06 Interpreting Assessment Results), the dilemma may be "Doctor, please don't mention that you found scoring errors that would help my opponent's case." As entire texts (Brodsky, 1999) have been written to provide extensive detail on how to prepare for and conduct oneself in giving expert testimony, this review gives details for just one component of testimony: giving full and honest opinions about one's findings. Testifying at deposition or in court can be very stressful and unnerving, especially if the retaining attorney attempts to coach or even bias your testimony beforehand.

In most cases, attorneys will ask to meet with their retained expert for 15 to 60 minutes prior to a deposition. This typically will involve some discussion of their expert's findings and opinions, including what the expert might say in response to likely questions from the deposing attorney. However, the occasional attorney might attempt to convince the expert to withhold certain opinions if possible. This could include the discovery of scoring errors made by another psychologist and the realization that accurate scoring could be seen as "helping the opposition." Of course, a forensic neuropsychologist cannot ignore these data and must inform the retaining attorney of his or her opinions, even if the opinions are based on errors not yet discovered by others in the case.

Protecting the Public

In the dilemma of protecting the public (ES 1.05 Reporting Ethical Violations), psychologists will sometimes encounter reports or opinions from colleagues whose work seems to be so riddled with error or without any reasonable scientific foundation that it raises a question as to whether that colleague is acting in a competent and ethical manner. Reaching a decision about whether to contact the colleague or perhaps eventually reporting the colleague to a regulatory or professional organization can be difficult. The psychologist should determine whether the perceived differences in opinions or work products simply reflect an honest difference in opinion or whether a colleague's work can be viewed by others as representing a significant threat to patients or the public good.

Previous reviews (Deidan & Bush, 2002; Grote, Lewin, Sweet, & van Gorp, 2000) have detailed when and how a psychologist might proceed in such situations. Obviously, frivolous or harassing complaints should never be made, but it is recommended that psychologists take appropriate steps when they perceive that a colleague has acted in a grossly incompetent or unethical manner.

It is also recommended that one not contact another psychologist, or file a complaint, until incident litigation has fully resolved. Although there may be emergent situations for which immediate reporting is required, more typically a complaint filed in the midst of ongoing litigation could be perceived as a tactic of intimidation or harassment. A position paper from the American Academy of Clinical Neuropsychology (2003) provides further discussion of this issue.

SUMMARY

This chapter reviews the potential impact of HIPAA, as well as the changes in the APA ethical principles that are of greatest relevance to the practice of forensic neuropsychology. Obstacles to the ethical practice of forensic neuropsychology are also reviewed. It is hoped that these reviews will serve as a helpful resource to those interested in practicing forensic neuropsychology in a way that will benefit the public.

REFERENCES

American Academy of Clinical Neuropsychology. (2001). Policy statement on the presence of third party observers in neuropsychological assessments. *The Clinical Neuropsychologist, 15*, 433–439.

American Academy of Clinical Neuropsychology. (2003). Official position of the American Academy of Clinical Neuropsychology on ethical complaints made against clinical neuropsychologists during adversarial proceedings. *The Clinical Neuropsychologist, 17*, 443–445.

American Psychological Association. (1953). *Ethical standards of psychologists.* Washington, DC: Author.

American Psychological Association. (2002). Ethical principles of psychologists and code of conduct. *American Psychologist, 57*, 1060–1073.

American Psychological Association. (2003). *1992–2002 Ethics codes comparison.* Retrieved March 15, 2003, from www.apa.org/ethics/codecomparison.html

Artiola, L., & Mullaney, H. (1998). Assessing patients whose language you do not know: Can the absurd be ethical? *The Clinical Neuropsychologist, 12*, 113–126.

Axelrod, B., Barth, J., Faust, D., Fisher, J., Heilbronner, R., Larrabee, G., et al. (2000). Presence of third party observers during neuropsychological testing: Official statement of the National Academy of Neuropsychology. *Archives of Clinical Neuropsychology, 15*, 379–380.

Binder, L. (1997). A review of mild head trauma: II. Clinical implications. *Journal of Clinical and Experimental Neuropsychology, 19*, 432–457.

Binder, L., Rohling, M., & Larrabee, G. (1997). A review of mild head trauma: I. Meta-analytic review of neuropsychological studies. *Journal of Clinical and Experimental Neuropsychology, 19*, 421–431.

Binder, L., & Thompson, L. (1995). The ethics code and neuropsychological assessment practices. *Archives of Clinical Neuropsychology, 10*, 27–46.

Brodsky, S. (1999). *The expert expert witness: More maxims and guidelines for testifying in court.* Washington, DC: American Psychological Association.

Bush, S. (in press). *A casebook of ethical challenges in neuropsychology.* Lisse, The Netherlands: Swets and Zeitlinger.

Bush, S., & Drexler, M. (Eds.). (2002). *Ethical issues in clinical neuropsychology.* Lisse, The Netherlands: Swets and Zeitlinger.

Butcher, J. N., Dahlstrom., W. G., Graham, J. R., Tellegen, A., & Kaemmer, B. (1989). *Minnesota Multiphasic Personality Inventory-2 (MMPI-2): Manual for administration and scoring.* Minneapolis: University of Minnesota Press.

Committee on Ethical Guidelines for Forensic Neuropsychologists. (1991). Specialty guidelines for forensic psychologists. *Law and Human Behavior, 15*, 655–665.

Constantinou, M., Ashendorf, L., & McCaffrey, R. (2002). When the third party of a neuropsychological evaluation is an audio-recorder. *The Clinical Neuropsychologist*, *16*, 407–412.

Daw Holloway, J. (2003a). A stop-gap in the flow of sensitive patient information. *Monitor on Psychology*, *34*, 22.

Daw Holloway, J. (2003b). What takes precedence: HIPAA or state law? *Monitor on Psychology*, *34*, 28.

Deidan, C., & Bush, S. (2002). Addressing perceived ethical violations in clinical neuropsychology. In S. Bush & M. Drexler (Eds.), *Ethical issues in clinical neuropsychology* (pp. 281–306). Lisse, The Netherlands: Swets and Zeitlinger.

Dikmen, S., Machamer, J., Winn, H., & Temkin, R. (1995). Neuropsychological outcome at 1-year post head injury. *Neuropsychology*, *9*, 80–90.

Division 40 of the American Psychological Association. (1989). Definition of a clinical neuropsychologist. *The Clinical Neuropsychologist*, *3*, 22.

Fisher, C. (2003, January/February). Test data standard most notable change in new APA ethics code. *The National Psychologist*, 12.

Grote, C., Kooker, E., Garron, D., Nyenhuis, D., Smith, C., & Mattingly, M. (2000). Performance of compensation seeking and non-compensation seeking samples on the Victoria Symptom Validity Test: Cross validation and extension of a standardization study. *Journal of Clinical and Experimental Neuropsychology*, *22*, 709–719.

Grote, C., Lewin, J., Sweet, J., & van Gorp, W. (2000). Responses to perceived unethical practices in clinical neuropsychology: Ethical and legal considerations. *The Clinical Neuropsychologist*, *14*, 119–134.

LaCalle, J. (1987). Forensic psychological evaluations through an interpreter: Legal and ethical issues. *American Journal of Forensic Psychology*, *5*, 29–43.

Lees-Haley, P. (1999). Commentary on Sweet and Moulthrop's debiasing procedures. *Journal of Forensic Neuropsychology*, *1*, 43–57.

Lezak, M. (1995). *Neuropsychological Assessment* (3rd ed.). New York: Oxford University Press.

Millard, Elizabeth (2002, November). *HIPAA compliance deadlines prompt questions, concerns*. Retrieved March 11, 2003, from www.masspsy.com/leading/0211_coverhipaa.html

National Academy of Neuropsychology. (2000). Test security. *Archives of Clinical Neuropsychology*, *15*, 383–386.

National Academy of Neuropsychology. (2001). *Definition of a neuro-psychologist. Official statement of the National Academy of Neuropsychology approved by the Board of Directors May 5, 2001*. Retrieved March 11, 2003, from www.nanonline.org

National Academy of Neuropsychology. (2003a). *Handling requests to release test data, recording and/or reproductions of test data*. Retrieved March 11, 2003, from www.nanonline.org

National Academy of Neuropsychology. (2003b). *Independent and court-ordered forensic neuropsychological examinations. Official statement of the National Academy of Neuropsychology approved by the Board of Directors October 14, 2003*. Retrieved March 11, 2003, from www.nanonline.org

National Academy of Neuropsychology. (2003c). *Informed consent in clinical neuropsychology practice. Official statement of the National Academy of Neuropsychology approved by the Board of Directors October 13, 2003*. Retrieved March 11, 2003, from www.nanonline.org

National Academy of Neuropsychology. (2003d). *Test security: An update. Official state-*

ment of the National Academy of Neuropsychology approved by the Board of Directors October 13, 2003. Retrieved March 11, 2003, from www.nanonline.org

Office of Legal Affairs, Rush-Presbyterian–St. Luke's Medical Center. (2001, September). Going, going . . . staying: The Bush administration finalizes the HIPAA Privacy Regulation. *Health Law Report, 9,* 2–3.

Ponton, M., & Leon-Carrion, J. (Eds.). (2001). *Neuropsychology and the Hispanic patient.* Mahwah, NJ: Erlbaum.

Smith, D. (2003, January). What you need to know about the new code. *Monitor on Psychology,* 62–65.

Sweet, J. (Ed.). (1999). *Forensic neuropsychology.* Lisse, The Netherlands: Swets and Zeitlinger.

Sweet, J., Grote, C. & van Gorp, W. (2002). Ethical issues in forensic neuropsychology. In S. Bush & M. Drexler (Eds.), *Ethical issues in clinical neuropsychology* (pp. 103–134). Lisse, The Netherlands: Swets and Zeitlinger.

Sweet, J., King, J., Malina, A., Bergman, M., & Simmons, A. (2002). Documenting the prominence of forensic neuropsychology at national meetings and in relevant professional journals from 1990 to 2000. *The Clinical Neuropsychologist, 16,* 481–494.

Sweet, J., Moberg, P., & Suchy, Y (2000). Ten-year follow-up survey of clinical neuropsychologists: Part I. Practices and beliefs. *The Clinical Neuropsychologist, 14,* 18–37.

Sweet, J., & Moulthrop, M. (1999a). Response to Lees-Haley's commentary: Debiasing techniques cannot be completely curative. *Journal of Forensic Neuropsychology, 1,* 49–57.

Sweet, J., & Moulthrop, M. (1999b). Self-examination questions as a means of identifying bias in adversarial assessment. *Journal of Forensic Neuropsychology, 1,* 73–88.

Wechsler, D. (1997). *Wechsler Adult Intelligence Scale* (3rd ed.). San Antonio, TX: The Psychological Corporation.

Wechsler, D. (1997). *Wechsler Memory Scale* (3rd ed.). San Antonio, TX: The Psychological Corporation.

Youngjohn, J., Lees-Haley, P., & Binder, L. (1999). Comment: Warning malingerers produces more sophisticated malingering. *Archives of Clinical Neuropsychology, 14,* 511–515.

Youngjohn, J., Spector, J., & Mapou, R. (1998). Failure to assess motivation, need to consider psychiatric disturbance, and absence of objectively verified physical pathology: Some common pitfalls in the practice of forensic neuropsychology. *The Clinical Neuropsychologist, 12,* 233–236.

4

Assessment of Malingering

GLENN J. LARRABEE

This chapter reviews definitions of malingering and research designs for investigation of malingering and discusses various procedures developed to identify the presence of malingering. The primary purpose is to provide a conceptual understanding of the construct of malingering rather than offer a detailed review of various procedures developed for detection of malingering. Detailed reviews of malingering procedures are provided by Sweet (1999); the two-part special series "Detection of Response Bias in Forensic Neuropsychology" (Hom & Denney, 2002a, 2002b) also offers a more extensive review of procedures specifically designed to detect the presence of malingering.

DEFINITION OF MALINGERING

Accurate neuropsychological evaluation is based on test procedures that are reliable, yielding consistent and stable scores, and valid, producing true measures of the abilities and traits that we assume we are measuring; thus, tests of attention should yield reliable and valid assessments of attention, and tests of memory should yield reliable and valid measurement of memory function.

Test procedures that have proven reliability and validity, however, may yield scores that are not reliable or valid measures for the individual examined. In these instances, questions about the accuracy of patient performance arise because of significant inconsistencies in test data (Iverson & Binder, 2000; Larrabee, 2000). These may include inconsistencies between neuropsychological domains (e.g., impaired attention with normal memory); inconsistencies between neuropsychological test scores and the suspected etiology of brain dysfunction (e.g., impaired IQ with normal memory in alleged hypoxic brain injury); inconsistencies between neuropsychological test scores and medically documented severity of injury (e.g., performance at levels characteristic of those associated with prolonged coma in a patient who had a blow to the head without loss of consciousness); and inconsistencies between neuropsychological test scores and behavioral presentation (e.g., failure on measures of recent and remote memory contrasted with the ability, during interview, to report an accurate clinical history).

Inconsistencies in test scores often are the result of variable effort and motivation. Variable motivation can be secondary to factors outside the patient's conscious intent or control, such as depression, anxiety, or conversion disorder, or may result from conscious, intentional response distortion such as occurs in factitious disorder or malingering (Iverson & Binder, 2000; Larrabee, 1990). Factitious disorder and malingering share intentional, volitional distortion or misrepresentation of symptoms, but differ in that the motivation for factitious disorder is the psychological need to assume a sick or disabled role (*Diagnostic and Statistical Manual of Mental Disorders*, fourth edition [*DSM-IV*], American Psychiatric Association, 1994). In contrast, *malingering* is the intentional production of false or grossly exaggerated physical and psychological symptoms for external incentives such as obtaining monetary compensation or avoiding criminal prosecution (*DSM-IV*, American Psychiatric Association, 1994; Rogers, 1997a).

Rogers (1997a) discussed various explanatory models of malingering, including (a) mentally disordered (pathological), (b) "bad" (criminological), and (c) attempting to meet objectives in adversarial circumstances (adaptational). The adaptational model, first proposed by Rogers in 1990 (1990a, 1990b) considers would-be malingerers as engaging in a cost–benefit analysis when confronted with an assessment perceived as indifferent or in opposition to their needs. In this model, malingering is more likely to occur when the context is adversarial, the personal stakes are very high, and there are no other perceived viable alternatives.

Rogers (1997a) noted that descriptive data generally support the adaptational model, with higher prevalence of malingering in adversarial settings (forensic vs. nonforensic) or when personal stakes are particularly high (e.g., avoiding military combat or succeeding in personal injury litigation). Rogers considered the adaptational model as providing "the broadest and least pejorative explanation of malingering" (Rogers, 1997a, page 8). As a consequence, clinicians may be less likely to ignore evidence of malingering because a person does not fit more judgmental criteria (Iverson & Binder, 2000). The cost–benefit analysis underlying the adaptational model also allows gradations of malingering (mild, moderate, severe) and better fits the definition of malingering as involving either fabricated or exaggerated deficits.

Malingering can occur in one of three patterns in neuropsychological settings (Iverson & Binder, 2000; Larrabee, 2000): (a) false or exaggerated reporting of symptoms (Berry et al., 1995; Larrabee, 1998); (b) intentionally poor performance on neuropsychological tests (Binder & Willis, 1991; Mittenberg, Rotholc, Russell, & Heilbronner, 1996); or (c) a combination of symptom exaggeration and intentional performance deficit (Heaton, Smith, Lehman, & Vogt, 1978). There has been a significant increase in research on developing specialized procedures to detect malingering, such as the Portland Digit Recognition Test (PDRT; Binder & Willis, 1991) and the Test of Memory Malingering (TOMM; Tombaugh, 1996), as well as research identifying patterns of malingering on standard clinical tests (Mittenberg, Aguila-Puentes, Patton, Canyock, & Heilbronner, 2002) and fabrication and exaggeration of symptoms on the Minnesota Multiphasic Personality Inventory 2 (MMPI-2; Butcher, Dahlstrom, Graham, Tellegen, & Kaemmer, 1989; Lees-Haley, 1992; Lees-Haley, English, & Glenn, 1991).

Drawing on the research of Rogers (1990a, 1990b), Pankratz and Binder (1997), and Greiffenstein and colleagues (Greiffenstein, Baker, & Gola, 1994; Greiffenstein, Gola, & Baker, 1995), Slick, Sherman, and Iverson (1999) have proposed diagnostic criteria for malingered neurocognitive dysfunction (MND). This is defined by Slick et al. (1999) as the volitional exaggeration or fabrication of cognitive dysfunction for the purpose of obtaining substantial material gain (e.g., compensation for injury) or avoiding or escaping legally obligated formal duty (e.g., prison, military) or responsibility (e.g., competency to stand trial).

The Slick et al. (1999) criteria require consideration of evidence from neuropsychological testing and self-report. Evidence from neuropsychological testing includes *definite negative response bias*, defined as below chance performance ($p < .05$) on one or more forced-choice measures of cognitive function, whereas *probable response bias* involves performance on one or more well-validated psychometric tests or indices consistent with feigning. Evidence from neuropsychological testing also includes discrepancies between test data and patterns of brain functioning, discrepancies between test data and observed behavior, discrepancies between test data and reliable collateral reports, and discrepancies between test data and documented background history.

The Slick et al. (1999) indicators of evidence from self-report include self-reported history discrepant with documented history, self-reported symptoms discrepant with known patterns of brain functioning, self-reported symptoms discrepant with behavioral observations, and self-reported symptoms discrepant with information obtained from collateral informants. Self-reported evidence of malingering also includes evidence of exaggerated or fabricated psychological dysfunction based on well-validated validity scales or indices from measures such as the MMPI-2.

The Slick et al. (1999) criteria for definite MND include (a) presence of a substantial external incentive, (b) definite negative response bias (e.g., worse-than-chance performance on forced-choice testing), and (c) behaviors that meet necessary criteria for definite negative response bias that are not fully accounted for by psychiatric, neurological, or developmental factors. The criteria for probable MND include (a) presence of a substantial external incentive; (b) two or more types of evidence from neuropsychological testing, excluding definite negative response bias or one type of evidence from neuropsychological testing, excluding definite negative response bias, and one or more types of evidence from self-report; and (c) behaviors that meet necessary neuropsychological testing criteria and self-report that are not fully accounted for by psychiatric, neurological, or developmental factors. The criteria for possible MND include (a) presence of a substantial external incentive; (b) evidence from self-report; and (c) evidence from self-report not fully accountable by psychiatric, neurological, or developmental factors.

Slick et al. (1999) urged thorough consideration of differential diagnoses before concluding that a person is malingering. They recommended that a "reasonable doubt" strategy be applied to decisions about the probability that a patient is malingering, keeping in mind the limitations of assessment methodology and the cost of false-positive errors.

RESEARCH DESIGNS FOR INVESTIGATION OF MALINGERING

Rogers (1997b) reviewed basic research designs for evaluation of malingering, including the case study approach, simulation studies, known-group designs, and differential prevalence designs. The case study approach was used by Pankratz, Fausti, and Peed (1975) in the evaluation of hysterical deafness and by Hiscock and Hiscock (1989) in their initial demonstration of the validity of their Digit Memory Test (DMT). Denney (1996) also employed a case study design in the evaluation of claimed remote memory loss in criminal defendants professing amnesia for the events contemporaneous with the alleged crime. Although these authors employed a single-case or multiple-single-case approach, all three investigations relied on the normal approximation to the binomial, applied to two-alternative, forced-choice testing, that could be used to generate probabilities of malingering (this approach is discussed in greater detail in the section on forced-choice symptom validity testing).

Simulation studies typically involve use of noninjured persons who are provided with instructions to attempt to feign deficit successfully in an imaginary litigation scenario. Rogers (1997b) noted the main problem with these types of studies is generalizability. That is, will the findings in normal individuals simulating malingering generalize to the real-world setting, in which the financial stakes are considerably larger and involve real potential for financial gain? Rogers (1997b) recommended a design strategy by which four groups are studied: (a) simulating nonclinical subjects, (b) honestly responding nonclinical subjects, (c) honestly responding clinical subjects, and (d) clinical subjects simulating greater impairment than they really experience. Note that this strategy should increase generalizability of the results over studies that merely employ simulating and nonsimulating, nonclinical subject groups.

A number of neuropsychological investigations have contrasted simulators with groups of subjects who have genuine clinical disorders, frequently suffering from moderate-to-severe traumatic brain injury (TBI). Heaton et al. (1978) used this approach, which has also been employed by Mittenberg and his group in their investigations of profiles of malingering on the Wechsler Adult Intelligence Scale–Revised (WAIS-R; Wechsler, 1981), Halstead-Reitan Battery (HRB; Reitan & Wolfson, 1993), and Wechsler Memory Scale–Revised (WMS-R; Mittenberg, Azrin, Millsaps, & Heilbronner, 1993; Mittenberg et al., 1996; Mittenberg, Theroux, Zielinski, & Heilbronner, 1995; Wechsler, 1987).

The differential prevalence design is rarely used and poses several problems of interpretation. In this design, a group known to have a higher base rate of malingering is investigated and contrasted with a group not suspected of having an elevated rate of malingering. As Rogers (1997b) pointed out, very little is learned from differential prevalence designs because we do not know *who* is dissimulating in each group and *how many* are dissimulating in each group.

The fourth type of research design is the known-groups design. This requires a two-part approach: establishing the criterion groups (bona fide patients and malingerers) and conducting a systematic analysis of similarities and differences between the criterion groups. This research design has benefited significantly from the specification of criteria for malingering by Slick et al. (1999), which provide stronger confidence in creating the criterion groups. These criteria for malingering have been employed by Greve, Bianchini, Mathias, Houston, and Crouch (2002) to contrast the performance of subjects who had probable MND with that of persons who had moderate-to-severe TBI. I (Larrabee, 2003b) employed the Slick et al. (1999) criteria to compare and contrast performance on the MMPI-2 as well as on a select number of standard neuropsychological test procedures in subjects with definite or probable MND and subjects who had suffered moderate and severe TBI (Larrabee, 2003a). As Rogers (1997b) noted:

Employment of known-groups comparisons addresses fully the clinical relevance of dissimulation research. First, the research typically is conducted in clinical or other professional settings where dissimulation is expected to occur. Second and more important, the persons engaging in dissimulation are doing so for real-world reasons. (p. 416)

When using a clinical comparison group to contrast performance either with a normal subject group simulating malingering or with a known group of malingerers, it is important that the clinical group not include malingering subjects. This is particularly problematic when the clinical group includes persons who themselves are in litigation. One cannot merely assume that a group of subjects with a bona fide condition such as moderate or severe TBI are performing at their best. Rohling, Binder, and Langhinrischen-Rohling (1995) found that patients in chronic pain in litigation averaged 0.48 pooled standard deviations higher on pain scales than those not in litigation, a value quite close to the .47 effect size found by Binder and Rohling (1996) in contrasting the neuropsychological performance of TBI patients in litigation versus the performance of nonlitigating TBI patients. Thus, when using a litigant clinical control group, this group must itself be screened for malingering.

SPECIALIZED TESTS OF MALINGERING
OF NEUROCOGNITIVE DEFICIT

Several specialized tests of malingered cognitive deficit have been devised, dating to Rey's 15-item and dot-counting procedures developed 40 years ago (Lezak, Howieson, & Loring, 2004; Rey, 1964). In modern times, these procedures fall in two categories: (a) tasks that appear to measure a cognitive ability, but are so simple that even persons with significant neuropsychological deficits can perform perfectly or near perfectly (e.g., Rey 15-Item Test); and (b) tests based on forced-choice testing, which can be evaluated for worse-than-chance performance using the normal approximation to the binomial theorem, usually referred to as symptom validity testing (SVT; e.g., PDRT, Binder & Willis, 1991).

Simplistic Tests Performed Normally by Brain-Injured Persons

The Rey 15-Item Test (Rey, 1964) is probably the best-known task typically performed normally by brain-injured persons, so that poor performance may be considered a result of reduced motivation. The 15 redundant stimuli (e.g., quantitatively equivalent roman and arabic numerals; upper- and lowercase identical letters of the alphabet; see Lezak et al., 2004) are presented for 10 seconds, then withdrawn, with the subject asked to draw as many of the items as he or she can recall. Various cutoffs have been recommended, but performance is typically considered motivationally suspect at 67% or less (Greiffenstein et al., 1994; Lee, Loring, & Martin, 1992; Lezak et al., 2004). The Rey 15-Item Test has been criticized as having poor sensitivity to the presence of malingering (Iverson & Binder, 2000; Sweet, 1999). Others have questioned both sensitivity and specificity (e.g., elevated level of false-positive errors in patients with genuine impairment secondary to amnestic disorder, dementia, or severe psychiatric disorder; Schretlen, Brandt, Krafft, & Van Gorp, 1991).

Because of these problems, it has been recommended that the test not be the sole measure of effort and motivation (Iverson & Binder, 2000), and that the test should not be used in truly amnestic populations or with patients suffering severe psychopathology (Schretlen et al., 1991). A meta-analysis of the 15-Item Test (Vickery, Berry, Inman, Harris, & Orey, 2001) reported an average specificity (i.e., correct identification of clinical patients as not malingering) of 92.5% (based on eight studies), average sensitivity (i.e., correct detection of malingerers as malingering) of 43.3% (based on seven studies), and average hit rate of 70.5% (based on six studies).

Two modifications of the 15-Item Test have appeared (Boone, Salazar, Lu, Warner-Chacon, & Razani, 2002; Griffin, Glassmire, Henderson, & McCann, 1997). Griffin et al. eliminated the sequence of three geometric patterns and three lowercase letters on the original Rey 15-Item Test and replaced them with two numerical sequence stimuli redundant with the numerical sequences on the original 15-Item Test. The sensitivity and specificity of the revised "Rey-II" were evaluated in honest and dissimulating college students and honest and dissimulating nonlitigating clinical groups of board-and-care residents (clinical groups included those with schizophrenia and developmental disability and elderly persons needing residential care). Performance on the Rey-II was contrasted with performance on the original 15-Item Test (with the exception of not having a condition of a dissimulating clinical group on the original 15-Item Test). Griffin et al. found that both quantitative and qualitative scores on the Rey-II were superior in discriminating genuine from poor effort in the college students (qualitative scores had 100% specificity and 69% sensitivity; quantitative scores had 97% specificity and 73% sensitivity). These values were lower in the college students for the original 15-Item Test for qualitative scores (100% specificity, 57% sensitivity) and quantitative scores (98% sensitivity, 40% specificity). In the clinical population administered the Rey-II, qualitative score specificity was 75%, with sensitivity of 71%.

The modification of the 15-Item Test developed by Boone, Salazar, et al. (2002) maintains the original stimuli and format of the 15-Item Test, but adds a recognition trial administered following the standard drawing-from-recall condition. The recognition trial presents Rey's 15 original stimuli with 15 numeric, geometric, and alphabetic foil stimuli on one page. The subject is then instructed to look at the page, which includes "the 15 things that I showed you as well as 15 items that were not on the page," and circle the things they remember from the page they previously viewed. Scoring includes (a) recall correct, (b) recognition correct, (c) false-positive recognitions, and (d) a combination score computed as recall correct plus recognition correct minus false-positive recognitions (combined score).

Boone, Salazar, et al. (2000) evaluated the sensitivity and specificity of the Rey 15-Item Plus Recognition trial in four groups of subjects: (a) a litigating group with independent evidence of suspect effort, (b) a clinic patient group (nondemented mixed neurological and psychiatric patients), (c) learning-disabled college students, and (d) normal control subjects (mean age 61.3 years). These authors found the best combination of sensitivity and specificity for the combined (recall plus recognition minus false-positive) score, yielding a sensitivity of 71.4% and specificity of 91.7–93.9%. In addition, Boone et al. identified four false-positive errors never made by clinic or learning-disabled patients and rarely (by one subject) by the normal controls.

Of suspect effort cases, 14% made at least one of the false-positive recognition errors compared with 0.02% of the three groups of normal-effort subjects. Boone, Salazar, et al. (2002) noted that, although these four errors were not frequent in the suspect-effort group, they may serve as virtual pathognomonic signs of noncredible performance when present (i.e., the presence of these signs would have nearly 100% positive predictive value for noncredible performance).

The Boone, Salazar, et al. (2002) investigation showed that addition of a recognition trial to the 15-Item Test improved both sensitivity and specificity compared to the traditional version of the test as well as to the other recent modification of the test stimuli (Griffin et al., 1997). Indeed, Boone, Salazar, et al. noted that the combined score raised sensitivity by 50% relative to recall alone and maintained high specificity.

Additional procedures for evaluation of effort that are sufficiently simple so that nonlitigating clinical patients can perform adequately include Rey's Dot-Counting Test (Boone et al., 2002; Lezak et al., 2004; Rey, 1964; Youngjohn, Burrows, & Erdal, 1995), and the b Test (Boone et al., 2000). The Dot-Counting Test requires the subject to count dots presented on index cards as quickly as possible. Some of the dots are grouped, whereas others are not grouped. A person taking as long or longer to count grouped dots as they did to count ungrouped dots is displaying motivationally suspect performance (Lezak et al., 2004).

Vickery et al. (2001) included the Dot-Counting Test as one of the tasks in their meta-analysis of measures of effort. These authors found that the Dot-Counting Test was equivalent in mean effect size to the 15-Item Test in separating subjects showing poor effort from those demonstrating adequate effort. Both the Dot-Counting Test and Rey 15-Item Test yielded smaller effect sizes than the DMT (Hiscock & Hiscock, 1989), the PDRT (Binder & Willis, 1991), and the 21-Item Test (Iverson, Franzen, & McCracken, 1991). Sensitivity and specificity values could not be computed for the Dot-Counting Test by Vickery et al. because of inconsistencies in scoring procedures.

Subsequent to the Vickery et al. (2001) meta-analysis, Boone, Lu, et al. (2002) published Dot-Counting Test data on large samples of persons with suspect effort, as well as on a large sample of clinical subjects. Using cutting scores based on ungrouped counting time plus grouped counting time and number of errors, sensitivity was 100% in a criminal forensic sample and 75% in a civil litigation sample, with specificity of at least 90% in the clinical groups.

The b Test (Boone et al., 2000) requires subjects to circle all the lowercase b's in a 15-page booklet, discriminating the b's from the q's, p's, d's, and those lowercase letters with diagonal stems. Boone et al. (2000) compared the b Test performance of litigating subjects suspected of malingering to the performance of nonlitigating learning-disabled subjects; older depressed subjects; nonlitigating individuals with moderate and severe closed head injury (CHI), left or right hemisphere cerebrovascular accident, or schizophrenia; and normal elderly. A cutoff of greater than two commission errors produced a sensitivity of 76.5%, and specificity for all comparison groups combined was 82.6%.

Measures of Effort and Motivation Based on Forced-Choice Testing

The application of forced-choice methodology and the normal approximation to the binomial to evaluate effort and validity of test performance represents a major advance in the evaluation of malingering (Binder, 1990; Binder & Pankratz, 1987; Hiscock & Hiscock, 1989). In a forced-choice task (e.g., identifying whether one has been touched once or twice; identifying which of two 5-digit numbers was presented previously), it is conceivable that someone could perform at chance level, consistent with zero ability. If, however, someone performs significantly worse than chance, based on application of the normal approximation to the binomial theorem, the assumption can be made that they had to know the correct answer to perform at such an improbably poor level. At extreme levels of probability (e.g., .05 or .01), it can be argued that such an improbable performance is tantamount to admission of malingering (Larrabee, 2000).

The formula for the uncorrected z approximation to the binomial is

$$z = (X - NP)/\sqrt{NPQ}$$

where X is the patient's score correct, N is the number of test items, and P and Q are the expected proportions of right and wrong answers, respectively. In a two-alternative task, $P = Q = .5$; in a four-alternative task, $P = .25$, $Q = .75$. A one-tail test is the most appropriate given the suspected intent of producing suppressed scores (Larrabee, 1992). Some recommend a correction factor of 0.5 in the numerator when N is less than 25 (for x falling below NP, the 0.5 is added to x; for x falling above NP, the 0.5 is subtracted from x; Siegel, 1956).

Note that, because the formula for the normal approximation to the binomial is based on the standard normal (z) distribution, forced-choice tests can be constructed "on the spot" for a particular patient. Pankratz et al. (1975) constructed a subject-specific forced-choice test for evaluating feigned deafness, and Pankratz, Binder, and Wilcox (1987) did the same for evaluation of exaggerated somatosensory deficits. Denney (1996) demonstrated that three criminal defendants suspected of malingering remote memory impairment in the context of evaluation for competency to proceed to trial performed at significantly worse-than-chance level on correct identification of facts relevant to the alleged offenses, presented in two-alternative, forced-choice format.

A variety of SVTs utilizing the forced-choice format have been published. Many used presentation of individual sequences of digits to the subject, who after some period of time must then "recognize" the multidigit number in a two-alternative, forced-choice format: DMT (Guilmette, Hart, & Giuliano, 1993; Hiscock & Hiscock, 1989); PDRT (Binder, 1993; Binder & Kelly, 1996; Binder & Willis, 1991); Victoria Symptom Validity Test (Grote et al., 2000; Slick, Hopp, Strauss, & Spellacy, 1996); or Computerized Assessment of Response Bias (CARB; Conder, Allen, & Cox, 1992).

Other procedures use words as test stimuli, including the 21-Item Test, in which the subject is presented with a list of 21 items they must freely recall, followed by two-alternative, forced-choice testing (Iverson, Franzen, & Mc-Cracken, 1991, 1994). The Word Memory Test (WMT) requires the subject to learn a list of several word pairs presented over two trials, followed by immediate and then delayed forced-choice recognition of one word from each word pair, with additional yes/no recognition and paired associate, followed by free-recall trials (Green, Iverson, & Allen, 1999; Green, Rohling, Lees-Haley, & Allen, 2001; Iverson, Green, & Gervais, 1999; Green, Lees-Haley, & Allen, 2002).

There is also a visual memory malingering measure based on two-alternative, forced-choice recognition of easily encoded visual stimuli, the Test of Memory Malingering (TOMM; Rees, Tombaugh, Gansler, & Moczynski, 1998; Tombaugh, 1996). Berry and colleagues (Inman et al. 1998) have developed the Letter Memory Test, a procedure for evaluating effort based on recognition of arrays of three, four, and five consonants presented in forced-choice format involving either two, three, or four choices (note that each stimulus length is tested in two-, three-, or four-alternative format so that stimulus length is fully crossed with number of alternatives). Last, Frederick (1997) developed a forced-choice measure of nonverbal and verbal abilities, the Validity Indicator Profile (VIP; also see Frederick, Crosby, & Wynkoop, 2000; Frederick, Sarfaty, Johnston, & Powel, 1994).

The two-alternative, forced-choice memory analog tests (CARB, DMT, PDRT, 21-Item Test, TOMM, Victoria Symptom Validity Test, and WMT) can be scored for worse-than-chance performance using the normal approximation to the binomial. In addition, these procedures can be scored on the basis of empirically derived cutting scores that minimize false-positive identification in nonlitigating groups of clinical patients because it has been found that many litigants suspected of malingering do not perform at levels that are significantly worse than chance. Typically, these tasks are sufficiently easy that the majority of nonlitigating neurological patients can perform extremely well (e.g., for the Letter Memory Test and DMT, the average correct scores for nonlitigating neurological patients were 99.5% and 99.3% correct, respectively, contrasted with 54.8% and 64.4% correct, respectively, for normal community volunteers faking head injury; see Inman et al., 1998; for the TOMM, the majority of nonlitigating neurological and psychiatric patients scored above the cutoff of 90% correct, see Rees et al., 1998; Tombaugh, 1996).

For the VIP, Frederick developed a more elaborate performance curve analysis based on item difficulty. On the VIP, items are randomly presented as to item difficulty level. In scoring, item difficulty is taken into account so that persons are expected to do less well as the task becomes more difficult. Departures from this expectation, particularly reversal of errors with better performance on more difficult than on easier items, are associated with a motivated performance deficit.

Studies of the comparative sensitivity of SVTs are beginning to appear. Vickery et al. (2001) conducted a meta-analysis of the DMT, PDRT, 21-Item Test, 15-Item Test, and Dot-Counting Test. The DMT was the most sensitive, separating honest and dissimulating responders by approximately 2 SD, whereas the 21-Item Test and PDRT had effect sizes of approximately 1.5 SD and 1.25 SD, respectively. In contrast, effect sizes were equivalent, and the smallest, for the 15-Item and Dot-Counting Tests, approximately 0.75 SD.

Vickery et al. (2000) also conducted sensitivity and specificity analyses. Based on four studies, the DMT had a specificity of 95.1% and a sensitivity of 83.4%; the PDRT had a specificity of 97.3%, sensitivity of 44%, and combined hit rate of 71.2% based on two studies. The 15-Item Test had a specificity of 92.5%, sensitivity of 43.3%, and combined hit rate of 70.5% based on a range of six to eight studies. The 21-Item Test had a specificity of 100%, sensitivity of 22%, and combined hit rate of 60.7% based on four to six studies.

Vickery et al. (2000) noted that the sensitivity of the 21-Item Test could be improved by using a more liberal cutting score than that originally proposed by the 21-Item Test authors. Vickery et al.'s study was weighted more heavily with noninjured dissimulators than studies using a known-group design employing actual clinical malingerers, which may limit the generalizability of their findings. These authors recommended *against* the use of any one measure, in isolation, as a malingering screening device because of the less-than-perfect sensitivities of the tests they reviewed.

Subsequent to the review by Vickery et al. (2001), Bianchini, Mathias, Greve, Houston, and Crouch (2001) reported a higher sensitivity (77%) for the PDRT, with a specificity of 100% in a known-group design discriminating clinical malingerers from subjects with moderate and severe CHI. Inman and Berry (2002) found that the Letter Memory Test and DMT attained the highest hit rates for identification of malingering in college students with and without history of mild head injury who took the tests following instructions for good effort versus instructions to deliberately perform poorly. The DMT had a specificity of 100%, sensitivity of 64%, and overall hit rate of 82%; the Letter Memory Test had a specificity of 100%, sensitivity of 73%, and overall hit rate of 87% compared to the 21-Item Test and 15-Item Test, which had sensitivities of 2% and 5%, respectively, and a specificity of 100% each. The classification results for the DMT and Letter Memory Test were also superior to the use of malingering cutting scores or formulas for Reliable Digit Span (RDS; cf. Greiffenstein et al., 1994; 100% specificity, 27% sensitivity, 65% combined hit rate); Seashore Rhythm Test (Reitan & Wolfson, 1993) errors greater than 8 (Trueblood & Schmidt, 1993; 98% specificity, 27% sensitivity, 64% combined hit rate); Rey Auditory Verbal Learning Test (AVLT; Rey, 1964) Recognition less than 8 (Greiffenstein et al., 1994; 100% specificity, 16% sensitivity, 60% combined hit rate); Digit Symbol (Wechsler, 1981) scale score less than 5 (cf. Trueblood, 1994; 100% specificity, 2% sensitivity, 53% combined hit rate); and the Bernard, McGrath, and Houston (1996) Wisconsin Card Sorting Test (WCST; Heaton, Chelune, Talley, Kay, & Curtiss, 1993) discriminant function (100% specificity, 9% sensitivity, 58% overall hit rate).

ASSESSMENT OF MALINGERING USING ATYPICAL PERFORMANCE PATTERNS ON STANDARD NEUROPSYCHOLOGICAL TESTS

Detection of malingering through the presence of atypical performance patterns on standard neuropsychological tests is the basis of the performance inconsistency approach discussed in the section on the definition of malingering (Larrabee, 1990; 2000; Slick et al., 1999). Test patterns should make "neuropsychological sense" (Larrabee, 1990); hence, a patient with impaired attention should not have above average memory (Mittenberg et al., 1993); a patient with impaired Wechsler Adult Intelligence Scale, Third Edition (WAIS-III; Wechsler, 1997a) Digit Span at a level characteristic of dementia should not have above average WAIS-III Vocabulary (Mittenberg et al., 1995, 2001); a patient with very poor Grip Strength (Reitan & Wolfson, 1993) should not perform above average on the Grooved Pegboard (Lafayette Instrument, P.O. Box 5729, Lafayette, IN; Greiffenstein, Baker, & Gola, 1996).

Mittenberg, Aguila-Puentes, et al. (2002) referred to multiple variable pattern analysis as neuropsychological profiling of symptom exaggeration and malingering. The authors credited Heaton et al. (1978) with the first demonstration that patterns of neuropsychological test performance could discriminate 16 noninjured dissimulators from 16 nonlitigating patients with moderate-to-severe

CHI. Using the WAIS (Wechsler, 1955) and HRB, discriminant function analysis correctly classified 100% of the dissimulators and patients with CHI. Based on the MMPI (Hathaway & McKinley, 1983) alone, only one subject in each group was misidentified. Significant univariate differences were found on the WAIS Digit Span, and for HRB tests including Category Test errors, Tactual Performance Test Total Time, Memory and Location, Finger Tapping, Finger Agnosia, suppressions, and the Hand Dynamometer.

Mittenberg et al. (1996) replicated the Heaton et al. results with an HRB discriminant function contrasting noninjured dissimulating subjects from nonlitigating subjects with CHI (mild, moderate, and severe TBI). Significant univariate differences were found on Category Test errors, Tactual Performance Test Total Time, Speech Sounds Perception Errors and Seashore Rhythm Correct, Trails B, Finger Tapping, Sensory Suppressions, Finger Agnosia, and Finger Tip Number Writing.

Patterns of performance indicative of poor effort have also been reported on individual neuropsychological tests, such as poor recognition memory on the AVLT (Binder, Villanueva, Howieson, & Moore, 1993); poor recognition memory on the California Verbal Learning Test (CVLT; Delis, Kramer, Kaplan, & Ober, 1987; Millis, Putnam, Adams, & Ricker, 1995); and atypical error patterns on problem-solving tests such as the WCST (Bernard et al., 1996; Suhr & Boyer, 1999) and Category Test (Tenhula & Sweet, 1996).

I (2003a) found that scores on Benton Visual Form Discrimination (VFD; Benton, Sivan, Hamsher, Varney, & Spreen, 1994), Finger Tapping (FT), RDS, Wisconsin Card Sorting Failure-to-Maintain Set (FMS), and the Lees-Haley Fake Bad Scale (FBS; Lees-Haley, English, & Glenn, 1991) on the MMPI-2 were useful in discriminating litigants with definite or probable MND from patients with moderate/severe TBI and various neurological and psychiatric disorders. Table 4-1 presents the test data for litigants with MND and for Clinical Patients (TBI, depression, and various neurological conditions). These data, the aforementioned studies, and the discriminant function analyses of Mittenberg and colleagues (Mittenberg et al., 1993, 1995, 1996) suggested that standard test procedures particularly sensitive to poor effort are tests of sensorimotor function, attention, recognition memory, and problem solving.

Motivational Impairment on Motor Function Tests

Binder and Willis (1991) contrasted the neuropsychological test performance of 10 subjects with mild CHI with low motivation on the PDRT (15 or less of 36 on the "hard" items or 30 or less of 72 total items) with that of 19 subjects with mild CHI scoring 23 or higher on the "hard" PDRT. The poorly motivated subjects with mild CHI performed significantly lower than the normally motivated subjects with mild CHI on the Finger Tapping and Grooved Pegboard Tests.

TABLE 4-1. Performance of Litigants With Definite or Probable Malingered Neurocognitive Dysfunction and Clinical Patients on Neuropsychological Tests Sensitive to Malingering

TEST	MND[a]	CLINICAL PATIENTS[b]	p	EFFECT SIZE[c]
VFD[d]				
M	26.39	29.89	.0005	1.02
SD	(4.58)	(2.25)		
FT[e]				
M	69.27	83.85	.005	0.70
SD	(27.95)	(13.78)		
RDS[f]				
M	7.15	9.78	.0005	1.33
SD	(1.82)	(2.11)		
FMS[g]				
M	1.29	.56	.005	0.67
SD	(1.36)	(.84)		
FBS[h]				
M	26.95	16.48	.0005	1.99
SD	(5.36)	(5.22)		

[a]MND (malingered neurocognitive dysfunction) = 24 litigants with definite and 17 litigants with probable MND.
[b]Clinical patients = 27 moderate/severe traumatic brain injury, 14 psychiatric, and 13 mixed neurologic diagnosis.
[c]Effect size: in pooled standard deviation units.
[d]VFD, Benton Visual Form Discrimination.
[e]FT, Finger Tapping combined right- and left-hand raw scores.
[f]RDS, Reliable Digit Span.
[g]FMS, Wisconsin Card Sorting Test Failure-to-Maintain Set.
[h]FBS, MMPI-2 Lees-Haley Fake Bad Scale.

Greiffenstein et al. (1996) compared the Grip Strength, Finger Tapping Test, and Grooved Pegboard performance of 54 subjects with moderate-to-severe CHI who also had unambiguous motor abnormalities on standard neurological examination (note that dense hemiplegics were excluded) with the performance of 131 litigating patients with postconcussion syndrome (PCS) who performed on at least one motor function score poorer than T40 using the normative data of Heaton, Grant, and Matthews (1991). The subjects with moderate-to-severe CHI showed the expected pattern of performing best on Grip Strength and worst on the Grooved Pegboard Test, whereas the PCS subjects performed poorest on Grip Strength and better on Finger Tapping and the Grooved Pegboard. In particular, the most significant PCS/CHI differences were on Grip Strength. Although the PCS subjects had higher scores on MMPI Scales 1, 2, 3, and 7 than the subjects with moderate-to-severe CHI, consistent with heightened reports of depression, anxiety, and physical symptoms in the PCS group, these MMPI scales did not correlate with motor performance in the PCS group. The authors suggested that the low Grip Strength scores of their PCS litigants were consistent with malingering, but not necessarily proof of malingering.

Rapport, Farchione, Coleman, and Axelrod (1998) attempted a replication of the Greiffenstein et al. (1996) motor function results with Grip Strength, Finger Tapping, and the Grooved Pegboard. These authors, using naïve and coached noninjured college student dissimulators and noninjured college student controls, did not replicate the Greiffenstein et al. results. Although the dissimulators were provided with descriptions of effects of spinal cord injury and mild head injury, they were not specifically advised to perform poorly on the motor function tests. This may explain the differences between the Rapport et al. (1998) results and those of Greiffenstein et al., who used actual litigating patients chosen for presence of reduced motor function scores.

Finger Tapping scores are also available from the Heaton et al. (1978) and Mittenberg et al. (1996) studies contrasting noninjured dissimulators with nonlitigating patients with CHI. Despite 18 years of difference between these two investigations, conducted in Denver, Colorado (Heaton et al., 1978), and Ft. Lauderdale, Florida (Mittenberg et al., 1996), there is a striking similarity in dominant plus nondominant raw score: The Heaton et al. dissimulators averaged 63.1 taps, and the Mittenberg et al. dissimulators averaged 63.0 taps. Table 4-2 displays average Finger Tapping data for dissimulating and head-injured subjects in the Heaton et al. (1978) and Mittenberg et al. (1996) studies; the Rapport et al. (1998) dissimulators; a group of dissimulators from Orey, Cragar, and Berry's (2000) study; a group of subjects with MND from Binder and Willis's (1991) study; and my (2003a) subjects with definite MND and moderate-to-severe TBI. These data suggest that scores in the low 60s and below are indicative of malingered Finger Tapping performance. Indeed, I (2003a) found that a combined (right plus left) raw Finger Tapping score less than 63 was optimal in discriminating litigants with definite MND from patients who had moderate-to-severe TBI.

Digit Span and Malingering

Mittenberg et al. (1995) found that the simple difference score between Vocabulary and Digit Span age-scaled scores worked almost as well as a discriminant function analysis employing seven WAIS-R/WAIS-III subtests in discriminating noninjured dissimulators from nonlitigating patients with CHI. Mittenberg et al. (2001) replicated this result using the WAIS-III, subjects with CHI, noninjured dissimulators, and a group of litigants identified as probable malingerers by

TABLE 4-2. Combined (Dominant Plus Nondominant) Finger Tapping
Speed for Head-Injured, Simulating, and Malingering Subjects

| | SUBJECT GROUP | | |
STUDY	TRAUMATIC BRAIN INJURY	SIMULATORS[a]	MND[b]
Heaton et al. (1978)[c]			
M	80.2	63.1	—
SD	(21.4)	(17.1)	—
Mittenberg et al. (1996)[d]			
M	75.6	63.0	—
SD	(20.4)	(32.7)	—
Binder & Willis (1991)[e]			
M	—	—	71.89
SD	—	—	(16.5)
Rapport et al. (1998)[f]			
M	—	60.0	—
SD	—	(19.2)	—
Orey et al. (2000)[g]			
M	—	64.19	—
SD	—	(18.67)	—
Larrabee (2003b)[h]			
M	78.37	—	70.97
SD	(13.64)	—	(26.72)

[a]Simulators, noninjured persons simulating impairment.

[b]MND, malingered neurocognitive deficit.

[c]Heaton et al. = 16 simulators, 16 traumatic brain injury (TBI).

[d]Mittenberg et al. = 80 simulators, 80 TBI.

[e]Binder & Willis = 10 probable MND.

[f]Rapport et al. = 31 simulators.

[g]Orey et al. = 26 simulators.

[h]Larrabee = 27 TBI, 24 definite MND.

virtue of current functioning IQ more than 15 points below estimated premorbid level of function. Trueblood and Schmidt (1993) recommended consideration of malingering when the age-scaled score for Digit Span was less than 7.

Greiffenstein et al. (1994) developed a procedure for evaluating effort based on the WAIS/WAIS-R/WAIS-III Digit Span Subtest: Reliable Digit Span (RDS). This is computed by summing the longest string of digits repeated without error over two trials under both forward and backward conditions. As an example, Greiffenstein et al. noted that a patient who passed both trials of three digits forward and both trials of two digits backward, but failed one trial at four digits forward and one trial at three digits reversed, would have an RDS of 5. Greif-fenstein et al. reported a sensitivity of 70% and specificity of 73% for an RDS of 7 or less in discriminating probable malingerers from patients with TBI and a sensitivity of 68% and specificity of 89% for an RDS of 7 or less in discrimi-nating probable malingerers from subjects with persistent PCS.

Meyers and Volbrecht (1998) replicated the RDS findings of Greiffenstein et al. (1994). In a comparison of 47 litigants with mild brain injury and 49 nonliti-gants with mild brain injury, only 4.1% of nonlitigants had an RDS of 7 or less, contrasted with 48.9% of litigants. In my (Larrabee, 2003a) investigation, a RDS score of 7 or less correctly identified 50% of litigants with definite MND and 93.5% of persons with moderate and severe TBI.

Measures of Recognition Memory

Several investigators have reported disproportionate impairment in recognition memory in probable malingerers. Binder et al. (1993) found significantly lower Rey AVLT recognition scores in litigants with mild TBI failing the PDRT than in nonlitigating head-injured patients. Suhr, Tranel, Wefel, and Barrash (1997) also reported poorer AVLT recognition scores for probable malingerers in com-parison to patients with head injury, depression, or somatization disorder. Binder, Kelly, Villanueva, and Winslow (2003) found that litigating subjects with mild TBI with good motivation outperformed litigating subjects with mild TBI who had poor motivation on the recognition trial of the AVLT. The poorly motivated litigants with mild TBI were also outperformed on AVLT recognition by a group of normally motivated nonlitigating patients with moderate-to-severe TBI.

Millis et al. (1995) found that litigants with mild TBI with poor motivation produced lower scores on CVLT Recognition Hits and Discriminability than did patients who had moderate or severe TBI. Coleman, Rapport, Millis, Ricker, and Farchione (1998) replicated these findings with a normal subject simulation design, although the effect was attenuated when the subjects were provided with cues on how to elude detection as a malingerer. Published research has yet to appear on the utility of the yes/no recognition task on the revision of the CVLT, the CVLT-II. Of note, the CVLT-II contains an additional, optional forced-choice task following completion of all other CVLT-II trials (Delis, Kramer, Kaplan, & Ober, 2000).

Poor performance on recognition memory in association with poor motivation has also been reported for the Rey Complex Figure Test (Corwin & Bylsma, 1993; Osterrieth, 1944; Rey, 1941); Warrington Recognition Memory Test (Warrington, 1984), and recognition tasks/scores on the Wechsler Memory Scale III (WMS-III; Wechsler, 1997b). Meyers and Volbrecht (1999), using a differential prevalence design, found that litigants (primarily those with mild TBI) produced memory error patterns characterized by poor recognition performance on the Rey Complex Figure Test, in contrast to nonlitigating individuals with mild TBI, who did not show evidence of poor recognition. Lu, Boone, Cozolino, and Mitchell (2003) found that a combination score based on copy plus true positive minus atypical recognition errors discriminated suspect effort cases from a variety of clinical cases. Millis (1992, 1994) and Millis and Putnam (1994) have shown that litigating subjects with mild TBI performed more poorly on the Recognition Memory Test, more so on Words than on Faces, in comparison to nonlitigating subjects with moderate and severe TBI.

Recognition memory procedures on the WMS-III are also sensitive to detection of poor effort. Killgore and DellaPietra (2000) found that simulating malingerers performed more poorly on five WMS-III Logical Memory recognition memory items than did persons with moderate-to-severe TBI. Of note, the five WMS-III Logical Memory items were items that naïve, noninjured persons who had not ever heard the WMS-III stories were able to identify by guessing the correct response at a level significantly better than chance. Glassmire et al. (2003) found that poor performance on WMS-III Faces I was characteristic of noninjured persons trying to simulate impairment, as well as characteristic of participants with moderate and severe TBI attempting to dissimulate impairment. Finally, Langeluddecke and Lucas (2003) found that WMS-III delayed auditory recognition memory tasks successfully discriminated a group of litigating subjects with mild TBI with probable MND from a group of litigating individuals with mild TBI with good motivation as well as from a group of litigating individuals with severe TBI.

Measures of Problem-Solving Ability

Persons identified as malingering also performed poorly and in neurologically atypical patterns of performance on measures of problem solving such as the WCST (Heaton, Chelune, Talley, Kay, & Curtiss, 1993) and the Category Test of the HRB. Bernard et al. (1996) found that noninjured simulators produced poorer performance ratios on Categories relative to Perseverative Errors on the WCST in comparison to patients with TBI or other central nervous system disorders.

Suhr and Boyer (1999) found that student simulators as well as probable malingerers could be discriminated from nonlitigating subjects with mild and moderate TBI on the basis of WCST Categories and FMS, with a lower ratio of Categories to FMS in the malingering groups. I (Larrabee, 2003a) found that FMS alone worked more effectively than the Suhr and Boyer discriminant score based on Categories and FMS in discriminating litigants with definite MND from patients with moderate and severe TBI.

Greve and Bianchini (2002) found an unacceptably high false-positive rate for both the Bernard et al. (1996) and Suhr and Boyer (1999) WCST discriminant function equations in discriminating simulating normal college students from patients with TBI, various neurological conditions, and substance abuse. In another investigation, Greve et al. (2002) improved the sensitivity and specificity of WCST malingering indicators by combining multiple indicators (e.g., Bernard et al., 1996, criteria and Suhr & Boyer, 1999, criteria), including "unique" errors on the WCST as another variable sensitive to malingering. These authors also provided different cutoffs for the Bernard et al. (1996) and Suhr and Boyer (1999) functions that minimized false-positive errors in discriminating probable malingerers from patients with TBI with adequate motivation.

Last et al. (2002) found varying degrees of classification accuracy for the Bernard et al. (1996) and Suhr and Boyer (1999) WCST classification formulas, as well as for a logistic regression formula developed by King et al. that employed FMS, Categories Achieved, and Percent Conceptual Responses. Overall, these formulas worked well; however, King et al. found classification limitations in association with chronicity and severity of the reported TBI and advised against use of any single WCST insufficient effort criterion in isolation.

Indicators of insufficient effort suggestive of malingering have also been developed for the Category Test. Tenhula and Sweet (1996) performed a double cross-validation study contrasting normal subjects simulating impairment on the Category Test with performance on the Category Test of normal subjects performing optimally and with nonlitigating patients with severe TBI. A number of Category Test indicators showed good discrimination of the simulating malingerers from the normal and severe TBI groups, including Total Number of Errors, Items from Subtests I and II, "Bolter et al." items (Bolter, Picano, & Zych, 1985; items rarely missed by patients with bona fide brain damage), Number of Errors on Subtest VII, and Number of "Easy" items (items rarely missed by the group with severe TBI, similar to the Bolter et al. items). The best sensitivity (75.6%) and specificity (98.1%) were associated with number of errors on Subtests I and II.

In a replication study that also investigated the effects of coaching on feigned performance, DiCarlo, Gfeller, and Oliveri (2000) also found that the number of errors on Subtests I and II was consistently the most accurate malingering indicator regardless of degree of coaching or presence of TBI. Sweet and King (2002) provided further review of Category Test validity indicators with case examples and recommendations for use.

DETECTION OF SYMPTOM EXAGGERATION

Forensic neuropsychological evaluation entails both direct examination of the litigant/defendant, including interview, testing, and behavioral observation, as well as record review. These sources of information are then integrated by the forensic neuropsychologist. The direct part of the evaluation includes interviewing, testing of neuropsychological abilities, and quantification of symptom report through interview (including structured interview); use of symptom checklists; and use of formal self-report instruments such as the MMPI-2 (Butcher, Dahlstrom, Graham, Tellegen, & Kaemmer, 1989) or pain scales such as the McGill Pain Questionnaire (MPQ; Melzack, 1975). Obviously, a litigant/defendant can control both the degree of effort exerted on testing and the number and magnitude of reported symptoms. Consequently, the forensic examiner must be able to discriminate legitimate from exaggerated symptom report.

The most widely used symptom report scale in forensic neuropsychology is the MMPI/MMPI-2 (Lees-Haley, Smith, Williams, & Dunn, 1996). The MMPI and MMPI-2 have long played a role in assessment of malingered symptom report (Berry, Baer, & Harris, 1991; Graham, 2000; Greene, 2000; Rogers, Sewell, & Salekin, 1994). The prototypic MMPI scale for detection of malingering is the Infrequency or F scale, which was originally derived by selecting items endorsed by 10% or fewer of the normal adult sample (Graham, 2000). The MMPI-2 (Butcher et al., 1989) includes the F scale, as well as the Fb scale, developed for items occurring on the second half of the MMPI-2, again endorsed by 10% or fewer of the normal adult sample using the same methodology as that used to develop F. In addition, the MMPI-2 includes measures of response inconsistency, including the Variable Response Inconsistency scale (VRIN), a measure designed to detect response inconsistency as the reason for significant elevations at a T score of 100 or more on F or 90 or more on Fb. A second consistency score, True Response Inconsistency scale (TRIN), measures the tendency to respond either "True" or "False" in an indiscriminant manner. The MMPI/MMPI-2 also include measures such as the F-minus-K index, Obvious–Subtle difference scores, and Dissimulation-revised scales, which are sensitive to malingering of psychiatric disorder (Greene, 2000). Of all the scales, F is one of the most effective in discriminating valid from invalid psychiatric profiles (see Berry et al., 1991).

Following the publication of the MMPI-2, Arbisi and Ben-Porath (1995) developed the Infrequency-Psychopathology Scale, F(p), by selecting MMPI-2 items endorsed by 20% or fewer of hospitalized psychiatric patients as well as infrequently endorsed by 20% or fewer of MMPI-2 normal subjects. In a subsequent investigation, Arbisi and Ben-Porath (1998) found that F(p) outperformed F in distinguishing between psychiatric patients performing honestly and those attempting to fake bad.

Gass and Luis (2001) demonstrated that the sensitivity of F(p) to symptom exaggeration was reduced by the presence of four items from the L scale of the MMPI-2. These authors showed that these four items actually measured defensiveness, not exaggeration, and recommended removal of the items from the F(p). A shortened version of F(p) that omitted the four L scale items was found to be superior to the original F(p) as a measure of symptom exaggeration.

Despite demonstration of the sensitivity of F, Fb, F(p), F minus K, and other MMPI-2 scores such as the sum of Obvious-Subtle difference, and Dissimulation-revised scores to detection of exaggerated psychiatric symptomatology (Rogers et al., 1994), these MMPI-2 validity scales may not be sensitive to exaggeration of symptoms in personal injury settings for litigants pursuing neuropsychological claims. Indeed, Greiffenstein et al. (1995) found that F, total sum of Obvious-Subtle difference, and F minus K did *not* discriminate probable malingerers from subjects with TBI and from those with persistent PCS despite the presence of significant group differences on several measures of neuropsychological malingering, including the Rey 15-Item Test, Recognition Word List, AVLT Recognition score, RDS, and PDRT-27.

Lees-Haley and colleagues (Lees-Haley et al., 1991; Lees-Haley, 1992) recognized a different pattern of symptom reporting in personal injury litigants and developed a scale that would be sensitive to personal injury exaggeration, the FBS. The FBS was constructed on a rational content basis, taking into consideration unpublished frequency counts of malingerer's MMPI-2 test data and responses that fit a model of goal-directed behavior with a focus of (a) appearing honest; (b) appearing psychologically normal except for the influence of the alleged cause of injury; (c) avoiding admitting preexisting psychopathology; (d) attempting to minimize the impact of previously disclosed preexisting complaints; (e) minimizing or hiding preinjury antisocial or illegal behavior; and (f) presenting a degree of injury or disability within perceived limits of plausibility. The FBS contains 18 items scored in the "True" direction and 25 items scored in the "False" direction.

Greene (1997) presented data to show that the FBS did not correlate strongly with F (.14), Fb (.26), or F(p) (.08), in contrast to significant correlations between F, Fb, and F(p) that averaged .75 for normal subjects and patients with mental disorders. Most of the FBS items occurred on MMPI-2 Scales 1 and 3, with six on Scale 1, seven on Scale 3, and seven appearing on Scales 1 and 3. One FBS item appeared on L, one on K, four on F, four on Scale 2, two on Scale 4, four on Scale 6, three on Scale 7, six on Scale 8, and three on Scale 0 (note that there is some item overlap on more than one scale).

Lees-Haley et al. (1991), using an FBS cutoff of 20 or higher, found that 24 of 25 (96%) of personal injury claimants assessed as malingering emotional distress were correctly classified, with 18 of 20 (90%) claimants assessed as presenting genuine injuries correctly classified. Subsequently, Lees-Haley (1992) found sensitivity and specificity values of 75% and 96%, respectively, using an FBS cutoff of 24 or higher for males and 74% and 92%, respectively, for a cutoff of 26 or higher for females, for discriminating pseudo-posttraumatic stress disorder (PTSD) claimants from claimants with legitimate emotional distress.

I (Larrabee, 1998) found that 11 of 12 litigants with independent objective evidence of malingering on tasks such as the Rey 15-Item Test and PDRT produced elevated scores (>23 for males, >26 for females), whereas only 3 had elevated F scales (T > 69 for the MMPI, T > 64 for the MMPI-2), despite T scores on Scales 1 and 3 that exceeded scores for chronic pain samples (Keller & Butcher, 1991). In addition, the sample of probable malingerers produced scores on Scale 3 that exceeded those produced by noninjured persons simulating somatoform disorder on the MMPI-2 (Sivec, Lynn, & Garske, 1994).

In a subsequent investigation, I (Larrabee, 2003c) found that the FBS was significantly more sensitive to detection of symptom exaggeration than F, Fb, or F(p) in 33 litigants with definite or probable MND. Moreover, the MMPI-2 profiles of the definite/probable malingerers were characterized by significantly higher elevations on Scales 1, 3, and 7 than scores produced by a variety of clinical groups, including those with nonlitigating severe CHI, multiple sclerosis, spinal cord injury, chronic pain, and depression. The definite and probable malingerers also produced significantly higher elevations on Scales 2 and 8 than were produced by all clinical groups, with the exception of the depressed clinical patient group. I (Larrabee, 2003c) contrasted the neuropsychological malingering profile obtained, with elevations on the FBS and Scales 1, 2, 3, 7, and 8, with the Graham, Watts, and Timbrook (1991) profile for simulated psychiatric disturbance, which was characterized by significantly elevated F and significant elevations on Scales 6 and 8. These data were interpreted as showing at least two patterns of malingering on the MMPI-2: malingered injury and malingered severe psychiatric disturbance.

Miller and Donders (2001) found that litigating patients with mild TBI produced higher FBS scores than nonlitigating patients with mild TBI and were twice as likely to produce FBS scores that fell beyond 23 for males and 25 for females. The finding that both the litigating and nonlitigating individuals with mild TBI produced more significant elevations on the FBS than nonlitigating patients with moderate-to-severe TBI led Miller and Donders to recommend caution in using the FBS solely as an indicator of symptom exaggeration. The authors recommended that elevated FBS scores be interpreted as suggesting the likelihood that something other than acquired cerebral dysfunction was accounting for maintaining the patient's symptomatology. In this vein, they recommended that elevated FBS scores be supplemented with other data demonstrating invalid performance before concluding that a person is malingering.

Martens, Donders, and Millis (2001) replicated the Miller and Donders (2001) results, demonstrating higher FBS scores for litigating subjects with mild TBI in comparison to subjects with moderate or severe TBI. They also showed a significant association between the FBS and measures of invalid effort derived from the CVLT. Again, prior psychiatric history was associated with elevations on the FBS in subjects with mild TBI, including those who were not litigating, indicating that invalid response set alone was not the sole explanation of elevated FBS scores. Not a single patient with moderate or severe TBI produced invalid scores on both the FBS and CVLT, reinforcing the suggestion that use of multiple independent criteria to determine the presence of invalid response set improved diagnostic accuracy for malingering (Slick et al., 1999; Sweet, 1999).

Greiffenstein, Baker, Gola, Donders, and Miller (2002) compared groups of litigating patients with mild TBI with atypical symptom history/outcome, litigating individuals with moderate-to-severe TBI, and nonlitigating individuals with moderate-to-severe TBI. Setting specificity at 80% for the litigating individuals with moderate-to-severe TBI resulted in an FBS cutting score above 23 and identified 57% of atypical litigants with mild TBI, but only 4% of nonlitigating individuals with moderate-to-severe TBI.

Although Greiffenstein et al. (2002) could not exclude litigation status as a potential factor in FBS elevation in their litigating group with moderate-to-severe TBI, there was some evidence that FBS scores were related to neurological abnormalities in the litigating patients with moderate-to-severe TBI (e.g., the FBS correlated positively with the presence of anosmia and residual motor impairment). Of interest, the FBS correlated significantly with three measures of invalid neuropsychological test performance, including the PDRT-27, Rey 15-Item Test, and Rey's Word Recognition List, in the litigating subjects with atypical mild TBI, but the FBS did not correlate with these measures in the litigating group with moderate-to-severe TBI. The FBS also correlated significantly with a Symptom Improbability Rating Scale score within the litigating sample with atypical mild TBI.

Meyers, Millis, and Volkert (2002) developed a composite, weighted validity index for the MMPI-2 based on the T score for F, the raw F-minus-K difference, F(p), Dissimulation Scale–Revised, Es (Ego Stength), sum difference of Obvious and Subtle scores, and the FBS. These authors were able to discriminate litigating patients with chronic pain with cognitive complaints from nonlitigating patients with chronic pain with cognitive complaints using their weighted index. Moreover, the empirically derived cutoff score that had 100% specificity (i.e., identified none of the nonlitigating patients with chronic pain) identified 36% of the litigating patients with chronic pain and 86% of noninjured persons attempting to simulate chronic pain impairment. The FBS scores greater than 24 identified 42% of the litigating patients with chronic pain, whereas only 16% of the nonlitigants scored in this range. No nonlitigating patient with chronic pain scored over 29 on the FBS.

I (Larrabee, 2003b) found that the FBS was superior to F, Fb, F(p), Meyers's Weighted Validity Index, F minus K, Dissimulation Scale–Revised, Obvious-

Subtle difference, and Es in discriminating 26 litigants with definite MND (worse than chance on the PDRT) from 29 patients with moderate or severe TBI. In a combined sample of definite and probable MND plus the TBI subjects, the FBS was the only MMPI-2 validity scale that correlated significantly with the PDRT. The FBS also correlated significantly with all other MMPI-2 validity scales except for F(p) and F minus K, but correlated most strongly with Es and Meyers's Index. The FBS correlated significantly with MMPI-2 clinical scales 1, 2, 3, 6, 7, 8, and 0, with the strongest correlations occurring with 1, 2, 3, and 7.

An FBS cutting score above 20 or 21 provided optimal classification of the malingering and head-injured groups, with a sensitivity of .808 and specificity of .862. None of the subjects with moderate-to-severe TBI scored higher than 30 on the FBS, with only 3% (one subject) scoring higher than 25. I concluded that the data were consistent with the presence of different dimensions of exaggeration on the MMPI-2, extending the findings in my (Larrabee, 2003c) investigation. These data were seen as consistent with the demonstration by Lanyon (2001) of MMPI-2 dimensions of (a) exaggerated psychiatric symptoms and (b) exaggerated health concerns in a mixed forensic sample (child custody evaluees, personal injury litigants, and criminal defendants; note that a third dimension not relevant to the present discussion was also obtained: exaggeration of virtue).

Ross, Millis, Krukowski, Putnam, and Adams (2004) reported a sensitivity of .90 and specificity of .90 using an FBS cutoff of 21 or higher or 22 or higher to discriminate 59 probable malingerers from 59 nonlitigating patients with moderate and severe TBI. None of their nonlitigating subjects with moderate-to-severe TBI scored higher than 26 on the FBS (100% specificity).

In an investigation that included the subjects from my studies (Larrabee, 1998, 2003b, 2003c) as well as additional clinical and malingering subjects, the FBS was the single most sensitive measure for discriminating definite MND from moderate and severe TBI compared with other measures of motivational impairment derived from Benton VFD, FT, RDS, and Wisconsin Card Sorting FMS (Larrabee, 2003a). The FBS remained the most frequently failed validity indicator in a cross-validation discriminating litigants with probable MND from groups of nonlitigating psychiatric and neurological patients (also see Table 4-1).

The FBS has also been shown by others to be sensitive to the presence of symptom exaggeration in mixed personal injury samples. Posthuma and Harper (1998) found the FBS was elevated in a sample of personal injury litigants contrasted with FBS scores produced by a child custody litigant sample. Tshushima and Tshushima (2001) found that only the FBS significantly discriminated a sample of personal injury litigants from a sample of clinical patients, and the FBS also had the largest effect size contrasting the personal injury group with a group of job applicants undergoing employment screening.

The sensitivity and specificity of the FBS decline when investigated in psychiatric settings. Rogers, Sewell, and Ustad (1995) found that F, Fb, F minus K, and F(p) were superior to the FBS in correct identification of psychiatric outpatients taking the MMPI-2 under honest or simulated malingering conditions. In the honest condition, the FBS had a 21.1% false-positive rate, with only a 48.5% sensitivity in the malingered condition. Rogers et al. (1995) commented that their results did not necessarily demonstrate the invalidity of the FBS, which they observed may be more sensitive in context-specific (e.g., personal injury) or diagnosis-specific (e.g., PTSD) circumstances.

Two studies have appeared that are critical of the FBS as a measure of symptom exaggeration. Butcher, Arbisi, Atlis, and McNulty (2003) concluded that the FBS had an unacceptably high rate of false-positive identification in clinical groups, overidentified malingering in a personal injury sample, and showed poor internal consistency. Butcher et al. studied six subject samples; four samples were obtained from the National Computer Systems (NCS) database (profiles sent in by clinicians for NCS scoring/interpretation), including psychiatric inpatients, individuals in a correctional facility, general medical patients, and those with chronic pain. Another sample was from a large tertiary care Veterans Affairs medical center, with a sixth sample that included personal injury litigants.

Butcher et al. (2003) did not report the percentage of subjects involved in compensation or litigation actions in the psychiatric, chronic pain, general medical, or Veterans Affairs samples and did not report the context in which the MMPI-2s were conducted in the correctional facility (e.g., competency to proceed to trial, criminal responsibility, consideration for early release). Moreover, Butcher et al. did not report results on measures of exaggeration and symptom validity that were independent of the MMPI-2 for their correctional facility or personal injury samples. Hence, specificity values based on true false positives cannot be computed; sensitivity values, absent independent assessment of malingering in the correctional facility and personal injury samples, also cannot be computed. At best, elevated scores in the personal injury sample can serve as base rate indications of the frequency of malingering, assuming the FBS is a valid indicator of symptom exaggeration. Considered in this light, the rates of exaggeration of 24.1% for males (FBS > 23) and 37.9% for females (FBS > 25) reported by Butcher et al. (2003) are well within previously reported base rates of malingering in neuropsychological personal injury evaluations (59%, Greiffenstein et al., 1994; 42%, Grote et al., 2000; 49%, Meyers & Volbrecht, 1998).

The Butcher et al. (2003) article actually contained data supporting the construct validity of the FBS. These authors performed a content analysis identifying five groups of items: (a) somatic symptoms, (b) sleep disturbance, (c) tension or stress, (d) low energy/anhedonia, and (e) denial of deviant attitudes or behaviors. Although Butcher et al. criticized the FBS as having poor internal consistency, the median Cronbach α of .62 for all six subject samples is quite similar to the Cronbach α of .64 for males and .63 for females for the F scale reported in the MMPI-2 manual (Table D-7, p. 97; Butcher et al., 1989). Of particular interest, the Cronbach α was .85 for the personal injury sample, showing that the five content areas of the FBS identified by Butcher et al. are *highly* interrelated in personal injury litigants compared to lower values in patients with chronic pain (.47) and general medical patients (.58). Last, Butcher et al., in their Table 4, showed that the FBS correlated most strongly with MMPI-2 Scales 1, 2, 3, 7, and 8, which are the MMPI-2 scales most likely to be elevated in personal injury probable malingerers (Boone & Lu, 1999; Larrabee, 1998, 2003b, 2003c; Ross et al., 2004).

Bury and Bagby (2002) compared the MMPI-2 validity scales of a sample of patients diagnosed with PTSD to samples of university students completing the MMPI-2 under standard instructions and under four conditions of exaggeration: (a) faking PTSD; (b) coached on PTSD symptoms only; (c) coached on MMPI-2 validity scales only; and (d) coached on both PTSD symptoms as well as MMPI-2 validity scales. These authors found that the family of F scales, particularly Fb and F(p), consistently produced the highest overall classification rates and relatively stable estimates of positive and negative predictive power (NPP) across the different malingering conditions. In contrast, the authors found that the FBS was ineffective and failed to produce significant group differences between the PTSD claimants and the research participants in each of the fake PTSD conditions.

The Bury and Bagby (2002) article suffers, however, from a "fatal" research design error: 100% of their clinical PTSD sample was seeking continuation or reinstatement of compensation from the Workplace Safety and Insurance Board of Toronto, Ontario, Canada. In addition, Bury and Bagby did not assess their clinical sample for evidence of symptom exaggeration/test performance invalidity on measures that were independent of the MMPI-2. This is a critical design error that invalidates their conclusions. Indeed, Bury and Bagby stated:

In the context of these incentives, symptom exaggeration is expected, and the comparatively low classification rates may be a result of the presence of individuals in the workplace PTSD comparison sample who were actually exaggerating or malingering their condition. (pp. 482–483)

The authors (Bury and Bagby, 2002) went on to state that there was evidence in their clinical PTSD sample that some of the claimants were likely exaggerating their symptoms. Hence, the FBS may well have been a poor discriminator of the clinical PTSD sample because a sizable proportion of the sample was malingering. This interpretation is supported by review of Table 1 on page 476 of the Bury and Bagby article, which shows a mean FBS of 26.31 for their clinical PTSD sample, a value that is well within the range of mean FBS scores produced by analogue malingerers and suspected malingerers (Lees-Haley, Iverson, Lange, Fox, & Allen, 2002; see Table 4-3).

TABLE 4-3. Lees-Haley Fake Bad Scale Endorsement by Clinical Patients, Simulators, and Malingerers

	SUBJECT GROUP		
STUDY	CLINICAL PATIENTS	SIMULATORS	MALINGERERS
Lees-Haley et al. (1991)[a]			
M	15.7	25.0	27.6
SD	(4.11)	(8.5)	(4.65)
Lees-Haley (1992)[b]			
M	18.2	—	27.2
SD	(5.3)	—	(5.2)
Larrabee (2003b)[c]			
M	15.67	—	26.15
SD	(6.02)	—	(5.41)
Ross et al. (2004)[d]			
M	14.61	—	28.61
SD	(4.65)	—	(5.12)

[a]Lees-Haley et al.: 25 clinical subjects with emotional distress following personal injury; 67 noninjured subjects simulating emotional reaction to injury; 25 subjects malingering after personal injury.

[b]Lees-Haley: 64 clinical subjects with emotional distress following injury; 55 subjects with malingering posttraumatic stress disorder.

[c]Larrabee: 29 clinical patients with moderate/severe traumatic brain injury (TBI); 26 litigants with definite malingered neurocognitive dysfunction.

[d]Ross et al.: 59 subjects with moderate/severe TBI, and 59 litigants with probable malingered neurocognitive dysfunction.

Greiffenstein, Baker, Peck, Axelrod, and Gervais (in press) found that the FBS had good sensitivity, specificity, and positive predictive power (PPP) in discriminating 48 nonlitigating patients suffering psychological trauma following events such as completed rape or serious injury (mutilation/traumatic amputation) from 57 litigants with atypical symptom report seeking compensation for psychological damages following relatively minor events (e.g., minor frights not meeting *DSM-IV* "gatekeeper" criteria for major trauma). In contrast, the F family (F, Fp, and F minus K) showed poor discriminant utility. Logistic regression yielded optimal FBS cutting scores of 21 for males and 26 for females. FBS scores greater than 30 for females and greater than 29 for males were associated with 100% positive predictive power for detection of implausible psychological trauma claims.

In summary, there appear to be at least two types of malingering detected by the MMPI-2. In the first, scores are elevated on F and the F scale derivatives, including Fb, F(p), F minus K, with extreme elevations on clinical Scales 6 and

8 (Graham, 2000; Greene, 2000). This pattern is consistent with exaggeration of severe psychopathology and likely occurs with greater frequency in settings in which suffering psychosis may mitigate external consequences such as conviction of crimes or compulsory military service.

The second type of malingering detected by the MMPI-2 is exaggeration of symptoms in the context of personal injury litigation in general and litigation for neuropsychological claims specifically. This is characterized by elevations on the FBS, as well as elevations on Scales 1, 2, 3, 7, and 8. Optimal cutting scores for personal injury litigants claiming neuropsychological impairments are in the low 20s (21 or higher, Ross et al., 2004; 22 or higher, Larrabee, 2003b). As with any cutting scores, there is always the risk of false-positive identification. False positive scores greater than 30 are highly unlikely as no scores fell in this range based on data collected on 236 clinical patients, including those with psychological trauma ($n = 48$, Greiffenstein et al., in press); moderate or severe TBI ($n = 29$, Larrabee, 2003b; $n = 59$, Ross et al., 2004); and chronic pain ($n = 100$, Meyers et al., 2002).

Last, as with any measure of exaggeration or performance invalidity, diagnostic certainty increases with the presence of abnormal scores on other independent indicators (Larrabee, 2003b; Martens et al., 2001; Slick et al., 1999; Sweet, 1999). Per the work of Donders and colleagues (Martens et al., 2001; Miller & Donders, 2001), preexisting psychiatric history can be a mitigating factor in nonlitigating individuals with mild TBI, and per Greiffenstein et al. (2002), presence of anosmia or residual motor impairment can be a mitigating factor in evaluating the FBS scores of litigating patients with moderate and severe TBI.

ADDITIONAL DIAGNOSTIC CONSIDERATIONS

The diagnosis of malingering in the individual case, using the Slick et al. (1999) criteria, involves relying on psychometric measures of response bias. These measures are associated with various degrees of sensitivity (to the true presence of response bias) and specificity (accurate detection of the absence of response bias). The diagnostic accuracy of response bias procedures in the individual case also depends on the base rate or frequency of malingering in the forensic population. Given information on sensitivity, specificity, and base rate, one can compute for individual measures of response bias the PPP, or probability that someone with a positive score is truly malingering, and NPP, or probability that someone with a negative score truly is not malingering (Baldessarini, Finklestein, & Arana, 1983; chapter 1, this volume).

Two articles provide converging support for a 40% prevalence of malingering in litigating claimants with mild TBI. Mittenberg, Patton, Canyock, and Condit (2002) surveyed members of the American Board of Clinical Neuropsychology who did forensic work and in personal injury litigants with mild TBI found base rates of malingering of 38.5% unadjusted for referral source, increasing slightly to 41.24% when adjusted for referral source. Additional information obtained in this survey showed that the board certified respondents typically employed several sources of information similar to the Slick et al. (1999) criteria for probable MND, strengthening the likely accuracy of the base rate obtained by Mittenberg, Patton, et al.

The base rate figures obtained by Mittenberg, Patton, et al. for litigants with mild TBI are quite close to the base rate of malingering in mild TBI as I reported (Larrabee, 2003a) based on my review of 11 studies (Binder & Kelly, 1996; Frederick et al., 1994; Greiffenstein et al., 1994; Grote et al., 2000; Heaton et al., 1978; Meyers & Volbrecht, 1998; Millis, 1992; Millis et al., 1995; Rohling, Green, Allen, & Iverson, 2002; Trueblood & Schmidt, 1993; Youngjohn et al., 1995), which identified 548/1,363 persons (40%) who showed motivated performance deficit suggestive of malingering. Of additional interest, Mittenberg, Patton, et al. (2002) also provided adjusted base rates of malingering for several other alleged conditions, including 38.61% for fibromyalgia (FM) or chronic fatigue, 33.51% for pain or somatoform disorders, 29.49% for neurotoxic disorders, and 25.63% for electrical injury.

The Mittenberg, Patton, et al. (2002) and my (Larrabee, 2003a) base rates for malingering of 40% for litigants with mild TBI and Mittenberg, Patton, et al.'s malingering base rate of 33.51% for pain or somatoform disorders are quite consistent with the results of the Carroll, Abrahamse, and Vaiana (1995) investigation of the costs of excess medical claims for automobile personal injuries. Carroll et al. analyzed "soft" (i.e., sprain/strain) and "hard" (i.e., fractures) injury claims as a function of compensation system per state (e.g., tort system, dollar no-fault, and verbal no-fault) and found that 35–42% of all medical costs submitted in support of auto injury claims were excessive.

The review of SVTs published by Vickery et al. (2001), covering data obtained on the DMT, PDRT, Rey 15-Item Test, 21-Item Test, and Dot-Counting Test, showed an average sensitivity of 56.0%, average specificity of 95.7%, and average hit rate of 76.8%. These data showed findings characteristic of most tests of malingering: The specificity is set at a high value to minimize the occurrence of false-positive errors, that is, misidentifying someone as a malingerer who is not truly malingering. The consequence of setting specificity high is that sensitivity is low; that is, using the Vickery et al. (2001) data, on average 44% of persons who truly are malingering go undetected.

Computation of PPP and NPP, using the average sensitivity and specificity values reported by Vickery et al. (2001) and malingering base rate of 40%, yields a PPP of .897 (proportion of true positives to true positives plus false positives) and an NPP of .765 (proportion of true negatives to true negatives plus false negatives). These data show that the probability of truly identifying malingering when test scores exceed the cutoff is higher than the probability of correctly detecting the absence of malingering. Consequently, negative findings on SVTs are poor at ruling out the presence of malingering; in contrast, greater confidence can be afforded positive findings on SVTs (Bianchini, Mathias, & Greve, 2001; Faust & Ackley, 1998; Slick et al., 1999). Thus, a clinician doing a forensic assessment does not merely tally the number of passes and failures on SVTs and conclude malingering or absence of malingering based on which outcome has the greatest number of tallies.

Actually, using multiple criteria for assessment of malingering is supported on a statistical basis, both for improving sensitivity and for keeping constant or increasing specificity (Iverson & Franzen, 1996; Larrabee, 2003a; Martens et al., 2001; Orey et al., 2000; Vickery et al., 2004). An example of this, using a known-group design, is one of my studies (Larrabee, 2003a). This investigation derived cutoff scores on five tests for discriminating litigants with definite MND from patients who had moderate or severe TBI: Benton VFD, FT, RDS, WCST FMS, and the Lees-Haley FBS from the MMPI-2. The sensitivity and specificity, respectively, of the individual tests at specific cutting scores were .48 and .931 for VFD, .40 and .935 for FT, .50 and .935 for RDS, .48 and .871 for FMS, and .808 and .862 for FBS. Evaluating all possible pairwise combinations of scores exceeding cutoff (e.g., FT and RDS; FMS and FBS; etc.) resulted in a sensitivity of .875 and specificity of .889. Evaluating all possible three-way combinations reduced sensitivity to .542 (still higher than the individual sensitivities for VFD, FT, RDS, and FMS), but resulted in 100% specificity (i.e., no false-positive scores), a value better than that achieved by any individual test.

Vickery et al. (2004) reported similar results in a simulation design in which noninjured persons and persons with moderate-to-severe TBI completed testing under conditions of standard as well as malingering instructions. Sensitivity dropped as a function of the number of scores falling in the range of motivational impairment increased, whereas specificity increased as a function of the number of motivationally impaired scores. Perfect specificity was achieved at three or more test failures, the same result I reported (Larrabee, 2003a). Subjects with three or more test failures had 100% PPP for malingering regardless of the base rate. Persons with two or more test failures had PPP of .952 and NPP of .808 at a malingering base rate of 40% in the Vickery et al. investigation. These values, obtained with a simulation design, can be compared to the PPP of .913 and NPP of .921 I reported (Larrabee, 2003a) in a known-group design for discriminating definite and probable MND from moderate-to-severe TBI, psychiatric, and neurological patients, employing two or more test failures at a malingering base rate of 40%.

My finding of improved sensitivity and constant or improved specificity (Larrabee, 2003a) by aggregating scores across multiple measures of malingering is understood as a function of the rarity of test scores exceeding malingering cutoffs for truly impaired patients in combination with regression to the mean. My

(Larrabee, 2003a) investigation included 27 subjects with moderate or severe TBI, 13 nonlitigating patients with various disorders affecting the central nervous system, and 14 patients with psychiatric disorders, primarily major depressive disorder, yielding a total of 54 clinical patients.

The performance of these 54 patients on VFD, FT, RDS, FMS, and FBS was analyzed for this chapter to determine mean performance and standard deviations for this mixed clinical sample. Then, z scores were determined, relative to the clinical sample, for scores on the five malingering indicators beyond the empirical cutoffs for malingering. The average z score for these cutoffs, collapsed across all five malingering indicators, was 1.57 SD beyond the clinical group mean (showing an average false-positive rate per test of 5.8%). The average intercorrelation (using Fisher's z transformation) of the five malingering indicators was .175. Thus, based on regression to the mean and the average z score associated with the malingering cutoffs, the predicted value of performance on any given test given a performance at a z score of 1.57 on another malingering indicator was (.175)(1.57) or a z score of .274, a value substantially *below* the average z score of 1.57 associated with performance invalidity. Thus, although a clinical patient may on rare occasion (5.8%) obtain a score beyond the cutoff for malingering on any one of the five malingering indicators I identified (Larrabee, 2003b), it is not likely that *two* scores will exceed the cutoff.

Boone and Lu (2003) made a similar point related to the probability of multiple scores exceeding cutoff for malingering in nonmalingering clinical patients. They observed that specificity is typically set at .90 to keep false-positive identification at a minimum. Assuming the tests are not strongly correlated (see the above discussion), Boone and Lu noted that the overall false-positive rate for six "failed" effort measures could be as low as 1 in 1 million (.1 × .1 × .1 × .1 × .1 × .1). Applying this reasoning to the Slick et al. (1999) criteria for probable response bias, the probability of a false-positive score for two tests exceeding cutoff for malingering, each with a specificity of .90 with no correlation between the two tests in a nonlitigating clinical sample, is (.1 × .1) or .01. Boone and Lu (2003) conclude that rather than inflating (false positive) error, administering several independent and well-validated effort techniques serves to substantially increase diagnostic accuracy.

My (Larrabee, 2003a) investigation also provided further support for the validity of the probable MND diagnostic category proposed by Slick et al. (1999). I derived the cutting scores by contrasting the performance of litigants with definite MND (worse-than-chance performance on the PDRT) with that of patients who had moderate-to-severe TBI. I also conducted a cross-validation of the malingering algorithm with a sample of litigants meeting the Slick et al. (1999) criteria for probable MND, contrasted with groups of nonlitigants with psychiatric or mixed neurological diagnoses. Of particular interest was the *absence* of significant differences on the five malingering indicators (VFD, FT,

RDS, FMS, and FBS) in a comparison of the probable MND subjects with the definite MND subjects, despite significant group differences on the PDRT. These data suggested that the diagnostic certainty associated with a conclusion of probable MND is essentially the same as that associated with the presence of definite MND.

The above line of reasoning can be extended to scores beyond cutoffs on individual tests associated with 100% specificity, that is, a performance exceeded by 100% of nonlitigating individuals with moderate and severe TBIs. If the cutoff score associated with 100% specificity is based on a large sample and particularly if the cutting score is cross-validated across different nonlitigating clinical samples, such scores have 100% PPP (i.e., 100% certainty of malingering because PPP is determined by dividing the true positive rate by the true positive rate plus a false positive rate of zero). Performance on tests/cut scores meeting the above conditions of 100% specificity are arguably equivalent, in terms of diagnostic certainty, to worse-than-chance performance.

FUTURE DIRECTIONS

The 1990s characterized a veritable explosion in research on malingering, culminating with the publication of the Slick et al. (1999) criteria for malingered neurocognitive dysfunction. The area of identification of poor effort on specialized tests of malingering (e.g., PDRT, CARB, WMT, TOMM) and identification of atypical performance patterns on standard clinical tests (e.g., Mittenberg's work on the WAIS-R/III, WMS-R, HRB) is better defined than the area of assessment of exaggerated symptom report, particularly in the area of personal injury litigation.

It is particularly noteworthy that there is very little research on malingering of chronic pain, despite the near total reliance on self-report instruments for assessment of chronic pain. Indeed, Turk and Melzack (2001) did not review malingering in the second edition of their *Handbook of Pain Assessment*. This is particularly important given Mittenberg et al.'s (2002) results showing a base rate of malingering of 38.61% for FM/chronic fatigue and 33.51% for pain/somatoform disorders, values consistent with Meyers et al.'s (2002) data that yielded a base rate for malingering of 36% determined from scores produced on their MMPI-2 weighted validity index by a large sample of litigating chronic pain patients.

Gervais et al. (2001) found that 30% of patients with FM receiving disability failed either the CARB or WMT, with the failure rate increasing to 44% in patients with FM seeking disability. These values were contrasted with CARB/WMT failure rates of 0% in rheumatoid arthritis and 4% in patients with FM not receiving disability.

I (Larrabee, 2003d) compared the pain scale endorsement of 29 litigants with definite or probable MND who also complained of pain and had FBS scores of at least 22 to published data on patients with chronic pain for the MPQ (Melzack, 1975; Mikail, Dubreuil, & D'Eon, 1993); Pain Disability Index (Tait, Chibnall, & Krause, 1990); and Modified Somatic Perception Questionnaire (MSPQ; Main, 1983). At a specificity of .90 (i.e., a score only achieved by fewer than 10% of patients with chronic pain, from samples that were not characterized by compensation-seeking versus noncompensation seeking status or screened for malingering), the sensitivities were .21 for the MPQ, .59 for the Pain Disability Index, and .90 for the MSPQ. In particular, the MSPQ showed high sensitivity at high specificities (sensitivity values were .86 and .69, respectively, at specificities of .95 and .99).

Modifications to the Slick et al. (1999) criteria for probable MND can be considered. My findings (Larrabee, 2003a) and those of Vickery et al. (2004) that multiple indicators of response bias more accurately discriminate malingerers from clinical patients suggest modification of the Slick et al. (1999) criteria for evidence from neuropsychological testing. Presently, the neuropsychological testing criterion cannot be met if an examinee only has multiple indicators of probable response bias, and does not show other Slick et al. (1999) test indicators such as *discrepancy between test data and known patterns of brain functioning*, *discrepancy between test data and observed behavior*, *discrepancy between test data and reliable collateral report*, or *discrepancy between test data and documented background history*. My data (Larrabee, 2003a) and those of Vickery et al. (2004) suggest that two or more indicators of probable response bias alone should meet the neuropsychological test evidence requirement for probable malingering.

Similarly, self-report and evidence of symptom exaggeration should play a larger role in the Slick et al. (1999) criteria. Presently, an examinee can meet the examination criterion for probable MND with two indicators from neuropsychological testing, or one indicator from neuropsychological testing and one from self-report, but multiple indicators from self-report can only provide evidence for possible MND. This creates an asymmetry in the examination criteria for test evidence and self-report evidence. Consequently, my recommendation that multiple indicators of probable response bias should be sufficient for a diagnosis of probable MND can be extended to consideration of multiple measures of symptom exaggeration, such as those on the MMPI-2, Structured Interview of Reported Symptoms (Rogers, Bagby, & Dickens, 1992), and indicators of exaggerated chronic pain as sufficient for diagnosis of probable MND.

Diagnostic statistics allow consideration of modification of the Slick et al. (1999) criteria for definite MND. Replicated studies defining cutting scores associated with 100% PPP yield information that could be viewed as consistent with the presence of definite MND. Because it is conceivable that the universe of nonmalingering patients can never be completely exhausted, and to minimize diagnostic error, the finding of two scores at values associated with zero false positives could be viewed as consistent with definite MND. Moreover, should my (Larrabee, 2003b) and Vickery et al.'s findings of 100% PPP associated with three or more scores exceeding cutoff be replicated, this finding also can be considered representative of definite MND. Applying the reasoning of Boone and Lu (2003), the probability of three or more scores over cutoff at a per-test false-positive rate of .10 for scores that are essentially independent in nonmalingering samples is ($.1 \times .1 \times .1$) or .001. At a per-test false-positive rate of .06 or less (Larrabee, 2003a; Vickery et al., 2001), this compound probability becomes ($.06 \times .06 \times .06$) or .0002.

Another area that has seen limited research is the area of subtypes of malingering. The majority of specialized tests of malingering follow memory paradigms (e.g., PDRT, CARB, WMT, TOMM), with the exception of the VIP. Yet, research investigations contrasting simulating or known groups of malingerers to patients with moderate or severe TBI showed atypical performance on measures of perception, motor function, attention, and problem solving (Greiffenstein et al., 1996; Heaton et al., 1978; Larrabee, 2003a; Mittenberg et al., 1993, 1995, 1996). I have identified subtypes of malingering through cluster analysis that showed specific impairment on (a) memory, perception, and motor function; (b) symptom exaggeration; (c) motor function and symptom exaggeration; (d) problem solving; and (e) perception and problem solving (Larrabee, 2004a). These data highlight the need for additional measures of malingering of motor dysfunction, impaired perception, and abnormal problem solving. I also identified, through cluster analysis, two basic types of MMPI-2 profiles present in a large sample of personal injury litigants with MND: subtype variations on a somatoform exaggeration profile (characterizing the majority, 88%, of profiles) and a subtype profile showing exaggeration of severe psychopathology (Larrabee, 2004b).

Since Slick et al.'s (1999) observation that almost no research exists on the coexistence of legitimate neuropsychological dysfunction with poor effort or malingering, cases have started to appear in the literature (Bianchini, Greve, & Love, 2003; Boone & Lu, 2003). Slick et al. noted that one of the most pressing questions is whether it is possible to tease apart legitimate from exaggerated impairment when both may be present.

I have encountered a case, referred by the attorneys for the defense, in which the plaintiff suffered a severe CHI (admission Glasgow Coma Scale of 3, with 1 month to follow commands and 3 months of posttraumatic amnesia). On direct evaluation, the plaintiff failed the Rey 15-Item Test with a Recognition score of 5, PDRT-27 correct total of 48%, and a Lees-Haley FBS of 28. On earlier testing with another examiner, the plaintiff performed poorly on the "Easy" items of the Category Test and had an RDS score of 7. These poor scores on measures of effort and malingering precluded confident interpretation of the plaintiff's very poor performance across a variety of tasks. He did appear to have a potentially valid pattern of motor impairment, with performance declining from Grip Strength to FT, to the Purdue and Grooved Pegboards (cf. Greif-fenstein et al., 1996). Because of his poor effort, other conclusions had to be based on base rate expectations. Per the results of Dikmen et al. (1994) regarding employment following TBI, it was pointed out that only 8% of patients with TBI who had time-to-follow commands of 29 days or more had returned to work within 2 years, making it unlikely that the plaintiff was going to return to gainful employment.

Thus, when poor effort and brain dysfunction coexist, it is possible to reach conclusions based on published outcome data in patient groups sharing similar injury severity characteristics (see Dikmen, Machamer, Winn, & Temkin, 1995; Dikmen et al., 1994; Rohling, Meyers, & Millis, 2003). Similarly, in the presence of evidence for poor effort, scores in the low end of the normal range should be given greater weight because these low normal scores themselves may well represent an underestimate of actual ability. Perhaps another approach to evaluating the presence of legitimate deficit co-occurring with poor motivation, can be derived from future research on subtypes of malingering, such that patterns of various cognitive performances that are valid can be discriminated from invalid patterns of performance (i.e., legitimate memory impairment accompanied by malingered motor function). Bianchini et al. (2003) provide additional discussion of these issues.

ACKNOWLEDGMENT

I acknowledge the assistance of Bridgette O'Brien in the preparation of this chapter.

REFERENCES

American Psychiatric Association. (1994). *Diagnostic and statistical manual of mental disorders* (4th ed.). Washington, DC: Author.

Arbisi, P. A., & Ben-Porath, Y. S. (1995). An MMPI-2 infrequent response scale for use with psychopathological populations: The Infrequency Psychopathology Scale, F(p). *Psychological Assessment, 7*, 424–431.

Arbisi, P. A., & Ben-Porath, Y. S. (1998). The ability of Minnesota Multiphasic Personality Inventory-2 validity scales to detect fake-bad responses in psychiatric inpatients. *Psychological Assessment, 10*, 221–228.

Baldessarini, R. J., Finklestein, S., & Arana, G. W. (1983). The predictive power of diagnostic tests and the effects of prevalence of disease. *Archives of General Psychiatry, 40*, 569–573.

Benton, A. L., Sivan, A. B., Hamsher, K. deS., Varney, N. R., & Spreen, O. (1994).

Contributions to neuropsychological assessment: A clinical manual (2nd ed.). New York: Oxford University Press.

Bernard, L. C., McGrath, M. J., & Houston, W. (1996). The differential effects of simulating malingering, closed head injury, and other CNS pathology on the Wisconsin Card Sorting Test: Support for the "pattern of performance" hypothesis. *Archives of Clinical Neuropsychology, 11,* 231–245.

Berry, D. T. R., Baer, R., & Harris, M. (1991). Detection of malingering on the MMPI: A meta-analysis. *Clinical Psychology Review, 11,* 19–45.

Berry, D. T. R., Wetter, M. W., Baer, R. A., Youngjohn, J. R., Gass, C. S., Lamb, D. G., et al. (1995). Over reporting of closed head injury symptoms on the MMPI-2. *Psychological Assessment, 7,* 517–523.

Bianchini, K. J., Greve, K. W., & Love, J. M. (2003). Definite malingered neurocognitive dysfunction in moderate/severe traumatic brain injury. *The Clinical Neuropsychologist, 17,* 574–580.

Bianchini, K. J., Mathias, C. W., & Greve, K. W. (2001). Symptom validity testing: A critical review. *The Clinical Neuropsychologist, 15,* 19–45.

Bianchini, K. J., Mathias, C. W., Greve, K. W., Houston, R. J., & Crouch, J. A. (2001). Classification accuracy of the Portland Digit Recognition Test in traumatic brain injury. *The Clinical Neuropsychologist, 15,* 461–470.

Binder, L. M. (1990). Malingering following minor head trauma. *The Clinical Neuropsychologist, 4,* 25–36.

Binder, L. M. (1993). Assessment of malingering after mild head trauma with the Portland Digit Recognition Test. *Journal of Clinical and Experimental Neuropsychology, 15,* 170–182.

Binder, L. M., & Kelly, M. P. (1996). Portland Digit Recognition Test performance by brain dysfunction patients without financial incentives. *Assessment, 3,* 403–409.

Binder, L. M., Kelly, M. P., Villanueva, M. R., & Winslow, M. M. (2003). Motivation and neuropsychological test performance following mild head injury. *Journal of Clinical and Experimental Neuropsychology, 25,* 420–430.

Binder, L. M., & Pankratz, L. (1987). Neuropsychological evidence of a factitious memory complaint. *Journal of Clinical and Experimental Neuropsychology, 9,* 167–171.

Binder, L. M., & Rohling, M. L. (1996). Money matters: A meta-analytic review of the effects of financial incentives on recovery after closed-head injury. *American Journal of Psychiatry, 153,* 7–10.

Binder, L. M., Villanueva, M. R., Howieson, D., & Moore, R. T. (1993). The Rey AVLT recognition memory task measures motivational impairment after mild head trauma. *Archives of Clinical Neuropsychology, 8,* 137–147.

Binder, L. M., & Willis, S. C. (1991). Assessment of motivation after financially compensable minor head trauma. *Psychological Assessment: A Journal of Consulting and Clinical Psychology, 3,* 175–181.

Bolter, J. F., Picano, J. J., & Zych, K. (1985, October). *Item error frequencies on the Halstead Category Test: An index of performance validity.* Paper presented at the annual meeting of the National Academy of Neuropsychology, Philadelphia, PA.

Boone, K. B., & Lu, P. H. (1999). Impact of somatoform symptomatology on credibility of cognitive performance. *The Clinical Neuropsychologist, 13,* 414–419.

Boone, K. B., & Lu, P. H. (2003). Noncredible cognitive performance in the context of severe brain injury. *The Clinical Neuropsychologist, 17,* 244–254.

Boone, K. B., Lu, P. H., Back, C., King, C., Lee, A., Philpott, L., et al. (2002). Sensitivity and specificity of the Rey Dot Counting Test in patients with suspect effort and various clinical samples. *Archives of Clinical Neuropsychology, 17,* 625–642.

Boone, K. B., Lu, P., Sherman, D., Palmer, B., Back, C., Shamieh, E., et al. (2000). Validation of a new technique to detect malingering of cognitive symptoms: The b Test. *Archives of Clinical Neuropsychology, 15,* 227–241.

Boone, K. B., Salazar, X., Lu, P., Warner-Chacon, K., & Razani, J. (2002). The Rey 15-Item Recognition Trial: A technique to enhance sensitivity of the Rey 15-Item Memorization Test. *Journal of Clinical and Experimental Neuropsychology, 24,* 561–573.

Bury, A. S., & Bagby, R. M. (2002). The detection of feigned uncoached and coached posttraumatic stress disorder with the MMPI-2 in a sample of workplace accident victims. *Psychological Assessment, 14,* 472–484.

Butcher, J. N., Arbisi, P. A., Atlis, M. M., & McNulty, J. L. (2003). The construct validity of the Lees-Haley Fake Bad Scale. Does this scale measure somatic malingering and feigned emotional distress? *Archives of Clinical Neuropsychology, 18,* 473–485.

Butcher, J. N., Dahlstrom, W. G., Graham, J. R., Tellegen, A., & Kaemmer, B. (1989). *Minnesota Multiphasic Personality Inventory (MMPI-2).* Minneapolis: University of Minnesota Press.

Carroll, S., Abrahamse, A., & Vaiana, M. (1995). *The costs of excess medical claims for automobile personal injuries.* Santa Monica, CA: RAND.

Coleman, R. D, Rapport, L. J., Millis, S. R., Ricker, J. H., & Farchione, T. J. (1998). Effects of coaching on detection of malingering on the California Verbal Learning Test. *Journal of Clinical and Experimental Neuropsychology, 20,* 201–210.

Conder, R., Allen, L., and Cox, D. (1992). *Computerized Assessment of Response Bias Test manual.* Durham, NC: Cognisyst.

Corwin, J., & Bylsma, F. W. (1993). Translations and commentary on excerpts from Andre' Rey's *Psychological examination of traumatic encephalopathy* and P. A. Osterrieth's *The Complex Figure Copy Test. The Clinical Neuropsychologist, 7,* 3–21.

Delis, D. C., Kramer, J. H., Kaplan, E., & Ober, B. A. (1987). *California Verbal Learning Test: Adult version.* San Antonio, TX: Psychological Corp.

Delis, D. C., Kramer, J. H., Kaplan, E., & Ober, B. A. (2000). *CVLT-II. California Verbal Learning Test* (2nd ed., adult version). San Antonio, TX: Psychological Corp.

Denney, R. L. (1996). Symptom validity testing of remote memory in a criminal forensic setting. *Archives of Clinical Neuropsychology, 11,* 589–603.

DiCarlo, M. A., Gfeller, J. D., & Oliveri, M. V. (2000). Effects of coaching on detecting feigned cognitive impairment with the Category Test. *Archives of Clinical Neuropsychology, 15,* 399–413.

Dikmen, S. S., Machamer, J. E., Winn, H. R., & Temkin, N. R. (1995). Neuropsychological outcome at 1-year post head injury. *Neuropsychology, 9,* 80–90.

Dikmen, S. S., Temkin, N. R., Machamer, J. E., Holubkov, A. L., Fraser, R. T., & Winn, H. R. (1994). Employment following traumatic head injuries. *Archives of Neurology, 51,* 177–186.

Faust, D., & Ackley, M. A. (1998). Did you think it was going to be easy? Some methodological suggestions for the investigation and development of malingering detection techniques. In C. R. Reynolds (Ed.), *Detection of malingering during head injury litigation* (pp. 1–54). New York: Plenum Press.

Frederick, R. I. (1997). *Validity Indicator Profile manual.* Minnetonka, MN: NCS Assessments.

Frederick, R. I., Crosby, R. D., & Wynkoop, T. F. (2000). Performance curve classification of invalid responding on the Validity Indicator Profile. *Archives of Clinical Neuropsychology, 15,* 281–300.

Frederick, R. I., Sarfaty, S. D., Johnston, J. D., & Powel, J. (1994). Validation of a detector of response bias on a forced-choice test of nonverbal ability. *Neuropsychology*, *8*, 118–125.

Gass, C. S., & Luis, C. A. (2001). MMPI-2 scale F(p) and symptom feigning: Scale refinement. *Assessment*, *8*, 425–429.

Gervais, R. O., Russell, A. S., Green, P., Allen, L. M., Ferrari, R., & Pieschl, S. D. (2001). Effort testing in patients with fibromyalgia and disability incentives. *The Journal of Rheumatology*, *28*, 1892–1899.

Glassmire, D. M., Bierley, R. A., Wisniewski, A. M., Greene, R. L., Kennedy, J. E., & Date, E. (2003). Using the WMS-III Faces subtest to detect malingered memory impairment. *Journal of Clinical and Experimental Neuropsychology*, *25*, 465–481.

Graham, J. R. (2000). *MMPI-2. Assessing personality and psychopathology* (3rd ed.). New York: Oxford University Press.

Graham, J. R., Watts, D., & Timbrook, R. E. (1991). Detecting fake-good and fake-bad MMPI-2 profiles. *Journal of Personality Assessment*, *57*, 264–277.

Green, P., Iverson, G. L., & Allen, L. M. (1999). Detecting malingering in head injury litigation with the Word Memory Test. *Brain Injury*, *13*, 813–819.

Green, P., Lees-Haley, P. R., & Allen, L. M. (2002). The Word Memory Test and the validity of neuropsychological test scores. *Journal of Forensic Neuropsychology*, *2*, 97–124.

Green, P., Rohling, M. L., Lees-Haley, P. R., & Allen, L. M. (2001). Effort has a greater effect on test scores than severe brain injury in compensation claimants. *Brain Injury*, *15*, 1045–1060.

Greene, R. L. (1997). Assessment of malingering and defensiveness by multiscale inventories. In R. Rogers (Ed.), *Clinical assessment of malingering and deception* (2nd ed.) (pp. 169–207). New York: Guilford Press.

Greene, R. L. (2000). *The MMPI-2. An interpretive manual* (2nd ed.). Boston: Allyn and Bacon.

Greiffenstein, M. F., Baker, W. J., & Gola, T. (1994). Validation of malingered amnesia measures with a large clinical sample. *Psychological Assessment*, *6*, 218–224.

Greiffenstein, M. F., Baker, W. J., & Gola, T. (1996). Motor dysfunction profiles in traumatic brain injury and post-concussion syndrome. *Journal of the International Neuropsychological Society*, *2*, 477–485.

Greiffenstein, M. F., Baker, W. J., Gola, T., Donders, J., & Miller, L. (2002). The Fake Bad Scale in atypical and severe closed head injury. *Journal of Clinical Psychology*, *58*, 1591–1600.

Greiffenstein, M. F., Baker, W. J., Peck, E., Axelrod, B., & Gervais, R. (in press). The Fake Bad Scale and MMPI-2 F-Family in detection of implausible trauma claims. *The Clinical Neuropsychologist*.

Greiffenstein, M. F., Gola, T., & Baker, W. J. (1995). MMPI-2 validity scales versus domain specific measures in detection of factitious traumatic brain injury. *The Clinical Neuropsychologist*, *9*, 230–240.

Greve, K. W., & Bianchini, K. J. (2002). Using the Wisconsin Card Sorting Test to detect malingering: An analysis of the specificity of two methods in nonmalingering normal and patient samples. *Journal of Clinical and Experimental Neuropsychology*, *24*, 48–54.

Greve, K. W., Bianchini, K. J., Mathias, C. W., Houston, R. J., & Crouch, J. A. (2002). Detecting malingered performance with the Wisconsin Card Sorting Test: A preliminary investigation in traumatic brain injury. *The Clinical Neuropsychologist*, *16*, 179–191.

Griffin, G. A. E., Glassmire, D. M., Henderson, E. A., & McCann, C. (1997). Rey II: Redesigning the Rey Screening Test of Malingering. *Journal of Clinical Psychology, 53*, 757–766.

Grote, C. L., Kooker, E. K., Garron, D. C., Nyenhuis, D. L., Smith, C. A., & Mattingly, M. L. (2000). Performance of compensation seeking and non-compensation seeking samples on the Victoria Symptom Validity Test: Cross-validation and extension of a standardization study. *Journal of Clinical and Experimental Neuropsychology, 23*, 709–719.

Guilmette, T., Hart, K., & Giuliano, A. (1993). Malingering detection: The use of a forced-choice method in identifying organic versus simulated memory impairment. *The Clinical Neuropsychologist, 7*, 59–69.

Hathaway, S. R., & McKinley, J. C. (1983). *Minnesota Multiphasic Personality Inventory manual.* New York: Psychological Corp.

Heaton, R. K., Chelune, G. J., Talley, J. L., Kay, G. G., & Curtiss, G. (1993). *Wisconsin Card Sorting Test manual.* Odessa, FL: Psychological Assessment Resources.

Heaton, R. K., Grant, I., & Matthews, C. G. (1991). *Comprehensive norms for an expanded Halstead-Reitan Battery: Demographic corrections, research findings, and clinical applications.* Odessa, FL: Psychological Assessment Resources.

Heaton, R. K., Smith, H. H., Jr., Lehman, R. A., & Vogt, A. J. (1978). Prospects for faking believable deficits on neuropsychological testing. *Journal of Consulting and Clinical Psychology, 46*, 892–900.

Hiscock, M., & Hiscock, C. K. (1989). Refining the forced-choice method for the detection of malingering. *Journal of Clinical and Experimental Neuropsychology, 11*, 967–974.

Hom, J., & Denney, R. L. (Eds.). (2002a). Detection of response bias in forensic neuropsychology. Part I. *Journal of Forensic Neuropsychology, 2*, 1–166.

Hom, J., & Denney, R. L. (Eds.). (2002b). Detection of response bias in forensic neuropsychology. Part II. *Journal of Forensic Neuropsychology, 3*, 167–314.

Inman, T. H., & Berry, D. T. R. (2002). Cross-validation of indicators of malingering. A comparison of nine neuropsychological tests, four tests of malingering, and behavioral observations. *Archives of Clinical Neuropsychology, 17*, 1–23.

Inman, T. H., Vickery, C. D., Berry, D. T. R., Lamb, D. G., Edwards, C. L., & Smith, G. T. (1998). Development and initial validation of a new procedure for evaluating adequacy of effort given during neuropsychological testing: The Letter Memory Test. *Psychological Assessment, 10*, 128–139.

Iverson, G. L., & Binder, L. M. (2000). Detecting exaggeration and malingering in neuropsychological assessment. *Journal of Head Trauma Rehabilitation, 15*, 829–858.

Iverson, G. L., & Franzen, M. D. (1996). Using multiple objective memory procedures to detect simulated malingering. *Journal of Clinical and Experimental Neuropsychology, 18*, 38–51.

Iverson, G. L., Franzen, M. D., & McCracken, L. M. (1991). Evaluation of an objective assessment technique for the detection of malingered memory deficits. *Law and Human Behavior, 15*, 667–676.

Iverson, G. L., Franzen, M. D., & McCracken, L. M. (1994). Application of a forced-choice memory procedure designed to detect experimental malingering. *Archives of Clinical Neuropsychology, 9*, 437–450.

Iverson, G. L., Green, P., & Gervais, R. (1999, March/April). Using the Word Memory Test to detect biased responding in head injury litigation. *The Journal of Cognitive Rehabilitation*, 2–6.

Keller, L. S., & Butcher, J. N. (1991). *Assessment of chronic pain patients with the MMPI-2*. Minneapolis: University of Minnesota Press.

Killgore, W. D. S., & DellaPietra, L. (2000). Using the WMS-III to detect malingering: Empirical validation of the Rarely Missed Index (RMI). *Journal of Clinical and Experimental Neuropsychology, 22,* 761–771.

King, J. H., Sweet, J. J., Sherer, M., Curtiss, G., & Vanderploeg, R. D. (2002). Validity indicators within the Wisconsin Card Sorting Test: Application of new and previously researched multivariate procedures in multiple traumatic brain injury samples. *The Clinical Neuropsychologist, 16,* 506–523.

Langeluddecke, P. M., & Lucas, S. K. (2003). Quantitative measures of memory malingering on the Wechsler Memory Scale–Third Edition in mild head injury litigants. *Archives of Clinical Neuropsychology, 18,* 181–197.

Lanyon, R. I. (2001). Dimensions of self-serving misrepresentation in forensic assessment. *Journal of Personality Assessment, 76,* 169–179.

Larrabee, G. J. (1990). Cautions in the use of neuropsychological evaluation in legal settings. *Neuropsychology, 4,* 239–247.

Larrabee, G. J. (1992). On modifying recognition memory tests for detection of malingering. *Neuropsychology, 6,* 23–27.

Larrabee, G. J. (1998). Somatic malingering on the MMPI and MMPI-2 in litigating subjects. *The Clinical Neuropsychologist, 12,* 179–188.

Larrabee, G. J. (2000). Forensic neuropsychological assessment. In R. D. Vanderploeg (Ed.), *Clinician's guide to neuropsychological assessment* (2nd ed., pp. 301–335). Mahwah, NJ: Lawrence Erlbaum.

Larrabee, G. J. (2003a). Detection of malingering using atypical performance patterns on standard neuropsychological tests. *The Clinical Neuropsychologist, 17,* 410–425.

Larrabee, G. J. (2003b). Detection of symptom exaggeration with the MMPI-2 in litigants with malingered neurocognitive dysfunction. *The Clinical Neuropsychologist, 17,* 54–68.

Larrabee, G. J. (2003c). Exaggerated MMPI-2 symptom report in personal injury litigants with malingered neurocognitive deficit. *Archives of Clinical Neuropsychology, 18,* 673–686.

Larrabee, G. J. (2003d). Exaggerated pain report in litigants with malingered neurocognitive dysfunction. *The Clinical Neuropsychologist, 17,* 395–401.

Larrabee, G. J. (2004a, February). *Identification of subtypes of malingered neurocognitive dysfunction.* Paper presented at the annual meeting of the International Neuropsychological Society, Baltimore, MD.

Larrabee, G. J. (2004b, February). *Subtypes of MMPI-2 profiles in litigants with malingered neurocognitive dysfunction.* Paper presented at the annual meeting of the International Neuropsychological Society, Baltimore, MD.

Lee, G., Loring, D., & Martin, R. (1992). Rey's 15-Item Visual Memory Test for the detection of malingering: Normative observations on patients with neurological disorders. *Psychological Assessment, 4,* 43–46.

Lees-Haley, P. R. (1992). Efficacy of MMPI-2 validity scales and MCMI-II modifier scales for detecting spurious PTSD claims: F, F-K, Fake Bad Scale, Ego Strength, Subtle-Obvious Subscales, Dis, and DEB. *Journal of Clinical Psychology, 48,* 681–688.

Lees-Haley, P. R., English, L. T., & Glenn, W. J. (1991). A Fake Bad Scale for the MMPI-2 for personal injury claimants. *Psychological Reports, 68,* 203–210.

Lees-Haley, P. R., Iverson, G. L., Lange, R. T., Fox, D. D., and Allen, L. M. (2002).

Malingering in forensic neuropsychology: *Daubert* and the MMPI-2. *Journal of Forensic Neuropsychology, 3,* 167–203.

Lees-Haley, P. R., Smith, H. H., Williams, C. W., & Dunn, J. T. (1996). Forensic neuropsychological test usage: An empirical survey. *Archives of Clinical Neuropsychology, 11,* 45–51.

Lezak, M. D., Howieson, D. B., & Loring, D. W. (2004). *Neuropsychological assessment* (4th ed.). New York: Oxford University Press.

Lu, P. H., Boone, K. B., Cozolino, L., & Mitchell, C. (2003). Effectiveness of the Rey-Osterrieth Complex Figure Test and the Meyers and Meyers Recognition Memory Trial in the detection of suspect effort. *The Clinical Neuropsychologist, 17,* 426–440.

Main, C. J. (1983). The Modified Somatic Perception Questionnaire (MSPQ). *Journal of Psychosomatic Research, 27,* 503–514.

Martens, M., Donders, J., & Millis, S. R. (2001). Evaluation of invalid response sets after traumatic head injury. *Journal of Forensic Neuropsychology, 2,* 1–18.

Melzack, R. (1975). The McGill Pain Questionnaire: Major properties and scoring methods. *Pain, 30,* 191–197.

Meyers, J. E., Millis, S. R., & Volkert, K. (2002). A validity index for the MMPI-2. *Archives of Clinical Neuropsychology, 17,* 157–169.

Meyers, J. E., & Volbrecht, M. (1998). Validation of reliable digits for detection of malingering. *Assessment, 5,* 303–307.

Meyers, J. E., & Volbrecht, M. (1999). Detection of malingerers using the Rey Complex Figure and recognition trial. *Applied Neuropsychology, 6,* 201–207.

Mikail, S. F., Dubreuil, S., & D'Eon, J. L. (1993). A comparative analysis of measures used in the assessment of chronic pain patients. *Psychological Assessment, 5,* 117–120.

Miller, L. J., & Donders, J. (2001). Subjective symptomatology after traumatic head injury. *Brain Injury, 15,* 297–304.

Millis, S. R. (1992). The Recognition Memory Test in the detection of malingered and exaggerated memory deficits. *The Clinical Neuropsychologist, 6,* 406–414.

Millis, S. R. (1994). Assessment of motivation and memory with the Recognition Memory Test after financially compensable mild head injury. *Journal of Clinical Psychology, 50,* 601–605.

Millis, S. R., & Putnam, S. H. (1994). The Recognition Memory Test in the assessment of memory impairment after financially compensable mild head injury: A replication. *Perceptual and Motor Skills, 70,* 384–386.

Millis, S. R., Putnam, S. H., Adams, K. M., & Ricker, J. H. (1995). The California Verbal Learning Test in the detection of incomplete effort in neuropsychological evaluation. *Psychological Assessment, 7,* 463–471.

Mittenberg, W., Aguila-Puentes, G., Patton, C., Canyock, E. M., & Heilbronner, R. L. (2002). Neuropsychological profiling of symptom exaggeration and malingering. *Journal of Forensic Neuropsychology, 3,* 227–240.

Mittenberg, W., Azrin, R., Millsaps, C., & Heilbronner, R. (1993). Identification of malingered head injury on the Wechsler Memory Scale-Revised. *Psychological Assessment, 5,* 34–40.

Mittenberg, W., Patton, C., Canyock, E. M., & Condit, D. C. (2002). Baserates of malingering and symptom exaggeration. *Journal of Clinical and Experimental Neuropsychology, 24,* 1094–1102.

Mittenberg, W., Rotholc, A., Russell, E., & Heilbronner, R. (1996). Identification of malingered head injury on the Halstead-Reitan Battery. *Archives of Clinical Neuropsychology, 11,* 271–281.

Mittenberg, W., Theroux, S., Aguila-Puentes, G., Bianchini, K., Greve, K., & Rayls, K. (2001). Identification of malingered head injury on the Wechsler Adult Intelligence Scale–3rd Edition. *The Clinical Neuropsychologist, 15*, 440–445.

Mittenberg, W., Theroux, S., Zielinski, R. E., & Heilbronner, R. L. (1995). Identification of malingered head injury on the Wechsler Adult Intelligence Scale–Revised. *Professional Psychology: Research and Practice, 26*, 491–498.

Orey, S. A., Cragar, D. E., & Berry, D. T. R. (2000). The effects of two motivational manipulations on the neuropsychological performance of mildly head-injured college students. *Archives of Clinical Neuropsychology, 15*, 335–348.

Osterrieth, P. A. (1944). Le test de copie d'une figure complexe. *Archives de Psychologie, 30*, 206–356.

Pankratz, L., & Binder, L. M. (1997). Malingering on intellectual and neuropsychological measures. In R. Rogers (Ed.) *Clinical assessment of malingering and deception* (2nd ed., pp. 223–236). New York: Guilford Press.

Pankratz, L., Binder, L. M., & Wilcox, L. (1987). Evaluation of an exaggerated somatosensory deficit with symptom validity testing. *Archives of Neurology, 44*, 798.

Pankratz, L., Fausti, S. A., & Peed, S. A. (1975). A forced choice technique to evaluate deafness in a hysterical or malingering patient. *Journal of Consulting and Clinical Psychology, 43*, 421–422.

Posthuma, A. B., and Harper, J. F. (1998). Comparison of MMPI-2 responses of child custody and personal injury litigants. *Professional Psychology: Research and Practice, 29*, 417–443.

Rapport, L. J., Farchione, T. J., Coleman, R. D., & Axelrod, B. N. (1998). Effects of coaching on malingered motor function profiles. *Journal of Clinical and Experimental Neuropsychology, 20*, 89–97.

Rees, L. M., Tombaugh, T. N., Gansler, D., & Moczynski, N. (1998). Five validation experiments of the Test of Memory Malingering (TOMM). *Psychological Assessment, 10*, 10–20.

Reitan, R. M., & Wolfson, D. (1993). *The Halstead-Reitan Neuropsychological Test Battery: Theory and clinical interpretation* (2nd ed.). South Tucson, AZ: Neuropsychology Press.

Rey, A. (1941). L'examen psychologique dans le cas d'encephalopathie traumatique. *Archives de Psychologie, 28*, 286–340.

Rey, A. (1964). *L'examen clinique en psychologie* [The clinical examination in psychology]. Paris: Presses Universitaires de France.

Rogers, R. (1990a). Development of a new classificatory model of malingering. *Bulletin of the American Academy of Psychiatry and Law, 18*, 323–333.

Rogers, R. (1990b). Models of feigned mental illness. *Professional Psychology: Research and Practice, 21*, 182–188.

Rogers, R. (1997a). Introduction. In R. Rogers (Ed.), *Clinical assessment of malingering and deception* (2nd ed., pp. 1–19). New York: Guilford Press.

Rogers, R. (1997b). Researching dissimulation. In R. Rogers (Ed.), *Clinical assessment of malingering and deception* (2nd ed., pp. 398–426). New York: Guilford Press.

Rogers, R., Bagby, R. M., & Dickens, S. E. (1992). *Structured Interview of Reported Symptoms* (*SIRS*) *and professional manual*. Odessa, FL: Psychological Assessment Resources.

Rogers, R., Sewell, K. W., & Salekin, R. T. (1994). A meta-analysis of malingering on the MMPI-2. A systematic examination of fake-bad indicators. *Assessment, 1*, 227–237.

Rogers, R., Sewell, K. W., & Ustad, K. L. (1995). Feigning among chronic outpatients on the MMPI-2: A systematic analysis of fake-bad indicators. *Assessment, 2*, 81–89.

Rohling, M. L., Binder, L. M., & Langhinrischen-Rohling, J. (1995). Money matters: A meta-analytic review of the association between financial compensation and the experience and treatment of chronic pain. *Health Psychology, 14*, 537–547.

Rohling, M. L., Green, P., Allen, L. M., & Iverson, G. L. (2002). Depressive symptoms and neurocognitive test scores in patients passing symptom validity tests. *Archives of Clinical Neuropsychology, 17*, 205–222.

Rohling, M. L., Meyers, J. E., & Millis, S. R. (2003). Neuropsychological impairment following traumatic brain injury: A dose–response analysis. *The Clinical Neuropsychologist, 17*, 289–302.

Ross, S. R., Millis, S. R., Krukowski, R. A., Putnam, S. H., & Adams, K. M. (2004). Detecting probable malingering on the MMPI-2: An examination of the Fake-Bad Scale in mild head injury. *Journal of Clinical and Experimental Neuropsychology, 26*, 115–124.

Schretlen, D., Brandt, J., Krafft, L., & Van Gorp, W. (1991). Some caveats in using the Rey 15-Item Memory Test to detect malingered amnesia. *Psychological Assessment, 3*, 667–672.

Siegel, S. (1956). *Nonparametric statistics for the behavioral sciences*. New York: McGraw-Hill.

Sivec, H. J., Lynn, S. J., & Garske, J. P. (1994). The effect of somatoform disorder and paranoid psychotic role-related dissimulations as a response set on the MMPI-2. *Assessment, 1*, 69–81.

Slick, D. J., Hopp, G., Strauss, E., & Spellacy, F. (1996). Victoria Symptom Validity Test: Efficiency for detecting feigned memory impairment and relationship to neuropsychological tests and MMPI-2 validity scales. *Journal of Clinical and Experimental Neuropsychology, 18*, 911–922.

Slick, D. J., Sherman, E. M. S., & Iverson, G. L. (1999). Diagnostic criteria for malingered neurocognitive dysfunction: Proposed standards for clinical practice and research. *The Clinical Neuropsychologist, 13*, 545–561.

Suhr, J. A., & Boyer, D. (1999). Use of the Wisconsin Card Sorting Test in the detection of malingering in student simulator and patient samples. *Journal of Clinical and Experimental Neuropsychology, 21*, 701–708.

Suhr, J., Tranel, D., Wefel, J., & Barrash, J. (1997). Memory performance after head injury: Contributions of malingering, litigation status, psychological factors, and medication use. *Journal of Clinical and Experimental Neuropsychology, 19*, 500–514.

Sweet, J. J. (1999). Malingering: Differential diagnosis. In J. J. Sweet (Ed.), *Forensic neuropsychology* (pp. 255–285). Lisse, The Netherlands: Swets and Zeitlinger.

Sweet, J. J., and King, J. H. (2002). Category Test validity indicators: Overview and practice recommendations. *Journal of Forensic Neuropsychology, 3*, 241–274.

Tait, R. C., Chibnall, J. T., & Krause, S. (1990). The Pain Disability Index: Psychometric properties. *Pain, 40*, 171–182.

Tenhula, W. N., & Sweet, J. J. (1996). Double cross-validation of the Booklet Category Test in detecting malingered traumatic brain injury. *The Clinical Neuropsychologist, 10*, 104–116.

Tombaugh, T. N. (1996). *TOMM. Test of memory malingering*. North Tonawanda, NY: Multi-Health Systems.

Trueblood, W. (1994). Qualitative and quantitative characteristics of malingered and other invalid WAIS-R and clinical memory data. *Journal of Clinical and Experimental Neuropsychology, 16,* 597–607.

Trueblood, W., & Schmidt, M. (1993). Malingering and other validity considerations in the neuropsychological evaluation of mild head injury. *Journal of Clinical and Experimental Neuropsychology, 15,* 578–590.

Tsushima, W. T., & Tsushima, V. G. (2001). Comparison of the Fake Bad Scale and other MMPI-2 validity scales with personal injury litigants. *Assessment, 8,* 205–212.

Turk, D. C., & Melzack, R. (Eds.). (2001). *Handbook of pain assessment* (2nd ed.). New York: Guilford Press.

Vickery, C. D., Berry, D. T. R., Dearth, C. S., Vagnini, V. L., Baser, R. E., Cragar, D. E., et al. (2004). Head injury and the ability to feign neuropsychological deficits. *Archives of Clinical Neuropsychology, 19,* 37–48.

Vickery, C. D., Berry, D. T. R., Inman, T. H., Harris, M. J., & Orey, S. A. (2001). Detection of inadequate effort on neuropsychological testing: A meta-analytic review of selected procedures. *Archives of Clinical Neuropsychology, 16,* 45–73.

Warrington, E. K. (1984). *Recognition Memory Test.* Windsor, U.K.: NFER-Nelson.

Wechsler, D. (1955). *WAIS manual.* New York: Psychological Corp.

Wechsler, D. (1981). *WAIS-R manual.* New York: Psychological Corp.

Wechsler, D. (1987). *Wechsler Memory Scale-Revised manual.* San Antonio, TX: Psychological Corp.

Wechsler, D. (1997a). *WAIS-III. Administration and scoring manual.* San Antonio, TX: Psychological Corp.

Wechsler, D. (1997b). *WMS-III. Administration and scoring manual.* San Antonio, TX: Harcourt Brace.

Youngjohn, J. R., Burrows, L., & Erdal, K. (1995). Brain damage or compensation neurosis? The controversial post-concussion syndrome. *The Clinical Neuropsychologist, 9,* 112–123.

5

Functional Neuroimaging
in Forensic Neuropsychology

JOSEPH H. RICKER

Technological advances in neuroimaging have had a significant impact on how the functions of the human brain are studied and understood. In addition to providing a useful adjunct to the psychometric approaches to understanding human brain–behavior function (i.e., neuropsychology and cognitive neuroscience), the techniques developed by physicists, engineers, and radiologists have provided ways of assessing brain–behavior relationships that cannot be realized through any other approaches.

This enthusiasm for new technologies, however, must be tempered by an appreciation for scientific rigor and the need to establish diagnostic utility of these techniques. Clinical neuropsychologists and others are increasingly encountering functional neuroimaging and electrophysiological techniques (e.g., single photon emission computed tomography [SPECT], positron emission tomography [PET], quantitative electroencephalography [QEEG], magnetoencephalography [MEG], functional magnetic resonance imaging [fMRI]) in individual clinical and forensic cases. The clinical application of these techniques, however, is more often than not still formally considered investigational by the field in the populations encountered in cases referred for forensic neuropsychological evaluations (Ricker & Zafonte, 2000). All tests, however, whether based in MRI physics, radioisotope emission, electrophysiology, or paper and pencil,

159

must demonstrate sensitivity, specificity, and acceptability within their relevant disciplines before application in clinical or forensic cases in a valid manner.

As with all types of tests and procedures, neuroimaging technologies have numerous and critical limitations. Many psychological and medical tests are quite sensitive to a variety of situations that exhibit statistical departure from "average." In other words, many tests will differentiate between a clinical group and a nonclinical control group. What is of much greater importance, however, and what *must* be established before a test has clinical validity, is whether the test has specificity: Is this test result *specific* or unique to a particular condition or clinical population, but not to others? Of particular concern in both forensic and clinical settings is the application of functional neuroimaging procedures to cases of questioned or questionable injury (e.g., mild brain trauma, toxic exposure).

This chapter provides an overview of several functional neuroimaging procedures and their applications in the context of populations routinely encountered in the practice of forensic neuropsychology. This chapter also addresses many clinical limitations of these procedures that have implications for exercising caution when they are utilized in any evaluation, forensic or otherwise.

The clinical responsibility for interpreting the content of neuroimaging data rests with radiologists, not neuropsychologists. It is important, however, for neuropsychologists, other clinicians, and triers of fact to consider the multitude of factors and conditions that may result in positive neuroimaging findings. It is not advisable simply to accept the findings from investigative techniques as evidence of neuropathology and subsequently, whether intentionally or unintentionally, draw forceful conclusions of causality based on other findings or the patient's self-report. This seems like it should go without saying, but stepping back from the visual and subjective impact that functional imaging can have can be difficult.

REVIEW OF CLASSES OF EVIDENCE
FOR NEURODIAGNOSTIC PROCEDURES

The U.S. Department of Health and Human Services holds medical tests and procedures to standards of evidence. The fact that a medical test or procedure exists, is available, or has validity within certain populations under certain conditions does not constitute evidence of its reliability or validity under other circumstances. Instead, experts in appropriate fields evaluate new and existing tests and technologies with reference to their technical reliability and validity and, most important, their utility in specific situations and with specific populations.

Technologies, of course, are evaluated for safety, but they are also rated in terms of their utility (i.e., "established," "promising," "investigational," "doubtful," or "unacceptable"). In addition, there are classes of evidence ratings. These include, in descending order of support, the following: Class I, supporting evidence is provided by one or more well-designed, randomized, controlled clinical trials; Class II, supporting evidence provided by one or more well-designed clinical studies (e.g., case control, cohort studies); and Class III, supporting evidence is provided by expert opinion, nonrandomized historic controls, or at least one case report. It is notable that the types of functional neuroimaging that are encountered in forensic cases (SPECT, PET, fMRI, QEEG) are all rated as investigational in terms of their application in potential forensic populations (e.g., mild brain injury; Therapeutics and Technology Subcommittee, 1996; American College of Radiology [ACR], 1999; M. Nuwer, 1997). Nonetheless, as empirical support is gradually established, their valid use is likely to become a future reality.

The ACR rates all neuroimaging and radiographic assessment and interventions in detail, using various criteria for clinically appropriate use (i.e., the technique or device has sufficient evidence to support its noninvestigational use for a specific clinical syndrome such as brain injury, or procedurally such as in mammography). Under current nomenclature, neuroimaging technologies are rated on a scale of 1 to 9, with 1 representing "least appropriate" and 9 representing "most appropriate." Detailed descriptions and downloadable full committee reports are available from the ACR at http://www.acr.org.

RESTING VERSUS DYNAMIC IMAGING

In functional neuroimaging, techniques can be conceptualized into two broad categories: resting and activated (Ricker, 2004). Resting paradigms are those that acquire images during nondynamic (i.e., "static" or baseline) conditions. There have been numerous studies using resting functional neuroimaging in various populations, most of which have examined chronic glucose uptake (exclusively with PET), resting cerebral blood flow (using PET or SPECT), or resting electrophysiological activity (e.g., EEG, QEEG, or MEG).

Essentially, resting studies are those that occur when a participant is ostensibly not engaged in any specific task. Resting studies, by design, have no explicit or systematic requirements of the participant other than those required to acquire a technically valid image successfully, such as having the participant lie still, minimize head movement, eliminate extraneous light and noise, and so forth (Raichle, 2001).

Unlike resting studies, activation studies require participants to receive sensory input (e.g., a visual array) or engage in an activity (either cognitive or motor) systematically to examine changes in some time- or stimulus-linked aspect of brain physiology (Roland, 1993). These tasks are usually administered in adherence to a strict protocol, typically with some form of overt response required to provide verification that the participant is actively engaged in the requested task. Because of the technologies related to, and physical properties of, the dependent variables examined, activation studies have much briefer time windows than resting studies. Some technologies are able to image changes across time in a relatively continuous manner (e.g., MEG and event-related fMRI). Given this degree of control, the experimenter is able to make more reliable inferences about cerebral activity underlying the cognitive process in question.

RADIOLIGAND-BASED IMAGING

Single-Photon Emission Computed Tomography

Radioligand-based imaging using SPECT is an approach to functional imaging with an emphasis on regional cerebral blood flow (rCBF), but specific neuroreceptor imaging studies are also possible (Holman & Devous, 1992). SPECT technology is based on the concept that regional changes in brain activity or chemistry can be indirectly measured via externally placed gamma radiation detectors ("cameras") that detect the regional accumulations of tracer flow or receptor-binding isotopes.

The dependent variable in SPECT derives from the well-established principle of increased cerebral activity correlating with increased blood flow. That is, when neural activity in a region of the brain increases, related glucose and oxygen requirements also increase. Because the blood supply carries glucose and oxygen to the brain, the flow of blood to the active area increases (Ingvar & Risberg, 1965). The radioisotopes themselves are absorbed into the glial cells, but are not readily excreted. Thus, the absorbed radioisotopes remain in greater concentration in the more active areas. Through normal radioactive decay, the isotope emits annihilated radioactive particles (i.e., photons), which are then detected by external processors ("cameras"). Computer-based reconstruction then permits representations to be made of differences in blood flow.

Relative to other functional imaging techniques, there are several advantages to SPECT. It is more widely available than PET or fMRI. Unlike with PET, the radioisotopes that are typically used with SPECT can be ordered and delivered in advance, thus precluding the necessity of an on-site cyclotron *and* chemist, as are required for PET.

There is limited use for SPECT in imaging change in blood flow from one point in time to another (e.g., from preictal to ictal state). It is not appropriate, however, for use in mapping blood flow that changes rapidly over time (such as those encountered in most states of cognitive activity) or for making direct inferences about brain metabolism (Roland, 1993). The most commonly used radioactive isotopes for SPECT are absorbed by the brain within 2 minutes, but may have half-lives of several hours. The effect of this is that once the tracer has been administered, the resulting images acquired will remain the same for the next several hours, thus making SPECT a poor tool for measuring rapid or fluctuating changes. It is also not as diverse as other imaging techniques, such as PET, but novel ligands are under continuous development.

The compound 123-I–paraiodoamphetamine (IAMP) provides a unique look at immediate and delayed perfusion. In addition, IAMP has amphetaminelike qualities, which allow for distinct presynaptic and postsynaptic imaging. Although IAMP is no longer available in the United States, a newer compound (99m-Technetium–hexamethylpropyleneamine [HMPAO]) is used for the same purposes. Technetium is a primary blood perfusion agent with the property of rapid cerebral uptake. It is retained in brain structures for several hours, allowing for image capture at various time points following ligand administration.

Recent technological advances have provided for multiple-head scanners, which have improved resolution. There are several sources of potential measurement error for SPECT, however (Zhang, Park, & Kim, 1994). Unlike PET, SPECT imaging requires that regional counts be normalized to an area that is presumably free of injury, and its resolution does not yet approach that of PET imaging. Color SPECT imaging software can produce visually striking—and potentially misleading—images, but reliable and valid interpretation is best accomplished through quantitative pixel counts (Loutfi & Singh, 1995). It must also be noted that although SPECT *can* be used quantitatively, this is not the case in most settings. Visual inspection of SPECT maps is a qualitative process, and interpretation may vary from clinician to clinician.

In addition, image reconstruction is typically based on presumptions about which brain regions are "normal." Relative flow values in SPECT are often based on a region such as the thalamus or cerebellum. Although such assumptions might be valid for some populations with focal lesions (e.g., stroke), they might not be valid for populations with involvement that is more diffuse (e.g., traumatic brain injury [TBI]). Although SPECT is very sensitive to detecting regional differences in resting blood flow, there is little specificity to the patterns obtained. Thus, the results of a series of SPECT images can be affected by many factors, including premorbid injury or illness, emotional disturbances, medications, or current substance use (Ricker & Zafonte, 2000).

Positron Emission Tomography

Positron emission tomography (PET) is another radioisotope-based approach to imaging. The variable of interest is usually glucose absorption (measured by uptake of fluorodeoxyglucose), although oxygen-15 PET scanning is also used for activated imaging studies (Buckner & Logan, 2001). In spite of the exponential growth in investigational fMRI publications (overwhelmingly conducted with healthy individuals), PET remains the "gold standard" for functional neuroimaging. It is also remains quite expensive, however (approximately U.S. $2,000 for a series of resting PET images), and requires a cyclotron to be present on site for most radioisotopes.

PET has been widely used as a research tool since the 1970s, but its application for persons with TBI has been minimally investigated. PET has the capability of demonstrating specific biochemical or physiological processes associated with cerebral blood flow and metabolism. The resulting PET image represents the spatial distribution of radioisotopes, which is usually portrayed on an actual or standardized anatomical (MRI) template.

PET studies typically utilize tracers such as $[^{18}F]$-fluorodeoxyglucose (FDG) for the quantification of resting (i.e., nonactivated) regional brain metabolism. Studies of blood flow changes associated with motor or cognitive activity can be accomplished using tracers such as oxygen-15-labeled water. Radiolabeled ligands that target dopaminergic, serotonergic, and other receptor systems have been developed and are seen as a potential area of future research. Genetically mediated transporter markers (e.g., for dopamine transport) are also available.

Functional Magnetic Resonance–Based Imaging

All magnetic resonance–based imaging techniques capitalize on the presence of hydrogen in all of the body's tissues. When the nuclei of hydrogen atoms are placed in a strong magnetic field, they align in parallel to the field's direction. In MRI, radiofrequency pulses are presented at a 90° angle relative to the magnetic field. When this occurs, the hydrogen nuclei realign and begin spinning in a different direction (*excitation*). The radiofrequency pulse is then stopped, and the nuclei return to their original alignment and spin. This process of resuming previous nuclei states results in the emission of an electronic signal that can be detected by the scanner.

It should be noted that only about 1% of the hydrogen atoms in the magnetic field emit a response, but this results in enough signal to permit the reconstruction of images. Because most of the atoms that are excited in this process are found within water molecules, water content and tissue density dictate the signal that is detected by the scanner and subsequently digitally reconstructed into an image (Springer, Patlak, Playka, & Huang, 2000).

Functional magnetic resonance imaging (fMRI) is a variant of conventional MRI. The critical difference, however, is that the dependent variable of interest in fMRI is alteration in signal intensity related to increases in blood flow resulting from changes in brain activity. Thus, fMRI is more concerned with changes in brain activity than anatomical structure per se. Although the primary goal of structural MRI is to generate high-resolution anatomical images of underlying brain structure, the goal of functional MRI is to allow the investigator to make inferences about regional changes in brain activity.

As discussed for other techniques dependent on blood flow, in fMRI specific tasks or stimuli are introduced to the individual in the scanner to elicit increased cerebral activity. When neural activity increases in a region, there is an increase in blood flow to that region. When the brain is at rest, there is a tight correlation between rCBF, regional cerebral metabolic rate for glucose, and regional cerebral metabolic rate for oxygen. With activity, however, rCBF can increase by over 50%, which is well beyond metabolic demands. The physiological basis for this is not clear (Weisskoff, 2000).

With the excess of blood flow to the region, particularly in light of only minimal increase in oxygen extraction, there is a resulting localized abundance of oxyhemoglobin relative to deoxyhemoglobin in the venous and capillary beds that perfuse the active regions of cortex. Oxyhemoglobin is naturally diamagnetic; deoxyhemoglobin is paramagnetic (i.e., becomes readily magnetized within a magnetic field). With increased neural activity and concomitant increased blood flow, there is a net increase in diamagnetic material (oxyhemoglobin) and a net decrease in paramagnetic material (deoxyhemoglobin).

This results in an increase in signal intensity that can be detected externally and is represented as higher signal intensity on T2* ("T2-star") weighted scans. This change in signal intensity is referred to as the blood oxygen level–dependent (BOLD) effect (Chen & Ogawa, 2000). In magnets of "average" strength (e.g., 1.5 tesla), the signal changes appear to emanate from veins and large venules. In high-field magnets (e.g., 3, 4, or even greater tesla, an index of magnitude in comparison to the magnetic field strength of the earth's gravity), signal is more likely obtained from microvessels, small venules, and capillaries. The signal changes obtained are very small, on the order of 1–6%, and occur over approximately a 2- to 6-second time frame (depending on brain region, age of the participant, and the task performed).

Because fMRI utilizes the body's natural physical responses to high-strength magnetism, no exogenous tracers, radioisotopes, or contrast agents are necessary. The anatomical resolution of fMRI is superior to that of SPECT or PET. There are numerous activation paradigms that can be carried out in fMRI, and it allows for greater flexibility in paradigm with reference to repeatability and brevity of overall session (Ricker, 2004).

As with any imaging procedure, however, fMRI can be impacted by numerous variables. Although publications discussing the use of fMRI in healthy individuals have appeared since 1990, very few fMRI studies exist in clinical populations, and there are particularly few in populations of primary interest in rehabilitation medicine. Movement can disrupt head alignment and may perturb the magnetic field itself. Thus, head movement must be eliminated, and other extraneous movements must be reduced. Overt responses to tasks must be minimal at most. Movements of the jaw required for talking are often considered too excessive during fMRI, but event-related paradigms do allow for some degree of overt verbal responding (Ishikawa, 2002).

The normal high-frequency noise within the scanner must be considered when evaluating individuals with possible acquired neuropathology or neuropsychiatric disturbance. The examiner or technician must also monitor for idiosyncratic responses such as claustrophobia, anxiety, boredom, disengagement, or actual onset of sleep while in the scanner.

Although virtually any contemporary MRI scanner can be adapted to functional imaging, fMRI is still investigational in many populations, including brain trauma (ACR, 1999), and is thus primarily a research tool at this time. This also limits its availability to primarily academic medical centers. Even a single fMRI session will generate a very large volume of data. Thus, computer hardware requirements must be considered, along with data storage and data security. Finally, fMRI protocols do not and cannot "automatically" or "objectively" yield brain maps, and at present there are no normative values for fMRI scans or activity levels. The resulting images must be carefully and skillfully reconstructed, and this reconstruction process should be considered as much art as science. The approach that taken in reconstructing and displaying the data in the form of brain image data will have an impact on the portrayal, and potentially the interpretation, of the end product.

ELECTROPHYSIOLOGICAL TECHNIQUES

Quantitative Electroencephalography

Electroencephalography (EEG) is a neurophysiological index of cerebral function that has widespread use. In medical rehabilitation populations, it is used to assess seizure activity, coma, and gross outcome. Data from traditional qualitative EEG analysis does not, however, allow for identification and quantification of the spectra of wave frequencies that occur in the human brain. Thus, conventional EEG is useful clinically only as a very gross monitor and has little utility in advance prediction of outcome. When Fourier transform analysis is applied to EEG, however, it allows continuous monitoring and quantification across all cerebral wave frequencies. This approach is more commonly referred to as quantitative electroencephalography (QEEG; Cantor, 1999).

The term QEEG is applied to a group of interrelated technologies centered on the mathematical concept of spectral analysis (Wallace, Wagner, Wagner, & McDeavitt, 2001). In essence, the EEG signal is digitally processed, and the relative contributions of each frequency are identified and quantified. When digitized, the individual component frequencies of a complex waveform (i.e., amount of alpha, beta, delta, and theta contained within the signal) can be discerned in a manner superior to that of traditional visual analysis of EEG printed output.

There are several approaches to displaying QEEG spectral data. In the *compressed spectral array* format, the frequency components from a series of epochs (e.g., 30-second blocks of time) are quantified. The output is then represented sequentially either in print or graphically, permitting interpretation of changes in the EEG signal over time (Luccas et al., 1999).

Another approach is *topographical mapping* (Skrandies, 1995). In this format, each electrode in the EEG montage is assigned a color value (or gray scale shading level) for each frequency range. The color or shading represents the frequency level underlying the electrode. The color map (or shading gradient) is then superimposed on an oval (representing the head). The resulting brain map resembles what might be obtained from a resting SPECT or PET. It is imperative, however, that to appreciate the fact that the topographical map is derived from a minimal number of data points, reflects only cortical surface activity, and has many interpolated color values (e.g., the colors or shadings between electrodes are interpolated).

A third approach to data representation is that of probability mapping (Nuwer, 1990). This approach utilizes topographic mapping as a basis, but compares the map to a normative database (i.e., a composite map). An individual's map may then be statistically compared to the normative map, and inferences based on the normal distribution are made in interpretation.

Magnetoencephalography

In addition to electrical activity, neurons also generate minute magnetic fields that can be measured using an approach known as magnetoencephalography (MEG), which involves the use of liquid helium to cool conducting coils to almost absolute zero. When cooled to such low temperatures, the electrical resistance of the conductor is greatly reduced, and very small changes in magnetic field can be detected (King, Park, Smith, & Wheless, 2000). The miniscule nature of these fields requires significant amplification to be useful. Using devices known as superconducting quantum-interference devices (SQUIDs), the changes in magnetic fields produced by neuronal activity can be detected. An array of conductors is situated around the head of the participant, which allows the placement of multiple detectors (Kado, Komuro, Shimogawara, & Uehara, 1996).

The physiological basis of MEG is that of normal neuronal membrane signal conduction. The flow of electrical current within an active neuron generates a magnetic field. When a synapse becomes active, there is a current flow across the neuronal membrane. This current diffuses intracellularly and then emerges extracelluarly at a fixed distance from where it began (i.e., from dendrite to synapse). This results in the opportunity for "sources" and "sinks" extracellularly. In the presence of an asymmetrically oriented neuron, the sources and sinks create dipolar electromagnetic fields that cancel one another out. The intracellular current between the region of synaptic activation and the point at which the current returns to extracellular space does not cancel out (Tang, Perlmutter, Malaszenko, Phung, & Reeb, 2002). This magnetic field can be recorded.

Although intuitively similar to EEG, MEG has some advantages. First, MEG frequencies are technically easier to record than those from EEG given that the detectors are located in a helmet for placement adjacent to the scalp and thus do not have to be individually applied (or interconnected). Second, magnetic fields are not affected by the variability in skull thickness over different regions of cortex. Third, in general, the component structure of the MEG response is actually simpler than that derived through EEG. There are, of course, disadvantages to MEG. MEG is very expensive and thus not widely available. MEG also does not detect deep (e.g., subcortical) sources of activity. MEG, along with EEG, lacks the anatomical precision of other neuroimaging techniques (Stern & Silbersweig, 2001).

DIAGNOSTIC GROUPS ENCOUNTERED IN FORENSIC CONTEXTS

Brain Injury

Single photon emission computed tomographic studies of brain injury

In chronic moderate and severe TBI (i.e., at least several months following acute injury), resting studies generally consistently demonstrated either hypometabolism or decreased resting blood flow, predominantly within prefrontal cortex (Bergsneider et al., 2001; Bergsneider, Hovda, & Shalmon, 1997; Fontaine, Azouvi, Remy, Bussel, & Samson, 1999; Gross, Kling, Henry, Herndon, & Lavretsky, 1996; Jansen, van der Naalt, & van Zomeren, 1996; Langfitt et al., 1986; Rao et al., 1984; Ricker et al., 2001; Tenjin, Ueda, & Mizukawa, 1990). In most of these studies, decreased blood flow and metabolism were generally in excess of what might be expected based solely on findings from structural scans (i.e., computerized tomography [CT] and MRI). The presence of decreased resting blood flow or metabolism is not, however, in and of itself evidence of compromised or nonfunctional brain tissue (e.g., Duara et al., 1992).

Numerous investigations have demonstrated that SPECT is better than structural imaging (i.e., CT and MRI) in the detection of the presence and extent of trauma-related lesions. Application has been made of SPECT to mild brain injury; it has demonstrated regionally decreased blood flow in the presence of normal acute CT scans, but there is tremendous variability across individuals (i.e., no pathognomonic profile has emerged). Positive SPECT findings have also sometimes been demonstrated in cases of below-average neuropsychological test scores in cases of mild brain trauma, but it should be noted that SPECT findings are usually not predictive of test performance (Umile, Plotkin, & Sandel, 1998).

In spite of advances in technology and data analysis, the utility of SPECT for characterizing specific illness and injury states or predicting outcome remains controversial. It has shown particular utility when correlating neuropsychological parameters with the chronic effects of severe brain injury (Ichise et al., 1994), but caution must be exercised given that systemic metabolic abnormalities, substance use, and emotional disorders can have an impact on SPECT results and interpretations. For example, the results of SPECT (and PET) studies have been abnormal in disorders such as depression (Sackheim, Prohovnik, & Moeller, 1990); manic–depressive disorder (Iidaka, Nakajima, Ogikubo, & Fukuda, 1995); obsessive–compulsive disorders (Adams, Warneke, McEwan, & Fraser, 1993); generalized anxiety disorders (Uchiyama, Sue, Fukumitsu, Mori, & Kawakami, 1997); and schizophrenia (Paulman, Devous, & Gregory, 1990). Frequently, SPECT demonstrates abnormalities in dementia (Read, Miler, Mena, & Kim, 1995) and cerebrovascular disease (Masdeu & Brass, 1995) and suggests decreased tracer uptake in normal aging (Mozley, Kim, & Gur, 1996).

Also, SPECT demonstrates positive functional neuroimaging findings in domains that frequently covary with (or are attributed to) TBI, such as learning disabilities (Wood, Flowers, Buchsbaum, & Tallal, 1991) and somatization disorder (Lazarus & Cotterell, 1989). Finally, SPECT often demonstrates abnormalities in aggression (Amen, Stubblefield, & Carmichael, 1996); alcohol dependence (Modell & Mountz, 1995) and alcohol withdrawal (Mampunza, Verbanck, Verhas, & Martin, 1995); opiate use (Krystal, Woods, Kosten, & Rosen, 1995); hallucinogenic drug use (Hertzman, Reba, & Kotlyarov, 1990); and cocaine abuse (Miller, Mina, Giombetti, & Villenueva-Meyer, 1992). In addition, at least 6% of noninjured, medically healthy individuals may demonstrate focal abnormalities on SPECT imaging (Umile et al., 1992).

Some investigators have noted that, when used in a prospective design, a negative SPECT scan is a good predictor of a favorable outcome after brain injury, and that SPECT overall correlates well with the severity of the initial trauma (Jacobs, Put, Ingels, & Bossuyt, 1994). Still lacking are prospective studies of SPECT (as well as PET and fMRI) in differential diagnosis, prognosis, and intervention.

SPECT has been useful in research studies following brain injury, but there is no particular SPECT profile that is pathognomonic or reliable for brain injury (Herscovitch, 1996; Ricker, 2004). Clinically, the literature does not support the routine use of SPECT for the evaluation of postconcussion syndrome specifically or for brain injury in general. The Therapeutics and Technology Subcommittee of the American Academy of Neurology (1996) rated SPECT as an investigational procedure for the study of brain trauma. The ACR (1999) rated

SPECT as inappropriate (a rating of 2 on a scale of 1 to 9, with 1 indicating "least appropriate") in the evaluation of postconcussive symptoms. In spite of the professional cautions and the present conclusions regarding the lack of scientific support for the routine use of SPECT in brain injury, SPECT appears to be used frequently in clinical and forensic contexts as a means of supporting a diagnosis of brain injury.

Positron emission tomographic studies of brain injury

Experimental studies of TBI have shown that cerebral hyperglycolysis is a pathophysiological response that occurs in response to injury-induced neurochemical cascades. Bergsneider and colleagues (Bergsneider et al., 1997, 2001) have shown, via FDG-PET, that hyperglycolysis occurs in both regional and global settings after severe brain injury in humans. Such abnormalities may also exist transiently after milder injury.

Several studies have demonstrated the ability of PET to detect abnormalities not seen on static imaging in cases of moderate and severe brain injury (see review by Ricker, 2004). In addition, data exist to suggest that functional imaging demonstrates areas of physiological dysfunction beyond the boundaries of static lesions seen on structural imaging. Langfitt and colleagues (Langfitt et al., 1986) presented some of the earliest functional imaging data from individuals who had sustained severe TBI. Also, FDG-PET was compared with CT, MRI, and SPECT studies. They were able to demonstrate with PET that cerebral hypometabolism extended beyond the morphometric boundaries of lesion as imaged with the structural methods of CT and MRI.

It has been demonstrated that the intermediate metabolic reduction phase begins to resolve approximately 1 month following injury regardless of injury severity (Bergsneider et al., 2001). The correlation between the extent of change in neurological disability and the change in cerebral metabolic rate for glucose from the early to late period is modest, however. Cobalt-55 PET can also demonstrate regional abnormalities beyond those shown by CT and MRI following severe TBI (Jansen et al., 1996).

In spite of the application of functional imaging studies in forensic situations when there is a question about the occurrence of, or disability resulting from, TBI, there are surprisingly few studies that have actually attempted to correlate functional imaging findings with cognition. In most of the studies that have attempted to correlate functional imaging with testing, the findings from psychometric assessment have been examined with those from functional imaging conducted either prior to or following memory evaluation. For example, Ruff and colleagues (1994) described FDG-PET and neuropsychological test findings among a selected series of nine individuals who had sustained mild brain trauma and whose static imaging (CT or MRI) studies were negative, but the findings have minimal generalizability given that the subjects were specifically selected for inclusion based on *outcome* rather that *a priori* criteria. In addition, scanning and neuropsychological evaluation were separated in time by an average of 11 months.

In a study of 20 persons with mild TBI, it was noted that local abnormal cerebral metabolic rates correlated with complaints and neuropsychological test results obtained during the chronic phase of recovery (Gross et al., 1996). In moderate and severe TBI, resting PET studies demonstrated frontal hypometabolism, with correlated poor performance on neuropsychological tests thought to be mediated by frontal lobe functioning (Fontaine et al., 1999).

PET activation studies are likely to be far more sensitive to the functional effects of brain injury or disease because such paradigms introduce in vivo cognitive challenges (Baron, 1995). The first PET study to apply a cognitive activation paradigm with individuals who sustained severe TBI (Ricker et al., 2001) demonstrated left frontal lobe rCBF changes in individuals with TBI during free recall when compared to controls, but rCBF increases were noted in more posterior brain regions during both free and cued recall in subjects with TBI. The change in allocation of neural resources during tasks with greater cognitive load may suggest greater frontal lobe involvement resulting from increased cognitive effort. Of additional note is the finding that, during recognition tasks, both the controls and the individuals with TBI performed at comparable behavioral levels (i.e., within normal limits), yet the individuals with TBI still demonstrated increased change in regional cerebral blood flow relative to the controls. This suggests that, after brain injury, individuals must exert more cognitive effort than controls to attain the same level of overt behavior. A subsequent oxygen-15 PET study in TBI by a different group of investigators also demonstrated similar findings on a verbal list-learning task (Levine et al., 2002).

Functional magnetic resonance imaging studies of brain injury

In the first fMRI studies of individuals with TBI (McAllister et al., 1999, 2001), the investigators examined individuals with a very recent history (i.e., within the previous 30 days) of mild brain injury. As in the Ricker et al. (2001) PET study of chronic severe TBI, the individuals with mild TBI in the McAllister studies demonstrated intact behavioral performance on a verbal working memory task, but they did show right hemisphere lateralized fMRI activation in response to increased working memory load. In an fMRI investigation of working memory following moderate and severe TBI (Christodoulou et al., 2001), increased blood flow and more widespread dispersion of cortical activation was noted during working memory tasks. This again suggested that increased cognitive effort is reflected in increased brain activation on fMRI.

Although PET and fMRI clearly represent more advanced approaches to brain imaging when compared to SPECT, none have reached a sufficient threshold of evidence for routine use in mild brain trauma. Currently, PET is classified at the same level of clinical appropriateness as SPECT (i.e., 2 on a scale of 9) by the ACR (1999). Given the paucity of fMRI research in TBI, the ACR has not fully evaluated fMRI and continues to classify this procedure as investigational in the examination of brain injury.

Quantitative electroencephalographic studies after traumatic brain injury

The literature regarding the utility of QEEG in brain injury is growing. Much of the investigational work in the area of QEEG and brain injury has been in the area of coma (Wallace et al., 2001). For example, previous work has shown poor outcome among a population of persons with severe TBI who continued to show slow pattern responses (Bricolo, Turazzi, & Faccioli, 1978). A poor prognosis is more likely among individuals with severe TBI who have silent or slow QEEG patterns; those who have active sleep–wake cycles and variation of pattern tend to have much better outcomes (Sironi, 1983).

The amount of QEEG slowing corresponds to reaction level scale scores in comatose individuals (Matousek, Takuchi, Starmark, & Stalhammer, 1996). The prognostic efficacy of QEEG spectral analysis has been compared to that of the Glasgow Coma Scale (Teasdale & Jennett, 1974), brain stem auditory evoked potentials, and CT in individuals in coma within 3 weeks of TBI (Thatcher, Walker, Gerson, & Geisler, 1989), although generalizability is limited (Ricker & Zafonte, 2000).

There has been less systematic evaluation of the efficacy of QEEG in discriminating individuals with mild TBI from controls, and there remains some question as to the clinical utility of this brain mapping approach in this type of differential diagnosis (Hagglund & Persson, 1990; Thatcher et al., 1989). In fact, although QEEG can demonstrate impressive statistical discriminant functions in mild brain injury, it has been demonstrated that it may actually have an *inferior* hit rate relative to simple clinical diagnosis (Ricker & Zafonte, 2000). Although still certainly holding promise, it can be concluded that, at present, QEEG remains more of a research tool than a diagnostic instrument in brain trauma.

The Therapeutics and Technology Assessment Subcommittee of the American Academy of Neurology along with the American Clinical Neurophysiology Society (formerly the American Electroencephalographic Society) have published a practice guideline report on the use of digital EEG that discusses the insufficiency of evidence for the use of digital EEG in the diagnosis and assessment of postconcussion syndrome or minor or moderate brain injury (M. Nuwer, 1997). Although certainly not everyone agrees with the conclusions of the American Academy of Neurology (e.g., Hoffmann et al., 1999), additional cross-validation with independent groups and appropriate experimental design will be needed to establish the utility of QEEG in clinical and forensic differential diagnosis.

Toxic Exposure

Neuroanatomical imaging techniques such as CT and MRI are often utilized in cases of known or suspected toxic exposure. Given the nature of possible neurotoxin effects, however, functional neuroimaging procedures are likely to be of greater validity in the detection of neurophysiological dysfunction.

Measures of neurotoxins in blood, urine, or occasionally hair may be more useful in confirming exposure if available within a period of recent exposure such that they would still be present. Examples of these are carboxyhemoglobin levels, blood lead levels, and 24-hour urinary mercury and arsenic (Armstrong, 2004).

Some toxic exposures (e.g., those from solvents) are associated with a non-specific finding of cortical atrophy on CT, which alone may not be considered sensitive to early subclinical signs (Triebig & Lang, 1993) and may be most useful to rule out mass lesions. Structural MRI (i.e., T1 and T2 weighted) may be useful to identify white matter changes, especially after solvent exposure. Magnetic resonance imaging has been more sensitive to chronic cortical effects of solvent exposure than CT (Filley, 1999; Hartman, 1995; Rosenberg, Spitz, Filley, Davis, & Schaumberg, 1988).

Advanced functional brain imaging tests are generally nonspecific and are more useful in ruling on other causes of cognitive dysfunction, for example, mass lesions or vascular changes.

Regional cerebral blood flow studies using SPECT or PET have demonstrated functional correlates of abnormal neuropsychological test results in occupational exposure cases with various etiologies. These approaches may not be very helpful in distinguishing neurotoxic from other abnormalities at present, however (Armstrong, 2004). The PET or SPECT studies of receptor binding may be of greater utility in demonstrating receptor system–specific effects of toxins (Edling et al., 1997).

There is a growing utilization of event-related potentials, especially in the experimental literature (Reinhardt et al., 1997). P300 and N250 latencies and P200 amplitude indicated significant differences between solvent-exposed painters and controls (Morrow, Steinhauer, & Hodgson, 1992). Visual-evoked potentials have been suggested as susceptible to alteration by exposure to solvents, metals, pesticides, and other neurotoxins such as carbon monoxide (Urban & Lukas, 1990).

Criminal Forensics

In the same manner that neuropsychological testing is used in the determination of mitigating brain-based factors in violence or even murder, functional neuroimaging is also increasingly used to defend individuals who have been charged with such criminal activity. Functional neuroimaging is also used when a defendant has been convicted, but mitigating factors might result in a reduction in penalty (e.g., avoidance of the death penalty). As has been pointed out by others (Intrator et al., 1997; Mayberg, 1996; Raine, Buchsbaum, & LaCasse, 1997; Raine, Meloy, & Bihrle, 1998), and should be quite obvious to any reader of this chapter, great caution must be used before inferring positive brain imaging findings as mitigating criminal behavior. The overwhelming majority of individuals who demonstrate a positive finding in a neuroimaging study will have no history of crime or violence and will not be at any increased probability of ever engaging in such behaviors.

Structural and functional neuroimaging studies of aggressive and violent individuals have generally demonstrated frontal lobe abnormalities (Brower & Price, 2001). The nature of these findings is not specific, however. Such findings may be neurodevelopmental, or they may be acquired through brain injury or substance abuse.

There have been several studies that have used SPECT to examine aggressive and antisocial behavior (e.g., Amen et al., 1996; Hirono, Mega, & Dinov, 2000; Kuruglu, Arikan, & Vural, 1996). Each study demonstrated some level of decreased blood flow in the frontal lobes. As with TBI, however, such a finding is not, in and of itself, pathognomonic for a propensity toward violence and may be the result of a variety of other factors. Of course, one must also consider the possibility that genuine frontal lobe dysfunction may result in disinhibition, emotional disruption, and deficient judgment, which may contribute to some aspects of violent or criminal behavior.

Studies with PET have contrasted forensic psychiatric patients with controls. Some studies have demonstrated decreased frontal blood flow and metabolism associated with violent behavior (Volkow & Tancredi, 1987; Volkow, Tancredi, & Grant, 1995). A PET investigation of "impulsive aggression" in patients with personality disorders (chiefly antisocial, borderline, and narcissistic) showed decreased anterior medial and left anterior orbitofrontal metabolism, which correlated with higher self-ratings of aggression (Goyer, Andreason, & Semple, 1994).

Raine and colleagues (Raine et al., 1997) presented PET data from 41 individuals charged with murder or manslaughter. Compared with controls matched for age, gender, and previous psychiatric diagnosis if applicable, individuals charged with murder or manslaughter demonstrated (as a group) statistically significant bifrontal hypometabolism while performing a cognitive task known to activate prefrontal cortex. A later examination of these data (Raine, Meloy, & Bihrle, 1998) involved separating this sample into either a "predatory" (operationalized as controlled, purposeful aggression) or "affective" (operationalized as impulsive, emotionally charged aggression) category. Affective murderers demonstrated lower prefrontal metabolism compared to controls. Predatory murderers actually resembled controls in terms of frontal metabolism.

Most imaging studies of violent or criminal behavior seem to demonstrate an association between aggression and prefrontal hypoactivity. Most studies in this arena focus on bifrontal (specifically prefrontal) decreases in activity, but there are often other regions of hypoactivity as well. Inconsistencies in findings are likely attributable to variability in experimental design and selection of participants. The finding of prefrontal hypoactivity cannot be interpreted as a chronic substrate for uncontrollable violent behavior, however, as such a finding can be experimentally induced.

For example, in a PET study of healthy volunteers, Pietrini, Guazelli, and Basso (2000) asked participants to imagine a scenario involving their own aggressive behavior. Such imagery was associated with significant focal reductions in ventromedial frontal blood flow compared to those elicited by neutral scenarios. Thus, frontal lobe hypoactivity may be more associated with affective changes that may be associated with aggression, but these do not necessarily represent an inability to avoid committing an act of violence (Mayberg, 1996).

With reference to competency, the contribution of functional imaging is less clear (in comparison to the examination of possible mitigating factors) and might in fact be inappropriate. Competency to stand trial, as one example, is based on a multitude of factors related more to cognitive capacity and behavior rather than a yes/no decision as to the presence or absence of a change in the brain. A defendant might certainly have a previous brain injury or chronic neurological illness (e.g., seizure disorder), but could still be quite competent to participate in trial proceedings and ultimately to be held accountable for his or her actions. A very detailed and thoughtful examination of these factors is presented in this volume in chapters 12 and 13.

As Brower and Price (2001) outlined, there are many methodological problems in this literature, including an absence of prospective data, small sample sizes, or inadequate controls. In particular, there are factors that can certainly have an impact on functional imaging that are not taken into account, including poverty, abuse, violence, emotional disruption (either preexisting or in reaction to involvement with the criminal justice system), and substance abuse.

FUTURE RESEARCH

The past few years have seen tremendous advances in functional neuroimaging technologies and approaches to data analysis. In addition, there have been exploratory studies in several clinical populations, including populations that might be encountered in the context of forensic neuropsychological practice. In spite of these technological advances, these techniques remain investigational in most clinical populations and do not, from a scientific perspective, appear ready for *routine* deployment in forensic evaluations. This should not be misinterpreted as an entirely negative statement, however. In fact, it is my opinion and expectation that functional neuroimaging will eventually achieve the same level of applicability in forensic contexts that neuropsychological assessment has already achieved. As with neuropsychological assessment, this will not occur overnight or solely from the publication of a handful of case studies or small investigations drawn only from preselected personal injury or criminal forensic cases. It will occur after years of additional systematic research, first with many independent samples of clinical populations and then in studies that directly compare clinical populations with litigating populations. This is the standard that has been successfully followed in forensic neuropsychology, and there is no reason to hold functional neuroimaging techniques to a lower standard. In addition, this standard is not solely restricted to forensic applications, as well-designed and controlled studies of functional imaging can only serve to improve diagnosis and treatment for all clinical populations regardless of the context or setting in which such studies are requested.

REFERENCES

Adams, B. L., Warneke, L. B., McEwan, A. J. B., & Fraser, B. A. (1993). Single photon emission computerized tomography in obsessive compulsive disorder: A preliminary study. *Journal of Psychiatry and Clinical Neuroscience, 18*, 109–112.

Alster, J., Pratt, H., & Feinsod, M. (1993). Density spectral array, evoked potentials, and temperature rhythms in the evaluation and prognosis of the comatose patient. *Brain Injury, 7*, 191–208.

Amen, D. G., Stubblefield, M., & Carmichael, B. (1996). Brain SPECT findings and aggressiveness. *Annals of Clinical Psychiatry, 8*, 129–137.

American College of Radiology. (1999). *American College of Radiology appropriateness criteria*: Head trauma (pp. 507–524). Reston, VA: American College of Radiology.

Armstrong, A. (2004). Neuropsychological differential diagnosis of toxic exposure. In J. H. Ricker (Ed.), *Differential diagnosis in adult neuropsychological assessment* (pp. 179–217). New York: Springer.

Baron, J. C. (1995). Étude de la neuroanatomis functionelle de la perception par la tomographie à positons. *Revue Neurologique, 151*, 511–517.

Bergsneider, M., Hovda, D. A., McArthur, D. L., Etchpare, M., Huang, S. C, Sehati, N., et al. (2001). Metabolic recovery following human traumatic brain injury based on FDG-PET: Time course and relationship to neurological disability. *Journal of Head Trauma Rehabilitation, 16*(2), 135–148.

Bergsneider, M., Hovda, D., & Shalmon, E. (1997). Cerebral hyperglycolosis following severe traumatic brain injury in humans; a positron emission tomography. *Journal of Neurosurgery, 86*, 241–251.

Bricolo, A., Turazzi, S., & Faccioli, F. (1978). Clinical application of compressed spectral array in long-term EEG monitoring of comatose patients. *Electroencephalography and Clinical Neurophysiology, 45*, 211–225.

Brower, M. C., & Price, B. H. (2001). Neuropsychiatry of frontal lobe dysfunction in violent and criminal behaviour: A critical review. *Journal of Neurology, Neurosurgery, and Psychiatry, 71*, 720–726.

Buckner, R. L., & Logan, J. M. (2001). Functional neuroimaging methods: PET and FMRI. In R. Cabeza & A. Kingstone (Eds.), *Handbook of functional neuroimaging of cognition*. Cambridge, MA: MIT Press.

Cantor, D. S. (1999). An overview of quantitative EEG. In J. R. Evans & A. Abarbanel (Eds.), *Introduction to quantitative EEG and neurofeedback* (pp. 3–27). San Diego, CA: Academic Press.

Chen, W., & Ogawa, S. (2000). Principles of BOLD functional MRI. In C. T. Moonen & P. A. Bandettini (Eds.). *Functional MRI* (pp. 103–112). Berlin: Springer-Verlag.

Christodoulou, C., DeLisa, J., Ricker, J. H., Madigan, N., Bly, B. M., Lange, G., et al. (2001). Functional magnetic resonance imaging of working memory impairment following traumatic brain injury. *Journal of Neurology, Neurosurgery, and Psychiatry, 71*, 161–168.

Duara, R., Barker, W. W., Chang, J., Yoshii, F., Lowenstein, D. A., & Pascal, S. (1992). Viability of neocortical function shown in behavioral activation state PET studies in Alzheimer disease. *Journal of Cerebral Blood Flow and Metabolism, 12*, 927–934.

Edling, C., Hellman, B., Arvidson, B., Andersson, J., Hartvig, P., Lilja, A., et al. (1997). Do organic solvents induce changes in the dopaminergic system? Positron emission tomography studies of occupationally exposed subjects. *International Archives of Occupational and Environmental Health, 70*, 180–186.

Filley, C. M. (1999). Toxic leukoencephalopathy. *Clinical Neuropharmacology, 22*, 249–260.

Fontaine, A., Azouvi, P., Remy, P., Bussel, B., & Samson, Y. (1999). Functional anatomy of neuropsychological deficits after severe traumatic brain injury. *Neurology, 53*, 1963–1968.

Goldstein, A. S. (1967). *The insanity defense*. New Haven, CT: Yale University Press.

Goyer, P. F., Andreason, P. J., & Semple, W. E. (1994). Positron emission tomography and personality disorders. *Neuropsychopharmacology, 10*, 21–28.

Gross, H., Kling, A., Henry, G., Herndon, C., & Lavretsky, H. (1996). Local cerebral glucose metabolism in patients with long-term behavioral and cognitive deficits following mild head injury. *Journal of Neuropsychiatry and Clinical Neuroscience, 8*, 324–334.

Hagglund, Y., & Persson, H. (1990). Does Swedish amateur boxing lead to chronic brain damage? *Acta Neurologica Scandinavica, 82*, 353–360.

Hartman, D. E. (Ed.). (1995). *Neuropsychological toxicology: Identification and assessment of human neurotoxic syndromes* (2nd ed., pp. 149–224). New York: Plenum Press.

Herscovitch, P. (1996). Functional brain imaging: Basic principles and application to head trauma. In M. Rizzo & D. Tranel (Eds.), *Head injury and the postconcussive syndrome* (pp. 89–118). New York: Churchill Livingstone.

Hertzman, M., Reba, R. C., & Kotlyarov, E. V. (1990). Single photon emission computed tomography in phencyclidine and related drug abuse. *American Journal of Psychiatry, 147*, 255–256.

Hirono, N., Mega, M., & Dinov, I. (2000). Left frontotemporal hypoperfusion is associated with aggression in patients with dementia. *Archives of Neurology, 57*, 861–866.

Hoffman, D. A., Lubar, J. F., Thatcher, R. W., Sterman, M. B., Rosenfeld, P. J., Striefel, S., et al. (1999). Limitations of the American Academy of Neurology and American Clinical Neurophysiology Society paper on QEEG. *Journal of Neuropsychiatry and Clinical Neuroscience, 11*, 401–407.

Holman, B. L., & Devous, M. D. (1992). Functional brain SPECT: The emergence of a powerful clinical method. *Journal of Nuclear Medicine, 33*, 1888–1904.

Ichise, M., Chung, D. G., Wang, P., Wortzman, G., Gray, B. G., & Franks, W. (1994). Technetium-99m-HMPAO SPECT, CT, and MRI in the evaluation of patients with chronic traumatic brain injury: A correlation with neuropsychological performance. *Journal of Nuclear Medicine, 35*, 1217–1226.

Iidaka, T., Nakajima, T., Ogikubo, T., & Fukuda, H. (1995). Correlations between regional cerebral blood flow and the Hamilton Rating Scale for Depression in mood disorders: A study using 123-iodoamphetamine single photon emission computerized tomography. *Clinical Psychiatry, 37*, 951–958.

Ingvar, G. H., & Risberg, J. (1965). Influence of mental activity upon regional blood flow in man. *Acta Neurologica Scandinavica, 14*, 183–186.

Intrator, J., Hare, R., Stritzke, P., Brichtswein, K., Dorfman, D., Harpur, T., et al. (1997). A brain imaging (single photon emission computerized tomography) study of semantic and affective processing in psychopaths. *Biological Psychiatry, 42*, 96–103.

Ishikawa, T. (2002). Brain regions activated during the mandibular movement tasks in functional magnetic resonance imaging. *Kokubyo Gakkai Zasshi, 69*, 39–48.

Jacob, S. A., Put, E., Ingels, M., & Bossuyt, A. (1994). Prospective evaluation of technetium 99m HMPAO-SPECT in mild and moderate traumatic brain injury. *Journal of Nuclear Medicine, 35*, 942–947.

Jansen, H. M. L., van der Naalt, J., & van Zomeren, A. H. (1996). Cobalt-55 positron emission tomography in traumatic brain injury: A pilot study. *Journal of Neurology, Neurosurgery, and Psychiatry, 60*, 221–224.

Kado, H., Komuro, T., Shimogawara, M., & Uehara, G. (1996). Development of a multichannel SQUID system for magnetoencephalogram applications. *Electroencephalography and Clinical Neurophysiology, 47*, 405–415.

King, D. W, Park, Y. D., Smith, J. R., & Wheless, J. W. (2000). Magnetoencephalography in neocortical epilepsy. *Advances in Neurology, 84*, 415–423.

Krystal, J. H., Woods, S.W., Kosten, T. R., & Rosen, M. I. (1995). Opiate dependence and withdrawal: Preliminary assessment using single photon emission computerized tomography (SPECT). *American Journal of Drug and Alcohol Abuse, 21*, 47–63.

Kuroglu, A. C., Arikan, Z., & Vural, G. (1996). Single photon emission computerized tomography in chronic alcoholism. *British Journal of Psychiatry, 169*, 348–354.

Langfitt, T. W., Obrist, W. D., Alavia, A., Grossman, R. I., Zimmerman, R., Jaggi, J., et al. (1986). Computerized tomography, magnetic resonance imaging, and positron emission tomography in the study of brain trauma. *Journal of Neurosurgery, 64*, 760–767.

Lazarus, A., & Cotterell, K. P. (1989). SPECT scan reveals abnormality in somatization disorder patient. *Journal of Clinical Psychiatry, 50*, 475–476.

Levine, B., Cabeza, R., McIntosh, A. R., Black, S. E., Grady, C. L., & Stuss, D. T. (2002). Functional reorganisation of memory after traumatic brain injury: A study with H_2-^{15}O positron emission tomography. *Journal of Neurology, Neurosurgery, and Psychiatry, 73*, 173–181.

Loutfi, I., & Singh, A. (1995). A comparison of quantitative methods for brain single photon emission computed tomography analysis in head trauma and stroke. *Investigative Radiology, 30*, 588–594.

Luccas, F. J., Anghinah, R., Braga, N. I., Fonseca, L. C., Frochtengarten, M. L., Jorge, M. S., et al. (1999). Guidelines for recording/analyzing quantitative EEG and evoked potentials. *Arquivas Neuropsiquiatras, 57*, 132–146.

Mampunza, S., Verbanck, P., Verhas, M., & Martin, P. (1995). Cerebral blood flow in just detoxified alcohol dependent patients: A 99mTc-HMPAO-SPECT study. *Acta Neurologia Belgica, 95*, 164–169.

Masdeu, J. C., & Brass, L. M. (1995). SPECT imaging of stroke. *Journal of Neuroimaging*, *5*(Suppl. 1), 14–22.

Matousek, M., Takuchi, I., Starmark, J., & Stalhammer, D. (1996). Quantitative EEG analysis as a supplement to the clinical coma scale. *Acta Anaesthesiologica Scandinavica*, *40*, 824–831.

Mayberg, H. (1996). Medical-legal inferences from functional neuroimaging evidence. *Seminars in Clinical Neuropsychiatry*, *1*, 195–201.

McAllister, T. W., Saykin, A. J., Flashman, L. A., Sparling, M. B., Johnson, S. C., Guerin, S. J., et al. (1999). Brain activation during working memory 1 month after mild traumatic brain injury: A functional MRI study. *Neurology*, *53*, 1300–1308.

McAllister, T. W., Sparling, M. B., Flashman, L. A., Guerin, S. J., Mamourian, A. C., & Saykin, A. J. (2001). Differential working memory load effects after mild traumatic brain injury. *NeuroImage*, *14*, 1004–1012.

Miller, B. L., Mina, I., Giombetti, R., & Villanueva-Meyer, J. (1992). Neuropsychiatric effects of cocaine: SPECT measurements. *Journal of Addictive Disorders*, *11*, 47–58.

Modell, J. G., & Mountz, J. M. (1995). Focal cerebral blood flow change during craving for alcohol measured by SPECT. *Journal of Neuropsychiatry and Clinical Neurosciences*, *7*, 15–22.

Morrow, L. A., Steinhauer, S. R., & Hodgson, M. J. (1992). Delay in P300 latency in patients with organic solvent exposure. *Archives of Neurology*, *49*, 315–320.

Mozley, P. D., Kim, H. J., & Gur, R. C. (1996). Iodine-123-IPT SPECT imaging of CNS dopamine transporters: Nonlinear effects of normal aging on striatal uptake values. *Journal of Nuclear Medicine*, *37*, 1965–1970.

Nuwer, M. (1997). Assessment of digital EEG, quantitative EEG, and EEG brain mapping. Report of the American Academy of Neurology and the American Clinical Neurophysiology Society. *Neurology*, *49*, 277–292.

Nuwer, M. R. (1990). On the controversies about clinical use of EEG brain mapping. *Brain Tomography*, *3*, 103–111.

Paulman, R. G., Devous, M. D., & Gregory, R. R. (1990). Hypofrontality and cognitive impairment in schizophrenia: Dynamic single photon tomography and neuropsychological assessment of schizophrenic brain function. *Biological Psychiatry*, *27*, 377–399.

Pietrini, P., Guazzelli, M., & Basso, G. (2000). Neural correlates of imaginal aggressive behavior assessed by positron emission tomography in healthy subjects. *American Journal of Psychiatry*, *157*, 1772–1781.

Raichle, M. E. (2001). Functional neuroimaging: A historical and physiological perspective. In R. Cabeza & A. Kingstone (Eds.), *Handbook of functional neuroimaging of cognition* (pp. 3–26). Cambridge, MA: MIT Press.

Raine, A., Buchsbaum, M., & LaCasse, L. (1997). Brain abnormalities in murderers indicated by positron emission tomography. *Biological Psychiatry*, *42*, 495–508.

Raine, A., Meloy, J. R., & Bihrle, S. (1998). Reduced prefrontal and increased subcortical brain functioning assessed using positron emission tomography in predatory and affective murderers. *Behavioral Sciences and the Law*, *16*, 319–332.

Rao, N., Turski, P. A., Polcyn, R. E., Nickels, R. J., Matthews, C. G., & Flynn, M. M. (1984). 18-F Positron emission computed tomography in closed head injury. *Archives of Physical Medicine and Rehabilitation*, *65*, 780–785.

Read, S. L., Miler, B. L., Mena, I., & Kim, R. (1995). SPECT in dementia: Clinical and pathological correlation. *Journal of the American Geriatrics Society*, *42*, 1243–1247.

Reinhardt, F., Drexler, H., Bickel, A., Claus, D., Ulm, K., Angerer, J., et al. (1997).

Electrophysiological investigation of central, peripheral and autonomic nerve function in workers with long-term low-level exposure to carbon disulphide in the viscose industry. *International Archives of Occupational and Environmental Health*, *70*, 249–256.

Ricker, J. H. (2004). Functional neuroimaging in medical rehabilitation populations. In J. DeLisa & B. Gans (Eds.), *Rehabilitation medicine* (4th ed., pp. 229–242). Philadelphia: Lippincott-Raven.

Ricker, J. H., Müller, R. A., Zafonte, R. D., Black, K., Millis, S. R., & Chugani, H. (2001). Verbal recall and recognition following traumatic brain injury: A [15O]-water positron emission tomography study. *Journal of Clinical and Experimental Neuropsychology*, *23*, 196–206.

Ricker, J. H., & Zafonte, R. D. (2000). Functional neuroimaging in traumatic head injury: Clinical applications and interpretive cautions. *Journal of Head Trauma Rehabilitation*, *15*(2), 859–868.

Roland, P. (1993). *Brain activation*. New York: Wiley-Liss.

Rosenberg, N. L., Spitz, M. C., Filley, C. M., Davis, K. A., & Schaumberg, H. H. (1988). Central nervous system effects of chronic toluene abuse—Clinical, brainstem evoked response and magnetic resonance imaging studies. *Neurotoxicology and Teratology*, *10*, 489–495.

Ruff, R., Crouch, J. A., Troester, A. I., Marshall, L. F., Buchsbaum, M. S., Lottenberg, S., et al. (1994). Selected cases of poor outcome following a minor brain trauma: Comparing neuropsychological and PET assessment. *Brain Injury*, *8*, 297–308.

Sackheim, H. A, Prohovnik, I., & Moeller, J. (1990). Regional cerebral blood flow in mood disorders: Comparison of major depressives and normal controls at rest. *Archives of General Psychiatry*, *47*, 60–70.

Sironi, V. (1983). Diagnostic and prognostic value of spectral analysis in posttraumatic coma. In R. Vilans (Ed.), *Advances in neurotraumatology* (pp. 329–330). Amsterdam: Excerpta Medica.

Skrandies, W. (1995). Visual information processing: Topography of brain electrical activity. *Biological Psychology*, *40*, 1–15.

Springer, C. S., Patlak, C. S., Playka, I., & Huang, W. (2000). Principles of susceptability contrast-based functional MRI: The sign of the functional response. In C. T. Moonen & P. A. Bandettini (Eds.), *Functional MRI* (pp. 91–102). Berlin: Springer-Verlag.

Stern, E., & Silbersweig, D. A. (2001). Advances in functional neuroimaging methodology for the study of brain systems underlying human neuropsychological function and dysfunction. *Journal of Clinical and Experimental Neuropsychology*, *23*, 3–18.

Tang, A. C., Pearlmutter, B. A., Malaszenko, N. A., Phung, D. B., & Reeb, B. C. (2002). Independent components of magnetoencephalography: Localization. *Neural Computation*, *14*, 1827–1858.

Teasdale, G., & Jennett, B. (1974). Assessment of coma and impaired consciousness. *Lancet*, *2*, 81–84.

Tenjin, H., Ueda, S., & Mizukawa, N. (1990). Positron emission tomographic studies on cerebral hemodynamics in patients with cerebral contusion. *Neurosurgery*, *26*, 971–979.

Thatcher, R. W., Walker, R. A., Gerson, I. & Geisler, F. H. (1989). EEG discriminant analysis of mild head trauma. *Electroencephalography and Clinical Neurophysiology*, *73*, 94–106.

Therapeutics and Technology Subcommittee of the American Academy of Neurology. (1996). Assessment of brain SPECT. *Neurology*, *46*, 278–285.

Triebig, G., & Lang, C. (1993). Brain imaging techniques applied to chronically solvent-exposed workers: Current results and clinical evaluation. *Environmental Research, 61*, 239–250.

Uchiyama, M., Sue, H., Fukumitsu, N., Mori, Y., & Kawakami, K. (1997). Assessment of cerebral benzodiazepine receptor distribution in anxiety disorders by 123-I iomazenil SPECT. *Nippon Acta Radiologica, 57*, 41–46.

Umile, E. M., Plotkin, R. C., & Sandel, M. E. (1998). Functional assessment of mild traumatic brain injury using SPECT and neuropsychological assessment. *Brain Injury, 12*, 577–594.

Urban, P., & Lukas, E. (1990). Visual evoked potentials in rotogravure printers exposed to toluene. *British Journal of Industrial Medicine, 47*, 819–823.

Volkow, N. D., & Tancredi, L. (1987). Neural substrates of violent behavior: A preliminary study with positron emission tomography. *British Journal of Psychiatry, 151*, 668–673.

Volkow, N. D., Tancredi, L. R., & Grant, C. (1995). Brain glucose metabolism in violent psychiatric patients: A preliminary study. *Psychiatry Research, 61*, 243–253.

Wallace, B. E., Wagner, A. K., Wagner, E. P., & McDeavitt, J. T. (2001). A history and review of quantitative electroencephalography in traumatic brain injury. *Journal of Head Trauma Rehabilitation, 16*, 165–190.

Weisskoff, R. M. (2000). Basic theoretical models of BOLD signal change. In C.T. Moonen & P. A. Bandettini (Eds.), *Functional MRI* (pp. 115–123). Berlin: Springer-Verlag.

Whitebread, C. H., & Slobogin, C. (1993). *Criminal procedure: An analysis of cases and concepts* (3rd ed.). New York: Foundation Press.

Wood, F., Flowers, L., Buschbaum, M., & Tallal, P. (1991). Investigation of abnormal left temporal functioning in dyslexia through rCBF, auditory evoked potentials, and positron emission tomography. Special issue: Genetic and neurological influences on reading disability. *Reading and Writing, 3*, 379–393.

Zhang, J. J., Park, C. H., & Kim, S. M. (1994). Brain SPECT artifact in multidetector SPECT systems. *Clinical Nuclear Medicine, 19*, 789–791.

6

Forensic Aspects of Pediatric Traumatic Brain Injury

JACOBUS DONDERS

Traumatic brain injury (TBI) is an acquired condition in which the head is subjected to acute external mechanical forces that cause alteration in the physiological functioning of the brain and possibly physical brain damage. Pediatric TBI is a significant public health problem, not only because about 30% of all childhood injury deaths result from TBI, but also because there is considerable neurobehavioral morbidity in the survivors of childhood TBI.

Although there are many other forms of acquired brain injury in children, such as stroke or tumor, as well as congenital (e.g., Down syndrome) and perinatal (e.g., hypoxia) forms of brain compromise, those conditions are outside the scope of this review. Furthermore, because several overviews of general aspects of pediatric TBI are available (Arffa, 1998; Donders & Kuldanek, 1998; Yeates, 2000), the main goal of this chapter is to provide an update of the most recent neurobehavioral research, with a specific focus on the forensic aspects of TBI in children.

EPIDEMIOLOGY AND PATHOPHYSIOLOGY

Incidence statistics vary considerably across studies because of differences in definition, such as the degree of equating any injury to the head as a "brain" injury. Furthermore, studies are inconsistent regarding the inclusion of those children who died prior to arrival at the emergency room. In one of the most comprehensive reviews of various studies to date, Kraus (1995) estimated an average incidence of 180 per 100,000 children per year. Rates for boys are about 1.3 to 2.0 times greater than those for girls (F. P. Rivara, 1994). Falls are a common cause in young children, but with increasing age, motor vehicle accidents account for the majority of the more severe injuries (DiScala, Osberg, Gans, et al., 1991).

It must be realized that many cases of childhood TBI are preventable. For example, alcohol abuse and perception of injury risk by parents are much more meaningful predictors of accidental injury in children than a developmental personality characteristic of being "accident prone" (F. P. Rivara, 1995). Furthermore, available protective measures are not used consistently or most effectively. For example, properly installed car seats or three-point restraints offer relative protection to young children against the risk of sustaining severe TBI, but only if the children travel in the back seat (Agran, Castillo, & Winn, 1992; Marshall, Koch, & Egelhoff, 1998). Similarly, although bicycle helmets can offer substantial protection against TBI, they do not work if they are not fitted or worn correctly (Attewell, Glase, & McFadden, 2001; F. P. Rivara, Astley, Clarren, et al., 1999; Thompson, Rivara, & Thompson, 1996). Improvements are also needed regarding the ability of health care professionals to recognize risks of serious child abuse TBI before it takes place (Hicks & Gaughan, 1995; L. Miller, 1999).

The majority of cases of pediatric TBI can likely be considered "mild" in nature in the sense that they are not associated with prolonged coma or intracranial lesions on neuroimaging. However, there are several systems for the classification of severity of TBI. Some of these were initially developed for use with adults, so some caution is necessary when applying them to children. For example, estimates of posttraumatic amnesia may be difficult to obtain for young children with limited verbal skills, and such estimates are notoriously unreliable when they are obtained retrospectively.

The Glasgow Coma Scale (GCS) is a widely used ordinal ranking of severity, with scores ranging from 3 to 15. Scores below 8 suggest severe injury, scores 9–12 reflect moderate injury, and scores 13–15 indicate mild injury (Teasdale & Jennett, 1974). However, reliability of this scale may be compromised when children are sedated or when they have compromise of other parts of the body, such as intubation or spinal cord injury. Furthermore, it is customary to classify an injury as either "complicated mild" or "moderate" when the GCS exceeds 12 but is accompanied by an intracranial lesion on neuroimaging, although skull fractures do not necessarily meet this criterion (Williams, Levin, & Eisenberg, 1990). In addition, focal neurological signs such as pupillary reflex abnormalities may also signify more serious injury (Capruso & Levin, 1992; Prasad, Ewing-Cobbs, Swank, et al., 2002).

For all of these reasons, exclusive reliance on the total score of the GCS is not advised with pediatric TBI. However, the time to which children follow verbal commands (equivalent to a score of 6 on the Motor subscale on the GCS) appears to be a fairly reliable and commonly used indicator of length of coma (Massagli, Michaud, & Rivara, 1996).

It also needs to be realized that, although computed tomography (CT) scan is the most common and appropriate technique to evaluate acute lesions on the day of impact, some lesions do not become apparent until days later. With severe TBI, longer term posttraumatic hydrocephalus or seizures can also occur (McLean, Kaitz, Kennan, et al., 1995) and some chronic neurodegenerative changes do not become fully stable until evaluated with magnetic resonance imaging months or years later (Bigler, 1999).

The mechanisms by which TBI causes brain impairment are multifactorial and involve both primary and secondary injuries. Most often, there is an accelerating or decelerating force to the skull that can cause primary disruption of the underlying brain matter at the time of trauma. Such forces include linear displacement, which causes focal lesions such as cortical contusions and subdural hemorrhage, and intracranial rotation, which may result in diffuse lesions such as axonal shearing (Ghajar & Hariri, 1992; Noah, Hahn, Rubenstein, et al., 1992). Focal lesions in the frontal areas are common, but studies are not entirely consistent regarding the unique role that such focal lesions play in neurobehavioral outcome (Dennis, Guger, Roncadin, et al., 2001; Levin, Song, Scheibel, et al., 2000; Mendelsohn, Levin, Bruce, et al., 1992; Slomine, Gerring, Grados, et al., 2002). Involvement of subcortical structures and white matter tracts has also been associated with an increased risk for long-term neurobehavioral deficits (Gerring, Brady, Chen, et al., 2000; Levin, Benavidez, Verger-Maestre, et al., 2000; Verger, Junque, Levin, et al., 2001).

Secondary injuries are those that arise indirectly from trauma and may continue to develop for several days after injury. In children, they are most often the result of disrupted cerebral circulation and an associated cascade of neurochemical events, leading to hypoxic–ischemic injury and diffuse edema. There is growing evidence that adequate management of cerebral homeostasis, especially cerebral perfusion pressure, is one of the most critical variables regarding survival after pediatric TBI (Downard, Hulka, Mullins, et al., 2000; Hackbarth, Rzeszutko, Sturm, et al., 2002).

COMMON NEUROBEHAVIORAL SEQUELAE

It has been well established that severe TBI is associated with an increased likelihood of deficits in speed of information processing, memory for new information, executive functioning, and interpersonal pragmatics (for reviews, see Donders & Kuldanek, 1998, and Yeates, 2000). There is also growing consensus that the majority of children who sustain uncomplicated mild TBI have an essentially unremarkable long-term recovery (Fay, Jaffe, Polissar, et al., 1993; Light, Asarnow, Satz, et al., 1998; Satz, Zaucha, McCleary, et al., 1997). It is also abundantly clear that there is no such thing as a unitary profile of cognitive and psychosocial strengths and weaknesses after pediatric TBI. In fact, various distinct subtypes of recovery have been identified in both domains and related to injury severity characteristics (Butler, Rourke, Fuerst, et al., 1997; Donders & Warschausky, 1997). Rather than discussing the entire literature on all the possible neurobehavioral consequences of TBI, this review focuses selectively on the most recent and methodically sound outcome research.

One of the most significant developments over the past decade has been an increased appreciation of the need to include a control group when considering the long-term outcome after pediatric TBI. Early studies (e.g., Jaffe, Fay, Polissar, et al., 1992; Massagli, Jaffe, Fay, et al., 1996) used control participants who were matched to children with TBI on the basis of demographic and premorbid achievement characteristics. This methodology was useful to demonstrate that comparisons with controls often demonstrated greater proportions or greater magnitudes of deficits in neurobehavioral sequelae than did comparisons with population-based test norms. For example, although the average Performance IQ of children with severe TBI appeared to be well within the average range at 3 years postinjury, statistically it was significantly below that of the matched control group (Fay, Jaffe, Polissar, et al., 1994).

A potential problem with exclusive reliance on healthy controls is that such children cannot be equated to children with TBI in terms of the experience of a traumatic injury, hospitalization, or medical treatment, all of which can be stressful and potentially interfere with psychological functioning. This is an important consideration because it has been shown that children with mild TBI may appear to have neurobehavioral impairments when compared to children without injuries, but they tend to be indistinguishable in this regard from children with injuries to other parts of the body not involving the head (Asarnow, Satz, Light, et al., 1995; Bijur & Haslum, 1995). This also holds true for children with a history of multiple mild head injuries, as long as these are spaced apart several months, when compared to children with a history of multiple orthopedic injuries (Bijur, Haslum, & Golding, 1996).

One of the most comprehensive recent series of longitudinal studies of neurobehavioral recovery after pediatric TBI was done by Taylor and his colleagues (Taylor, Yeates, Wade, et al. 2001, 2002; Wade, Taylor, Drotar, et al., 2002; Yeates, Taylor, Wade, et al., 2002). These studies included baseline measures of premorbid status as well as a control group with orthopedic injuries. Moreover, the children were followed for an average of 4 years, which is considerably longer than many other studies. In addition, the investigators included a wide range of assessments of cognitive, behavioral, and psychosocial factors, and they employed multivariate statistical procedures to consider the additive and interactive effects of multiple potential predictor variables.

Yeates, Taylor, Wade, and colleagues (2002) found that, from a cognitive point of view, children with severe TBI continued to demonstrate considerable deficits at extended follow-up compared to both children with orthopedic injuries and children with moderate TBI. The effect sizes for these differences were largest on tasks requiring speed of information processing and explicit delayed recall of new information. These are areas that appear to be especially vulnerable to the effects of severe TBI in children (Anderson, Catroppa, Rosenfeld, et al., 2000; Hoffman, Donders, & Thompson, 2000; Levin, Song, et al., 2000; Roman, Delis, Willerman, et al., 1998; Tremont, Mittenberg, & Miller, 1999).

Taylor and colleagues (2002) also demonstrated that behavioral adjustment changes persist years after injury in children with severe TBI. However, these outcomes were moderated strongly by family characteristics, unlike the cognitive recovery, which was predicted more directly by injury severity. Other prospective studies by Max and colleagues have confirmed that severe TBI is a direct risk factor for a range of novel psychiatric disorders (Max, Koele, Castillo, et al., 2000; Max, Koele, Smith, et al., 1998). Furthermore, a moderating effect of psychosocial factors (e.g., socioeconomic status, preinjury family functioning) was found for symptoms such as oppositional-defiant behavior, but not for novel attention-deficit/hyperactivity disorder (ADHD; Max, Castillo, Bokura, et al., 1998; Max, Lindgren, Knudsen, et al., 1998). Although the psychiatric disorders covered a wide spectrum, the most common and most disabling symptoms were affective instability, aggression, and impaired social judgment. Children with severe TBI also demonstrated difficulties with social problem solving, even in the absence of overt psychiatric malfunction, which can contribute to difficulties with peer integration (Bohnert, Parker, & Warschausky, 1997; Janusz, Kirkwood, Yeates, et al., 2002; Warschausky, Cohen, Parker, et al., 1997).

Impairment in high-level language skills is another area that has been studied extensively over the past few years in children with TBI. It has been well established that even severe TBI typically does not result in lasting impairments of tests of overlearned and lower-level language skills, such as reflected in Verbal IQ scores and traditional language tests (Chapman, Watkins, Gustafson, et al., 1997; Donders, 1997). However, children with severe TBI do tend to have significant difficulties with the organizational and abstraction aspects of verbal discourse (Chapman, McKinnon, Levin, et al., 2001; Ewing-Cobbs, Brookshire, Scott, et al., 1998) and with the semantic and pragmatic aspects of language (Dennis & Barnes, 2001).

The work by Dennis and colleagues has clearly illustrated the difficulties that children with severe TBI have with inferencing and detecting intentionality in the speech of others (Barnes & Dennis, 2001; Dennis, Purvis, Barnes, et al., 2001), as well as with producing pragmatic speech acts of their own (Dennis &

Barnes, 2000). These problems also extend to text comprehension, for which children with severe TBI may not have impairments in literal comprehension, but have difficulties with inferencing and intentionality aspects (Dennis & Barnes, 2001).

SPECIAL EDUCATION SERVICES

In light of the significant neurobehavioral sequelae that have been described with severe pediatric TBI, it is no surprise that considerable proportions of these children need special education services for extended periods of time (Clark, Russman, & Orme, 1999; Ewing-Cobbs, Fletcher, Levin, et al., 1998; Kinsella, Prior, Sawyer, et al., 1997). Recently, L. J. Miller and Donders (2003) demonstrated that scores on the California Verbal Learning Test–Children's Version (Delis, Kramer, Kaplan, et al., 1994), obtained at an average of 3 months after injury, were more accurate in the prediction of special education placement 2 years later than a host of demographic (age, gender, parental occupational status) and injury (length of coma and lesions on neuroimaging) variables. This predictive power, as illustrated in Figure 6-1, reinforces the criterion validity of neuropsychological assessment in children with TBI.

Longitudinal research has also demonstrated that a considerable minority of children with residual neurobehavioral sequelae of TBI who could profit from

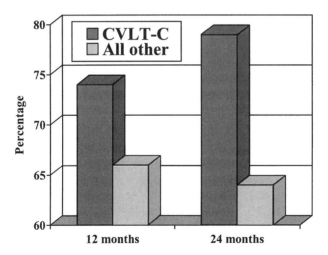

FIGURE 6-1. Proportions of all children at 12 and 24 months after traumatic brain injury ($n = 58$), correctly classified by initial level of performance on the California Verbal Learning Test–Children's Version (CVLT-C) and by combined demographic and injury variables (All other). From L. J. Miller & Donders (2003). Copyright © by the American Psychological Association. Reprinted with permission.

special education support are not receiving adequate services (Taylor, Yeates, Wade, et al., 2003). Thus, even when neuropsychological assessment is helpful in establishing risks and characterizing the problems that contribute to academic difficulties in children with TBI, this does not automatically guarantee efficient or adequate service delivery. For this reason, knowledge of federal and state guidelines regarding eligibility for special education services is important.

Under U.S. public law enacted as part of the Individuals With Disabilities Education Act (1990), TBI was defined as a separate category of special education in 1991. The following definition of TBI was included in this legislation:

Traumatic brain injury means an acquired injury to the brain caused by an external physical force, resulting in total or partial functional disability or psychosocial impairment, or both, that adversely affects a child's educational performance. The term applies to open or closed head injuries resulting in impairments in one or more areas, such as cognition; language; memory; attention; reasoning; abstract thinking; judgment; problem solving; sensory, perceptual, and motor abilities; psychosocial behavior; physical functions; information processing; and speech. The term does not apply to brain injuries that are congenital or degenerative or brain injuries induced by birth.

It is important to realize that states differ widely in their level of embracement or expansion of this federal definition. States cannot use a definition of TBI that is more restrictive than the federal one, but they are at liberty to adopt a more inclusive definition. For example, some states have added provisions to include children under the definition of TBI who acquired their brain injury as the result of vascular (e.g., stroke) or hypoxic (e.g., near-drowning) conditions (Katsiyannis & Conderman, 1994). Therefore, it is crucial that both families and providers be aware of their local state laws in this regard. This kind of information can typically be obtained from the state's Department of Education.

Regardless of the state or local jurisdiction, there are federal principles under the Individuals With Disabilities Education Act regarding the special education process (for a review, see Savage, Lash, Bennett, et al., 1995). These principles govern that any student with TBI should be able to receive a free and appropriate public education based on a nondiscriminatory evaluation, and that this education should take place in the environment that is the least restrictive for the child. Parents should be active participants in this process, and there should be a set of procedures regarding accountability, generally known as due process.

To be considered for any kind of special education placement (whether this is for TBI or not), the child must be referred to the school system's special education services committee. For many children with TBI who receive hospital-based rehabilitation services, such a referral can often be made (with parental consent) by treating professionals. In other instances, the parents may need to request an evaluation or meeting on their own. By law, schools cannot ignore such a referral.

The most appropriate services for a child with TBI will be determined by an individualized educational planning committee (IEPC), which should include an individual with some specialized training in the area of the suspected disability (i.e., sequelae of TBI). Parents have the right to be members of this team, and they are allowed to have assistance in this regard. For example, many states have "parent advocacy" programs.

The IEPC should result in a statement regarding eligibility for services, specific goals, a delineation of the accommodations and adaptations for the child, as well as a recommendation for specific placement. If parents do not agree with the decision of the IEPC, they have the right to request an arbitration or mediation hearing. State laws differ widely on time frames in this regard and regarding the degree to which parents can request a free independent evaluation for a second opinion. However, the mediation process cannot be used to deny or delay a due process hearing, and the results of the mediation are not binding (Lorber & Yurk, 1999). A due process hearing is administered by an impartial hearing officer of the court, and pediatric neuropsychologists may be called on as expert witnesses in this context. Rulings from due process hearings are binding to all parties involved.

Especially with children with TBI, who tend to change in their performance and needs over time, IEPC plans may need to be reviewed more frequently than the yearly (or sometimes once every 3 years) customary standard. More detailed reviews about special education procedures that have been written in language intelligible to most teachers and many parents include the work of Glang, Singer, and Todis (1997), Savage and Wolcott (1994), and Semrud-Clikeman (2001).

DEMOGRAPHIC MODERATING VARIABLES

There is no doubt that the likelihood of long-term neurobehavioral sequelae of pediatric TBI increases with greater injury severity. However, even among children with severe TBI, outcomes tend to vary considerably. There are several demographic variables that may play a moderating role in this regard. A *moderator* is defined as a variable that specifies the circumstances under which a condition results in a particular outcome (Holmbeck, 2002). In this case, the nature of the relationship between severity of TBI and neurobehavioral outcome varies as a function of some demographic characteristics of the child and family.

One of the most significant demographic influences on recovery after TBI is age. There are three distinct but interrelated dimensions of age that need to be considered in this regard (Dennis & Barnes, 1994; Taylor & Alden, 1997): age at injury, time since injury, and age at assessment of outcome.

Until the early 1990s, there was a common lore that the earlier in life the TBI occurred, the better it was because of a presumed great degree of plasticity in children's brains. This myth has clearly been debunked. There is strong evidence that TBI acquired early in life interferes with skills that are still in a phase of rapid development, which puts young children at increased risk for long-term deficits (Anderson, Morse, Klug, et al., 1997; Chapman & McKinnon, 2000; Ewing-Cobbs, Fletcher, Levin, et al., 1997; Woodward, Winterhalter, Donders, et al., 1999). Longitudinal research has suggested that children with severe TBI tend to show partial recovery during the first year after injury, but that this recovery reaches a plateau after that time, and there remain considerable residual neurobehavioral deficits at extended follow-up (Yeates, Taylor, Wade, et al., 2002). It is important to realize that this recovery trend was much more apparent for cognitive than for behavioral adjustment characteristics (Taylor et al., 2002). Other researchers have demonstrated that some neurobehavioral deficits may not become fully manifest until the child gets older (Fay et al., 1994). This may reflect an interaction of delayed maturation of specific (especially frontal) brain regions with an increase in the complexity of environmental demands on the child.

Investigations have also suggested that, in gender groups who were equated for injury and other demographic characteristics, boys tended to have more significant difficulties with speed of information processing and recall after TBI than girls (Donders & Hoffman, 2002; Donders & Woodward, 2003). This suggests that the effects of TBI may also be moderated by gender. Furthermore, several studies have suggested that socioeconomic status is important regarding the long-term neurobehavioral outcome after pediatric TBI, with more significant negative consequences in children from disadvantaged backgrounds (Kirkwood, Janusz, Yeates, et al., 2000; Max, Castillo, et al., 1998). However, the exact influence of socioeconomic status, independent of other factors is somewhat difficult to determine in light of the relatively higher attrition rates for children from less-advantaged backgrounds over extended follow-up (Taylor et al., 2003; Woodward et al., 1999).

FAMILY CHARACTERISTICS

When children sustain severe TBI, family life gets interrupted, and yet parents often need to be the most important long-term advocates for their children. Research over the past decade has provided important information about family dynamics and family outcomes as related to pediatric TBI. Family factors account for variability in children's neurobehavioral outcomes over and above that explained by injury-related variables, and a more adaptive preinjury family environment may act as a buffer regarding the impact of TBI (Anderson, Catroppa, Haritou, et al., 2001; Kinsella, Ong, Murtagh, et al., 1999; Max, Roberts,

Koele, et al., 1999; J. B. Rivara, Jaffe, Polissar, et al., 1996; Taylor, Yeates, Drotar, et al., 1997; Wade, Borawski, Taylor, et al., 2001; Yeates, Taylor, Drotar, et al., 1997). Examples of more adaptive family coping include open communication, lack of rigidity, equitable and efficient role distributions, and acceptance.

A good example of the moderating influence of family environment on neurobehavioral recovery from TBI comes from the work by Taylor and colleagues (Taylor et al., 2002). Figure 6-2 shows how recovery of mathematics skills was moderated by family stressors. Specifically, the group with severe TBI showed a rapid rate of recovery, compared to the other two groups, but only when the children's families did not experience a great degree of stress.

Longitudinal research has confirmed that substantial proportions of families of children who have experienced a severe TBI continue to report high levels of injury-related stress associated with some aspect of the child's recovery or the family's reactions many years later (Wade et al., 2002). However, it is important to realize that the influences between child neurobehavioral problems and family adjustment are bidirectional in nature. This was clearly illustrated by Taylor and colleagues, who used path analysis to model these reciprocal influences over time (Taylor et al., 2001). More child behaviors at 6 months after moderate-to-severe TBI predicted higher parental distress at 12 months, controlling for earlier family outcomes at 6 months; and higher parental distress at 6 months was associated with more child behaviors at 12 months, controlling for earlier behavior problems.

It has also been suggested that differences in ratings of parental distress and burden between groups with pediatric orthopedic versus brain injuries may be less pronounced for parents of African American children than for parents of Caucasian children at baseline, but that these negative consequences became more pronounced at follow-up (Yeates, Taylor, Woodrome, et al., 2002). However, the overall influence of ethnicity on children's outcome remains underexplored in the research on pediatric TBI.

COMPLICATING PREMORBID HISTORIES

Most studies of pediatric TBI have excluded children with premorbid complicating histories to avoid potential confounding of results. However, neuropsychologists are often asked to determine whether persistent postinjury neurobehavioral complaints or symptoms are caused by TBI, preexisting conditions such as ADHD, or both.

Several studies have documented that lower levels of preinjury functioning increase the risk for less-favorable outcome after pediatric TBI, both for the child (Ponsford, Wilmott, Rothwell, et al., 1999; Woodward et al., 1999) and for the family (J. B. Rivara et al., 1996; Wade, Taylor, Drotar, et al., 1996).

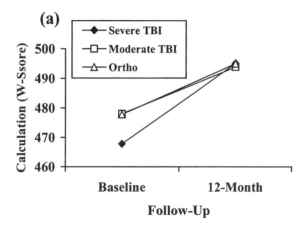

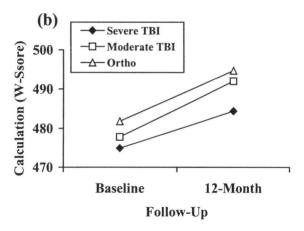

FIGURE 6-2. Model estimates of group mean W scores on the Calculation subtest of the Woodcock-Johnson Tests of Academic Achievement–Revised (Woodcock & Mather, 1989) at the baseline and the 12-month follow-up for children with (a) low and (b) high levels of family stressors (i.e., those from unstressed vs. stressed families) as defined by scores 1 *SD* below and 1 *SD* above the sample mean. The plots show catch-up in math skills in the group with severe traumatic brain injury (TBI) relative to the group with orthopedic injury (Ortho), but only when family stressors were low. From Taylor et al. (2002). Copyright © by the American Psychological Association. Adapted and reprinted with permission.

However, such group studies do not allow easy determination of which children with prior complicating histories do or do not have additional problems after TBI. Another interpretive problem is because some of the neurobehavioral symptoms that children may demonstrate after TBI are not specific to that condition. For example, children with mood disorders but without TBI may demonstrate difficulties with attention or memory (Livingston, Stark, Haak, et al., 1996; Moradi, Doost, Taghavi, et al., 1999), and children with ADHD and no history of TBI often have difficulties with executive skills (Barkley, 1997; Bayliss & Roodenrys, 2000; Seidman, Biederman, Faraone, et al., 1997). Differences were also found between children with and those without maltreatment-related posttraumatic stress disorder (excluding cases of TBI) on measures of attention and executive function (Beers & De Bellis, 2002).

Thus, it cannot be assumed on the basis of the presence of symptoms that are known to be common after TBI that the associated cause must be TBI. This kind of reverse reasoning would amount to a logical fallacy with a high likelihood of misattribution, particularly when dealing with children with mild TBI, for whom the preponderance of the studies does not suggest persistent injury-related sequelae (Satz et al., 1997).

Although things may appear to be less complicated with moderate-to-severe TBI, diagnostic inferences are not a panacea with increasing injury severity either. Specifically, it has been suggested that moderate-to-severe TBI with subcortical involvement may result in "secondary" ADHD that mimics closely the profile of children with preexisting ADHD, and that this is more likely to happen with children from maladjusted families, again suggesting a moderating influence of family environment (Gerring, Brady, Chen, et al., 1998, 2000). For all of these reasons, it is imperative that clinicians obtain premorbid academic and health records for children with TBI.

Several studies have indicated that the postinjury neuropsychological test scores of children with learning disabilities or psychiatric disorders who subsequently sustained a moderate-to-severe TBI were virtually undistinguishable from those of demographically matched children who sustained TBI of similar severity, but who did not have complicating premorbid histories (Donders & Strom, 1997, 2000). It was only through formal comparison with premorbid test results that a further deterioration in functioning as the result of TBI could be demonstrated in the children with preexisting conditions.

CHILD ABUSE

Child abuse TBI affects primarily children under 3 years of age (J. K. Brown & Minns, 1993). In fact, it has been suggested that the less-favorable neurobehavioral outcome after infant or preschool TBI compared to other age groups in epidemiological studies may be at least partly because of the high rate of inflicted injury in the youngest children (Ewing-Cobbs, Duhaime, & Fletcher, 1995). Of these, the shaken-baby condition, in which the child is subjected to rapid angular acceleration–deceleration forces that are sometimes compounded by actual impact, has the greatest mortality and morbidity (Duhaime, Christian, Moss, et al., 1996). However, the extent and implications of child abuse TBI are uncertain for various reasons.

First, it is difficult to obtain exact estimates of the prevalence of the problem. The most recently available statistics suggest that child abuse occurs in at least 13–15 per 1,000 children, but this may be a gross underestimation because of inconsistencies in definition and underreporting by perpetrators (Ammerman & Galvin, 1998; Knutson & DeVet, 1995). A second problem is that family instability and confidentiality restrictions make it difficult to follow many children longitudinally (Duhaime et al., 1996). Furthermore, nonabusive experiences such as parental neglect, poverty, and a highly stressed family environment are common comorbid factors that can confound measurement of the incremental significance of the physical trauma (G. W. Brown, 2002).

Despite all of these difficulties, there have been important new developments in the field of child abuse brain injury over the past several years. Several studies have identified hypoxic–ischemic injury as one of the most damaging factors affecting mortality and neurobehavioral morbidity after inflicted childhood TBI, with a possible secondary augmenting effect of neurotoxicity because of a sharp increase in excitatory amino acids (Geddes, Vowles, Hackshaw, et al., 2001; Ruppel, Kochanek, Adelson, et al., 2001; Stoodley, 2002). After controlling for other demographic variables, minority status and substance abuse appear to be risk factors for child abuse TBI, and such type of injury is in turn a risk factor for more severe brain compromise (Wagner, Sasser, Hammond, et al., 2000).

The specific findings associated with inflicted TBI in childhood have also become clearer. It is important to realize that children who have been physically or sexually abused have been reported to have smaller cerebral volume, reduced midsagittal callosal size, and increased lateral ventricles compared to demographically matched controls, even in the absence of known trauma to the head (De Bellis, Keshavan, Clark, et al., 1999). This may be caused by stress-induced hormonal influences that adversely affect brain structure and function (Bremmer, 2002).

However, the work by Ewing-Cobbs and colleagues clarified neuroimaging and other physical findings that appear to be unique to inflicted brain injury. Most specifically, in addition to nonspecific brain atrophy, the hallmarks of inflicted TBI include extra-axial (e.g., subdural) hemorrhages, seizures, and retinal hemorrhages (Ewing-Cobbs, Kramer, Prasad, et al., 1998; Ewing-Cobbs, Prasad, Kramer, et al., 2000). All these factors are associated with greater overall injury severity, with resulting poorer outcome in motor, cognitive, and behavioral domains (Ewing-Cobbs, Prasad, Kramer, et al., 1999).

The role for the neuropsychologist in the evaluation of children with child abuse TBI may be twofold. First, whenever child abuse is suspected, medical and health care professionals in virtually all states are subject to mandatory reporting laws (Kalichman, 1999). Second, a long-term developmental perspective is needed regarding these children (Finkelhor & Dziuba-Leatherman, 1994; L. Miller, 1999). There is currently no evidence for a unique "signature" neuropsychological profile associated with child abuse TBI. However, because these children typically are injured at an early age (when many skills are still emerging or in a stage of rapid development) and are more likely to grow up in a stressful or unstable family environment, they are at increased risk for long-term neurobehavioral deficits. Consequently, many of these children may need to be followed for a considerable number of years postinjury.

NEUROPSYCHOLOGICAL EVALUATION

Several recent reviews of the general aspects of pediatric neuropsychological assessment are available (Baron, 2000a; Fennell, 2000; Hooper, 2000). Some even address specific issues of the evaluation of children with TBI (Farmer, Clippard, Luehr-Wiemann, et al., 1997; Semrud-Clikeman, 2001). Therefore, this review focuses on some of the most critical issues as they pertain to forensic aspects of assessing children with TBI.

A careful review of medical and school records is important. For example, parental retrospective estimates of their child's duration of coma or premorbid academic achievement are not always accurate, and datings of onset of psychopathological symptoms are particularly unreliable (Angold, Erkanli, Costello, et al., 1996). In addition, a careful interview and history are essential. This should address in particular any factors that might augment or interact with the direct organic influence of TBI, such as preexisting problems or the postinjury family environment (Donders & Strom, 2000).

Other stressors should be reviewed that may have occurred at the time of injury (e.g., witnessing the accidental fatal injuries to a family member) or that are unrelated but still potentially relevant for the outcome of the child (e.g., range of resources of the local school district). For example, subjective anxiety may contribute to the maintenance of nonspecific somatic, cognitive, and behavioral symptoms after mild TBI (Mittenberg, Wittner, & Miller, 1997). Obtaining knowledge of the contextual demands of the children's academic environment is also needed to optimize recommendations for interventions (Bernstein, 2000).

There are multiple approaches to neuropsychological assessment (e.g., flexible vs. fixed batteries), and none have been proven to be more accurate than the others in the evaluation of sequelae of pediatric TBI. It is important, however, to include in the evaluation measures that tap into the abilities most commonly affected by severe TBI. For example, an evaluation that includes no or few tasks with a speeded component may miss the difficulties with processing speed that many of these children have and the associated potentially helpful adaptations and accommodations that could be considered in the classroom (Ylvisaker, Szekers, Haarbauer-Krupa, et al., 1994; Ylvisaker, Todis, Glang, et al., 2001). In addition, it is crucial to avoid overreliance on measures of academic achievement and psychometric intelligence because those tests rely heavily on overlearned skills that are often relatively preserved after TBI. The evaluation should be supplemented with measures with sufficient reliability that tap into new learning and that have established criterion validity. A good example is the California Verbal Learning Test–Children's Version (Delis et al., 1994). This task is not only sensitive to severity of TBI (Levin, Song, et al., 2000; Roman et al., 1998), but also has considerable predictive accuracy regarding long-term educational placement (L. J. Miller & Donders, 2003).

Clinicians should also be cognizant of the psychometric strengths and weaknesses of the instruments that they use. It has been well established that age is of considerable importance when considering neuropsychological test scores (Forster & Leckliter, 1994). Yet, norms for a variety of commonly used instruments are often based on samples that are either too small or insufficiently stratified to capture these age effects adequately (Kizilbash, Warschausky, & Donders, 2001). In addition, clinicians should be knowledgeable about the clinical validation of psychometric tests for the specific populations with which they intend to use them (American Educational Research Association, 1999). For example, the fact that a certain test has a specific factor structure in the standardization sample is no guarantee that it is able to differentiate the same constructs in children with TBI (Woodward & Donders, 1998).

Awareness of the differences in versions of specific tests is also important. For example, several studies have reported sensitivity of the Tower of London, a measure of executive functioning, to severity and lesion characteristics in children with TBI (Levin, Song, Scheibel, et al., 1997; Shum, Short, Tunstall, et al., 2000). However, very different versions of the task and different scoring methods were used across investigations, which is potentially problematic (Baker, Segalowitz, & Ferlisi, 2001; Berg & Byrd, 2002). There are currently available at least two very different versions of this task that have been standardized and normed for use with children as young as 7 years (Culbertson & Zillmer, 2001) and 8 years (Delis, Kaplan, & Kramer, 2001) of age. Future research will need to determine the degree to which they are interchangeable or which version has better criterion validity regarding the sequelae of pediatric TBI.

Particularly regarding higher-level executive abilities, it is also important to avoid exclusive reliance on psychometric instruments administered in the type of structured, distractor-free environment typical of most neuropsychological evaluations. In fact, the ecological validity of that practice has been challenged, specifically in reference to the evaluation of children with TBI (Silver, 2000). In this context, a promising addition to the assessment arsenal for the pediatric neuropsychologist has been the Behavior Rating Inventory of Executive Function (BRIEF; Baron, 2000b; Gioia, Isquith, Guy, et al., 2000). This rating scale, completed by parents or teachers, appears to offer incremental information that cannot be accounted for by laboratory tests alone about the daily functioning of children with TBI (Mangeot, Armstrong, Colvin, et al., 2002; Vriezen & Pigott, 2002).

Finally, it is important to include formal measures of emotional and psychosocial adjustment in the evaluation instead of focusing on cognitive variables only. In light of the research on behavioral and interpersonal sequelae of pediatric TBI (Bloom, Levin, Ewing-Cobbs et al., 2001; Max, Robertson, & Lansing, 2001; Taylor et al., 2002), it is essential to address these areas of functioning. Several rating scales offer global screening of adjustment from the perspective of the child, the parent, or the teacher (Achenbach, 1991a, 1991b, 1991c; Reynolds & Kamphaus, 1992). More in-depth measures of coping style and personality that offer both parent and child versions are available in the Personality Inventory for Children–Second Edition (Lachar & Gruber, 1999) and the Personality Inventory for Youth (Lachar & Gruber, 1995).

EFFORT AND MOTIVATION

There has been an explosion of investigations of effort and motivation affecting the performance of adults with TBI. Much of this research has focused on the effects of financial compensation seeking and complicating premorbid or comorbid psychosocial factors (Bordini, Chaknis, Ekman-Turner, et al., 2002; Green, Rohling, Lees-Haley, et al., 2001; Grote, Kooker, Garron, et al., 2000; Larrabee, chapter 4, this volume; Martens, Donders, & Millis, 2001; Sweet, Wolfe, Sattlberger, et al., 2000). Until recently, relatively little attention was paid to this issue in the evaluation of children with TBI. However, even young children have the capability to use deception (Polak & Harris, 1999), and they are not always willing to do their best on neuropsychological tests (Mantynen, Poikkeus, Ahonen, et al., 2001).

There are several studies that explored the feasibility of using forced-choice measures of effort and motivation in the clinical assessment of children. Constantinou and McCaffrey (2003) evaluated the performance of 5- to 12-year-old children on the Test of Memory Malingering (TOMM), a task that had originally been developed for use with adults (Rees, Tombaugh, Gansler, et al., 1998; Tombaugh, 1996). The results indicated that almost all children were more than

90% accurate on the second trial of this instrument, clearly "passing" the cutoff point for invalid performance. Others have cautioned, however, that some measures of effort designed for adults need to be interpreted with caution when used with children under the age of 11 years (Courtney, Dinkins, Allen, et al., 2003) or with children who do not have at least a third-grade reading level (Green & Flaro, 2003).

To date, there are no large-scale studies that have included measures of effort and motivation in the assessment of children with TBI. The only scales that include standard validity checks are typically those that pertain to self-report of emotional and social adjustment, such as the Personality Inventory for Youth (Lachar & Gruber, 1995). More research is needed before firm conclusions can be reached about the use of measures of effort and motivation in the evaluation of cognitive performance after pediatric TBI.

SUMMARY

Research over the past decade has provided important new insights into the sequelae of TBI in children, with specific relevance to application in a forensic context. It is clear that premorbid characteristics of both the child and the family need to be considered in the evaluation of outcome. Furthermore, the postinjury family environment is of significant influence on both the cognitive and the behavioral outcome of these children, although in the long run more so on the latter. Important changes have taken place in federal and state criteria regarding eligibility for special education services under the TBI qualification, and practitioners need to be aware of local guidelines and regulations for due process in this regard. There have also been advances in the area of psychometric assessment and an increased appreciation of the associated ecological and criterion validity, which will likely continue to help qualify and quantify the range of effects of TBI on children.

Mild, uncomplicated pediatric TBI is typically not associated with significant permanent neurobehavioral sequelae. At the same time, there is no doubt that a long-term developmental perspective is necessary regarding the evaluation of moderate-to-severe TBI in children. Even the best prospective longitudinal studies of TBI in children to date have typically been limited to considerably less than a decade after injury. Particularly for TBI that is sustained early in life, additional follow-up is needed to delineate individual recovery into the teen and adolescent years and the various influences on variability in outcome.

Future research should also explore the possible contributions of functional neuroimaging in the evaluation of sequelae of TBI because most studies to date have focused exclusively on structural imaging methods. Finally, more research is needed concerning the effectiveness of various intervention methods with children with TBI, all the way from acute care medical management through subacute rehabilitation to long-term educational and vocational training.

REFERENCES

Achenbach, T. M. (1991a). *Manual for the Child Behavior Checklist/4–18 and 1991 Profile.* Burlington: University of Vermont.

Achenbach, T. M. (1991b). *Manual for the Teachers Report Form and 1991 Profile.* Burlington: University of Vermont.

Achenbach, T. M. (1991c). *Manual for the Youth Self Report and 1991 Profile.* Burlington: University of Vermont.

Agran, P. F., Castillo, D. N., & Winn, D. G. (1992). Comparison of motor vehicle occupant injuries in restrained and unrestrained 4- to 14-year-olds. *Accident Analysis and Prevention, 24,* 349–355.

American Educational Research Association, American Psychological Association, and National Council on Measurement in Education. (1999). *Standards for educational and psychological testing.* Washington, DC: Author.

Ammerman, R. T., & Galvin, M. R. (1998). Child maltreatment. In R. T. Ammerman & J. V. Campo (Eds.), *Handbook of pediatric psychology and psychiatry, Vol. II: Disease, injury, and illness* (pp. 31–69). Boston: Allyn and Bacon.

Anderson, V. A., Catroppa, C., Haritou, F., et al. (2001). Predictors of acute child and family outcome following traumatic brain injury in children. *Pediatric Neurosurgery, 34,* 138–148.

Anderson, V. A., Catroppa, C., Rosenfeld, J., et al. (2000). Recovery of memory function following traumatic brain injury in pre-school children. *Brain Injury, 14,* 679–692.

Anderson, V. A., Morse, S. A., Klug, G., et al. (1997). Predicting recovery from head injury in young children: A prospective analysis. *Journal of the International Neuropsychological Society, 3,* 568–580.

Angold, A., Erkanli, A., Costello, E. J., et al. (1996). Precision, reliability and accuracy in the dating of symptom onsets in child and adolescent psychopathology. *Journal of Child Psychology and Psychiatry and Allied Disciplines, 37,* 657–664.

Arffa, S. (1998). Traumatic brain injury. In C. E. Coffey & R. A. Brumback (Eds.), *Textbook of pediatric neuropsychiatry* (pp. 1093–1140). Washington, DC: American Psychiatric Association.

Asarnow, R. F., Satz, P., Light, R., et al. (1995). The UCLA study of mild closed head injury in children and adolescents. In S. H. Brown & M. E. Michel (Eds.), *Traumatic head injury in children* (pp. 117–146). New York: Oxford University Press.

Attewell, R. G., Glase, K., & McFadden, M. (2001). Bicycle helmet safety: A meta-analysis. *Accident Analysis and Prevention, 33,* 345–352.

Baker, K., Segalowitz, S. J., & Ferlisi, M. C. (2001). The effect of differing scoring methods for the Tower of London task on developmental patterns of performance. *The Clinical Neuropsychologist, 15,* 309–313.

Barkley, R. A. (1997). Attention-deficit/hyperactivity disorder, self-regulation, and time: Toward a more comprehensive theory. *Journal of Developmental and Behavioral Pediatrics, 18,* 271–279.

Barnes, M. A., & Dennis, M. (2001). Knowledge-based inferencing after childhood head injury. *Brain and Language, 76,* 253–265.

Baron, I. S. (2000a). Clinical implications and practical applications of child neuropsychological evaluations. In K. O. Yeates, M. D. Ris, & H. G. Taylor (Eds.), *Pediatric neuropsychology: Research, theory, and practice* (pp. 439–456). New York: Guilford Press.

Baron, I. S. (2000b). Test review: Behavior Rating Inventory of Executive Function. *Child Neuropsychology, 6,* 235–238.

Bayliss, D. M., & Roodenrys, S. (2000). Executive processing and attention deficit hyperactivity disorder: An application of the supervisory attentional system. *Developmental Neuropsychology, 17,* 161–180.

Beers, S. R., & De Bellis, M. D. (2002). Neuropsychological function in children with maltreatment-related posttraumatic stress disorder. *American Journal of Psychiatry, 159,* 483–486.

Berg, W. K., & Byrd, D. L. (2002). The Tower of London spatial problem-solving task: Enhancing clinical and research implementation. *Journal of Clinical and Experimental Neuropsychology, 24,* 586–604.

Bernstein, J. H. (2000). Developmental neuropsychological assessment. In K. O. Yeates, M. D. Ris, & H. G. Taylor (Eds.), *Pediatric neuropsychology: Research, theory, and practice* (pp. 405–438). New York: Guilford.

Bigler, E. D. (1999). Neuroimaging in pediatric traumatic head injury: Diagnostic considerations and relationships to neurobehavioral outcome. *Journal of Head Trauma Rehabilitation, 14,* 406–423.

Bijur, P. E., & Haslum, M. (1995). Cognitive, behavioral, and motoric sequelae of mild head injury in a national birth cohort. In S. H. Brown & M. E. Michel (Eds.), *Traumatic head injury in children* (pp. 147–164). New York: Oxford University Press.

Bijur, P. E., Haslum, M., & Golding, J. (1996). Cognitive outcomes of multiple head injuries in children. *Journal of Developmental and Behavioral Pediatrics, 17,* 143–148.

Bloom, D. R., Levin, H. S., Ewing-Cobbs, L., et al. (2001). Lifetime and novel psychiatric disorders after pediatric traumatic brain injury. *Journal of the American Academy of Child and Adolescent Psychiatry, 40,* 572–579.

Bohnert, A. M., Parker, J. G., & Warschausky, S. A. (1997). Friendship and social adjustment of children following a traumatic brain injury: An exploratory investigation. *Developmental Neuropsychology, 13,* 477–486.

Bordini, E. J., Chaknis, M. M., Ekman-Turner, R. M., et al. (2002). Advances and issues in the diagnostic differential of malingering versus brain injury. *Neurorehabilitation, 17,* 93–104.

Bremmer, J. D. (2002). Neuroimaging of childhood trauma. *Seminars in Clinical Neuropsychiatry, 7,* 104–112.

Brown, G. W. (2002). Measurement and the epidemiology of childhood trauma. *Seminars in Clinical Neuropsychiatry, 7,* 66–79.

Brown, J. K., & Minns, R. A. (1993). Non-accidental head injury, with particular reference to whiplash shaking injury and medicolegal aspects. *Developmental Medicine and Child Neurology, 35,* 849–869.

Butler, K., Rourke, B. P., Fuerst, D. R., et al. (1997). A typology of psychosocial functioning in pediatric closed-head injury. *Child Neuropsychology, 3,* 98–133.

Capruso, D. X., & Levin, H. S. (1992). Cognitive impairment following closed head injury. *Neurologic Clinics, 10,* 879–893.

Chapman, S. B., & McKinnon, L. (2000). Discussion of developmental plasticity: Factors affecting cognitive outcome after pediatric traumatic brain injury. *Journal of Communication Disorders, 33,* 333–344.

Chapman, S. B., McKinnon, L., Levin, H. S., et al. (2001). Longitudinal outcome of verbal discourse in children with traumatic brain injury: Three-year follow-up. *Journal of Head Trauma Rehabilitation, 16*, 441–455.

Chapman, S. B., Watkins, R., Gustafson, C., et al. (1997). Narrative discourse in children with closed head injury, children with language impairment, and typically developing children. *American Journal of Speech and Language Pathology, 6*, 66–75.

Clark, E., Russman, S., & Orme, S. (1999). Traumatic brain injury: Effects on school functioning and intervention strategies. *School Psychology Review, 28*, 242–250.

Constantinou, M., & McCaffrey, R. J. (2003). Using the TOMM for evaluating children's effort to perform optimally on neuropsychological measures. *Child Neuropsychology, 9*, 81–90.

Courtney, J. C., Dinkins, J. P., Allen, L. M., et al. (2003). Age related effects in children taking the Computerized Assessment of Response Bias and Word Memory Test. *Child Neuropsychology, 9*, 109–116.

Culbertson, W. C., & Zillmer, E. A. (2001). *Tower of London—Drexel University (TOL^{DX})*. Toronto: Multi-Health Systems.

De Bellis, M. D., Keshavan, M. S., Clark, D. B., et al. (1999). Developmental traumatology part II: Brain development. *Biological Psychiatry, 45*, 1271–1284.

Delis, D. C., Kaplan, E., & Kramer, J. H. (2001). *Delis-Kaplan Executive Function System*. Austin, TX: Psychological Corporation.

Delis, D. C., Kramer, J. H., Kaplan, E., et al. (1994). *California Verbal Learning Test—Children's Version*. Austin, TX: Psychological Corporation.

Dennis, M., & Barnes, M. A. (1994). Developmental aspects of neuropsychology: Childhood. In D. Zaidel (Ed.), *Handbook of perception and cognition, Vol. 15: Neuropsychology* (pp. 219–246). New York: Academic Press.

Dennis, M., & Barnes, M. A. (2000). Speech acts after mild or severe childhood head injury. *Aphasiology, 14*, 391–405.

Dennis, M., & Barnes, M. A. (2001). Comparison of literal, inferential, and intentional text comprehension in children with mild or severe closed head injury. *Journal of Head Trauma Rehabilitation, 16*, 456–468.

Dennis, M., Guger, S., Roncadin, C., et al. (2001). Attentional-inhibitory control and social-behavioral regulation after childhood closed head injury: Do biological, developmental, and recovery variables predict outcome? *Journal of the International Neuropsychological Society, 7*, 683–692.

Dennis, M., Purvis, K., Barnes, M. A., et al. (2001). Understanding literal truth, ironic criticism, and deceptive praise following childhood head injury. *Brain and Language, 78*, 1–16.

DiScala, J. A., Osberg, J. S., Gans, B., et al. (1991). Children with traumatic head injury: Morbidity and postacute management. *Archives of Physical Medicine and Rehabilitation, 72*, 662–666.

Donders, J. (1997). Sensitivity of the WISC-III to injury severity in children with traumatic head injury. *Assessment, 4*, 107–109.

Donders, J., & Hoffman, N. M. (2002). Gender differences in learning and memory after pediatric traumatic brain injury. *Neuropsychology, 16*, 491–499.

Donders, J., & Kuldanek, A. (1998). Traumatic brain injury. In R. T. Ammerman & J. V. Campo (Eds.), *Handbook of pediatric psychology and psychiatry, Vol. 2: Disease, injury, and illness* (pp. 166–190). Boston: Allyn and Bacon.

Donders, J., & Strom, D. (1997). The effect of traumatic brain injury on children with learning disability. *Pediatric Rehabilitation, 1*, 179–184.

Donders, J., & Strom, D. (2000). Neurobehavioral recovery after pediatric head trauma:

Injury, pre-injury, and post-injury issues. *Journal of Head Trauma Rehabilitation, 15,* 792–803.

Donders, J., & Warschausky, S. (1997). WISC-III factor index score patterns after traumatic head injury in children. *Child Neuropsychology, 3,* 71–78.

Donders, J., & Woodward, H. (2003). Gender as a moderator of memory after traumatic brain injury in children. *Journal of Head Trauma Rehabilitation, 18,* 106–115.

Downard, C., Hulka, F., Mullins, R. J., et al. (2000). Relationship of cerebral perfusion pressure and survival in pediatric brain-injured patients. *Journal of Trauma, 49,* 654–658.

Duhaime, A. C., Christian, C., Moss, E., et al., 1996. Long-term outcome in infants with the shaken-impact syndrome. *Pediatric Neurosurgery, 24,* 292–298.

Ewing-Cobbs, L., Brookshire, B., Scott, M. A., et al. (1998). Children's narratives following traumatic brain injury: Linguistic structure, cohesion, and thematic recall. *Brain and Language, 61,* 395–419.

Ewing-Cobbs, L., Duhaime, A. C., & Fletcher, J. M. (1995). Inflicted and noninflicted traumatic brain injury in infants and preschoolers. *Journal of Head Trauma Rehabilitation, 10,* 13–24.

Ewing-Cobbs, L., Fletcher, J. M., Levin, H. S., et al. (1997). Longitudinal neuropsychological outcome in infants and preschoolers with traumatic brain injury. *Journal of the International Neuropsychological Society, 3,* 581–591.

Ewing-Cobbs, L., Fletcher, J. M., Levin, H. S., et al. (1998). Academic achievement and academic placement following traumatic brain injury in children and adolescents: A two-year longitudinal study. *Journal of Clinical and Experimental Neuropsychology, 20,* 769–781.

Ewing-Cobbs, L., Kramer, L., Prasad, K., et al. (1998). Neuroimaging, physical, and developmental findings after inflicted and noninflicted traumatic brain injury in young children. *Pediatrics, 102,* 300–307.

Ewing-Cobbs, L., Prasad, M., Kramer, L., et al. (1999). Inflicted traumatic brain injury: Relationship of developmental outcome to injury severity. *Pediatric Neurosurgery, 31,* 251–258.

Ewing-Cobbs, L., Prasad, M., Kramer, L., et al. (2000). Acute neuroradiologic findings in young children with inflicted or noninflicted traumatic brain injury. *Child's Nervous System, 16,* 25–33.

Farmer, J. E., Clippard, D. S., Luehr-Wiemann, Y., et al. (1997). Assessing children with traumatic brain injury during rehabilitation: Promoting school and community reentry. In E. D. Bigler, E. Clark, & J. E. Farmer (Eds.), *Childhood traumatic brain injury: Diagnosis, assessment, and intervention* (pp. 33–61). Austin, TX: PRO-ED.

Fay, G. C., Jaffe, K. M., Polissar, N. L., et al. (1993). Mild pediatric traumatic brain injury: A cohort study. *Archives of Physical Medicine and Rehabilitation, 74,* 895–901.

Fay, G. C., Jaffe, K. M., Polissar, N. L., et al. (1994). Outcome of pediatric traumatic brain injury at 3 years: A cohort study. *Archives of Physical Medicine and Rehabilitation, 75,* 733–741.

Fennell, E. B. (2000). Issues in child neuropsychological assessment. In R. D. Vanderploeg (Ed.), *Clinician's guide to neuropsychological assessment* (2nd ed., pp. 357–381). Mahwah, NJ: Erlbaum.

Finkelhor, D., & Dziuba-Leatherman, J. (1994). Victimization of children. *American Psychologist, 49,* 173–183.

Forster, A. A., & Leckliter, I. N. (1994). The Halstead-Reitan neuropsychological test battery for older children: The effects of age versus clinical status on test performance. *Developmental Neuropsychology*, *10*, 299–312.

Geddes, J. F., Vowles, G. H., Hackshaw, A. K., et al. (2001). Neuropathology of inflicted head injury in children. II. Microscopic brain injury in infants. *Brain*, *124*, 1299–1306.

Gerring, J. P., Brady, K. D., Chen, A., et al. (1998). Premorbid prevalence of ADHD and development of secondary ADHD after closed head injury. *Journal of the American Academy of Child and Adolescent Psychiatry*, *37*, 647–654.

Gerring, J. P., Brady, K. D., Chen, A., et al. (2000). Neuroimaging variables related to development of secondary attention deficit hyperactivity disorder after closed head injury in children and adolescents. *Brain Injury*, *14*, 205–218.

Ghajar, J., & Hariri, R. (1992). Management of pediatric head injury. *Pediatric Clinics of North America*, *39*, 1093–1125.

Gioia, G. A., Isquith, P. K., Guy, S. C., et al. (2000). *Behavior Rating Inventory of Executive Function*. Odessa, FL: Psychological Assessment Resources.

Glang, A., Singer, G. H., & Todis, B. (1997). *Students with acquired brain injury: The school's response*. Baltimore: Brookes.

Green, P., & Flaro, L. (2003). Word Memory Test Performance in children. *Child Neuropsychology*, *9*, 189–207.

Green, P., Rohling, M. L., Lees-Haley, P. R., et al. (2001). Effort has a greater effect on test scores than severe brain injury in compensation claimants. *Brain Injury*, *15*, 1045–1060.

Grote, C. L., Kooker, E. K., Garron, D. C., et al. (2000). Performance of compensation seeking and non-compensation seeking samples on the Victoria Symptom Validity Test: Cross-validation and extension of a standardization study. *Journal of Clinical and Experimental Neuropsychology*, *22*, 709–719.

Hackbarth, R. M., Rzeszutko, K. M., Sturm, G., et al. (2002). Survival and functional outcome in pediatric traumatic brain injury: A retrospective review and analysis of predictive factors. *Critical Care Medicine*, *30*, 1630–1635.

Hicks, R. A., & Gaughan, D. C. (1995). Understanding fatal child abuse. *Child Abuse and Neglect*, *19*, 855–863.

Hoffman, N., Donders, J., & Thompson, E. H. (2000). Novel learning abilities after traumatic head injury in children. *Archives of Clinical Neuropsychology*, *15*, 47–58.

Holmbeck, G. N. (2002). Post-hoc probing of significant moderational and mediational effects in studies of pediatric populations. *Journal of Pediatric Psychology*, *27*, 87–96.

Hooper, S. R. (2000). Neuropsychological assessment of the preschool child. In B. A. Bracken (Ed.), *The psychoeducational assessment of preschool children* (3rd ed., pp. 383–411). Needham Heights, MA: Allyn and Bacon.

Individuals With Disabilities Education Act (IDEA) of 1990, 20 U.S.C. § 1400 *et seq.* (1990).

Jaffe, K. M., Fay, G. C., Polissar, N. L., et al. (1992). Severity of pediatric brain injury and early neurobehavioral outcome: A cohort study. *Archives of Physical Medicine and Rehabilitation*, *73*, 540–547.

Janusz, J. A., Kirkwood, M. W., Yeates, K. A., et al. (2002). Social problem-solving skills in children with traumatic brain injury: Long-term outcomes and prediction of social competence. *Child Neuropsychology*, *8*, 179–194.

Kalichman, S. C. (1999). *Mandated reporting of suspected child abuse: Ethics, law, and policy*. Washington, DC: American Psychological Association.

Katsiyannis, A., & Conderman, G. (1994). Serving individuals with traumatic brain injury: A national survey. *Remedial and Special Education*, *15*, 319–325.

Kinsella, G., Ong, B., Murtagh, D., et al. (1999). The role of the family for behavioral outcome in children and adolescents following traumatic brain injury. *Journal of Consulting and Clinical Psychology, 67,* 116–123.

Kinsella, G. J., Prior, M., Sawyer, M., et al. (1997). Predictors and indicators of academic outcome in children 2 years following traumatic brain injury. *Journal of the International Neuropsychological Society, 3,* 608–616.

Kirkwood, M., Janusz, J., Yeates, K. O., et al. (2000). Prevalence and correlates of depressive symptoms following traumatic brain injury in children. *Child Neuropsychology, 6,* 195–208.

Kizilbash, A., Warschausky, S., & Donders, J. (2001). Assessment of speed of processing after pediatric head trauma: Need for better norms. *Pediatric Rehabilitation, 4,* 71–74.

Knutson, J. F., & DeVet, K. A. (1995). Physical abuse, sexual abuse, and neglect. In M. C. Roberts (Ed.), *Handbook of pediatric psychology* (2nd ed., pp. 589–616). New York: Guilford Press.

Kraus, J. F. (1995). Epidemiological features of brain injury in children: Occurrence, children at risk, causes, and manner of injury, severity, and outcomes. In S. H. Broman & M. E. Michel (Eds.), *Traumatic head injury in children* (pp. 22–39). New York: Oxford University Press.

Lachar, D., & Gruber, C. P. (1995). *Personality Inventory for Youth (PIY).* Los Angeles: Western Psychological Services.

Lachar, D., & Gruber, C. P. (1999). *Personality Inventory for Children—Second Edition (PIC-2).* Los Angeles: Western Psychological Services.

Levin, H. S., Benavidez, D. A., Verger-Maestre, K., et al. (2000). Reduction of corpus callosum growth after severe traumatic brain injury in children. *Neurology, 54,* 647–653.

Levin, H. S., Song, J., Scheibel, R. S., et al. (1997). Concept formation and problem-solving following closed head injury in children. *Journal of the International Neuropsychological Society, 3,* 598–607.

Levin, H. S., Song, J., Scheibel, R. S., et al. (2000). Dissociation of frequency and recency processing from list recall after severe closed head injury in children and adolescents. *Journal of Clinical and Experimental Neuropsychology, 22,* 1–15.

Light, R., Asarnow, R., Satz, P., et al. (1998). Mild closed-head injury in children and adolescents: Behavior problems and academic outcomes. *Journal of Consulting and Clinical Psychology, 66,* 1023–1029.

Livingston, R. B., Stark, K. D., Haak, R. A., et al. (1996). Neuropsychological profiles of children with depressive and anxiety disorders. *Child Neuropsychology, 2,* 48–62.

Lorber, R., & Yurk, H. (1999). Special pediatric issues: Neuropsychological applications and consultations in schools. In J. Sweet (Ed.), *Forensic neuropsychology: Fundamentals and practice* (pp. 369–418). Lisse, The Netherlands: Swets and Zeitlinger.

Mangeot, S., Armstrong, K., Colvin, A. N., et al. (2002). Long-term executive function deficits in children with traumatic brain injuries: Assessment using the Behavior Rating Inventory of Executive Function (BRIEF). *Child Neuropsychology, 8,* 271–284.

Mantynen, H., Poikkeus, A. M., Ahonen, T., et al. (2001). Clinical significance of test refusal among young children. *Child Neuropsychology, 7,* 241–250.

Marshall, K. W., Koch, B. L., & Egelhoff, J. C. (1998). Air bag-related deaths and serious injuries in children: Injury patterns and imaging findings. *American Journal of Neuroradiology, 19,* 1599–1607.

Martens, M., Donders, J., & Millis, S. R. (2001). Evaluation of invalid response sets after traumatic head injury. *Journal of Forensic Neuropsychology, 2,* 1–18.

Massagli, T. L., Jaffe, K. M., Fay, G. C., et al. (1996). Neurobehavioral sequelae of severe traumatic brain injury: A cohort study. *Archives of Physical Medicine and Rehabilitation, 77,* 223–231.

Massagli, T. L., Michaud, L. J., & Rivara, F. P. (1996). Association between injury indices and outcome after severe traumatic brain injury in children. *Archives of Physical Medicine and Rehabilitation, 77,* 125–132.

Max, J. E., Castillo, C. S., Bokura, H., et al. (1998). Oppositional defiant disorder symptomatology after traumatic brain injury: A prospective study. *Journal of Nervous and Mental Disease, 186,* 325–332.

Max, J. E., Koele, S. L., Castillo, C. C., et al. (2000). Personality change disorder in children and adolescents following traumatic brain injury. *Journal of the International Neuropsychological Society, 6,* 279–289.

Max, J. E., Koele, S. L., Smith, W. L., et al. (1998). Psychiatric disorders in children and adolescents after severe traumatic brain injury: A controlled study. *Journal of the American Academy of Child and Adolescent Psychiatry, 37,* 832–840.

Max, J. E., Lindgren, S. D., Knutson, C., et al. (1998). Child and adolescent traumatic brain injury: Correlates of disruptive behavior disorders. *Brain Injury, 12,* 41–52.

Max, J. E., Roberts, M. A., Koele, S. L., et al. (1999). Cognitive outcome in children and adolescents following severe traumatic brain injury: Influence of psychosocial, psychiatric, and injury-related variables. *Journal of the International Neuropsychological Society, 5,* 58–68.

Max, J. E., Robertson, B. A. M., & Lansing, A. E. (2001). The phenomenology of personality change due to traumatic brain injury in children and adolescents. *Journal of Neuropsychiatry and Clinical Neurosciences, 13,* 161–170.

McLean, D. E., Kaitz, E. S., Kennan, C. J., et al. (1995). Medical and surgical complications of pediatric brain injury. *Journal of Head Trauma Rehabilitation, 10,* 1–12.

Mendelsohn, D., Levin, H. S., Bruce, D., et al. (1992). Later MRI after head injury in children: Relationship to clinical features and outcome. *Child's Nervous System, 8,* 445–452.

Miller, L. (1999). Child abuse brain injury: Clinical, neuropsychological, and forensic considerations. *Journal of Cognitive Rehabilitation, 17,* 10–19

Miller, L. J., & Donders, J. (2003). Prediction of educational outcome after pediatric traumatic brain injury. *Rehabilitation Psychology, 48,* 237–241.

Mittenberg, W., Wittner, M. S., & Miller, L. J. (1997). Postconcussion syndrome occurs in children. *Neuropsychology, 11,* 447–452.

Moradi, A. R., Doost, H. T. N., Taghavi, M. R., et al. (1999). Everyday memory deficits in children and adolescents with PTSD: Performance on the Rivermead Behavioural Memory Test. *Journal of Child Psychology and Psychiatry and Allied Disciplines, 40,* 357–361.

Noah, Z. L., Hahn, Y. S., Rubenstein, J. S., et al. (1992). Management of the child with severe brain injury. *Critical Care Clinics, 8,* 59–77.

Polak, A., & Harris, P. L. (1999). Deception by young children following noncompliance. *Developmental Psychology, 35,* 561–568.

Ponsford, J., Wilmott, C., Rothwell, A., et al. (1999). Cognitive and behavioral outcome following mild traumatic brain injury in children. *Journal of Head Trauma Rehabilitation, 14,* 360–372.

Prasad, M. R., Ewing-Cobbs, L., Swank, P. R., et al. (2002). Predictors of outcome following traumatic brain injury in young children. *Pediatric Neurosurgery, 36,* 64–74.

Rees, L. M., Tombaugh, T. N., Gansler, D. A., et al. (1998). Five validation experiments of the Test of Memory Malingering (TOMM). *Psychological Assessment, 10,* 10–20.

Reynolds, C. R., & Kamphaus, C. W. (1992). *Behavior Assessment System for Children (BASC).* Circle Pines, MN: American Guidance Service.

Rivara, F. P. (1994). Epidemiology and prevention of pediatric traumatic brain injury. *Pediatric Annals, 23,* 12–17.

Rivara, F. P. (1995). Developmental and behavioral issues in childhood injury prevention. *Journal of Developmental and Behavioral Pediatrics, 16,* 362–370.

Rivara, F. P., Astley, S. J., Clarren, S. K., et al. (1999). Fit of bicycle safety helmets and risk of head injuries in children. *Injury Prevention, 5,* 194–197.

Rivara, J. B., Jaffe, K. M., Polissar, N. L., et al. (1996). Predictors of family functioning and change 3 years after traumatic brain injury in children. *Archives of Physical Medicine and Rehabilitation, 77,* 754–764.

Roman, M. J., Delis, D. C., Willerman, L., et al. (1998). Impact of pediatric traumatic brain injury on components of verbal memory. *Journal of Clinical and Experimental Neuropsychology, 20,* 245–258.

Ruppel, R. A., Kochanek, P. M., Adelson, P. D., et al. (2001). Excitatory amino acid concentrations in ventricular cerebrospinal fluid after severe traumatic brain injury in infants and children: The role of child abuse. *Journal of Pediatrics, 138,* 1–3.

Satz, P., Zaucha, K., McCleary, C., et al. (1997). Mild head injury in children and adolescents: A review of studies (1970–1995). *Psychological Bulletin, 122,* 107–131.

Savage, R. C., Lash, M., Bennett, K., et al. (1995). Special education for students with brain injury. *TBI Challenge, 3*(2), 3–7.

Savage, R. C., & Wolcott, B. (1994). *Educational dimensions of acquired brain injury.* Austin, TX: PRO-ED.

Seidman, L. J., Biederman, J., Faraone, S. V., et al. (1997). Toward defining a neuropsychology of attention deficit hyperactivity disorder: Performance of children and adolescents from a large, clinically referred sample. *Journal of Consulting and Clinical Psychology, 65,* 150–160.

Semrud-Clikeman, M. (2001). *Traumatic brain injury in children and adolescents: Assessment and intervention.* New York: Guilford Press.

Shum, D., Short, L., Tunstall, J., et al. (2000). Performance of children with traumatic brain injury on a four-disk version of the Tower of London and the Porteus Maze. *Brain and Cognition, 44,* 59–62.

Silver, C. H. (2000). Ecological validity of neuropsychological assessment in childhood traumatic brain injury. *Journal of Head Trauma Rehabilitation, 15,* 973–988.

Slomine, B. S., Gerring, J. P., Grados, M. A., et al. (2002). Performance on measures of executive function following pediatric traumatic brain injury. *Brain Injury, 16,* 759–772.

Stoodley, N. (2002). Non-accidental head injury in children: Gathering the evidence. *Lancet, 360,* 271–272.

Sweet, J. J., Wolfe, P., Sattlberger, E., et al. (2000). Further investigation of traumatic brain injury versus insufficient effort with the California Verbal Learning Test. *Archives of Clinical Neuropsychology, 15,* 105–113.

Taylor, H. G., & Alden, J. (1997). Age-related differences in outcomes following childhood brain insults: An introduction and overview. *Journal of the International Neuropsychological Society, 3,* 555–567.

Taylor, H. G., Yeates, K. O., Drotar, D., et al. (1997). Preinjury family environment as a determinant of recovery from traumatic brain injuries in school-age children. *Journal of the International Neuropsychological Society*, *3*, 617–630.

Taylor, H. G., Yeates, K. O., Wade, S. L., et al. (2001). Bidirectional child–family influences on outcomes of traumatic brain injury in children. *Journal of the International Neuropsychological Society*, *7*, 755–767.

Taylor, H. G., Yeates, K. O., Wade, S. L., et al. (2002). A prospective study of short- and long-term outcomes after traumatic brain injury in children: Behavior and achievement. *Neuropsychology*, *16*, 15–27.

Taylor, H. G., Yeates, K. O., Wade, S. L., et al. (2003). Long-term educational interventions after traumatic brain injury in children. *Rehabilitation Psychology*, *48*, 227–236.

Teasdale, G., & Jennett, B. (1974). Assessment of coma and impaired consciousness: A practical scale. *Lancet*, *2*, 81–84.

Thompson, D. C., Rivara, F. P., & Thompson, R. S. (1996). Effectiveness of bicycle safety helmets in preventing head injuries: A case–control study. *Journal of the American Medical Association*, *276*, 1968–1973.

Tombaugh, T. N. (1996). *Test of Memory Malingering*. Toronto: Multi-Health Systems.

Tremont, G., Mittenberg, W., & Miller, L. J. (1999). Acute intellectual effects of pediatric head trauma. *Child Neuropsychology*, *5*, 104–114.

Verger, K., Junque, C., Levin, H. S., et al. (2001). Correlation of atrophy measures on MRI with neuropsychological sequelae in children and adolescents with traumatic brain injury. *Brain Injury*, *15*, 211–221.

Vriezen, E. R., & Pigott, S. E. (2002). The relationship between parental report on the BRIEF and performance-based measures of executive function in children with moderate to severe traumatic brain injury. *Child Neuropsychology*, *8*, 296–303.

Wade, S. L., Borawski, E. A., Taylor, H. G., et al. (2001). The relationship of caregiver coping to family outcomes during the initial year following pediatric traumatic injury. *Journal of Consulting and Clinical Psychology*, *69*, 406–415.

Wade, S. L., Taylor, H. G., Drotar, D., et al. (1996). Childhood traumatic brain injury: Initial impact on the family. *Journal of Learning Disabilities*, *29*, 652–661.

Wade, S. L., Taylor, H. G., Drotar, D., et al. (2002). A prospective study of long-term caregiver and family adaptation following brain injury in children. *Journal of Head Trauma Rehabilitation*, *17*, 96–111.

Wagner, A. K., Sasser, H. C., Hammond, F. M., et al. (2000). Intentional traumatic brain injury: Epidemiology, risk factors, and associations with injury severity and mortality. *Journal of Trauma*, *49*, 404–410.

Warschausky, S., Cohen, E. H., Parker, J. G., et al. (1997). Social problem-solving skills of children with traumatic brain injury. *Pediatric Rehabilitation*, *1*, 77–81.

Williams, D. H., Levin, H. S., & Eisenberg, H. M. (1990). Mild head injury classification. *Neurosurgery*, *27*, 422–428.

Woodcock, R., & Mather, N. (1989). *Woodcock-Johnson Tests of Achievement–Revised: Standard and supplemental batteries*. Allen, TX: DLM Teaching Resources.

Woodward, H., & Donders, J. (1998). The performance of children with traumatic head injury on the Wide Range Assessment of Memory and Learning—Screening. *Applied Neuropsychology*, *5*, 113–119.

Woodward, H., Winterhalter, K., Donders, J., et al. (1999). Prediction of neurobehavioral outcome 1–5 years post pediatric traumatic head injury. *Journal of Head Trauma Rehabilitation*, *14*, 351–359.

Yeates, K. O. (2000). Closed-head injury. In K. O. Yeates, M. D. Ris, & H. G. Taylor

(Eds.), *Pediatric neuropsychology: Research, theory, and practice* (pp. 92–116). New York: Guilford Press.

Yeates, K. O., Taylor, H. G., Drotar, D., et al. (1997). Preinjury family environment as a determinant of recovery from traumatic brain injuries in school-age children. *Journal of the International Neuropsychological Society, 3*, 617–630.

Yeates, K. O., Taylor, H. G., Wade, S. L., et al. (2002). A prospective study of short- and long-term neuropsychological outcomes after traumatic brain injury in children. *Neuropsychology, 16*, 514–523.

Yeates, K. O., Taylor, H. G., Woodrome, S. E., et al. (2002). Race as a moderator of parent and family outcomes following pediatric traumatic brain injury. *Journal of Pediatric Psychology, 27*, 393–403.

Ylvisaker, M., Szekers, S. F., Haarbauer-Krupa, J., et al. (1994). Speech and language intervention. In R. C. Savage & G. F. Wolcott (Eds.), *Educational dimensions of acquired brain injury* (pp. 185–235). Austin, TX: PRO-ED.

Ylvisaker, M., Todis, B., Glang, A., et al. (2001). Educating students with TBI: Themes and recommendations. *Journal of Head Trauma Rehabilitation, 16*, 76–93.

7

Mild Traumatic Brain Injury

GLENN J. LARRABEE

Mild traumatic brain injury (MTBI) accounts for 72% of all traumatic brain injury, with an incidence of 145.4 per 100,000 (Kraus & Arzemanian, 1989). Based on the U.S. Census of 281,421,906 individuals as of April 1, 2000, this amounts to a little over 409,000 new cases of MTBI each year. Not surprisingly, MTBI is the most frequent type of case seen by neuropsychologists doing forensic work in personal injury settings (Ruff & Richardson, 1999).

Despite the frequency with which MTBI occurs, and despite the significant research that has occurred on sequelae of MTBI over the past 25 years, the issue of the incidence, cause, and persistence of deficits following MTBI remains controversial (Mittenberg & Strauman, 2000). Zasler (2000) wrote of two "extreme camps": one that generally believes that mild brain injury or postconcussive disorders do not occur or do not cause long-term impairment or disability and the other that tends to overdiagnose or "overtreat" MTBI and postconcussive disorders, with inadequate consideration of alternative causes. There has been a spirited exchange between Bigler and Lees-Haley and colleagues regarding the issue of persistent deficits and persistent neurological damage in MTBI (Bigler, 2001, 2003; Fox & Allen, 2003; Green, 2003; Lees-Haley, Green, Rohling, Fox, & Allen, 2003).

The continuing debate over the incidence, cause, and persistence of deficits in MTBI likely results from several factors. One factor involves the criteria used to diagnose MTBI. Another factor is the sophistication of research design for evaluation of the consequences of MTBI. A third factor is the confusion of symptomatic complaint with neurological dysfunction. A fourth factor, related to the first factor, is the lack of proper differential diagnosis. In the following sections of this chapter, I review the diagnosis of MTBI, the outcome of MTBI, the role of symptomatic complaint in MTBI, and last, the workup of the individual MTBI case.

DIAGNOSTIC CRITERIA

Diagnostic criteria for MTBI have evolved from research criteria, as well as from the recommendations of committees of learned clinicians. Mittenberg and Strauman (2000) observed that inconsistencies in the definition of MTBI complicate comparison and generalization across studies. These authors did observe that there is a general consensus across studies that MTBI is defined by an admission Glasgow Coma Scale (GCS) of 13 to 15. Yet, one of the largest outcome studies of the full range of TBI severity identified the MTBI group by the measure of less than 1 hour for time to follow a doctor's commands (Dikmen, Machamer, Winn, & Temkin, 1995). Levin, Mattis, et al. (1987) specified MTBI by criteria that included loss of consciousness for less than 20 minutes, postresuscitation GCS of 13–15, absence of focal neurological abnormalities, and no evidence of intracranial mass lesion. In the Levin, Mattis, et al. (1987) investigation, there was no evidence of persistent neuropsychological deficit on 3-month follow-up for patients meeting their MTBI diagnostic criteria. In a subsequent investigation, Williams, Levin, and Eisenberg (1990) found that those TBI patients with admission GCS values of 13–15 who had evidence of intracranial lesion, characterized as "complicated" MTBI, had poorer 6-month outcomes than did those subjects who had GCS values of 13–15 without evidence of intracranial pathology. The Williams et al. complicated MTBI patients had outcomes more similar to the moderate TBI (GCS 9–12) than the MTBI patients. In contrast, Dikmen et al.'s (1995) MTBI group was classified by time to follow commands less than 1 hour, including patients with potential structural lesions or secondary complications, and showed no evidence of persistent neuropsychological deficits at 1-year posttrauma in comparison to an orthopedic trauma control group.

The Mild Traumatic Brain Injury Committee of the Head Injury Interdisciplinary Special Interest Group of the American Congress of Rehabilitation has proposed a definition of MTBI (American Congress of Rehabilitation Medicine [ACRM], 1993). These criteria define MTBI by traumatically induced physiological disruption of brain function, as manifested by *at least* one of the following: (a) any period of loss of consciousness; (b) any loss of memory for events immediately before or after the accident; (c) any alteration in mental state at the time of the accident (e.g., feeling dazed, disoriented, or confused); (d) focal neurological deficit(s) that may or may not be transient, but for which the severity of the injury does not exceed the following: (e) loss of consciousness of approximately 30 minutes or less; (f) after 30 minutes, an initial GCS of 13–15; and (g) posttraumatic amnesia (PTA) not greater than 24 hours.

The ACRM definition includes the head being struck, the head striking an object, and the brain undergoing an acceleration–deceleration movement (i.e., whiplash) without direct external trauma to the head. The ACRM does not include specific symptoms as part of the primary criteria for MTBI, but does state that physical symptoms (e.g., dizziness, headache), cognitive deficits (e.g., attention, memory), and behavioral changes or alterations in degree of emotional responsivity (e.g., irritability, emotional lability) are additional evidence that an MTBI has occurred.

A potential problem with the ACRM criteria is that they allow for determination of criteria beyond the acute (i.e., day of injury) status of the patient. For example, I have seen several cases of alleged MTBI with no evidence of loss of consciousness, disorientation, or PTA based on emergency medical service (EMS) or emergency room (ER) records or based on detailed interview (e.g., the patient accurately recalls the events of the accident and postaccident treatment, verified against Department of Motor Vehicles, EMS, and ER records), but on examination 1 to 2 months later are diagnosed as having MTBI based on their report to a physician that they were "dazed" and because they endorsed symptoms of headache, irritability, and forgetfulness, typically on a history/record form completed in the physician's office. This goes counter to the recommended practice of defining MTBI by acute injury characteristics rather than by severity of symptoms at random points after trauma (see Alexander, 1995).

Indeed, Lees-Haley, Fox, and Courtney (2001), studying groups of litigating individuals with MTBI and other injury (nonbrain injury) trauma, found, during retrospective questioning, that although 67% of those with MTBI reported confusion and 71% reported feeling dazed immediately after trauma, high proportions of the non-TBI group also reported being dazed (51%) and confused (65%). These data highlight the limited utility of self-reported feelings of being dazed and confused as a marker of the occurrence of MTBI. By contrast, EMS or ER records documenting independently observed confusion or disorientation can provide evidence consistent with MTBI.

Another problem posed by various diagnostic criteria for MTBI is that the criteria themselves do not provide much information for assessing gradations in severity of MTBI. This is particularly important when attempting to assess or conduct research on the group of patients with MTBI who do not show the characteristic pattern of full recovery, a group characterized by Ruff and Richardson (1999) as the "miserable minority."

Subdividing MTBI by severity was supported by Culotta, Sementelli, Gerold, and Watts (1996), who found greater need for neurosurgical intervention, more computed tomography (CT) scan abnormalities, and increased incidence of skull fractures in patients with GCS of 13 compared to GCS of 14. Patients with GCS of 14 had greater morbidity than patients with GCS of 15. Culotta et al. recommended segregating MTBI patients with GCS of 15 from those with scores of 14 and 13. Although these data showed the benefits of grading severity of MTBI relative to acute injury characteristics, Culotta et al. did not study long-term neuropsychological outcome for these different levels of GCS.

Ruff and Richardson (1999) proposed subdividing MTBI by three categories of severity, proceeding from less to more severe: Type I, altered state or transient loss of consciousness, PTA of 1 to 60 seconds, and one or more neurological symptom; Type II, definite loss of consciousness, with time either unknown or less than 5 minutes, PTA of 60 seconds to 12 hours, and one or more neurological symptom; and Type III, loss of consciousness of 5 to 30 minutes, PTA greater than 12 hours, and one or more neurological symptom.

Published standards for gradation of concussion in sports also allow for assessment of the severity of MTBI (American Neurological Association, 1997). *Concussion* is defined as a trauma-induced alteration in mental status that may or may not involve loss of consciousness, with confusion and amnesia identified as the hallmarks of concussion. The American Academy of Neurology (1997) proposed three different grades of concussion: Grade I, characterized by transient confusion, no loss of consciousness, and concussion symptoms or mental status abnormalities on examination that resolve in less than 15 minutes; Grade II, characterized by transient confusion, no loss of consciousness, and concussion symptoms or mental status abnormalities on examination that last more than 15 minutes; and Grade III, characterized by any loss of consciousness, either brief (seconds) or prolonged (minutes).

Hinton-Bayre and Geffen (2002) investigated concussion severity grades in 21 professional rugby league players who suffered concussion. Testing concussed athletes at 2 and 10 days posttrauma, Hinton-Bayre and Geffen found no relationship between concussion severity, using the American Academy of Neurology (AAN) criteria, and two other sets of criteria (Colorado Medical Society, 1990; Cantu, 1986) and performance on Speed of Comprehension, Digit Symbol, and the Symbol Digit Test. Similarly, Lovell, Iverson, Collins, McKeag, and Maroon (1999) found no differences in neuropsychological test performance as a function of positive loss of consciousness, no loss of consciousness, or uncertain loss of consciousness in persons admitted to the ER for evaluation of uncomplicated MTBI.

In contrast, McCrea, Kelly, Randolph, Cisler, and Berger (2002), in an investigation of immediate neurocognitive effects of sports concussion, found that subjects with loss of consciousness were most severely impaired immediately after injury, whereas those without loss of consciousness or PTA were least impaired. All of the McCrea et al. subjects returned to preinjury baseline levels of performance within 48 hours of injury.

The investigations of Culotta et al. (1996), Hinton-Bayre and Geffen (2002), and Lovell et al. (1999) did not provide consistent evidence either supporting or contradicting the value of grading severity of MTBI. In contrast, the study by McCrea et al. (2002) demonstrated differences between MTBI subjects as a function of presence/absence of loss of consciousness both immediately following and 15 minutes after trauma. The McCrea et al. (2002) data clearly support the value of grading severity of MTBI in the first hour posttrauma, providing support for the utility of these criteria regarding return-to-play decisions (American Academy of Neurology, 1997). Additional research is needed to establish the value of grading severity of MTBI relative to long-term outcome of MTBI.

APPROPRIATE RESEARCH DESIGNS

One significant factor that has contributed to the apparent contradictory findings in the MTBI literature is the use of samples of convenience as opposed to prospective outcome research or sports concussion research utilizing preinjury baseline testing followed by repeated measures examination subsequent to MTBI. Certainly, subject-as-own-control designs, with repeated measures studies of nonconcussed persons to control for practice effects, are the strongest designs for investigation of the outcome of MTBI. The weakest designs are those employing clinical samples of convenience, such as might be aggregated from a clinic specializing in treatment of persons with persisting symptoms 1 to 2 years post-MTBI.

Differences in study outcome as a function of research design can be very significant. Dikmen et al. (1995) conducted what is arguably the best prospective outcome study of the complete range of TBI severity. Dikmen et al. compared patients with TBI with six different levels of severity, defined by time to follow commands (the highest level of function on the motor component of the GCS; this score is not affected by the presence of intubation, which can affect the verbal component of the GCS and consequently have an impact on the total GCS score). The mildest level of injury was represented by the group that took less than 1 hour to follow commands, whereas the most severely injured group took 29 days or more to follow commands.

In addition, Dikmen et al. (1995) collected a large trauma control sample that had been admitted to the hospital because of traumatic injuries not involving the head. By using such a control group, Dikmen et al. controlled for socioeconomic status as well as for psychosocial factors associated with suffering traumatic injury, the experience of being injured sufficiently to be transported to the hospital, and the potentially confounding effects of pain. The trauma control and TBI patients did not differ on age, education, or gender. Also, by using a trauma control group, Dikmen et al. indirectly controlled for effects related to litigation. Although Dikmen et al. did not report percentage involved in litigation for the trauma control group, there is no reason to expect a significant difference in litigation for the trauma control and the more mildly injured patients with TBI, particularly those who followed commands within less than 1 hour. Both the TBI and trauma control subjects were examined at 1 month and 1 year posttrauma. At 1 year posttrauma, the MTBI group (those taking less than 1 hour to follow commands) did not differ significantly from the trauma control group in performance on a comprehensive neuropsychological test battery.

   Results from studies using samples of convenience that did not control for effects of nonhead traumatic injury can be quite different. For example, Leininger, Gramling, Farrell, Kreutzer, and Peck (1990) found significant neuropsychological performance differences comparing 31 patients with MTBI and brief loss of consciousness and 22 MTBI patients experiencing "dazing" injuries without loss of consciousness to the performance of a group of 23 control subjects who were friends and family of inpatients with head injury at the Medical College of Virginia. The MTBI patients were tested, on average, 7 months posttrauma. In another study, Guilmette and Rasile (1995) compared the verbal memory performance of 16 patients with MTBI to the performance of 16 controls who were community volunteers matched on age, education, and gender to the MTBI patients. On testing done a mean of 16.4 months posttrauma, the MTBI patients performed significantly less well than the control subjects on all three memory tests.

   The differences in outcome between the prospective investigation using trauma controls conducted by Dikmen et al. (1995) and the nonprospective investigations of Leininger et al. (1990) and Guilmette and Rasile (1995) that did not use trauma control subjects are more obvious when the study results are examined for effect sizes. These effect sizes, represented in terms of d, the difference between the MTBI and control group mean, in pooled standard deviation units (i.e., the pooled MTBI/control group standard deviation) are shown in Table 7-1.

   As can be seen in Table 7-1, the effect size for the Dikmen et al. MTBI group, tested 1 year posttrauma, is essentially zero, consistent with complete overlap of the MTBI and trauma control group score distributions. In contrast, the 0.57 effect size for the Leininger et al. (1990) MTBI group is most similar

TABLE 7-1. Effect Size as a Function of Severity of Brain Injury

STUDY	MINOR BRAIN INJURY	1–24 HOURS	2–5 DAYS	6–13 DAYS	14–28 DAYS	29+ DAYS
Dikmen et al. (1995)	0.02	0.23	0.45	0.69	1.33	2.30
Leininger et al. (1990)	0.57	—	—	—	—	—
Guilmette and Rasile (1995)	1.10	—	—	—	—	—

Note. Severity of injury is Glasgow Coma Scale of 13–15 or time to follow commands less than 1 hour for minor brain injury; other values are time to follow commands.

to the effect size for the Dikmen et al. (1995) group who took between 6 and 13 days to follow commands. Even more significant is the 1.10 effect size for the Guilmette and Rasile (1995) MTBI group, which is most similar to the effect size for the Dikmen et al. (1995) group who took between 14 and 28 days to follow commands. Clearly, the results of the work of Leininger et al. (1990) and Guilmette and Rasile (1995) cannot be accepted as representative of outcome from MTBI when considered in terms of a dose–response analysis of TBI (Dikmen et al., 1995; Rohling, Meyers, & Millis, 2003).

The above differences in study outcome may be partly a consequence of motivational factors secondary to litigation. In the Leininger et al. (1990) study, 39 patients were pursuing litigation, and 14 were not pursuing litigation. Leininger et al. did compare the two groups and found that the litigating group performed significantly less well on the copy portion of the Complex Figure Test, but this difference did not remain significant when the Bonferroni correction procedure was applied. However, the litigating/nonlitigating contrasts suffered from both an imbalance of subjects (over twice as many litigant as nonlitigant subjects) and low power, given the sample size of the nonlitigating group. Leininger et al. did not report the mean performances and standard deviations for the litigating and nonlitigating subjects, so the reader is unable to see whether there is a consistent pattern of lower mean score for the litigants. Guilmette and Rasile (1995) did not specify the proportion of their MTBI sample who had a potentially compensable injury, but did note that they screened subjects who had ongoing Workman's Compensation or personal injury litigation with forced-choice symptom validity testing. They did not, however, match their MTBI and control group subjects on symptom validity test performance or use analysis of covariance with symptom validity performance as the covariate.

Litigation effects are significant. Binder and Rohling (1996) found an effect size of 0.47 between litigating and nonlitigating TBI patients, with the effect particularly strong for those with MTBI. Moreover, Binder and Kelly (1996) found that, on the Portland Digit Recognition Test (a measure of symptom validity and malingering), up to 47% of a series of individuals with MTBI performed at the level of the bottom 2% of a sample of nonlitigating patients with severe TBI. Green, Rohling, Lees-Haley, and Allen (2001) found that measures of effort sensitive to malingering accounted for 50% of the variance in neuropsychological test performance, in contrast to 10% accounted for by TBI severity. Last, Mittenberg, Patton, Canyock, and Condit (2002), in a survey of American Board of Clinical Neuropsychology (ABCN) board-certified neuropsychologists who did forensic work, found a base rate of malingering of approximately 40% in litigating MTBI subjects.

Thus, future outcome research on MTBI optimally should be based on prospective investigations using trauma control subjects (Dikmen et al., 1995; Satz et al., 1999), and symptom validity testing (Green et al., 2001). Satz et al. also advocated using a noninjury reference group as a third group, so that MTBI versus other injury and MTBI versus no injury comparisons can be made. Per their Table 1, Satz et al.'s design with three subject groups allows evaluation of four separate conclusions: (a) no effect, head injury or other injury; (b) general injury effect, body and head; (c) specific head injury effect; and (d) other injury, not head injury, must be the causal factor.

Studies involving MTBI clinical samples of convenience can still yield potentially useful information if they employ an orthopedic trauma control group matched on age, education, and gender and screened and matched for performance on sensitive symptom validity tests such as the Word Memory Test (Green, Iverson, & Allen, 1999) or the Portland Digit Recognition Test (Binder & Kelly, 1996). Alternatively, studies that have a primary focus other than MTBI, such as Bornstein et al.'s (1993) study of HIV-positive patients with and without history of MTBI or Alterman, Goldstein, Shelly, and Bober's (1985) investigation of alcoholic subjects with and without history of MTBI, can be considered "pseudoprospective" (cf. Binder, Rohling, & Larrabee, 1997) because the primary focus is the clinical condition (HIV status or alcohol abuse) with the presence or absence of MTBI on a historic basis.

THE TYPICAL OUTCOME

Cumulative research on the outcome of a single, uncomplicated MTBI shows that neuropsychological deficits may persist for up to 3 months, but the norm is full recovery, with no long-term residual deficits (Binder, 1997; Binder et al., 1997; Dikmen et al., 1995; Levin, Mattis, et al., 1987; Ruff et al., 1989). Binder et al. (1997) conducted a meta-analysis of eight published studies of adult MTBI, with 11 total samples studied at least 3 months posttrauma and selected on the basis of a history of MTBI rather than because they were symptomatic; the study had a subject attrition rate on follow-up of less than 50%. The total aggregated sample included 314 patients with MTBI and 308 control subjects. Using the g statistic (MTBI and control pooled standard deviation), the overall effect size of 0.07 was nonsignificant, but the d statistic (control group standard deviation) of 0.12 was significant at $p < .03$. Measures of attention had the largest effect sizes, with $g = 0.17$, $p < .02$, and $d = 0.20$, $p < .006$. Binder et al. (1997) observed that these small effect sizes were equivalent to 2 points for the WAIS-R (Wechsler Adult Intelligence Scale–Revised) IQ or WMS-R (Wechsler Memory Scale–Revised) General Memory score (for $d = 0.12$) and 3 points on the Attention/Concentration Index of the WMS-R (for $d = 0.20$). These values are smaller than the measurement errors for these WAIS-R and WMS-R scores (Wechsler, 1981, 1987).

Binder et al. (1997) computed an estimated prevalence of persistent neuropsychological impairment of 5% based on their effect-size analysis. At such a low base rate of impairment, the positive predictive value of neuropsychological test scores (true positives divided by true positives plus false positives) was .32 at a sensitivity of .90 and specificity of .90 (note that lower sensitivity of .80 and specificity of .88, values based on the Heaton, Grant, and Matthews, 1991, data, yield a positive predictive value of only .26). In contrast, negative predictive values (true negatives divided by true negatives plus false negatives) were .98 to .99. Binder et al. (1997) concluded that at these low positive but high negative predictive values, the clinician would more likely be correct when not diagnosing rather than diagnosing brain injury in patients reporting chronic disability after MTBI.

The likelihood of full recovery from single, uncomplicated MTBI is further supported by data emerging from sports concussion research. Macciocchi, Barth, Alves, Rimel, and Jane (1996) followed collegiate athletes who were tested preseason and then within 1, 5, and 10 days post-MTBI; these individuals were contrasted with control athletes tested preseason and at 1, 5, and 10 days posttrauma. Inspection of group mean performance showed no significant performance difference compared to baseline at 24 hours posttrauma; however, the MTBI group did differ when their change scores (pre- to postinjury) were compared to the change scores of the noninjured control group. At 10 days, there were essentially no differences in the MTBI group versus the control group.

Collins et al. (1999) found that college football players who were concussed showed significantly poorer Hopkins Verbal Learning Test performance compared to noninjured players at 24 hours after injury. Moderate differences in performance persisted until at least 5 days posttrauma.

Echemendia, Putukian, Mackin, Julian, and Shoss (2001) found significant differences in neuropsychological test performance for athletes sustaining MTBI in comparison to nonconcussed control athletes at 2 hours and 48 hours posttrauma. There were no multivariate group differences at 1 week posttrauma, although univariate differences were seen on a few measures. At 1 month postinjury, a statistically significant difference was found on one measure, with the injured athletes marginally outperforming the noninjured athlete control subjects.

McCrea et al. (2003) found that concussed collegiate football players showed recovery over the first week posttrauma. Symptoms of concussion (e.g., headache, dizziness) gradually resolved by Day 7. Directly measured cognitive function improved to baseline (preinjury) levels within 5 to 7 days following concussion, and balance deficits dissipated within 3 to 5 days posttrauma. The mild impairments in cognitive processing and verbal memory that were apparent on neuropsychological testing 2 days posttrauma resolved by Day 7. McCrea et al. (2003) found no significant differences in symptoms or functional impairments in the concussed and nonconcussed athlete controls 90 days following concussion. The good long-term outcome of a single, uncomplicated MTBI appears to extend across the age range. Full recovery from MTBI is generally expected for children (Bijur, Haslam, & Golding, 1996; Satz et al., 1997). Very young children, aged 3 to 7 years, also make good recovery for intellectual skills, receptive language, and everyday and spatial memory, although they may have persistent problems in higher linguistic skills (Anderson, Catroppa, Morse, Haritou, & Rosenfeld, 2001).

Older adults also showed good outcome from a single, uncomplicated MTBI. Goldstein, Levin, Goldman, Clark, and Altonen (2001) found that older adults (average age 62.3 years) suffering MTBI performed at similar levels to older adults not suffering MTBI; this was examined on measures of attention, memory, and executive function when tested, on average, 25 days posttrauma. The only difference between the older adults with MTBI and control subjects was seen on the Controlled Oral Word Association test. Both the individuals with MTBI and noninjured controls outperformed a group of older adults suffering moderate TBI on all measures of language, attention, memory, and executive dysfunction.

In a subsequent article, Goldstein and Levin (2001) reviewed extensive literature on cognitive outcome following mild and moderate TBI in adults over 50 years of age. These authors concluded that patients suffering MTBI, unlike those suffering moderate TBI, exhibited cognitive functioning similar to noninjured controls by 1 to 2 months posttrauma. Despite evidence of full neuropsychological recovery, MTBI patients continued to report significant anxiety, depression, and somatic preoccupation. Goldstein and Levin found that the lowest postresuscitation GCS and the presence of intracranial pathology were more strongly associated with outcome than durations of PTA and impaired consciousness.

In a recent meta-analysis, Schretlen and Shapiro (2003) included sports concussion studies with traditional prospective clinical studies and found that persons with MTBI essentially returned to a baseline level of performance within 1 to 3 months posttrauma. Indeed, there was a 97% overlap of control and MTBI test performance by 1 month posttrauma, and the 95% confidence intervals of effect size estimates at both 30–89 days and more than 89 days posttrauma included zero. Schretlen and Shapiro interpreted these data as showing that the overall cognitive test performance of those with MTBI was essentially indistinguishable from that of matched controls by 1 month posttrauma.

The above findings showing essentially full neuropsychological recovery following a single, uncomplicated MTBI for most patients also appear to extend to return to work following MTBI. Dikmen et al. (1994) found that 82% of TBI patients who took 5 or fewer hours to follow commands had returned to work by 12 months, with 84% back to work by 24 months, compared to 87% of orthopedic trauma controls who had returned to work in the first year post-trauma.

FACTORS POTENTIALLY RELATED TO PERSISTENT PROBLEMS FOLLOWING MILD TRAUMATIC BRAIN INJURY

Wilson, Teasdale, Hadley, Wiedman, and Lang (1994) demonstrated the need to consider GCS *and* PTA in evaluating MTBI. These investigators found a close association between GCS and PTA for those patients who experienced 6 hours or more of coma following TBI (note that 6 hours of coma is beyond what would be considered MTBI). Eight patients had coma less than 6 hours with PTA greater than 7 days, and three of these eight were only briefly unconscious, if at all. These data demonstrated the importance of basing diagnosis of MTBI on both circumscribed loss of consciousness and circumscribed PTA.

Williams et al. (1990) found that patients with GCS of 13–15 *and* CT evidence of structural lesion were more similar in neuropsychological outcome to patients with moderate TBI (GCS 9–12) than they were similar to those with MTBI (GCS 13–15 without CT scan abnormalities). The GCS 13–15 group with CT-identified lesions was identified as mild/complicated by Williams et al. (1990).

Magnetic resonance imaging (MRI) is more sensitive than CT scan in detecting lesions following mild-to-moderate TBI (Levin, Amparo, et al., 1987; Levin, Williams, Eisenberg, High, & Guinto, 1992). Levin et al. (1992) found that although MRI-identified lesions were more prevalent than those identified by CT in mild-to-moderate head injury and more prominent in moderate (GCS 9–12) relative to mild (GCS 13–15) TBI, these lesions resolved over 1 to 3 months follow-up, paralleling the recovery seen in neuropsychological test scores. For some of the subjects with acute MRI-identified lesions, however, neuropsychological impairment persisted despite resolution of the lesion on MRI.

Dikmen, Machamer, and Temkin (2001) further addressed factors related to presence and persistence of deficits following MTBI, including patients with complicated MTBI. Four groups of subjects were formed, characterized by decreasing sample size as a function of stringency of definition of the groups. The most inclusive group was identified by GCS of 13–15, followed by a group defined by GCS and time-to-follow commands of less than 1 hour, followed by a group who met the prior conditions with the added condition of normal CT scan, followed by the most restrictive classification that met all preceding criteria plus had PTA less than or equal to 24 hours. At 1 month posttrauma, the group defined by GCS 13–15 alone differed on the Verbal Selective Reminding Test from all other MTBI groups, which did not differ from one another or from a group of control patients with non-TBI trauma. There were no 1-month group differences on measures of attention, psychomotor speed, or Performance IQ. At 1 year posttrauma, there were no group differences on any measures.

In a subsequent investigation, Dikmen, Machamer, and Temkin (2003) found that TBI patients with GCS of 13–15 who also had abnormal CT scans differed from TBI patients with GCS of 13–15 without abnormal CT scans for both level of consciousness and neuropsychological outcome. The individuals with GCS 13–15 with positive CT scans had fewer cases with GCS of 15, with a corresponding greater number of cases with GCS 13 and 14; had longer time to follow commands; and had longer PTA than the group with GCS 13–15 without CT scan abnormality. Similarly, the GCS 13–15 CT-positive group had lower verbal memory (Selective Reminding), Performance IQ, Trail Making B, and Halstead Impairment Index at testing 1 month posttrauma than the group of GCS 13–15 with normal CT, which itself did not differ from a control group with non-TBI trauma. At 1 year posttrauma follow-up, the CT-positive group had lower Selective Reminding than the trauma control group, with no differences between the CT-negative and trauma control group.

Based on the research of Levin and colleagues (Levin et al., 1992; Williams et al., 1990) and Dikmen and colleagues (Dikmen et al., 2001, 2003), TBI patients with GCS of 13–15 who also have CT scan or MRI abnormalities may not have a truly MTBI. Moreover, the Dikmen et al. (2001, 2003) and Wilson et al. (1994) investigations showed the importance of considering duration of PTA in differentiating true MTBI from those with apparent cases of MTBI who actually have more severe injuries.

Some investigators have presented data suggesting that MTBI results in a reduction in cerebral reserve (see Satz, 1993, for a general discussion of brain reserve capacity following brain injury). Ewing, McCarthy, Gronwall, and Wrightson (1980) found evidence for persisting cognitive deficits in apparently recovered MTBI patients who were subjected to hypoxic stress. This finding appears consistent with evidence from the same laboratory demonstrating a longer recovery time for persons following MTBI if there was a history of prior concussion (Gronwall, 1989; Gronwall & Wrightson, 1975).

Reduced cerebral reserve was also suggested by the Collins et al. (1999) sports concussion investigation, which found that collegiate football players with one or more prior concussions who also had preexisting learning disability had poorer baseline (preseason) test results on the Trail Making Test Part B and on the Symbol Digit Modalities Test than did football players without history of prior concussion. Guskiewicz et al. (2003) found that football players with a history of three or more concussions were three times more likely to experience a subsequent concussion than football players without history of prior concussion. There was a dose effect of prior concussion with length of recovery: 30% of players with history of three or more prior concussions had symptoms lasting greater than 1 week compared to 14.6% of players with one previous concussion.

Data also exist that challenge the hypothesis of reduced cerebral reserve. Alterman et al. (1985) found no significant neuropsychological performance differences between alcoholic patients with and without history of a prior MTBI. Dikmen, Donovan, Loberg, Machamer, and Temkin (1993) found no significant interactions between alcohol use and head trauma severity in relation to neuropsychological outcome in their study of the full range of head trauma severity (i.e., MTBI, moderate and severe TBI).

Bornstein et al. (1993) found no significant neuropsychological differences between those HIV-positive patients with a history of MTBI and those without history of MTBI. Bijur et al. (1996) did not find evidence for cumulative effects of MTBI in comparing children with a history of one, two, or three MTBIs with non-head-injured orthopedic controls with history of one, two, or three orthopedic injuries. Bijur et al. suggested that cognitive deficits associated with multiple MTBI were secondary to social and personal factors related to multiple injuries rather than resulting from damage to the head. Last, Cullum and Thompson (1999) referenced an ongoing investigation that found that MTBI patients with and without history of prior MTBI did not differ from one another or from a group of non-TBI trauma control subjects when tested within 1 week and within 2 months of the accident.

SYMPTOMATIC COMPLAINT IN MILD TRAUMATIC BRAIN INJURY: THE POSTCONCUSSION SYNDROME

Postconcussion syndrome (PCS) refers to a constellation of somatic (e.g., headache), cognitive (e.g., memory), and emotional (e.g., irritability) symptoms following MTBI (Alexander, 1995; Axelrod et al., 1996). There has been a longstanding controversy over whether PCS results from neurological or physiogenic factors versus nonneurological or psychogenic factors (Gasquoine, 1997; Lishman, 1988). Physiogenic factors are likely operative in the first 1 to 3 months posttrauma, during the time when ongoing neuropsychological deficits are resolving, whereas psychogenic factors are more likely related to chronic PCS, also known as persistent postconcussion syndrome (PPCS), persisting several months after MTBI (Alexander, 1995; Binder, 1997).

For example, Dikmen, McLean, and Temkin (1986) found that, 1 month after trauma, 3 of 12 PCS symptoms (bothered by noise, insomnia, and memory difficulties) discriminated MTBI from control subjects, but at 1 year, there were no differences in symptom endorsement. Binder (1997) reported that 7–8% of MTBI patients remained symptomatic on a chronic basis, a value slightly higher than the 5% rate of persistent neuropsychological deficit reported by Binder et al. (1997).

There is increasing evidence that questions the validity of the PCS symptom constellation. To qualify as a syndrome, a condition must demonstrate a set of specifically associated symptoms broadly present in persons who have the condition and absent in those who do not have it (note the relevance to sensitivity and specificity). Symptoms thought to be representative of PCS, such as headache, memory difficulty, and irritability, are also seen in persons with suspected neurotoxic exposure (Larrabee, 1990; Lees-Haley & Brown, 1993) and in persons who have chronic pain but no history of TBI (Iverson & McCracken, 1997). Level of depression is more strongly associated with PCS report than is head injury status (Brulot, Strauss, & Spellacy, 1997; Suhr & Gundstad, 2002; Trahan, Ross, & Trahan, 2001). These symptoms occur frequently in the non-brain-injured population; for example, Lees-Haley and Brown (1993) found that 62% of outpatient family practice patients endorsed headache, 20% endorsed memory problems, and 38% endorsed irritability. Moreover, Lees-Haley and Brown found very high endorsement of these symptoms in persons in litigation for emotional distress or industrial stress, without neurological claims or injuries, with 89% reporting headaches, 53% reporting memory problems, and 77% reporting irritability. In this vein, litigating MTBI subjects endorsed more symptoms than nonlitigants, despite not differing on demographic characteristics, TBI severity ratings, or premorbid risk factors for poor outcome (Feinstein, Ouchterlony, Somerville, & Jardine, 2001). PCS-type symptoms increase in relation to stress, independent of presence or absence of history of MTBI (Gouvier, Cubic, Jones, Brantley, & Cutlip, 1992).

Table 7-2 displays PCS-type complaints for the Lees-Haley and Brown (1993) outpatient medical patients, nonneurological litigants, and a sample of individuals with MTBI reported by Mittenberg, DiGuilio, Perrin, and Bass (1992). These data clearly demonstrate the poor specificity for purported PCS symptomatic complaints, which can occur with high frequency in nonconcussed persons, such that relying on these symptoms as indicative of PCS would result in abnormally high false-positive diagnoses. In this vein, it is noteworthy that of the eight symptoms proposed in the *Diagnostic and Statistical Manual of Mental Disorders*, fourth edition (*DSM-IV*; American Psychiatric Association, 1994) as part of the research criteria for PCS, only one, disordered sleep, discriminated individuals with MTBI from control subjects at 1 month posttrauma in the Dikmen et al. (1986) study. This same symptom of disturbed sleep was endorsed by 59% of the Iverson and McCracken (1997) non-TBI chronic pain patients. All eight *DSM-IV* PCS symptoms also had high rates of occurrence in the Lees-Haley and Brown (1993) non-head-injured litigants, ranging from 44% (dizziness) to over 80% (disordered sleep, 92%; headache, 88%; anxiety, 93%).

TABLE 7-2. Complaint Base Rates

	PERCENTAGE ENDORSING COMPLAINT		
SYMPTOM	MILD TRAUMATIC BRAIN INJURY[a]	MEDICAL OUTPATIENTS[b]	NONNEUROLOGICAL LITIGANTS[b]
Headache	59.1	62	88
Anxiety	58.3	54	93
Depression	63.2	32	89
Poor concentration	70.5	26	78
Dizziness	52.0	26	44
Visual problems	45.4	22	32
Irritability	65.9	38	77
Fatigue	63.9	58	79
Trouble thinking	57.6	16	59[c]
Poor memory	50.6[d]	20	53

[a]Mittenberg et al. (1992); 100 persons with mild traumatic brain injury.
[b]Lees-Haley and Brown (1993); 50 nonlitigating medical outpatients and 170 persons in litigation for psychological stress or distress and without neurological claims or injuries.
[c]"Confusion" in Lees-Haley and Brown (1993).
[d]"Forgets why they entered a room," the most frequent of 20 memory complaints in Mittenberg et al. (1992).

Postconcussion syndrome and other "neurological" symptoms are poorly correlated with actual neuropsychological test performance for a variety of clinical samples. Patients with severe TBI, Alzheimer-type dementia, and nontraumatic focal hemispheric brain disease frequently demonstrate anosognosia or denial or minimization of deficit (Feher, Larrabee, Sudilovsky, & Crook, 1994; Prigatano, 1996; Prigatano & Altman, 1990). Conversely, persons without neuropsychological deficit may misreport memory dysfunction secondary to depression (Larrabee & Levin, 1986; Larrabee, West, & Crook, 1991; Williams, Little, Scates, & Blockman, 1987) or secondary to somatization (Hanninen et al., 1994). Brulot et al. (1997) found no correlation between Minnesota Multiphasic Personality Inventory 2 (MMPI-2) neurocorrection items (i.e., those items purportedly related to neurological dysfunction) and initial GCS, duration of PTA, or neuropsychological test performance in a large sample of TBI patients comprised primarily of subjects with MTBI. Rather, the purported neurocorrection items were significantly associated with elevations on the MMPI-2 Depression Content Scale.

Mittenberg et al. (1992) found that head trauma-naïve normal subjects, when asked to imagine they had sustained an MTBI, endorsed the same set of PCS symptoms as did persons with actual MTBI. Of particular interest, the subjects with MTBI underestimated the frequency at which these symptoms occurred prior to their trauma. Mittenberg et al. related their results to a process of selective attentional bias to common internal states, stress, and arousal. Putnam and Millis (1994) provided a similar explanation, characterized PPCS as a somatoform disorder, and drew parallels between selective attentional bias in persons with MTBI and the self-directed selective attention to bodily sensations in persons with elevated health concerns (see Watson & Pennebaker, 1989).

Failure to appreciate the nonspecificity of PCS symptoms can lead to misdiagnosis and iatrogenesis of persistent complaints (Larrabee, 1997; Newcombe, Rabbitt, & Briggs, 1994). If a patient is prone to attend selectively to common phenomenon and incorrectly attribute these to "brain injury," then "diagnosing" these symptoms as "PCS" can be quite damaging. Such a patient, who on a premorbid basis manifests tendencies toward excessive health concerns, may focus excessively on common daily symptoms such as irritability and forgetfulness and become more anxious regarding these "symptoms," fearing that these are the result of their recent MTBI. The problem is compounded if these individuals are informed by a variety of health care professionals that they have suffered TBI.

Consistent with the above conceptualization of PPCS, Mittenberg, Tremont, Zielinski, Fichera, and Rayls (1996) found that providing a patient with MTBI with a printed cognitive behavioral manual and having the patient meet with a therapist prior to hospital discharge resulted in shorter duration of symptoms and lower symptom endorsement rates at 6-month follow-up in comparison to a nontreatment control group who received routine hospital treatment and discharge recommendations. The cognitive behavioral manual reviewed the nature and incidence of expected symptoms, the cognitive behavioral model of symptom maintenance and treatment, as well as techniques for reducing symptoms and instructions for gradual resumption of premorbid activities (see Mittenberg, Zielinski, & Fichera, 1993).

Negative expectations about outcome of MTBI can also affect neuropsychological test performance in addition to maintaining or increasing PCS symptom report. Suhr and Gunstad (2002) found that those MTBI subjects who had their attention called to their prior head injury history and who were advised of the potential effects of head injury on cognition ("diagnosis threat") performed less well on measures of general intellect and memory than did a group of MTBI subjects provided with neutral test instructions. Moreover, the diagnosis threat group rated themselves as putting forth less effort on the tests, and their self-rated degree of effort correlated with their performance on the Rey Auditory Verbal Learning Test and with their performance on the Complex Figure Test. Although Suhr and Gunstad did not administer symptom validity testing, the scores reported in their Table 2 are not consistent with the presence of malingering in the diagnosis threat group (e.g., their mean age-scaled score on Digit Span was 11.1). Hence, the motivational factors affecting the diagnosis threat group's performance appear to be unintentional and outside their conscious control.

DIFFERENTIAL DIAGNOSIS OF THE PATIENT WITH MILD TRAUMATIC BRAIN INJURY

As noted by Binder et al. (1997), the low base rate (5%) of persistent impairment following MTBI, results in positive predictive power of less than 50%, indicating a clinician is more likely to be incorrect than correct in diagnosing brain damage as the cause of persistent impairment. These data do not indicate that persistent impairment cannot occur, but do strongly underscore the need for the clinician to perform a careful differential diagnosis of the individual MTBI patient because the risk of false-positive diagnosis is high (Binder, 1997).

Risk factors for persistent problems following MTBI were reviewed in the section, "Factors Potentially Related to Persistent Problems Following Mild Traumatic Brain Injury." These factors include the possible effects of prior MTBIs on increased symptoms or prolonged recovery time following a subsequent MTBI. If such effects do occur, they should be manifested early on, with demonstration of prolonged confusion/disorientation immediately following an MTBI. Conversely, a very rapid return to orientation and processing of ongoing memory following an MTBI would appear to contradict any potential additive effects of a prior MTBI.

As noted, individuals with apparent MTBI who may have admission GCS values in the MTBI range of 13 to 15, who have CT or MRI abnormalities, focal neurological findings on day of injury, or PTA lasting longer than 24 hours are not actually individuals with MTBI. Rather, these are cases of complicated MTBI. Such cases may have recovery patterns more similar to moderate TBI as opposed to MTBI; that is, these cases may have persistent neuropsychological deficits on a chronic basis.

Thus, the careful differential diagnosis of the patient with MTBI must begin with the acute injury characteristics (Alexander, 1995). Records from EMS rescue runs and hospital ER records are important for characterizing day-of-injury TBI severity. These records will provide information on level of orientation, GCS rating, time of accident, and time spent in the hospital, as well as procedures conducted in the hospital. The memory and orientation of the patient with MTBI can be evaluated during clinical interview and later cross-checked against the EMS and ER records. Statements characterizing a patient as "oriented times three" actually describe the highest level of verbal response on the GCS. Moreover, orientation to time is typically the last component of orientation to recover during the resolution of PTA (High, Levin, & Gary, 1990). Hence, someone who is oriented times three (time, place, and person) is most likely no longer in PTA. The ER records will also contain information on presence/absence of focal neurological signs and whether a CT scan was done, as well as the results of any CT scan.

The section on PCS, which reviewed the nonspecificity of symptoms for MTBI, demonstrated the relationship of these symptoms to factors of depression, stress, and somatization. Consequently, any careful differential diagnosis of the individual MTBI case should also consider the possibility of symptom expression and maintenance because of a diagnosable psychiatric disorder. Binder (1997) cited Symonds (1937), who stated that, "It is not only the kind of injury that matters, but the kind of head" (p. 1092). As Binder observed, the kind of head is virtually as broad as the *DSM-IV*.

In addition to being sensitive to neurological dysfunction, performance on neuropsychological tests is also affected by a variety of psychiatric disorders, particularly disorders such as depression that affect attention and effortful processing (Cohen, Weingartner, Smallberg, Pickar, & Murphy, 1982; Cohen, 1993). Several *DSM-IV* disorders, including schizophrenia, mood disorders, anxiety disorders, and particularly posttraumatic stress disorder (PTSD), are characterized by accompanying cognitive symptoms (American Psychiatric Association, 1994).

Levin et al. (2001) found no neuropsychological differences when examined at 3 months posttrauma between trauma controls and a group of patients with mild-to-moderate TBI. In contrast, when the trauma control and MTBI groups were combined, then divided on the basis of presence/absence of either PTSD or major depressive disorder (MDD), differences emerged on neuropsychological testing. Patients with PTSD performed significantly less well on the Wisconsin Card Sorting Test than did patients without PTSD. Patients with MDD performed significantly less well on the Symbol Digit Modality Test, Rey Complex Figure, Verbal Selective Reminding Test, and Wisconsin Card Sorting Test than did patients without MDD. In particular, Levin et al. found that MDD was comorbid with PTSD, in addition to the aforementioned neuropsychological abnormalities, and associated with disability measured by the Glasgow Outcome Scale and Community Integration Questionnaire.

Chapter 10 in this volume reviews somatoform stress disorders, which must also be considered in any differential diagnosis of suspected MTBI. Mittenberg and Strauman (2000) considered PPCS following MTBI as a unique somatoform disorder specific to concussion. Alternatively, significant overlap of PCS symptoms with other disorders not characterized by history of concussion (e.g., chronic pain, Iverson & McCracken, 1997; litigants claiming psychological injuries, Lees-Haley & Brown, 1993) suggests that PPCS may be one of many exemplars of a more general category of somatoform stress disorder rather than specific to MTBI. This conclusion was supported in particular by Gouvier et al. (1992), who found no difference in rates of PCS symptom endorsement in college students who had history of MTBI compared with students who did not have history of MTBI. Moreover, both the MTBI and non-MTBI students experienced increased PCS symptom endorsement under periods of heightened daily stress.

Developmental disorders (Spreen, Risser, & Edgell, 1995) and substance abuse (see chapter 9, this volume) can also affect symptomatic complaints and neuropsychological test performance. Developmental learning disorders can present with specific reduction in verbal cognitive and memory skills (Rourke, 1991). Developmental nonverbal learning disability can result in significant social interaction difficulties in addition to specific reductions in nonverbal visual perceptual skills (Rourke, 1995). Persons with preexisting diagnoses of attention-deficit/hyperactivity disorder can show neuropsychological deficits in attention, as well as problems in impulse control (Barkley, 1998).

Chronic pain and pharmacological treatment of pain are also related to symptomatic complaints similar to those in PCS (Iverson & McCracken, 1997) as well as to changes in neuropsychological test performance (Taylor, Cox, & Mailis, 1996; Uomoto & Esselman, 1993). Chronic pain complaints, particularly headache and neck/shoulder and back pain, are significantly more frequent in those with MTBI relative to moderate or severe TBI; for instance, 95% of those with MTBI in one series had pain complaints, in contrast to only 22% of individuals with moderate-to-severe TBI with pain complaints (Uomoto & Esselman, 1993).

Taylor et al. (1996) compared the information-processing performance of three groups of patients, those with (a) whiplash, (b) chronic pain without history of whiplash or head injury, and (c) moderate-to-severe TBI. The whiplash and chronic pain groups were carefully matched on IQ, WMS-R Digit and Visual Span, pain severity ratings, and MMPI-2 profiles. Taylor et al. found no group differences on either the Paced Auditory Serial Addition Test (PASAT) or Auditory Consonant Trigrams procedures. Both the chronic pain and whiplash groups had higher pain ratings and MMPI-2 Depression scales than the moderate-to-severe TBI group, but did not differ from one another. These data clearly demonstrate the effects of chronic pain on neuropsychological test performance. Moreover, these data contradict the association between whiplash and brain dysfunction secondary to MTBI claimed by some investigators (Sweeney, 1992). Indeed, Taylor et al. (1996) concluded that their results demonstrated poor specificity for detecting subtle effects of brain trauma and did not support the theory of neuronal degeneration as the etiology of whiplash-related cognitive complaints.

Substance abuse, particularly alcohol abuse, is a significant differential diagnostic consideration, particularly given the known association of alcohol use with motor vehicle accidents. As reviewed, alcohol use does not appear to affect outcome adversely in MTBI (Alterman et al., 1985; Dikmen et al., 1993). Alcohol abuse, in and of itself, however, is certainly associated with neuropsychological deficits (Parsons, Butters, & Nathan, 1987). Data also exist demonstrating that nonalcoholic progeny of alcoholic parents perform more poorly on neuropsychological testing than do nonalcoholic progeny of nonalcoholic parents (see Parsons, 1987, for a review of these findings). Bolla reviews the neuropsychological effects of drugs of abuse in chapter 9 of this volume.

A major consideration in any differential diagnosis of MTBI is the possibility that deficits and complaints are the result of malingering. Malingering, the exaggeration or fabrication of symptoms or deficits for external incentives in adversarial circumstances, is reviewed by Larrabee in chapter 4 of this volume. Malingering is a frequent occurrence in litigated MTBI cases. Larrabee (2003) and Mittenberg et al. (2002) found, using different methodologies, an approximate 40% base rate of malingering in litigated MTBI cases, suggesting that this is a reliable estimate of malingering base rate on average. The base rate of 40% is eight times the 5% frequency of persistent neuropsychological deficits in individuals with MTBI who were followed prospectively since the time of their injury and reported by Binder et al. (1997). Indeed, Mittenberg et al. (2002) argued that, given Binder et al.'s 5% base rate of persistent deficit following MTBI and their survey data indicating a malingering base rate of 40%, the actual base rate of malingering in litigants showing neuropsychological deficits following MTBI may be as high as 88%. Refer to chapter 4 in this volume for further discussion of the evaluation and diagnosis of malingering.

FUTURE DIRECTIONS

There are two main areas for which additional research will be of interest: (a) developing a better understanding of the persons falling in the miserable minority who have less than the expected full recovery following MTBI and (b) additional research into the consequences of multiple MTBIs. Do persons in the miserable minority have preexisting problems that predispose to experiencing less than full recovery from MTBI? Following how many MTBIs does someone need to become concerned about potential permanent neuropsychological deficits?

Research on identification of persons who are going to fall in the miserable minority needs to be conducted on a prospective basis from the time of injury forward, rather than on the basis of samples of convenience collected from persons presenting for clinical services 1 or 2 years posttrauma. As discussed in this chapter, following patients prospectively, from the time they enter the emergency room, ensures a study of a representative sample of MTBI.

Given the strong evidence emerging from the sports concussion research of full recovery from a single MTBI (Collins et al., 1999; Echemendia et al., 2001; Macciocci et al., 1996; McCrea et al., 2003) and the strong evidence, in prospective research, of full recovery (Binder et al., 1997; Dikmen et al., 1995; Schretlen & Shapiro, 2003), it may develop that persons falling in the miserable minority have persisting complaints and problems on a psychological basis as part of a somatoform equivalent disorder (Mittenberg et al., 1992, 1996; Putnam & Millis, 1994; Suhr & Gundstad, 2002), as a consequence of posttraumatic stress disorder (Levin et al., 2001), or as a consequence of preexisting psychiatric or neurological conditions (Dikmen et al., 2001; Luis, Vanderploeg, & Curtiss, 2003).

Alternatively, it may develop that, as a function of greater neurological insult, persons with GCS of 13 are at greater risk for less-than-full recovery than are persons who have GCS of 15 (Culotta et al., 1996). Thus, efforts directed at grading the severity of MTBI, such as have been developed for sports concussion (American Neurological Association, 1997) or criteria developed by Ruff and Richardson (1999) that emphasize duration of PTA and persistence of neurological symptoms in the first 24 hours posttrauma, may yield information useful in predicting who will become part of the miserable minority. Last, the role of litigation in persistence of MTBI symptomatology must be explored further (Binder & Rohling, 1996).

Additional research is needed on the relationship of multiple MTBIs to the likelihood of persistent neuropsychological deficits. Gronwall's laboratory (Gronwall, 1989; Gronwall & Wrightson, 1975) showed that persons with a history of prior MTBI took longer to recover than persons with a single MTBI. The issue of persistence of deficit was not addressed. Collins et al. (2002) reported that concussed high school athletes with three or more prior concussions were 9.3 times more likely than concussed athletes with no prior history of concussion to demonstrate three to four abnormal on-field markers of concussion severity. McCrea et al. (2003) found greater risk of sustaining a subsequent concussion in football players with history of preexisting concussion and longer time for symptom resolution in patients with history of three as opposed to one prior concussion.

Of particular interest in relation to evaluating the effects of multiple MTBIs is the work of Bijur et al. (1996), who found that an apparent cumulative effect of multiple MTBIs in children did *not* reflect cumulative neuropsychological deficit; rather, the lower performance of children with multiple MTBI paralleled the performance of children with multiple orthopedic injuries. In other words, children at risk for multiple injuries (head or orthopedic) had lower neuropsychological scores than those children with a single injury (head or orthopedic), showing Satz et al.'s (1999) "general injury effect, head and body," but *not* showing evidence for head injury effect.

The optimal "laboratories" for evaluation of the effects of multiple MTBIs are the sports concussion programs currently in place in professional and collegiate sports programs. Preseason baseline neuropsychological testing allows more accurate measurement of post-MTBI cognitive change. Per Bijur et al.'s

(1996) research, a control group of athletes suffering one or more significant orthopedic injuries would be of interest as a control for general injury (head and nonhead) effects on neuropsychological test performance.

ACKNOWLEDGMENT

I acknowledge the assistance of Bridgette O'Brien in the preparation of this chapter.

REFERENCES

Alexander, M. P. (1995). Mild traumatic brain injury: Pathophysiology, natural history, and clinical management. *Neurology, 45,* 1253–1260.

Alterman, A. I., Goldstein, G., Shelly, C., & Bober, B. (1985). The impact of mild head injury on neuropsychological capacity in chronic alcoholics. *International Journal of Neuroscience, 28,* 155–162.

American Academy of Neurology. (1997). Practice parameter: The management of concussion in sports (summary statement). *Neurology, 48,* 581–585.

American Congress of Rehabilitation Medicine. (1993). Definition of mild traumatic brain injury. *Journal of Head Trauma Rehabilitation, 8,* 86–87.

American Psychiatric Association. (1994). *Diagnostic and statistical manual of mental disorders* (4th ed.). Washington, DC: Author.

Anderson, V., Catroppa, C., Morse, S., Haritou, F., & Rosenfeld, J. (2001). Outcome from mild head injury in young children: A prospective study. *Journal of Clinical and Experimental Neuropsychology, 23,* 705–717.

Axelrod, B. N., Fox, D. D., Lees-Haley, P. R., Earnes, K., Dolezal-Wood, S., & Goldman, R. S. (1996). Latent structure of the Postconcussion Syndrome Questionnaire. *Psychological Assessment, 8,* 422–427.

Barkley, R. A. (Ed.). (1998). *Attention-deficit hyperactivity disorder. A handbook for diagnosis and treatment* (2nd ed.). New York: Guilford Press.

Bigler, E. D. (2001). The lesion(s) in traumatic brain injury: Implications for clinical neuropsychology. *Archives of Clinical Neuropsychology, 16,* 95–131.

Bigler, E. D. (2003). Neurobiology and neuropathology underlie the neuropsychological deficits associated with traumatic brain injury. *Archives of Clinical Neuropsychology, 18,* 595–621.

Bijur, P. E., Haslum, M., & Golding, J. (1996). Cognitive outcomes of multiple mild head injuries in children. *Developmental and Behavioral Pediatrics, 17,* 143–148.

Binder, L. M. (1997). A review of mild head trauma. Part II: Clinical implications. *Journal of Clinical and Experimental Neuropsychology, 19,* 432–457.

Binder, L. M., & Kelly, M. P. (1996). Portland Digit Recognition Test performance by brain dysfunction patients without financial incentives. *Assessment, 3,* 403–409.

Binder, L. M., & Rohling, M. L. (1996). Money matters: A meta-analytic review of the effects of financial incentives on recovery after closed head injury. *American Journal of Psychiatry, 153,* 5–8.

Binder, L. M., Rohling, M. L., & Larrabee, G. J. (1997). A review of mild head trauma.

Part I: Meta-analytic review of neuropsychological studies. *Journal of Clinical and Experimental Neuropsychology, 19*, 421–431.

Bornstein, R. A., Podraza, A. M., Para, M. F., Whitacre, C. C., Fass, R. J., Rice, R. R., et al. (1993). Effect of minor head injury on neuropsychological performance in asymptomatic HIV-1 infection. *Neuropsychology, 7*, 228–234.

Brulot, M. M., Strauss, E., & Spellacy, F. (1997). Validity of the Minnesota Multiphasic Personality Inventory-2 correction factors for use with patients with suspected head injury. *The Clinical Neuropsychologist, 11*, 391–401.

Cantu, R. C. (1986). Guidelines for return to contact sports after a cerebral concussion. *Physical Sports Medicine, 14*, 10.

Cohen, R. A. (1993). *The neuropsychology of attention.* New York: Plenum Press.

Cohen, R. M., Weingartner, H., Smallberg, S. A., Pickar, D., & Murphy, D. L. (1982). Effort and cognition in depression. *Archives of General Psychiatry, 39*, 593–597.

Collins, M. W., Grindel, S. H., Lovell, M. R., Dede, D. E., Moser, D. J., Phalin, B. R., et al. (1999). Relationship between concussion and neuropsychological performance in college football players. *Journal of the American Medical Association, 282*, 964–970.

Collins, M. W., Lovell, M. R., Iverson, G. L., Cantu, R. C., Maroon, J. C., & Field, M. (2002). Cumulative effects of concussion in high school athletes. *Neurosurgery, 51*, 1175–1181.

Colorado Medical Society. (1990). *Report of the sports medicine committee. Guidelines for the management of concussion in sports.* Denver, CO: Author.

Cullum, C. M., & Thompson, L. L. (1999). Evaluation of neuropsychological status following mild traumatic brain injury. In M. J. Raymond, T. L. Bennett, L. C. Hartlage, & C. M. Cullum (Eds.), *Mild traumatic brain injury* (pp. 31–47). Austin, TX: Pro-Ed.

Culotta, V. P., Sementilli, M. E., Gerold, K., & Watts, C. C. (1996). Clinicopathological heterogeneity in the classification of mild head injury. *Neurosurgery, 38*, 245–250.

Dikmen, S. S., Donovan, D. M., Loberg, T., Machamer, J. E., & Temkin, N. R. (1993). Alcohol use and its effects on neuropsychological outcome in head injury. *Neuropsychology, 7*, 296–305.

Dikmen, S. S., Machamer, J. E., & Temkin, N. R. (2001). Mild head injury: Facts and artifacts. *Journal of Clinical and Experimental Neuropsychology, 23*, 729–738.

Dikmen, S. S., Machamer, J. E., & Temkin, N. R. (2003, February). *Mild traumatic brain injury with and without CT abnormalities.* Paper presented at the annual meeting of the International Neuropsychological Society, Honolulu, HI.

Dikmen, S. S., Machamer, J. E., Winn, H. R., & Temkin, N. R. (1995). Neuropsychological outcome at 1-year post head injury. *Neuropsychology, 9*, 80–90.

Dikmen, S., McLean, A., & Temkin, N. (1986). Neuropsychological and psychosocial consequences of minor head injury. *Journal of Neurology, Neurosurgery, and Psychiatry, 49*, 1227–1232.

Dikmen, S. S., Temkin, N. R., Machamer, J. E., Holubkov, A. L., Fraser, R. T., & Winn, H. R. (1994). Employment following traumatic head injuries. *Archives of Neurology, 51*, 177–186.

Echemendia, R. J., Putukian, M., Mackin, R. S., Julian, L., & Shoss, N. (2001). Neuropsychological test performance prior to and following sports-related mild traumatic brain injury. *Clinical Journal of Sports Medicine, 11*, 23–31.

Ewing, R., McCarthy, C., Gronwall, D., & Wrightson, P. (1980). Persisting effects of minor head injury observable during hypoxic stress. *Journal of Clinical Neuropsychology, 2*, 147–155.

Feher, E. P., Larrabee, G. J., Sudilovsky, A., & Crook, T. H. (1994). Memory self-report in Alzheimer's disease and in age-associated memory impairment. *Journal of Geriatric Psychiatry and Neurology, 7,* 58–65.

Feinstein, A., Ouchterlony, D., Somerville, J., & Jardine, A. (2001). The effects of litigation on symptom expression: A prospective study following mild traumatic brain injury. *Medical Science and the Law, 41,* 116–121.

Fox, D. D., & Allen, L. M. (2003). Discussion. Rebuttal to Bigler's response to our commentary on "The lesion(s) in traumatic brain injury": Let's stick to science. *Archives of Clinical Neuropsychology, 18,* 623–624.

Gasquoine, P. G. (1997). Postconcussion symptoms. *Neuropsychology Review, 7,* 77–85.

Goldstein, F. C., & Levin, H. S. (2001). Cognitive outcome after mild and moderate traumatic brain injury in older adults. *Journal of Clinical and Experimental Neuropsychology, 23,* 739–753.

Goldstein, F. C., Levin, H. S., Goldman, W. P., Clark, B. A., & Altonen, T. K. (2001). Cognitive and neurobehavioral function after mild versus moderate traumatic brain injury in older adults. *Journal of the International Neuropsychological Society, 7,* 373–383.

Gouvier, W. D., Cubic, B., Jones, G., Brantley, P., & Cutlip, Q. (1992). Postconcussion symptoms and daily stress in normal and head-injured college populations. *Archives of Clinical Neuropsychology, 7,* 193–211.

Green, P. (2003). Discussion. Welcoming a paradigm shift in neuropsychology. *Archives of Clinical Neuropsychology, 18,* 625–627.

Green, P., Iverson, G. L., & Allen, L. (1999). Detecting malingering in head injury litigation with the Word Memory Test. *Brain Injury, 13,* 813–819.

Green, P., Rohling, M. L., Lees-Haley, P. R., & Allen, L. M. (2001). Effort has a greater effect on test scores than severe brain injury in compensation claimants. *Brain Injury, 15,* 1045–1060.

Gronwall, D. (1989). Cumulative and persisting effects of concussion on attention and cognition. In H. S. Levin, H. M. Eisenberg, & A. L. Benton (Eds.), *Mild head injury* (pp. 153–162). New York: Oxford University Press.

Gronwall, D., & Wrightson, P. (1975). Cumulative effect of concussion. *Lancet, 2,* 995–997.

Guilmette, T. J., & Rasile, D. (1995). Sensitivity, specificity, and diagnostic accuracy of three verbal memory measures in the assessment of mild brain injury. *Neuropsychology, 9,* 338–344.

Guskiewicz, K. M., McCrea, M., Marshall, S. W., Cantu, R. C., Randolph, C., Barr, W., et al. (2003). Cumulative effects associated with recurrent concussion in collegiate football players. The NCAA concussion study. *Journal of the American Medical Association, 290,* 2549–2555.

Hanninen, T., Reinikainen, K. J., Helkala, E.-L., Koivisto, K., Mykkanen, L., Laakso, M., et al. (1994). Subjective memory complaints and personality traits in normal elderly subjects. *Journal of the American Geriatric Society, 42,* 1–4.

Heaton, R. K., Grant, I., & Matthews, C. G. (1991). *Comprehensive norms for an expanded Halstead-Reitan battery. Demographic corrections, research findings, and clinical applications.* Odessa, FL: Psychological Assessment Resources.

High, W. M., Levin, H. S., & Gary, H. E. (1990). Recovery of orientation following closed-head injury. *Journal of Clinical and Experimental Neuropsychology, 12,* 703–714.

Hinton-Bayre, A. D., & Geffen, G. (2002). Severity of sports-related concussion and neuropsychological test performance. *Neurology, 59,* 1068–1070.

Iverson, G. L., & McCracken, L. M. (1997). "Postconcussive" symptoms in persons with chronic pain. *Brain Injury, 11,* 783–790.

Kraus, J. F., & Arzemanian, S. (1989). Epidemiologic features of mild and moderate brain injury. In J. T. Hoff, T. E. Anderson, & T. M. Cole (Eds.), *Mild to moderate head injury* (pp. 9–28). Boston, MA: Blackwell.

Larrabee, G. J. (1990). Cautions in the use of neuropsychological evaluation in legal settings. *Neuropsychology, 4,* 239–247.

Larrabee, G. J. (1997). Neuropsychological outcome, postconcussion symptoms, and forensic considerations in mild closed head trauma. *Seminars in Clinical Neuropsychiatry, 2,* 196–206.

Larrabee, G. J. (2003). Detection of malingering using atypical performance patterns on standard neuropsychological tests. *The Clinical Neuropsychologist, 17,* 410–425.

Larrabee, G. J., & Levin, H. S. (1986). Memory self-ratings and objective test performance in a normal elderly sample. *Journal of Clinical and Experimental Neuropsychology, 8,* 275–284.

Larrabee, G. J., West, R. L., & Crook, T. H. (1991). The association of memory complaint with computer-simulated everyday memory performance. *Journal of Clinical and Experimental Neuropsychology, 13,* 466–478.

Lees-Haley, P. R., & Brown, R. S. (1993). Neuropsychological complaint baserates of 170 personal injury claimants. *Archives of Clinical Neuropsychology, 8,* 203–209.

Lees-Haley, P. R., Fox, D. D., & Courtney, J. C. (2001). A comparison of complaints by mild brain injury claimants and other claimants describing subjective experiences immediately following their injury. *Archives of Clinical Neuropsychology, 16,* 689–695.

Lees-Haley, P. R., Green, P., Rohling, M. L., Fox, D. D., & Allen, L. M. (2003). Commentary. The lesion(s) in traumatic brain injury: Implications for clinical neuropsychology. *Archives of Clinical Neuropsychology, 18,* 585–594.

Leininger, B. E., Gramling, S. E., Farrell, A. D., Kreutzer, J. S., & Peck, E. A. (1990). Neuropsychological deficits in symptomatic minor head injury patients after concussion and mild concussion. *Journal of Neurology, Neurosurgery, and Psychiatry, 53,* 293–296.

Levin, H. S., Amparo, E., Eisenberg, H. M., Williams, D. H., High, W. M., McCardle, C., et al. (1987). Magnetic resonance imaging and computerized neurobehavioral sequelae of mild and moderate head injuries. *Journal of Neurosurgery, 66,* 706–713.

Levin, H. S., Brown, S. A., Song, J. X., McCauley, S. R., Boake, C., Contant, C. F., et al. (2001). Depression and posttraumatic stress disorder at 3 months after mild to moderate traumatic brain injury. *Journal of Clinical and Experimental Neuropsychology, 23,* 754–769.

Levin, H. S., Mattis, S., Ruff, R. M., Eisenberg, H. M., Marshall, L. F., Tabaddor, K., et al. (1987). Neurobehavioral outcome following minor head injury: A three-center study. *Journal of Neurosurgery, 66,* 234–243.

Levin, H. S., Williams, D. H., Eisenberg, H. M., High, W. M., & Guinto, F. C. (1992). Serial MRI and neurobehavioral findings after mild to moderate closed head injury. *Journal of Neurology, Neurosurgery, and Psychiatry, 55,* 255–262.

Lishman, W. A. (1988). Physiogenesis and psychogenesis in the "post-concussional syndrome." *British Journal of Psychiatry, 153,* 460–469.

Lovell, M. R., Iverson, G. L., Collins, M. W., McKeag, D., & Maroon, J. C. (1999).

Does loss of consciousness predict neuropsychological decrements after concussion. *Clinical Journal of Sports Medicine, 9,* 193–198.

Luis, C. A., Vanderploeg, R. D., & Curtiss, G. (2003). Predictors of postconcussion symptom complex in community dwelling male veterans. *Journal of the International Neuropsychological Society, 9,* 1001–1015.

Macciocchi, S. N., Barth, J. T., Alves, W., Rimel, R. W., & Jane, J. A. (1996). Neuropsychological functioning and recovery after mild head injury in collegiate athletes. *Neurosurgery, 39,* 510–514.

McCrea, M., Guskiewicz, K. M., Marshall, S. W., Barr, W., Randolph, C., Cantu, R. C., et al. (2003). Acute effects and recovery time following concussion in collegiate football players. The NCAA concussion study. *Journal of the American Medical Association, 290,* 2556–2563.

McCrea, M., Kelly, J. P., Randolph, C., Cisler, R., & Berger, L. (2002). Immediate neurocognitive effects of concussion. *Neurosurgery, 50,* 1032–1042.

Mittenberg, W., DiGiulio, D. V., Perrin, S., & Bass, A. E. (1992). Symptoms following mild head injury: Expectation as aetiology. *Journal of Neurology, Neurosurgery, and Psychiatry, 55,* 200–204.

Mittenberg, W., Patton, C., Canyock, E. M., & Condit, D. C. (2002). Base rates of malingering and symptom exaggeration. *Journal of Clinical and Experimental Neuropsychology, 24,* 1094–1102.

Mittenberg, W., & Strauman, S. (2000). Diagnosis of mild head injury and the postconcussion syndrome. *Journal of Head Trauma Rehabilitation, 15,* 783–791.

Mittenberg, W., Tremont, G., Zielinski, R. F., Fichera, S., & Rayls, K. R. (1996). Cognitive behavioral prevention of postconcussion syndrome. *Archives of Clinical Neuropsychology, 11,* 139–145.

Mittenberg. W., Zielinski, R., & Fichera, R. (1993). Recovery from mild head injury: A treatment manual for patients. *Psychotherapy in Private Practice, 12,* 37–52.

Newcombe, F., Rabbitt, P., & Briggs, M. (1994). Minor head injury: Pathophysiological or iatrogenic sequelae? *Journal of Neurology, Neurosurgery, and Psychiatry, 57,* 709–716.

Parsons, O. A. (1987). Neuropsychological consequences of alcohol abuse: Many questions—some answers. In O. A. Parsons, N. Butters, & P. E. Nathan (Eds.), *Neuropsychology of alcoholism: Implications for diagnosis and treatment* (pp. 153–175). New York: Guilford.

Parsons, O. A., Butters, N., & Nathan, P. E. (Eds.). (1987). *Neuropsychology of alcoholism: Implications for diagnosis and treatment.* New York: Guilford Press.

Prigatano, G. P. (1996). Behavioral limitations TBI patients tend to underestimate: A replication and extension to patients with lateralized cerebral dysfunction. *The Clinical Neuropsychologist, 10,* 191–201.

Prigatano, G. P., & Altman, I. M. (1990). Impaired awareness of behavioral limitations after traumatic brain injury. *Archives of Physical Medicine and Rehabilitation, 71,* 1058–1064.

Putnam, S. H., & Millis, S. R. (1994). Psychosocial factors in the development and maintenance of chronic somatic and functional symptoms following mild traumatic brain injury. *Advances in Medical Psychotherapy, 7,* 1–22.

Rohling, M. L., Meyers, J. E., & Millis, S. R. (2003). Neuropsychological impairment following traumatic brain injury: A dose–response analysis. *The Clinical Neuropsychologist, 17,* 289–302.

Rourke, B P. (Ed.). (1991). *Neuropsychological validation of learning disability subtypes*. New York: Guilford Press.

Rourke, B. P. (Ed.). (1995). *Syndrome of nonverbal learning disabilities. Neurodevelopmental manifestations*. New York: Guilford Press.

Ruff, R. M., Levin, H. S., Mattis, S., High, W. M., Marshall, L. F., Eisenberg, H. M., et al. (1989). Recovery of memory after mild head injury: A three-center study. In H. S. Levin, H. M. Eisenberg, & A. L. Benton (Eds.), *Mild head injury* (pp. 176–188). New York: Oxford University Press.

Ruff, R. M., & Richardson, A. M. (1999). Mild traumatic brain injury. In J. J. Sweet (Ed.), *Forensic neuropsychology. Fundamentals and practice* (pp. 313–338). Lisse, The Netherlands: Swets and Zeitlinger.

Satz, P. (1993). Brain reserve capacity on symptom onset after brain injury. A formulation and review of evidence for threshold theory. *Neuropsychology, 7*, 273–295.

Satz, P., Alfano, M. S., Light, R., Morgenstern, H., Zaucha, K., Asarnow, R. F., et al. (1999). Persistent post-concussive syndrome: A proposed methodology and literature review to determine the effects, if any, of mild head and other bodily injury. *Journal of Clinical and Experimental Neuropsychology, 21*, 620–628.

Satz, P., Zaucha, K., McCleary, C., Light, R., Asarnow, R., & Becker, D. (1997). Mild head injury in children and adolescents: A review of studies (1970–1995). *Psychological Bulletin, 122*, 107–131.

Schretlen, D. J., & Shapiro, A. M. (2003). A quantitative review of the effects of traumatic brain injury on cognitive functioning. *International Review of Psychiatry, 15*, 341–349.

Spreen, O., Risser, A. T., & Edgell, D. (1995). *Developmental neuropsychology*. New York: Oxford University Press.

Suhr, J. A., & Gunstad, J. (2002). "Diagnosis threat": The effect of negative expectations on cognitive performance in head injury. *Journal of Clinical and Experimental Neuropsychology, 24*, 448–457.

Sweeney, J. E. (1992). Non-impact brain injury: Grounds for clinical study of the neuropsychological effects of acceleration forces. *The Clinical Neuropsychologist, 6*, 443–457.

Symonds, C. P. (1937). Mental disorder following head injury. *Proceedings of the Royal Society of Medicine, 30*, 1081–1092.

Taylor, A. E., Cox, C. A., & Mailis, A. (1996). Persistent neuropsychological deficits following whiplash: Evidence for chronic mild traumatic brain injury? *Archives of Physical Medicine and Rehabilitation, 77*, 529–535.

Trahan, D. E., Ross, C. E., & Trahan, S. L. (2001). Relationships among postconcussional-type symptoms, depression, and anxiety in neurologically normal young adults and victims of mild brain injury. *Archives of Clinical Neuropsychology, 16*, 435–445.

Uomoto, J. M., & Esselman, P. C. (1993). Traumatic brain injury and chronic pain: Differential types and rates by head injury severity. *Archives of Physical Medicine and Rehabilitation, 74*, 61–64.

Watson, D., & Pennebaker, J. W. (1989). Health complaints, stress, and distress: Exploring the central role of negative affectivity. *Psychological Review, 96*, 234–254.

Wechsler, D. (1981). *Wechsler Adult Intelligence Scale–Revised*. San Antonio, TX: Psychological Corporation.

Wechsler, D. (1987). *Wechsler Memory Scale–Revised*. San Antonio, TX: Psychological Corporation.

Williams, D. H., Levin, H. S., & Eisenberg, H. M. (1990). Mild head injury classification. *Neurosurgery, 27*, 422–428.

Williams, J. M., Little, M. M., Scates, S., & Blockman, N. (1987). Memory complaints
and abilities among depressed older adults. *Journal of Consulting and Clinical Psychology, 55*, 595–598.

Wilson, J. T., Teasdale, G. M., Hadley, D. M., Wiedman, K. D., & Lang, D. (1994).
Post-traumatic amnesia: Still a valuable yardstick. *Journal of Neurology, Neurosurgery, and Psychiatry, 57*, 198–201.

Zasler, N. (2000). Medical aspects. In S. A. Raskin & C. A. Mateer (Eds.), *Neuropsychological management of mild traumatic brain injury* (pp. 23–38). New York: Oxford
University Press.

8

Moderate and Severe Traumatic Brain Injury

MARK SHERER
CHARLENE F. MADISON

Mortality and morbidity caused by trauma are major public health problems in the United States. Data from the National Center for Health Statistics (Hoyert, Arias, Smith, Murphy, & Kochanek, 2001) indicate that trauma is the fifth leading cause of death for all Americans. Trauma is the leading cause of death for Americans from ages 1 to 34 years and the third leading cause of death from ages 35 to 54 years. The majority of trauma deaths are caused by traumatic brain injury (TBI).

Based on the 2000 U.S. Census population of 281,421,906, approximately 1,250,000 Americans were treated in hospital emergency departments (Jager, Weiss, Coben, & Pepe, 2000), 250,000 were hospitalized, and 56,000 died as a result of TBI in 2000 (Thurman, Alverson, Dunn, Guerrero, & Sniezek, 1999). Estimates indicate that 80,000 to 90,000 persons have new onset of disability each year caused by TBI (Thurman, Alverson, Dunn, et al., 1999). More than a million Americans live with disability caused by TBI (Thurman, Alverson, Browne, et al., 1999). Although the emotional cost of TBI is incalculable, the lifetime cost for persons who sustain TBI each year is estimated to be $37 billion (Max, MacKenzie, & Rice, 1991).

Given this high incidence and the likelihood of persistent impairments, neuropsychologists often evaluate and treat persons with TBI. Patients with moderate and severe TBI are much more likely to require inpatient (Harrison-Felix,

Newton, Hall, & Kreutzer, 1996) or postacute rehabilitation (Malec & Moessner, 2001; Sherer, Bergloff, High, & Nick, 1999) services compared to patients with mild TBI. Patients with mild TBI may be more likely to be seen in forensic or other compensation-related settings for which determination of whether the patient has any brain impairment or persisting sequelae is the focus of the evaluation (Binder, 1997; Binder & Willis, 1991).

The long-term effects of mild TBI remain controversial. Most consecutive series of trauma center patients with uncomplicated mild TBI showed that cognitive symptoms and deficits are resolved by 3 months postinjury (Dikmen, McLean, & Temkin, 1986; Levin, Mattis, et al., 1987; Williams, Levin, & Eisenberg, 1990). However, other investigators have found significant self-report of neurobehavioral symptoms in samples of patients with mild TBI who are referred for services in the postacute period (Alexander, 1992; Cicerone & Kalmar, 1995). These persistent complaints have been referred to as *postconcussion syndrome*, which is viewed by some as maintained by psychological rather than neurological factors (Mittenberg & Strauman, 2000). As a group, patients with moderate and severe TBI have poorer outcome in terms of both mortality and morbidity than patients with mild TBI (Dikmen et al., 1994; Dikmen, Machamer, Winn, & Temkin, 1995; Levin, 1993, 1995; Zhang, Jiang, Zhong, Yu, & Zhu, 2001).

Forensic issues in mild TBI are addressed in chapter 7 in the current volume. This chapter reviews (a) classification of TBI; (b) incidence of moderate and severe TBI; (c) course of recovery after moderate and severe TBI; (d) neuropsychological assessment of patients with moderate and severe TBI; (e) outcome after moderate and severe TBI including mortality, as well as physical, cognitive, neurobehavioral, and functional status outcomes; (f) prediction of outcome after TBI; and (g) life care planning for persons with continuing impairments after TBI.

CLASSIFICATION OF TRAUMATIC BRAIN INJURY SEVERITY

According to the Traumatic Brain Injury Model Systems National Data Center (1999), TBI can be defined as follows:

Damage to brain tissue caused by an external mechanical force as evidenced by: Loss of consciousness due to brain trauma, post-traumatic amnesia (PTA), skull fracture, or objective neurological findings attributed to TBI on physical examination or mental status examination.

Other authors (Williams et al., 1990) did not find that skull fracture is always associated with brain impairment. TBI severity is generally determined based on the depth of impaired consciousness or duration of impaired consciousness.

The most commonly used measure of depth of impaired consciousness is the Glasgow Coma Scale (GCS) (Teasdale & Jennett, 1974). The GCS measures

levels of responsiveness in eye opening, motor movement, and verbal communication. Scores range from 3 to 15, with higher scores indicating more intact
functioning. Patients with scores of 7 and below are definitely in coma, and
over 50% of those with scores of 8 are in coma (Jennett & Teasdale, 1977).
The GCS scores used for classification of TBI severity should be obtained immediately postresuscitation or at admission to the emergency department. Patients with postresuscitation GCS scores of 3 to 8 are classified as having had
severe TBI, and those with scores from 9 to 12 are classified as having had
moderate injuries (Clifton, Hayes, Levin, Michel, & Choi, 1992; Hannay &
Sherer, 1996; Levin & Eisenberg, 1991). Some researchers further divide the
severe group into very severe (GCS 3 to 5) and severe (GCS 6 to 8) (Zhang et
al., 2001).

Patients with GCS scores between 13 and 15 are classified as having had
mild injuries, but outcomes of these patients depend on the presence or absence
of depressed skull fracture or intracranial pathology as shown on the initial
computed tomographic (CT) scan. Patients with GCS scores between 13 and 15
with no depressed skull fracture or pathology on initial CT scan have uncomplicated mild TBI and have very favorable outcomes (Dikmen, Machamer, & Temkin, 2003; Williams et al., 1990). Patients with initial GCS scores between 13
and 15 who do have depressed skull fractures or CT scan abnormalities have
complicated mild TBI, and their outcomes are more similar to patients with
moderate TBI (Dikmen et al., 2003; Williams et al., 1990).

Return to a conscious or responsive state after TBI is indicated by ability to
follow simple commands, indicate yes/no reliably through words or gestures,
give intelligible verbalizations, or provide other purposeful behaviors (Giacino
et al., 2002). Most studies of recovery from TBI have used ability to follow
commands as the primary indication of return to a conscious state, but some
have used purposeful withdrawal from a painful stimulus (Levin, 1995; Whyte,
Cifu, Dikmen, & Temkin, 2001). Whyte and colleagues (Whyte et al., 2001)
found that ability to follow commands was the more useful of the two indices.

The interval from onset of injury to recovery of ability to follow commands
has proven to be a useful index in determining injury severity. Although time
to follow commands is the most accurate term for this interval, some authors
use the term *duration of unconsciousness.* This term may be inaccurate as some
aphasic patients may clearly be "conscious," but fail to demonstrate command
following (Levin, 1995).

Time to follow commands has been predictive of global outcome, neuropsychological functioning, personal independence, and employment outcome after
TBI (Dikmen, McLean, Temkin, & Wyler, 1986; Dikmen & Machamer, 1995;
Dikmen et al., 1994). Poorer outcomes are associated with longer intervals from
time of injury to time of recovery of ability to follow commands. The usefulness
of this index of TBI severity is limited by the lack of a commonly agreed-on

classification scheme. Further research is needed to determine the time to follow commands intervals that correspond to severe, moderate, or mild TBI.

Another index of TBI severity is duration of posttraumatic amnesia (PTA), which refers to the phase of recovery from TBI during which the patient is responsive, but is acutely confused and disoriented and is unable to form and retain new memories (Russell, 1932; Symonds, 1937). Although disorientation and memory disturbance are hallmarks of this phase of recovery, researchers have noted the similarity of this state to delirium and have recommended use of the term posttraumatic confusional state (Nakase-Thompson, Sherer, Yablon, Nick, & Trzepacz, 2004; Sherer, Nakase-Thompson, Nick, & Yablon, 2003; Stuss et al., 1999). Numerous studies have shown that duration of PTA is predictive of various aspects of outcome after TBI, including neuropsychological outcome, independent living status, and return to work (Dikmen et al., 1994; Ellenberg, Levin, & Saydjari, 1996; Sherer, Sander, et al., 2002).

Duration of PTA can be assessed retrospectively by waiting until the patient is no longer confused and asking him or her to report the first memory that he or she can recall following the brain injury (Symonds & Russell, 1943). More commonly, duration of PTA is determined prospectively by serial assessment of the patient's degree of disorientation. The most commonly used measure for this purpose is the Galveston Orientation and Amnesia Scale (GOAT) (Levin, O'Donnell, & Grossman, 1979). Other similar scales include the Orientation Log (Jackson, Novack, & Dowler, 1998), the Oxford Scale (Artiola I Fortuny, Briggs, Newcombe, Ratcliff, & Thomas, 1980), and the Westmead Scale (Shores, Marosszeky, Sandanam, & Batchelor, 1986).

As with time to follow commands, the usefulness of duration of PTA as an index of TBI severity is limited by the lack of commonly agreed on criteria for intervals indicating severe, moderate, and mild injuries. Perhaps the most commonly used criteria were developed by Russell and Smith (1961). In this scheme, patients with PTA less than 1 hour are classified as having had slight concussion, patients with PTA of 1 to 24 hours are classified as having had moderate concussion, patients with PTA of 1 to 7 days are classified as having had severe concussion, and patients with PTA over 7 days are classified as having had very severe concussion. Use of this scheme will result in misclassification of mild or moderate injuries as severe injuries because PTA of up to 2 weeks is not uncommon after complicated mild and moderate TBI (as classified by GCS criteria).

INCIDENCE OF MODERATE AND SEVERE TRAUMATIC BRAIN INJURY

The overall incidence rate of TBI is difficult to determine. This is because many individuals with mild TBI may not seek medical care, and if they do seek care, they may not be admitted to a hospital. Data from the National Hospital Ambulatory Medical Care Survey (Jager et al., 2000) indicated that 444 persons per 100,000 seek medical care for TBI each year. Based on a year 2000 U.S. census population of 281,421,906, this would indicate that approximately 1,250,000 persons sought medical care following TBI in 2000. The majority of these injuries would have been mild and would not have required hospitalization. Older series of patients hospitalized with TBI indicated that even of this group, 80% had mild injuries (Kraus, McArthur, Silverman, & Jayaraman, 1996).

With changes in health care provision, there has been a trend for fewer patients with mild TBI to be admitted to hospitals (Thurman & Guerrero, 1999). However, the hospitalization rates for patients with moderate and severe TBI remain largely unchanged from earlier reports. The Centers for Disease Control and Prevention estimated that 98 persons per 100,000 are hospitalized because of TBI each year (Thurman & Guerrero, 1999). Over 50% of these have mild injuries; 21% have moderate injuries, and 19% have severe injuries. The hospitalization rate for moderate TBI is 21 per 100,000, indicating about 59,000 injuries in 2000, and the hospitalization rate for severe TBI is 19 per 100,000, indicating about 53,500 injuries in 2000 for a total of about 102,500 moderate and severe TBIs per year. These rates do not include patients who expired prior to hospitalization. The Centers for Disease Control and Prevention estimated that approximately 56,000 persons die from TBI each year, and 80,000 to 90,000 are left with persistent disability caused by TBI each year (Thurman, Alverson, Dunn, et al., 1999).

COURSE OF RECOVERY

Significant TBI results in some degree of impaired consciousness (Levin, 1992; Ommaya & Gennarelli, 1974). Patients with severe injuries have coma (Ommaya & Gennarelli, 1974). Coma is a temporary nonresponsive state in which the patient has closed eyes, follows no instructions, gives no communication, and shows no purposeful movements (Teasdale & Jennett, 1974). Large consecutive series of patients admitted to emergency departments with severe TBI indicated that 23% to 49% of patients do not recover from coma (Murray et al., 1999; Zhang et al., 2001). Those patients who do survive almost always recover to a more responsive state. A small percentage of surviving patients, 1% to 5%, may remain in a nonresponsive vegetative state (Murray et al., 1999), but even these patient show recovery of some brain stem functioning and have return of sleep/wake cycles with periods of eye opening.

Surviving, nonvegetative patients recover to some degree of responsiveness to the environment. This level of responsiveness may be markedly reduced at first, as in the minimally conscious state (Giacino et al., 2002). Patients in this state show minimal, but definite, evidence of awareness of self or the environment. Examples include localized motor responses to noxious stimuli or sounds, sustained visual fixation, vocalization in response to a stimulus, smiling or crying in response to a stimulus, and inconsistent command following. Resolution of the minimally conscious state is indicated by consistent command following, verbal or gestural yes/no responding, intelligible verbalization, or some other evidence of consistent purposeful behavior, such as functional use of objects. This state is generally temporary, but may be permanent in a small subset of patients.

Most commonly, resolution of coma is followed by a responsive but markedly confused state. Patients with moderate TBI may have loss of consciousness at the time of injury, but (by definition) are responsive but confused at presentation to the emergency department. The period of acute confusion following TBI is a temporary phase of recovery (Levin, 1993). Most patients recover from the confused state, at least to some degree, although they may be left with persistent cognitive and behavioral impairments (Levin, 1992). Duration of confusion is a commonly used index of injury severity (Russell & Smith, 1961).

The confused phase of recovery after TBI is a complex state that manifests in a variety of neurobehavioral impairments. Early writers (Russell, 1932; Symonds, 1937) described deficits in arousal, memory, orientation, attention, language, behavior, mood, and perception. The period of confusion is now commonly called PTA, but early writers used many terms, including acute traumatic psychosis, aftereffects of concussion, traumatic confusion, and delirium.

Many previous investigations of the period of confusion after TBI have primarily focused on disorientation and memory impairment. High and colleagues (High, Levin, & Gary, 1990) found that orientation after TBI recovers sequentially, with initial recovery of orientation to person followed by orientation to place and time. Memory disturbance after head trauma is characterized by some loss of ability to recall events immediately preceding injury (retrograde amnesia) as well as a period of inability to encode and later recall new memories (anterograde amnesia) (Levin, 1992). Memory impairment during posttraumatic confusion is greatest for explicit, episodic memory with some sparing of implicit and procedural memory (Ewert, Levin, Watson, & Kalisky, 1989).

Attentional impairments during early recovery from TBI include difficulties focusing attention on the examiner, sustaining attention, processing information, and excessive distractibility (Levin, 1993). In their investigation of attentional functions in confused patients, Stuss and colleagues (1999) demonstrated that attentional abilities recover in an orderly manner after TBI. Performance on attentional tasks improved prior to obtaining a GOAT score in target range or ability to recall three words at a 24-hour delay (Stuss et al., 1999). Stuss and colleagues argued that attentional disturbance is a key aspect of impaired consciousness after TBI. They noted the similarity of this state to delirium and proposed the term *posttraumatic confusional state* (PTCS) to replace the more commonly used PTA.

Other investigators have studied motor restlessness (agitation) in confused patients after TBI. These investigations have found an association of restlessness with cognitive impairment. Agitation is common in patients with low levels of cognitive function, but rare in patients with higher levels of cognitive function (Corrigan & Mysiw, 1988). Patients with intermediate levels of cognitive function are equally likely to be agitated or nonagitated. Patients experience cognitive improvement prior to resolution of agitation as opposed to resolution of agitation followed by cognitive recovery.

Additional support has been provided for considering the period of confusion after TBI to be a complex neurobehavioral state similar to delirium, as opposed to a state primarily characterized by memory impairment, as suggested by the term PTA. Nakase-Thompson and colleagues (2004) found that 59 (69%) of 85 consecutive TBI patients admitted for inpatient rehabilitation met diagnostic criteria for delirium (American Psychiatric Association, 1994) at some point during their hospitalizations. Delirium in TBI is associated with poorer functional outcome at discharge from inpatient rehabilitation (Thompson, Sherer, Yablon, Kennedy, & Nick, 2002). Sherer, Nakase-Thompson, and colleagues (2003) found that seven key symptoms characterize the confused state after TBI: (a) disorientation, (b) impaired cognition, (c) restlessness, (d) fluctuation of symptom presentation, (e) sleep disturbance, (f) decreased daytime level of arousal, and (g) psychotic-type symptoms.

Preliminary cluster analysis of data from 62 consecutive TBI admissions for inpatient rehabilitation revealed two subtypes of confusional state. One type was characterized by high rates of restlessness and psychotic-type symptoms in conjunction with disorientation, cognitive impairment, and sleep disturbance. The second type was also characterized by disorientation and cognitive impairment, but these patients showed higher rates of daytime drowsiness and lower rates of restlessness, psychotic-type symptoms, and sleep disturbance (Sherer, Nakase-Thompson, et al., 2003). These two clusters appeared to indicate that post-TBI confusion can take an agitated form and a nonagitated form. These findings support the position of Stuss and colleagues (1999) that this phase of recovery after TBI is better characterized as PTCS as opposed to PTA.

After resolution of PTA (or PTCS), patients continue to show progressive resolution of physical, cognitive, and behavioral impairments. There is general agreement that recovery continues for up to 18 months after moderate or severe TBI (Dikmen, Reitan, & Temkin, 1983; Levin, 1995; Tabaddor, Mattis, & Zazula, 1984), and there is some evidence that some cognitive functions may continue to recover after this 18-month time frame (Millis et al., 2001; van Zomeren & Deelman, 1978).

In a few patients, recovery may be compromised by late complications such as posttraumatic epilepsy or posttraumatic hydrocephalus. Late seizures (greater than 2 weeks postinjury) occur in only about 4% to 7% of survivors of nonpenetrating TBI, but the incidence may be as high as 50% for patients with penetrating TBI (Annegers, Hauser, Coan, & Rocca, 1998; Yablon, 1996). The incidence of posttraumatic hydrocephalus is not well known because of wide variation in the degree of monitoring for this condition. One prospective series in which all patients with moderate or severe TBI admitted for inpatient rehabilitation received head CT scans found an incidence of 13% (Yu, Yablon, Ivanhoe, & Boake, 1995).

The TBI patients with large focal hemispheric lesions or certain subcortical, brain stem, or cerebellar lesions may have persistent motor impairments (Bontke, Zasler, & Boake, 1996; Horn & Sherer, 1999). Such impairments may include spasticity, dysphagia (impaired swallowing), dysarthria, balance disturbances, or hemiparesis. Most patients with moderate or severe TBI show good resolution of motor impairments.

The prognosis for recovery of cognitive abilities after moderate and severe TBI is less favorable than for motor functions. Risk for persistent cognitive impairment is related to initial injury severity, as indicated by postresuscitation GCS score or time to follow commands (Dikmen, Machamer, Winn, & Temkin, et al., 1995; Tabaddor et al., 1984). Even at 1 year postinjury, all patients with very severe TBI (time to follow commands 14 days or longer) have residual cognitive impairments, and more than half of those with time to follow commands between 1 hour and 13 days have residual deficits (Dikmen et al., 1995). Although the general course of recovery of cognitive abilities is for continuing improvements for about 18 months postinjury, a subgroup of patients shows improvement beyond this period (Millis et al., 2001). There is limited evidence that another subgroup of patients may show late decline (Millis et al., 2001; Ruff et al., 1991). Age at time of injury appears to be a risk factor for late decline, with older age at time of injury indicating greater risk for late decline.

The typical pattern of impairments after blunt head trauma includes slowed fine motor movements, decreased attention, decreased cognitive speed, memory impairment, impaired complex language skills and discourse, and impaired executive functions (Levin, 1993). Severe persistent aphasia or visual perceptual impairment are uncommon after diffuse injuries, but may occur in patients with focal injuries (Levin, 1993).

Patients with moderate and severe TBI may also show persistent neurobehavioral impairments, such as increased irritability, headache, anxiety, difficulty concentrating, fatigue, restlessness, and depression (Oddy, Humphrey, & Uttley, 1978; Satz et al., 1998). Patients and family members are more likely to report these neurobehavioral impairments than either cognitive or physical impairments in the postacute period (Brooks, Campsie, Symington, Beattie, & McKinlay, 1987; Lezak, 1987, 1989). Family members reported that these neurobehavioral symptoms, particularly personality change and threats of violence, cause more stress than cognitive or physical impairments (Brooks, Campsie, Symington, Beattie, & McKinlay, 1986). There is some evidence that family member report of these symptoms may actually increase with the passage of time (Brooks et al., 1986). It is unclear whether this is because of an actual increase in the frequency or severity of behavioral problems as opposed to a greater sensitivity to the effects of these problems.

One factor in family member stress associated with residual neurobehavioral impairments is the tendency for some TBI survivors to be partially or totally unaware of these problems (Prigatano, Altman, & O'Brien, 1990; Sherer, Boake, et al., 1998). Impaired self-awareness is common after moderate and severe TBI, both in the acute (Sherer, Hart, et al., 2003) and the postacute periods (Sherer, Bergloff, et al., 1998). Patients with poor self-awareness have poor motivation to change as they do not perceive the need to change (Malec & Moessner, 2001).

NEUROPSYCHOLOGICAL ASSESSMENT OF PATIENTS WITH MODERATE AND SEVERE TRAUMATIC BRAIN INJURY

There are a number of contributions that neuropsychological assessment can make to the care of persons with moderate and severe TBI. Such evaluations provide documentation of cognitive, behavioral, and emotional status and may assist with determination of patients' ability to function independently (Sherer & Novack, 2003). Documentation of status is useful to provide feedback to family members, improve patient self-awareness, guide treatment efforts, and assess the effectiveness of medication trials. Areas of functional ability that may be assessed include decision-making capacity, capacity for safe and independent home functioning, driving capacity, and ability to return to work.

The focus of neuropsychological assessment is determined both by the goals of the assessment and by the stage of recovery of the patient. Early neuropsychological assessment may focus on determining level of responsiveness and documenting changes in level of responsiveness in minimally conscious patients. Measures such as the Coma Recovery Scale (Giacino, Kezmarsky, DeLuca, & Cicerone, 1991) provide a structured repeatable protocol for assessing low-level patients. Areas assessed include arousal and attention, auditory perception, visual perception, motor function, oromotor ability, communication, and initiation.

With responsive but confused patients, assessment focuses on orientation, attentional skills, ability to form new memories, and level of agitation. Measures such as the GOAT (Levin et al., 1979) or Orientation Log (Jackson et al., 1998) can be used to assess orientation. The Toronto Test of Acute Recovery After

TBI (Stuss et al., 1999) includes simple measures of attentional skills and ability to form and retain new memories. The Agitated Behavior Scale (Corrigan, 1989) is the most commonly used measure of agitation after TBI. A new measure, the Confusion Assessment Protocol (Sherer, Nakase-Thompson, et al., 2003), includes elements of all these areas, and preliminary findings indicated that it may be useful in assessing a wide range of symptoms of confusion after TBI.

Some writers recommended delaying administration of formal neuropsychological tests until the patient has emerged from PTA (Clifton et al., 1992). This recommendation is based on the assumption that confused, disoriented patients will perform poorly on all tests, and thus little additional information will be obtained. Nonetheless, there is some evidence that administration of selected neuropsychological measures to patients still in PTA can result in useful data that are predictive of later functional status (Hannay & Sherer, 1996).

Initial and follow-up comprehensive neuropsychological evaluations of persons with moderate or severe TBI should assess a wide range of abilities, including orientation, fine motor skills, divided and sustained attention, cognitive speed, memory, language skills, visual-perceptual skills, and executive functions (Hannay & Sherer, 1996).

Two sample core neuropsychological batteries are presented in Table 8-1. Additional tests can be added to either of these batteries based on clinical judgment. Neurobehavioral problems such as mental flexibility, planning, unusual

TABLE 8-1. Sample Core Neuropsychological Assessment Batteries for Traumatic Brain Injury (TBI)

HOUSTON CONFERENCE BATTERY[a]	TBI MODEL SYSTEMS BATTERY[b]
Digit Symbol Substitution	Galveston Orientation and Amnesia Test
Paced Auditory Serial Addition Test	Grooved Peg Board Test
Rey Complex Figure Test	Digit Span
Selective Reminding Test	Symbol Digit Modalities Test
Controlled Oral Word Association Test	Trail Making Test
Trail Making Test, Part B	Benton Visual Form Discrimination Test
Wisconsin Card Sorting Test	Block Design Test
Grooved Peg Board Test	Controlled Oral Word Association Test
Neurobehavioral Rating Scale	Token Test
	Rey Auditory Verbal Learning Test
	Logical Memory Test
	Wisconsin Card Sorting Test
	Neurobehavioral Functioning Inventory

Note. Descriptions of these tests can be found in reference volumes on neuropsychological assessment such as Lezak (1995) and Spreen and Strauss (1998).
[a]Clifton et al. (1992).
[b]Traumatic Brain Injury Model Systems National Data Center (1999).

thought content, agitation, disinhibition, emotional withdrawal, hostility, depression, anxiety, and motor slowing should also be assessed (McCauley et al., 2001). Measures such as the Neurobehavioral Rating Scale (Levin, High, et al., 1987) and the Neurobehavioral Functioning Inventory (Kreutzer, Marwitz, Seel, & Serio, 1996) are helpful with assessment of neurobehavioral impairments.

The relationship between cognitive functioning and personal independence and employment is complex. Although neuropsychological findings are related to functional outcomes such as personal independence (Hart et al., 2003) and employment (Dikmen et al., 1994; Sherer, Sander, et al., 2002; Sherer, Novack, et al., 2002), these functional outcomes are also influenced by a variety of other factors, such as premorbid functioning, demographic variables, environmental supports, and family support (Sherer, Nick, et al., 2003). There are a number of instruments that can be used to rate patient functioning directly in these areas. Three scales that have been included in the TBI Model Systems protocol (Traumatic Brain Injury Model Systems National Data Center, 1999) are described next.

The Disability Rating Scale (DRS) (Rappaport, Hall, Hopkins, Belleza, & Cope, 1982) was developed to track patient progress after TBI from coma to return to community activities. The DRS is a 30-point scale that rates eight areas of functioning: eye opening; verbalization; motor response; level of cognitive ability for daily activities of feeding, toileting, and grooming; overall level of dependence; and employability. Higher scores indicate greater disability. Interrater reliability has ranged from 0.97 to 0.98 (Gouvier, Blanton, LaPorte, & Nepomuceno, 1987; Rappaport et al., 1982). The DRS has been sensitive to improvements in functioning between 2 and 6 months postinjury, as well as between 6 months and 1 year (Hall, Cope, & Rappaport, 1985).

The Supervision Rating Scale (SRS) (Boake, 1996) can be used to quantify the level of personal independence. The level of supervision received is rated on a 13-point ordinal scale, ranging from "independent" to "full-time direct supervision (with patient in physical restraints)." The SRS has satisfactory interrater reliability (Boake, 1996). The SRS scores are related to patient living arrangement and to skills in activities of daily living.

The Community Integration Questionnaire (Willer, Rosenthal, Kreutzer, Gordon, & Rempel, 1993) was developed to assess degree of community integration after TBI. Community functioning is rated in three areas: home integration, social integration, and productive activity. Studies of interrater reliability have found moderate to strong reliability (Sander et al., 1997; Willer, Ottenbacher, & Coad, 1994). Validity studies have shown that Community Integration Questionnaire scores are correlated with other measures of functional status, such as the DRS (Sander et al., 1999).

In an attempt to provide some guidance regarding timing of neuropsychological evaluations for patients with TBI of different severities, Sherer and Novack

TABLE 8-2. Schedule for Neuropsychological Evaluations After Traumatic Brain Injury (TBI)

TIME OF EVALUATION	SEVERE TBI	MODERATE TBI	MILD TBI
At resolution of posttraumatic amnesia	X	X	X
1 week to 1 month postinjury			X
3 months postinjury	X	X	X
6 months postinjury	X	X	
1 year postinjury	X	X	X
2 years postinjury	X	X	

(2003) conducted a survey of 41 neuropsychologists. Survey participants were selected based on board certification, published research on TBI, and current participation in TBI research. Of those surveyed, 33 responded. These respondents reported a median of 20 years of clinical experience with patients with TBI (range 7 to 35 years). Guidelines for timing of assessments based on this survey are summarized in Table 8-2. These guidelines provide general suggestions. Timing of testing for any specific patient should be determined by clinician judgment based on evaluation of factors unique to that patient.

In cases of moderate or severe TBI, there will generally be clear-cut medical evidence indicating that the patient sustained brain injury. This may be in the form of radiological findings, medical documentation of loss of consciousness, coma, sustained confusion, or operative reports. Nonetheless, such patients may occasionally exaggerate symptoms when seen for follow-up evaluations, particularly if they are engaged in litigation. Consequently, the symptom validity measures described by Larrabee in chapter 4 of this volume should also be administered for those patients with moderate or severe TBI who are involved in litigation or compensation actions.

OUTCOME AFTER MODERATE AND SEVERE
TRAUMATIC BRAIN INJURY

Outcome after moderate and severe TBI can be assessed in many ways. Neurosurgical studies may focus on early survival, and rehabilitation studies may focus on return to work or independent living. The Glasgow Outcome Scale (GOS; Jennett & Bond, 1975) is the most commonly used measure of overall outcome after TBI. With the GOS, outcomes are rated in five categories: (a) death; (b) vegetative state (unable to follow commands or communicate); (c) severe disability (conscious but requiring assistance to meet basic physical and cognitive needs such feeding, toileting, grooming, or personal safety); (d) moderate disability (able to meet basic physical and cognitive needs and use public transportation and work in a sheltered workshop, but unable to return to nonsheltered work or resume other major societal roles); and (e) good recovery (able to return to nonsheltered work, although perhaps in a decreased capacity, and resume social roles, although some neurological or psychological impairments may remain).

Death is a common outcome after severe TBI. Death rates for patients with severe TBI who have been hospitalized range from 23% to 50% (Braakman, Gelpke, Habbema, Maas, & Minderhoud, 1980; Jiang, Gao, Li, Yu, & Zhu, 2002; Marion, 1996; Murray et al., 1999; Zhang et al., 2001). The most typical death rate is about 40%. Causes of early death after TBI include brain swelling, diffuse axonal injury, increased intracranial pressure, and intracranial hematomas (Graham, Adams, & Gennarelli, 1993; Marion, 1996).

Only a few patients remain in a vegetative state after severe TBI. At 3 months postinjury, fewer than 10% of patients are in a vegetative state (Choi & Barnes, 1996; Choi et al., 1994), and by 6 months, only 4% remain vegetative (Murray et al., 1999). Of those who are vegetative at 3 months, 50% improve, 25% expire, and 25% remain in a vegetative state, so that, by 1 year postinjury, the incidence of vegetative state ranges from less than 1% (Jiang et al., 2002) to 2% or 3% (Choi et al., 1994; Choi & Barnes, 1996) of severe TBI survivors.

Outcome proportions for patients with severe disability, moderate disability, and good recovery given next are for patients with severe TBI who survived their acute hospitalizations, excluding those who expired. At 3 months postinjury, approximately 31% to 32% of surviving patients initially hospitalized with severe TBI remained with severe disability (Choi & Barnes, 1996; Choi et al., 1994). By 6 months postinjury, only about 22% remained with severe disability (Choi & Barnes, 1996; Choi et al., 1994; Murray et al., 1999). By 1 year postinjury, many patients who experienced severe disability at 3 months postinjury recovered to moderate disability or good recovery. Only about 17% of surviving patients remained with severe disability (Choi & Barnes, 1996; Choi et al., 1994).

Approximately 30% of patients with severe TBI have moderate disability at 3 and 6 months postinjury (Choi & Barnes, 1996; Choi et al., 1994; Murray et al., 1999). However, some of the patients who had moderate disability at 3 months have achieved good recovery by 6 months; some patients who were vegetative or had severe disability at 3 months have recovered to moderate disability by 6 months. By 1 year postinjury, 17% to 22% of patients with severe TBI remain with moderate disability (Choi et al., 1994; Zhang et al., 2001).

Good recovery is achieved by only 22% of patients with severe TBI by 3 months postinjury (Choi & Barnes, 1996; Choi et al., 1994). By 6 months postinjury, this has increased to over 35% (Choi et al., 1994; Murray et al., 1999). At 1 year after severe TBI, 46% to 54% of patients with severe TBI have reached good recovery (Choi et al., 1994; Zhang et al., 2001). Thus, for patients who survive severe TBI, good recovery is the most likely GOS outcome by 1 year postinjury. Note that these patients may remain with significant cognitive or neurobehavioral problems even though they have recovered well enough to return to work.

Death is a rare outcome after moderate TBI, occurring in fewer than 10% of cases (Murray et al., 1999; Stein, 1996). When death does occur, it is likely to be caused by associated trauma or medical complications (Signorini, Andrews, Jones, Wardlaw, & Miller, 1999). Vegetative state is even a rarer outcome after moderate TBI, with some large trauma series reporting no cases (Murray et al., 1999).

Severe disability does occur after moderate TBI, although it is uncommon. Some reports indicated that no moderately injured patients remained with severe disability at 6 months postinjury (Williams et al., 1990); others found that 6% (Stein, 1996) to 14% (Murray et al., 1999) had severe disability. Moderate disability is a more common outcome and is seen in about 25% of patients at 6 months postinjury (Jain, Layton, & Murray, 2000; Stein, 1996; Williams et al., 1990). Good recovery is by far the most common outcome after moderate TBI, with 53% (Murray et al., 1999) to 73% (Williams et al., 1990) of cases showing good recovery by 6 months postinjury. As with patients with severe TBI, good recovery cannot be taken to mean complete recovery.

Although data on GOS outcome categories are informative, clinicians, family, and patients are more likely to be concerned about the likelihood that a patient will return to work or to independent living. Employment outcomes have been studied more intensively than independent living outcomes. Perhaps this is because of the greater ease of characterizing employment status as opposed to degree of personal independence.

Reported return to work rates following TBI range from 22% to 66% (Sander, Kreutzer, Rosenthal, Delmonico, & Young, 1996). The wide range of rates is contributed to by interstudy differences in injury classification, populations sampled, time from injury to follow-up, and definition of employment. Previous investigations have focused on two populations of patients with TBI, consecutive cases seen at trauma centers and patients seen for inpatient rehabilitation. Both populations are important, but findings based on one population should not be generalized to the other. The subset of TBI patients admitted for inpatient rehabilitation excludes those with very poor outcomes, such as patients in a vegetative state and those with very good outcomes, such as those who are oriented and independent with activities of daily living prior to discharge from the acute care hospital.

Brooks and colleagues (Brooks, McKinlay, Symington, Beattie, & Campsie, 1987) reported on a series of 134 patients with severe TBI seen on an acute neurosurgical service. Most patients (75%) were employed at time of injury, but only 25% were employed at follow-up. Follow-up evaluations were performed ranging from 2 to 7 years postinjury. Dikmen and colleagues (1994) reported on a series of 366 patients with TBI who were admitted to a trauma center. Patients who were not employed at time of injury were excluded from study. At 1 year postinjury, 26% of patients with severe injuries had returned to work, and 56% of patients with moderate injuries had returned to work. By 2 years postinjury, 37% of patients with severe injuries were working, and 64% of patients with moderate injuries were working.

Sherer and colleagues (Sherer, Nick, et al., 2003) reported on 1,615 patients with TBI who were admitted to 17 TBI Model Systems sites for inpatient rehabilitation. Of this population, 72% were employed at time of injury. The 1-year employment outcome data were available for 1,083 patients. Of these 1,083 patients, 63% had severe injuries, 16% had moderate injuries, and 20% had complicated mild injuries. Patients who were available at follow-up had a higher preinjury employment rate (76%) than those lost to follow-up (68%). This suggests that the 1-year postinjury employment rate for the 1,083 patients is likely to overestimate the overall 1-year postinjury employment rate. For the 1,083 patients with available 1-year postinjury employment data, the employment rate was 35%.

We were unable to find a report of independent living status based on a consecutive series of patients seen at a trauma center. Hart and colleagues (Hart et al., 2003) reported on a series of 563 patients with TBI who were seen for inpatient rehabilitation. Patients who could not complete a neuropsychological evaluation during inpatient rehabilitation were excluded from study, meaning that patients with more severe injuries may be underrepresented in the study sample. Of this sample, 69% were rated as receiving no supervision at 1-year follow-up. There were 24% who received varying degrees of part-time supervision, and 7% received full-time supervision. Amount of supervision received at follow-up was generally related to initial injury severity as determined by GCS rating, with those having more impaired initial GCS ratings receiving more supervision at follow-up. However, initial GCS scores for those who were independent at follow-up ranged from 3 to 15, as did initial GCS scores for those receiving the highest levels of supervision at follow-up.

PREDICTION OF OUTCOME

There is a very large body of literature on prediction of outcome after moderate and severe TBI. Interpretation of this literature is complicated by the wide variety of populations sampled, time frames of outcomes, and outcomes studied. Factors predictive of a given outcome in a particular population over a specified time frame may not be at all predictive of apparently related outcomes in a different population over a different time frame. This is particularly the case for subpopulations who are highly selected (e.g., patients admitted for postacute rehabilitation services). We briefly review predictors of death after TBI and functional status at follow-up.

Factors most predictive of death after TBI are those that directly indicate neurological and physiological status early after injury. Such factors include (a) level of responsiveness as indicated by admission GCS score (Eisenberg & Weiner, 1987; Mosenthal et al., 2002); (b) pupillary responses (Andrews et al., 2002; Jiang et al., 2002; Wardlaw, Easton, & Statham, 2002); (c) initial CT scan findings (particularly presence of subarachnoid blood or mass lesion such as subdural hematoma) (Eisenberg & Weiner, 1987; Mataro et al., 2001; Wardlaw et al., 2002); (d) elevated temperature (Andrews et al., 2002; Jiang et al., 2002); (e) electrophysiological findings (Claassen & Hansen, 2001; Vespa et al., 2002); (f) elevated intracranial pressure (Eisenberg & Weiner, 1987; Jiang et al., 2002); and (g) hypoxia (Andrews et al., 2002; Eisenberg & Weiner, 1987; Jiang et al., 2002). Of demographic variables, age is most predictive of death, with older age associated with greater risk of death (Jiang et al., 2002; Mosenthal et al., 2002; Susman et al., 2002). Early neurosurgical management also affects death rates. Centers that managed patients aggressively, as indicated by intra-cranial monitor placement, had 40% lower mortality rates than centers with less-aggressive management (Bulger et al., 2002).

Late functional status (return to work and personal independence) after TBI is affected by even more factors than early outcome. As time from injury to outcome becomes greater, injury characteristics become less important, and other factors such as premorbid functioning and environmental supports become more important. Factors predictive of functional outcome can be categorized as preinjury factors (including demographic variables), injury severity variables, cognitive and neurobehavioral impairments, and environmental supports. Find-ings for these variables are presented in Table 8-3.

LIFE CARE PLANNING

As the review here describes, some individuals who sustain TBI experience significant, long-lasting residual impairments. These patients often require con-tinuing medical and rehabilitation interventions as well as environmental adapta-tions to minimize their residual disabilities and enhance their quality of life (Sherer, Madison, & Hannay, 2000). The costs associated with meeting these needs are usually quite high, and many are not time limited. Thus, as with many other chronic medical conditions, patients with the most severe injuries have the greatest long-term impairments and therefore the largest costs associated with their care (Putnam & Adams, 1992). Life care planning is a service that can benefit these patients both in clinical settings and when litigation is involved.

A life care plan delineates the services and items required for the current and long-term care of the person with moderate or severe TBI as well as the costs

TABLE 8-3. Factors Predictive of Functional Outcome After
Traumatic Brain Injury (TBI)

	REFERENCES
Preinjury Factors	
Age	Keyser-Marcus et al. (2002); Sherer, Nick, et al. (2003)
Years of education	Hart et al. (2003); Sherer, Sander, et al. (2002)
Preinjury employment	Keyser-Marcus et al. (2002); Sherer, Sander, et al. (2002)
Substance use	MacMillan, Hart, Martelli, and Zasler (2002); Sherer et al. (1999)
Injury Severity Variables	
Initial Glasgow Coma Scale	Dikmen et al. (1994); Levin et al. (1990)
Time to follow commands	Dikmen et al. (1994); Hart et al. (2003)
Duration of posttraumatic amnesia	Boake et al. (2001); Sherer, Sander, et al. (2002)
Cognitive and Neurobehavioral Impairments	
Early cognitive status	Boake et al. (2001); Dikmen et al. (1994); Sherer, Sander, et al. (2002)
Postinjury depression	Ruff et al. (1993); Seel et al. (2003)
Impaired self-awareness	Sherer, Bergloff, et al. (1998); Trudel, Tryon, and Purdum (1998)
Early functional status	Gollaher et al. (1998); Ponsford, Olver, Curran, and Ng (1995)
Environmental Supports	
Family support	Prigatano et al. (1994)
Access to postacute brain injury rehabilitation	Malec and Basford (1996)

for this care (Deutsch & Sawyer, 1985). In the clinical setting, the life care plan provides a working guideline for the appropriate allocation and provision of resources needed for care recommended by the rehabilitative team. In the legal setting, the life care plan aids the person with TBI, family members, and attorneys in the determination of an appropriate settlement that will provide for the lifetime needs of the injured person.

Historically, the professional training of life care planners has been varied (Barker, 1999; Evans, 1997; Rice, Hicks, & Wiehe, 2000), but most have a strong background in rehabilitation. Currently, there are no state or federal educational guidelines or licensure requirements for self-identified life care planners. Rehabilitation professionals practicing as life care planners can work individually or in concert with a life care planning team. However, all benefit from physician input to anticipate and recommend all necessary medical services.

This process preferably includes direct consultation with a physician during the development of the comprehensive plan (Katz & Delaney, 2002; Zuckerman & Wollner, 1999). Life care plans developed without direct medical consultation should be considered preliminary or pending physician review (Cassidy & Madison, 2003). Information needed for preparation of the life care plan may be obtained through (a) thorough review of available medical records; (b) interview of the person with TBI or the family regarding current and preinjury functioning; (c) interview of care providers or other medical personnel; (d) knowledge of standards and methods of provision of medical, rehabilitation, and attendant care; (e) knowledge of appropriate vendors of medical equipment and health care providers; (f) knowledge of long-term care options, including home and facility placements; and (g) knowledge of the sequelae and course of recovery expected for the type and severity of injury suffered.

Types of care, services, and other issues to be considered in developing the description of the patient's current and long-term needs are routine medical care, nonroutine medical care, therapeutic modalities, facility care, attendant/supervisory care, aids for independent function, home services, medications, wheelchair needs, orthotics/prosthetics, other equipment, supplies, transportation, architectural renovations, counseling, vocational services, educational services, case management, and potential complications. Following delineation of these needs, research is conducted to establish costs associated with the respective items and services. Existing providers and vendors are used whenever possible, and anticipated providers and vendors are identified as needed with consideration to geographic suitability. The information gathered in the aforementioned procedures is presented in narrative form and tables in the life care plan.

The format of the life care plan can vary. The total cost format is typically a brief letter that identifies only the total annual cost and the total one-time cost associated with the individual's overall care requirements. The category-of-care format is typically a short report that identifies the categories of care required by an individual with associated annual and one-time costs for each category, as well as the total annual cost and the total one-time cost associated with the individual's overall care. The report may also include a brief description of the items contained within each category. The comprehensive format is typically a lengthy report that identifies the categories of care required by an individual and further identifies the specific items contained within each category. Information for each item is provided regarding purpose, frequency of care/replacement schedule, estimated unit cost, provider/vendor, and annual/one-time cost. This format also typically provides the annual and one-time costs for each category of care, as well as the total annual cost and the total one-time cost associated with the individual's overall care.

Tables 8-4, 8-5, 8-6, and 8-7 are examples of charts that could be found in the comprehensive format to define routine medical care, nonroutine medical

TABLE 8-4. Routine Medical Care

DESCRIPTION	PURPOSE	FREQUENCY	ESTIMATED UNIT COST	YEARS	ANNUAL COST	PROVIDER
Physiatrist	To monitor functional status	1–2 times per year	$75 per visit	Current year to life	$112.50	Name of physician
Neuropsychiatrist	For medication management	1–2 times per year	$125 per visit	Current year to life	$187.50	Name of physician
General practitioner	To monitor medical status	4 times per year	$40 per visit	Current year to life	$160.00	Name of physician
Laboratory diagnostics	Used in conjunction with medical status	4 times per year	$70 per workup	Current year to life	$280.00	Name of physician
Total annual cost					$740.00	

TABLE 8-5. Nonroutine Medical Care

DESCRIPTION	PURPOSE	FREQUENCY/ DURATION	ESTIMATED UNIT COST	YEARS	ONE-TIME COST
Postacute day treatment program	To maximize independent functioning	5 days per week for 12 weeks	$725 per day	One time	$43,500
Ophthalmological evaluation	To assess visual functioning	1 time	$150 per evaluation	One time	$150
Magnetic resonance imaging of the brain	To assess brain function	1 time	$2,200 per study	One time	$2,200
Total one-time cost					$45,850

care, attendant/facility care, and wheelchair needs for a person with TBI. Table 8-8 is a sample chart summarizing the categories and costs associated with the individual's overall care.

Although the life care plan focuses on the patient's probable needs (those needs deemed to be more likely required than not), potential needs are also considered. Probable needs are the patient's expected needs based on current medical and functional status; potential needs consider possible changes in the patient's medical status (e.g., late development of posttraumatic seizures) or life circumstances (e.g., unexpected incapacitation or death of the primary caretaker).

Projection of costs for the life care plan is typically based on an assumption of private pay and nonnegotiated rates. Reference to collateral resources, such as personal health care insurance or governmental programs (e.g., Medicare, Medicaid, etc.) may not be permitted from the legal perspective, and the ongoing availability of collateral resources as well as negotiated discounted rates from specific providers are typically not presumed. However, under some circumstances, with a specific request and permission, collateral resources and negotiated rates may be considered. This last approach is more typical for life care plans developed for clinical rather than legal purposes and constitutes a major difference between life care plans prepared within the legal and clinical settings. In the clinical arena, current and reasonably anticipated funding sources, as well as negotiated rates, are taken into consideration and identified. Items recommended by the physician for which no viable funding source can be found at the time of the life care plan's development are nevertheless included in the

TABLE 8-6. Attendant/Facility Care

DESCRIPTION	PURPOSE	SCHEDULE	ESTIMATED UNIT COST	YEARS	ANNUAL COST	PROVIDER
Home placement with assistive care services	To provide assistance and supervision with family participation within the home environment	8–12 hours per day, 335 days per year of privately hired home health aide services and	$7.50 per hour for private hire	Current year to life	$29,025	State workforce commission
		8–12 hours per day, 30 days per year of agency-hired home health aide services	$13.00 per hour for agency hire			Name of agency
Residential facility placement	To provide assistance and supervision within a residential setting for the brain injured	365 days per year	$250.00 per day	Current year to life	$91,250	Name of facility
Total annual cost						
Home placement					$29,025	
Facility placement					$91,250	

TABLE 8-7. Wheelchair Needs

DESCRIPTION	PURPOSE	REPLACEMENT SCHEDULE	ESTIMATED UNIT COST	YEARS	ANNUAL COST	VEND«
Manual wheel-chair	To facilitate mobility	Every 3–5 years	$2,300	Current year to life	$575	Name (vend
Wheelchair maintenance	To maintain function of wheel-chair	Every year	$250	Current year to life	$250	Name (vend
Bac-Pac	To transport personal care items	Every year	$50	Current year to life	$25	Name (vend«
Total annual cost					$850	

TABLE 8-8. Summary of Costs

AREA OF NEED	YEARS	ANNUAL COST	ONE-TIME COST
Routine medical care	Current year to life	$740.00	—
Nonroutine medical care	One time	—	$45,850
Therapeutic	Current year to life	$600	—
Evaluations/intervention	One time	—	$2,400
Medications	Current year to life	$1,500	—
Aids for independent function	Current year to life	$800	—
Attendant/facility care	Current year to life		—
Home placement		$29,025	
Residential facility placement		$91,250	
Wheelchair needs	Current year to life	$850	—
Transportation	Current year to life	$100	—
Architectural renovations	One time	—	$30,695
Family counseling	One time	—	$6,500
Medical case management	Current year to life	$675	—
	One time	—	$1,200
Total costs			$86,645
Home placement		$34,290	
Facility placement		$96,515	

plan. However, the funding source to provide for this need is designated as unknown (Cassidy & Madison, 2003).

Life care plans in both legal and clinical settings typically identify present-day costs. For purposes involving litigation, projection of changes in costs for outlying years is typically deferred to an economist. In clinical settings, some insurance carriers make the necessary economic adjustments to anticipate future increases in the costs associated with the recommendations. When working directly with disabled individuals or their families, the plan is reviewed on an annual basis, and cost adjustments, if necessary, are made at the time (Cassidy & Madison, 2003). An estimate of life expectancy may be incorporated within the life care plan. This estimate typically reflects statistical information or the opinion of a physician based on reasonable medical probability and current epidemiological literature.

Clinical issues that are pertinent to long-term care planning and resultant economic considerations include the following: (a) time since injury and stability of status, (b) prognosis for change with time or treatment, (c) age, (d) respiratory status, (e) mobility, (f) nutritional status, (g) bowel and bladder management, and (h) behavioral issues. For moderate and severe brain injury, the major cost for care is often attendant/supervisory care, and this is presented as an annual cost in the life care plan.

Options for long-term placement include home or facility placement. Factors to be considered that can exert a significant impact on cost projections with home placement include the following: (a) level of nursing care, (b) number of care hours required, (c) hourly versus live-in personnel, (d) privately hired versus agency hired personnel, (e) family participation, (f) school or work placement, and (g) respite care.

Care considerations that can affect cost projections for facility placement include the following: (a) ventilator care, (b) skilled nursing care, (c) assisted living, (d) traditional group home, (e) specialized group home, (f) comprehensive living community, (g) residential neurobehavioral program, and (h) long-term subacute care. Determination of the appropriate long-term placement setting for the person with TBI is crucial to his or her care well-being and is a key issue in financial planning for the patient and family.

Life care planning incorporates information from many sources, but one of the most important is the neuropsychological evaluation. The neuropsychologist, by virtue of training and experience, can play a key role in the determination of appropriate long-term placement and other issues (Evans, 1997). Cognitive, emotional, and behavioral functioning are often the leading factors considered when determining placement options and parameters. By evaluating these areas, as well as considering current social supports and the prognosis for change with time or treatment, the neuropsychologist can assist the life care planner in identifying suitable placement options over the lifetime of the individual. In this regard, the life care plan can only be as good as the accuracy of data from the neuropsychological evaluation and other sources. Hence, a neuropsychological report that overestimates the severity of residual impairment will lead to an inappropriate life care plan.

Historically, the discipline of life care planning has assisted attorneys in evaluating the needs and associated costs related to the care of disabled individuals in litigation (Schuster, 1994; Weed, 1996; Whitmore, 1996). Clinical applications of life care planning are becoming more prominent (Barker, 1999; Blackwell, Millington, & Guglielmo, 1999; Creasey & Dahlberg, 2001; Dahlberg, 2003; Evans, 1996; Harrell & Krause, 2002; Kreutz, 2002; Voogt, 1996). Advances in emergency transport and medical technology have contributed to increasing survival rates and life expectancy following catastrophic injuries and devastating illnesses. Survivors are often left with profound impairments that impede activities of daily living and social reintegration. This growing population often requires lifelong specialized care. Funding to meet these special needs is, at best, complicated, and at worst, nonexistent (Cassidy & Madison, 2003).

Discharge planning offered by treatment facilities has been historically limited in its scope, especially regarding long-term follow-up and attention to funding issues. Over time, the disabled individual and his or her family are often left with no professional guidance to address these lifelong functional and financial obstacles. In some specialized settings, comprehensive life care planning is gradually being incorporated into rehabilitation treatment and discharge planning. In this clinical model, the life care planner is a member of the rehabilitation team, which typically includes representatives from physical therapy, occupational therapy, speech therapy, vocational therapy, social services, nursing, neuropsychology, and case management. The team is headed by a physician with a focused interest in life care planning and experience in caring for individuals with chronic handicapping conditions.

The life care plan produced in this setting provides a long-term medical plan with delineation of providers and available funding. This model emphasizes the importance of a team approach, including physician input, to carry out development and ensure follow up of the plan. A case manager from the clinical setting or life care planning team or hired independently plays a pivotal role in its initial implementation and in following the evolution of the plan over time. This individual becomes the contact person for the family in the event problems develop, the individual's needs change, or revision of cost estimates is required. Significant changes may require reinvolving the clinical team to reevaluate the individual's needs in the face of these changing circumstances (Cassidy & Madison, 2003).

Other benefits of clinical life care planning include facilitating the exchange of information among health care professionals and realistic communication with all stakeholders about the long-term or age-related needs of the disabled individual, including the associated costs necessary to fund these requirements. It is hoped that this frank style of communication will foster the relationship of all involved, enhancing continuity of care and long-range planning.

This focus also directs attention to the prioritization of needs and the concomitant resources required to provide them, rather than the shortsighted "frontloading" of care and equipment on first encounter discharge with little regard for the future. Furthermore, this approach helps lead to the "in time" provision of services and equipment when they are needed most in the individual's rehabilitation rather than haphazard implementation on the first encounter after discharge. This preparation also focuses needed attention on long-term financial planning to avoid a lack of resources when expected complications arise or when the natural history of a disorder predicts changes in care necessary to avoid recidivism to acute treatment settings.

Additional benefits to the disabled individual and his or her family include pragmatic and emotional preparation for the future. Such preparation helps produce a sense of security that enhances quality of life for all concerned. Problematic funding may be confronted early in the rehabilitation process, and possible solutions to the obstacles may be pursued before a crisis in management occurs (Cassidy & Madison, 2003).

The cornerstones of clinical life care planning are development of a plan through a team approach that includes physician input, attention to public and private funding sources, and implementation and follow-up of the plan through aggressive case management. This approach will undoubtedly raise questions about the scope and cost of lifelong care required by individuals with long-term disabilities and chronic illnesses.

Based on current research, comprehensive responses to these critical questions are not readily available. Research in this area is only beginning. Efforts identified to date include investigation of the accuracy of life expectancy estimates in life care plans (Krause, 2002); investigation of the economic consequences of neuroprosthesis implantation for bowel and bladder management (Creasey & Dahlberg, 2001); investigation of the long-term survival, prognosis, and life care planning for patients with chronic locked-in syndrome (Katz, Haig, Clark, & DiPaola, 1992); and investigation of the lifetime costs after TBI associated with levels of the DRS (Robinson, 2001). Additional research is needed to address these issues as our society confronts an ever-expanding population of individuals with long-term impairments after TBI.

Thus, as a society we must confront these problems if we are to provide appropriate long-term care for this growing population (Zuckerman & Wollner, 1999). To this end, the broader application of clinical life care planning coupled with sound research will ensure that "discharge planning" provides a comprehensive plan to address patients' long-term health care and support needs.

ACKNOWLEDGMENT

Completion of this chapter was partially supported by the National Institute on Disability and Rehabilitation Research (H133A020514), the TBI Model System of Mississippi.

REFERENCES

Alexander, M. P. (1992). Neuropsychiatric correlates of persistent postconcussive syndrome. *Journal of Head Trauma Rehabilitation, 7,* 60–69.

American Psychiatric Association. (1994). *Diagnostic and statistical manual of mental disorders* (4th ed.) Washington, DC: Author.

Andrews, P. J., Sleeman, D. H., Statham, P. F., McQuatt, A., Corruble, V., Jones, P. A., et al. (2002). Predicting recovery in patients suffering from traumatic brain injury by using admission variables and physiological data: A comparison between decision tree analysis and logistic regression. *Journal of Neurosurgery, 97,* 326–336.

Annegers, J. F., Hauser, W. A., Coan, S. P., & Rocca, W. A. (1998). A population based study of seizures after traumatic brain injuries. *New England Journal of Medicine, 338,* 20–24.

Artiola I Fortuny, L., Briggs, M., Newcombe, F., Ratcliff, G., & Thomas, C. (1980). Measuring the duration of post traumatic amnesia. *Journal of Neurology, Neurosurgery, and Psychiatry, 43,* 377–379.

Barker, E. (1999). Life care planning. *RN, 62,* 58–61.

Binder, L. M. (1997). A review of mild head trauma. Part II: Clinical implications. *Journal of Clinical and Experimental Neuropsychology, 19,* 432–457.

Binder, L. M., & Willis, S. C. (1991). Assessment of motivation after financially compensable minor head trauma. *Psychological Assessment, 3,* 175–181.

Blackwell, T. L., Millington, M. J., & Guglielmo, D. E. (1999). Vocational aspects of life care planning for people with spinal cord injury. *Work, 13,* 13–19.

Boake, C. (1996). Supervision Rating Scale: A measure of functional outcome from brain injury. *Archives of Physical Medicine and Rehabilitation, 77,* 765–772.

Boake, C., Millis, S. R., High, W. M., Jr., Delmonico, R. L., Kreutzer, J. S., Rosenthal, M., et al. (2001). Using early neuropsychological testing to predict long-term productivity outcome from traumatic brain injury. *Archives of Physical Medicine and Rehabilitation, 82,* 761–768.

Bontke, C. F., Zasler, N. D., & Boake, C. (1996). Rehabilitation of the head-injured patient. In R. K.Narayan, J. E. Wilberger, & J. T. Povlishock (Eds.), *Neurotrauma* (pp. 841–858). New York: McGraw-Hill.

Braakman, R., Gelpke, G. J., Habbema, J. D. F., Maas, A. I. R., & Minderhoud, J. M. (1980). Systematic selection of prognostic features in patients with severe head injury. *Neurosurgery, 6,* 362–370.

Brooks, N., Campsie, L., Symington, C., Beattie, A., & McKinlay, W. (1986). The 5 year outcome of severe blunt head injury: A relative's view. *Journal of Neurology, Neurosurgery, and Psychiatry, 49,* 764–770.

Brooks, N., Campsie, L., Symington, C., Beattie, A., & McKinlay, W. (1987). The effects of severe head injury on patient and relative within seven years of injury. *Journal of Head Trauma Rehabilitation, 2,* 1–13.

Brooks, N., McKinlay, W., Symington, C., Beattie, A., & Campsie, L. (1987). Return to work within the first seven years of severe head injury. *Brain Injury, 1*, 5–19.

Bulger, E. M., Nathens, A. B., Rivara, F. P., Moore, M., MacKenzie, E. J., & Jurkovich, G. J. (2002). Management of severe head injury: Institutional variations in care and effect on outcome. *Critical Care Medicine, 30*, 1870–1876.

Cassidy, J. W., & Madison, C. F. (2003). Clinical life care planning: A physician led team approach. *Nexus News, 1*, 1–2.

Choi, S. C., & Barnes, T. Y. (1996). Predicting outcome in the head-injured patient. In R. K. Narayan, J. E. Wilberger, & J. T. Povlishock (Eds.), *Neurotrauma* (pp. 779–792). New York: McGraw-Hill.

Choi, S. C., Barnes, T. Y., Bullock, R., Germannson, T. A., Marmarou, A., & Young, H. F. (1994). Temporal profile of outcomes in severe head injury. *Journal of Neurosurgery, 81*, 169–173.

Cicerone, K. D., & Kalmar, K. (1995). Persistent postconcussion syndrome: The structure of subjective complaints after mild traumatic brain injury. *Journal of Head Trauma Rehabilitation, 10*, 1–17.

Claassen, J., & Hansen, H. C. (2001). Early recovery after closed traumatic head injury: Somatosensory evoked potentials and clinical findings. *Critical Care Medicine, 29*, 494–502.

Clifton, G. L., Hayes, R. L., Levin, H. S., Michel, M. E., & Choi, S. C. (1992). Outcome measures for clinical trials involving traumatically brain-injured patients: Report of a conference. *Neurosurgery, 31*, 975–978.

Corrigan, J. D. (1989). Development of a scale for assessment of agitation following traumatic brain injury. *Journal of Clinical and Experimental Neuropsychology, 11*, 261–277.

Corrigan, J. D., & Mysiw, W. J. (1988). Agitation following traumatic head injury: Equivocal evidence for a discrete stage of cognitive recovery. *Archives of Physical Medicine and Rehabilitation, 69*, 487–492.

Creasey, G. H., & Dahlberg, J. E. (2001). Economic consequences of an implanted neuroprosthesis for bladder and bowel management. *Archives of Physical Medicine and Rehabilitation, 82*, 1520–1525.

Dahlberg, J. (2003). The life care plan: A prediction of the future. *Topics in Spinal Cord Injury Rehabilitation, 6*, 20–26.

Deutsch, P. M., & Sawyer, H. M. (1985). *A guide to rehabilitation* (vols. 1 and 2). New York: Bender.

Dikmen, S. S., & Machamer, J. E. (1995). Neurobehavioral outcomes and their determinants. *Journal of Head Trauma Rehabilitation, 10*, 74–86.

Dikmen, S., Machamer, J., & Temkin, N. (2003). Mild TBI with or without CT abnormalities. *Journal of the International Neuropsychological Society, 9*, 172–173.

Dikmen, S. S., Machamer, J. E., Winn, R., & Temkin, N. R. (1995). Neuropsychological outcome at 1-year post head injury. *Neuropsychology, 9*, 80–90.

Dikmen, S., McLean, A., & Temkin, N. (1986). Neuropsychological and psychosocial consequences of minor head injury. *Journal of Neurology, Neurosurgery, and Psychiatry, 49*, 1227–1232.

Dikmen, S., McLean, A., Temkin, N. R., & Wyler, A. R. (1986). Neuropsychologic outcome at one-month postinjury. *Archives of Physical Medicine and Rehabilitation, 67*, 507–513.

Dikmen, S., Reitan, R. M., & Temkin, N. R. (1983). Neuropsychological recovery in head injury. *Archives of Neurology, 40*, 333–338.

Dikmen, S. S., Temkin, N. R., Machamer, J. E., Holubkov, A. L., Fraser, R. T., & Winn, R. (1994). Employment following traumatic head injuries. *Archives of Neurology, 51,* 177–186.

Eisenberg, H. M., & Weiner, R. L. (1987). Input variables: How information from the acute injury can be used to characterize groups of patients for studies of outcome. In H. S.Levin, J. Grafman, & H. M. Eisenberg (Eds.), *Neurobehavioral recovery from head injury* (pp. 13–29). New York: Oxford University Press.

Ellenberg, J. H., Levin, H. S., & Saydjari, C. (1996). Posttraumatic amnesia as a predictor of outcome after severe closed head injury. *Archives of Neurology, 53,* 782–791.

Evans, R. W. (1996). Commentary and an illustration on the use of outcome data in life care planning for persons with acquired neurological injuries. *NeuroRehabilitation, 7,* 157–162.

Evans, R. W. (1997). The role of the neuropsychologist in life care planning for brain injured populations. *Journal of Care Management, 3,* 46–47.

Ewert, J., Levin, H. S., Watson, M. G., & Kalisky, Z. (1989). Procedural memory during posttraumatic amnesia in survivors of severe closed head injury. Implications for rehabilitation. *Archives of Neurology, 46,* 911–916.

Giacino, J. T., Ashwal, S., Childs, N., Cranford, R., Jennett, B., Katz, D. I., et al. (2002). The minimally conscious state: Definition and diagnostic criteria. *Neurology, 58,* 349–353.

Giacino, J. T., Kezmarsky, M. A., DeLuca, J., & Cicerone, K. D. (1991). Monitoring rate of recovery to predict outcome in minimally responsive patients. *Archives of Physical Medicine and Rehabilitation, 72,* 897–901.

Gollaher, K., High, W. M., Jr., Sherer, M., Bergloff, P., Boake, C., Young, M. E., et al. (1998). Prediction of employment outcome one to three years following traumatic brain injury (TBI). *Brain Injury, 12,* 255–263.

Gouvier, W. D., Blanton, P. D., LaPorte, K. K., & Nepomuceno, C. (1987). Reliability and validity of the Disability Rating Scale and the Levels of Cognitive Functioning Scale in monitoring recovery from severe head injury. *Archives of Physical Medicine and Rehabilitation, 68,* 94–97.

Graham, D. I., Adams, J. H., & Gennarelli, T. A. (1993). Pathology of brain damage in head injury. In P. R. Cooper (Ed.), *Head injury* (3rd ed., pp. 91–113). Baltimore: Williams and Wilkins.

Hall, K. M., Cope, D. N., & Rappaport, M. (1985). Glasgow Outcome Scale and Disability Rating Scale: Comparative usefulness in following recovery in traumatic head injury. *Archives of Physical Medicine and Rehabilitation, 66,* 35–37.

Hannay, H. J., & Sherer, M. (1996). Assessment of outcome from head injury. In R. K. Narayan, J. E. Wilberger, & J. T. Povlishock (Eds.), *Neurotrauma* (pp. 723–747). New York: McGraw-Hill.

Harrell, T. W., & Krause, J. S. (2002). Personal assistance services in patients with SCI: Modeling an appropriate level of care in a life care plan. *Topics in Spinal Cord Injury Rehabilitation, 7,* 38–48.

Harrison-Felix, C., Newton, C. N., Hall, K. M., & Kreutzer, J. S. (1996). Descriptive findings from the Traumatic Brain Injury Model Systems National Data Base. *Journal of Head Trauma Rehabilitation, 11,* 1–14.

Hart, T., Millis, S., Novack, T., Englander, J., Fidler-Sheppard, R., & Bell, K. R. (2003). The relationship between neuropsychologic function and level of caregiver supervision at 1 year after traumatic brain injury. *Archives of Physical Medicine and Rehabilitation, 84,* 221–230.

High, W. M., Levin, H. S., & Gary, H. E. (1990). Recovery of orientation following closed-head injury. *Journal of Clinical and Experimental Neuropsychology, 12*, 703–714.

Horn, L. J., & Sherer, M. (1999). Rehabilitation of traumatic brain injury. In M. Grabois, S. J. Garrison, K. A. Hart, & L. D. Lehmkuhl (Eds.), *Physical medicine and rehabilitation: The complete approach* (pp. 1281–1304). Cambridge, MA: Blackwell Science.

Hoyert, D. L., Arias, E., Smith, B. L., Murphy, S. L., & Kochanek, K. D. (2001). Deaths: Final data for 1999. *National Vital Statistics Reports, 49*, 1–113.

Jackson, W. T., Novack, T. A., & Dowler, R. N. (1998). Effective serial measurement of cognitive orientation in rehabilitation: The Orientation Log. *Archives of Physical Medicine and Rehabilitation, 79*, 718–720.

Jager, T. E., Weiss, H. B., Coben, J. H., & Pepe, P. E. (2000). Traumatic brain injuries evaluated in U.S. emergency departments, 1992–1994. *Academic Emergency Medicine, 7*, 134–140.

Jain, N., Layton, B. S., & Murray, P. K. (2000). Are aphasic patients who fail the GOAT in PTA? A modified Galveston Orientation and Amnesia Test for persons with aphasia. *The Clinical Neuropsychologist, 14*, 13–17.

Jennett, B., & Bond, M. R. (1975). Assessment of outcome after severe brain damage. *Lancet*, 480–484.

Jennett, B., & Teasdale, G. (1977). Aspects of coma after severe head injury. *Lancet*, 878–881.

Jiang, J. Y., Gao, G. Y., Li, W. P., Yu, M. K., & Zhu, C. (2002). Early indicators of prognosis in 846 cases of severe traumatic brain injury. *Journal of Neurotrauma, 19*, 869–874.

Katz, R. T., & Delaney, G. A. (2002). Life care planning. *Physical Medicine and Rehabilitation Clinics of North American, 13*, ix, 287–308.

Katz, R. T., Haig, A. J., Clark, B. B., & DiPaola, R. J. (1992). Long-term survival, prognosis, and life-care planning for 29 patients with chronic locked-in syndrome. *Archives of Physical Medicine and Rehabilitation, 73*, 403–408.

Keyser-Marcus, L. A., Bricout, J. C., Wehman, P., Campbell, L. R., Cifu, D. X., Englander, J., et al. (2002). Acute predictors of return to employment after traumatic brain injury: A longitudinal follow-up. *Archives of Physical Medicine and Rehabilitation, 83*, 635–641.

Kraus, J. F., McArthur, D. L., Silverman, T. A., & Jayaraman, M. (1996). Epidemiology of brain injury. In R. K. Narayan, J. E. Wilberger, & J. T. Povlishock (Eds.), *Neurotrauma* (pp. 13–30). New York: McGraw-Hill.

Krause, J. S. (2002). Accuracy of life expectancy estimates in life care plans: Consideration of nonbiographical and noninjury factors. *Topics in Spinal Cord Injury Rehabilitation, 7*, 59–68.

Kreutz, D. (2002). Life care planning for spinal cord injury: Seating and mobility considerations. *Topics in Spinal Cord Injury Rehabilitation, 7*, 28–37.

Kreutzer, J. S., Marwitz, J. H., Seel, R., & Serio, C. D. (1996). Validation of a Neurobehavioral Functioning Inventory for adults with traumatic brain injury. *Archives of Physical Medicine and Rehabilitation, 77*, 116–124.

Levin, H. S. (1992). Neurobehavioral recovery. *Journal of Neurotrauma, 9*, S359–S373.

Levin, H. S. (1993). Neurobehavioral sequelae of closed head injury. In P. R. Cooper (Ed.), *Head injury* (pp. 525–551). Baltimore: Williams and Wilkins.

Levin, H. S. (1995). Prediction of recovery from traumatic brain injury. *Journal of Neurotrauma, 12*, 913–922.

Levin, H. S., & Eisenberg, H. M. (1991). Neurobehavioral outcome. *Neurosurgery Clinics of North America*, 2, 457–472.

Levin, H. S., Gary, H. E., Eisenberg, H. M., Ruff, R. M., Barth, J. T., Kreutzer, J. S., et al. (1990). Neurobehavioral outcome 1 year after severe head injury: Experience of the Traumatic Coma Data Bank. *Journal of Neurosurgery*, 73, 699–709.

Levin, H. S., High, W. M., Goethe, K. E., Sisson, R. A., Overall, J. E., Rhoades, H. M., et al. (1987). The Neurobehavioural Rating Scale: Assessment of the behavioural sequelae of head injury by the clinician. *Journal of Neurology, Neurosurgery, and Psychiatry*, 50, 183–193.

Levin, H. S., Mattis, S., Ruff, R. M., Eisenberg, H. M., Marshall, L. F., Tabaddor, K., et al. (1987). Neurobehavioral outcome following minor head injury: A three-center study. *Journal of Neurosurgery*, 66, 234–243.

Levin, H. S., O'Donnell, V. M., & Grossman, R. G. (1979). The Galveston Orientation and Amnesia Test: A practical scale to assess cognition after head injury. *Journal of Nervous and Mental Disease*, 167, 675–684.

Lezak, M. D. (1987). Relationships between personality disorder, social disturbances, and physical disability following traumatic brain injury. *Journal of Head Trauma Rehabilitation*, 2, 57–69.

Lezak, M. D. (1989). Assessment of psychosocial dysfunctions resulting dysfunctions resulting from head trauma. In M. D. Lezak (Ed.), *Assessment of behavioral consequences of head trauma* (pp. 113–143). New York: Liss.

Lezak, M. D. (1995). *Neuropsychological assessment* (3rd ed.) New York: Oxford University Press.

MacMillan, P. J., Hart, R. P., Martelli, M. F., & Zasler, N. D. (2002). Pre-injury status and adaptation following traumatic brain injury. *Brain Injury*, 16, 41–49.

Malec, J. F., & Basford, J. S. (1996). Postacute brain injury rehabilitation. *Archives of Physical Medicine and Rehabilitation*, 77, 198–207.

Malec, J. F., & Moessner, A. M. (2001). Self-awareness, distress, and postacute rehabilitation outcome. *Rehabilitation Psychology*, 45, 227–241.

Marion, D. W. (1996). Outcome from severe head injury. In R. K. Narayan, J. E. Wilberger, & J. T. Povlishock (Eds.), *Neurotrauma* (pp. 767–777). New York: McGraw-Hill.

Mataro, M., Poca, M. A., Sahuquillo, J., Pedraza, S., Ariza, M., Amoros, S., et al. (2001). Neuropsychological outcome in relation to the traumatic coma data bank classification of computed tomography imaging. *Journal of Neurotrauma*, 18, 869–879.

Max, W., MacKenzie, E. J., & Rice, D. P. (1991). Head injuries: Costs and consequences. *Journal of Head Trauma Rehabilitation*, 6, 76–91.

McCauley, S. R., Levin, H. S., Vanier, M., Mazaux, J. M., Boake, C., Goldfader, P. R., et al. (2001). The neurobehavioural rating scale-revised: Sensitivity and validity in closed head injury assessment. *Journal of Neurology, Neurosurgery, and Psychiatry*, 71, 643–651.

Millis, S. R., Rosenthal, M., Novack, T. A., Sherer, M., Nick, T. G., Kreutzer, J. S., et al. (2001). Long-term neuropsychological outcome after traumatic brain injury. *Journal of Head Trauma Rehabilitation*, 16, 343–355.

Mittenberg, W., & Strauman, S. (2000). Diagnosis of mild head injury and the postconcussion syndrome. *Journal of Head Trauma Rehabilitation*, 15, 783–791.

Mosenthal, A. C., Lavery, R. F., Addis, M., Kaul, S., Ross, S., Marburger, R., et al. (2002). Isolated traumatic brain injury: Age is an independent predictor of mortality and early outcome. *Journal of Trauma*, 52, 907–911.

Murray, G. D., Teasdale, G. M., Braakman, R., Cohadon, F., Dearden, M., Iannotti, F., et al. (1999). The European Brain Injury Consortium Survey of head injuries. *Acta Neurochir (Wien)*, *141*, 223–236.

Nakase-Thompson, R., Sherer, M., Yablon, S. A., Nick, T. G., & Trzepacz, P. T. (2004). Acute confusion following traumatic brain injury. *Brain Injury*, *18*, 131–142.

Oddy, M., Humphrey, M., & Uttley, D. (1978). Subjective impairment and social recovery after closed head injury. *Journal of Neurology, Neurosurgery, and Psychiatry*, *41*, 611–616.

Ommaya, A. K., & Gennarelli, T. A. (1974). Cerebral concussion and traumatic unconsciousness. Correlation of experimental and clinical observations of blunt head injuries. *Brain*, *97*, 633–654.

Ponsford, J. L., Olver, J. H., Curran, C., & Ng, K. (1995). Prediction of employment status 2 years after traumatic brain injury. *Brain Injury*, *9*, 11–20.

Prigatano, G. P., Altman, I. M., & O'Brien, K. P. (1990). Behavioral limitations that traumatic-brain-injured patients tend to underestimate. *The Clinical Neuropsychologist*, *4*, 163–176.

Prigatano, G. P., Klonoff, P. S., O'Brien, K. P., Altman, I. M., Amin, K., Chiapello, D. A., et al. (1994). Productivity after neuropsychologically oriented milieu rehabilitation. *Journal of Head Trauma Rehabilitation*, *9*, 91–102.

Putnam, S. H., & Adams, K. M. (1992). Regression-based prediction of long-term outcome following multidisciplinary rehabilitation for traumatic brain injury. *The Clinical Neuropsychologist*, *6*, 383–405.

Rappaport, M., Hall, K. M., Hopkins, K., Belleza, T., & Cope, D. N. (1982). Disability Rating Scale for severe head trauma: Coma to community. *Archives of Physical Medicine and Rehabilitation*, *63*, 118–123.

Rice, J., Hicks, P. B., & Wiehe, V. (2000). Life care planning: A role for social workers. *Social Work in Health Care*, *31*, 85–94.

Robinson, K. W. (2001). *Lifetime costs after traumatic brain injury associated with levels of the disability rating scale*. Unpublished doctoral dissertation, University of Houston.

Ruff, R. M., Marshall, L. F., Crouch, J., Klauber, M. R., Levin, H. S., Barth, J. T., et al. (1993). Predictors of outcome following severe head trauma: Follow-up data from the Traumatic Coma Data Bank. *Brain Injury*, *7*, 101–111.

Ruff, R. M., Young, D., Gautille, T., Marshall, L. F., Barth, J., Jane, J. A., et al. (1991). Verbal learning deficits following severe head injury: Heterogeneity in recovery over 1 year. *Journal of Neurosurgery*, *75*, S50–S58.

Russell, W. R. (1932). Cerebral involvement in head injury. A study based on the examination of two hundred cases. *Brain*, *55*, 549–603.

Russell, W. R., & Smith, A. (1961). Post-traumatic amnesia in closed head injury. *Archives of Neurology*, *5*, 16–29.

Sander, A. M., Fuchs, K. L., High, W. M., Jr., Hall, K. M., Kreutzer, J. S., & Rosenthal, M. (1999). The Community Integration Questionnaire revisited: An assessment of factor structure and validity. *Archives of Physical Medicine and Rehabilitation*, *80*, 1303–1308.

Sander, A. M., Kreutzer, J. S., Rosenthal, M., Delmonico, R., & Young, M. E. (1996). A multicenter longitudinal investigation of return to work and community integration following traumatic brain injury. *Journal of Head Trauma Rehabilitation*, *11*, 70–84.

Sander, A. M., Seel, R. T., Kreutzer, J. S., Hall, K. M., High, W. M., Jr., & Rosenthal, M. (1997). Agreement between persons with traumatic brain injury and their relatives regarding psychosocial outcome using the Community Integration Questionnaire. *Archives of Physical Medicine and Rehabilitation, 78,* 353–357.

Satz, P., Zaucha, K., Forney, D. L., McCleary, C., Asarnow, R. F., Light, R., et al. (1998). Neuropsychological, psychosocial, and vocational correlates of the Glasgow Outcome Scale at 6 months post-injury: A study of moderate to severe traumatic brain injury patients. *Brain Injury, 12,* 555–567.

Schuster, R. (1994). Life care planning and vocational assessment for the spinal cord injured population: An overview. *SCI Psychosocial Process, 7,* 165–169.

Seel, R. T., Kreutzer, J. S., Rosenthal, M., Hammond, F. M., Corrigan, J. D., & Black, K. (2003). Depression after traumatic brain injury: A National Institute on Disability and Rehabilitation Research Model Systems multicenter investigation. *Archives of Physical Medicine and Rehabilitation, 84,* 177–184.

Sherer, M., Bergloff, P., High, W., Jr., & Nick, T. G. (1999). Contribution of functional ratings to prediction of longterm employment outcome after traumatic brain injury. *Brain Injury, 13,* 973–981.

Sherer, M., Bergloff, P., Levin, E., High, W. M., Jr., Oden, K. E., & Nick, T. G. (1998). Impaired awareness and employment outcome after traumatic brain injury. *Journal of Head Trauma Rehabilitation, 13,* 52–61.

Sherer, M., Boake, C., Levin, E., Silver, B. V., Ringholz, G. M., & High, W. M., Jr. (1998). Characteristics of impaired awareness after traumatic brain injury. *Journal of the International Neuropsychological Society, 4,* 380–387.

Sherer, M., Hart, T., Nick, T. G., Whyte, J., Thompson, R. N., & Yablon, S. A. (2003). Early impaired self-awareness after traumatic brain injury. *Archives of Physical Medicine and Rehabilitation, 84,* 168–176.

Sherer, M., Madison, C. F., & Hannay, H. J. (2000). A review of outcome after moderate and severe closed head injury with an introduction to life care planning. *Journal of Head Trauma Rehabilitation, 15,* 767–782.

Sherer, M., Nakase-Thompson, R., Nick, T. G., & Yablon, S. A. (2003). Patterns of neurobehavioral deficits in TBI patients at rehabilitation admission. *Journal of the International Neuropsychological Society, 9,* 251–252.

Sherer, M., Nick, T. G., Sander, A. M., Hart, T., Hanks, R., Rosenthal, M., et al. (2003). Race and productivity outcome after traumatic brain injury: Influence of confounding factors. *Journal of Head Trauma Rehabilitation, 18,* 408–424.

Sherer, M., & Novack, T. A. (2003). Neuropsychological assessment after traumatic brain injury in adults. In G. P. Prigatano & N. H. Plishkin (Eds.), *Clinical neuropsychology and cost outcome research: A beginning* (pp. 39–60). New York: Psychology Press.

Sherer, M., Novack, T. A., Sander, A. M., Struchen, M. A., Alderson, A., & Thompson, R. N. (2002). Neuropsychological assessment and employment outcome after traumatic brain injury: A review. *The Clinical Neuropsychologist, 16,* 157–178.

Sherer, M., Sander, A. M., Nick, T. G., High, W. M., Jr., Malec, J. F., & Rosenthal, M. (2002). Early cognitive status and productivity outcome after traumatic brain injury: Findings from the TBI model systems. *Archives of Physical Medicine and Rehabilitation, 83,* 183–192.

Shores, E. A., Marosszeky, J. E., Sandanam, J., & Batchelor, J. (1986). Preliminary validation of a clinical scale for measuring the duration of post-traumatic amnesia. *Medical Journal of Australia, 144,* 569–572.

Signorini, D. F., Andrews, P. J. D., Jones, P. A., Wardlaw, J. M., & Miller, J. D. (1999). Predicting survival using simple clinical variables: A case study in traumatic brain injury. *Journal of Neurology, Neurosurgery, and Psychiatry, 66,* 20–25.

Spreen, O., & Strauss, E. (1998). *A compendium of neuropsychological tests* (2nd ed.) New York: Oxford University Press.

Stein, S. C. (1996). Outcome from moderate head injury. In R. K. Narayan, J. E. Wilberger, & J. T. Povlishock (Eds.), *Neurotrauma* (pp. 755–765). New York: McGraw-Hill.

Stuss, D. T., Binns, M. A., Carruth, F. G., Levine, B., Brandys, C. E., Moulton, R. J., et al. (1999). The acute period of recovery from traumatic brain injury: posttraumatic amnesia or posttraumatic confusional state? *Journal of Neurosurgery, 90,* 635–643.

Susman, M., DiRusso, S. M., Sullivan, T., Risucci, D., Nealon, P., Cuff, S., et al. (2002). Traumatic brain injury in the elderly: Increased mortality and worse functional outcome at discharge despite lower injury severity. *Journal of Trauma, 53,* 219–223.

Symonds, C. P. (1937). Mental disorder following head injury. *Proceedings of the Royal Society of Medicine, 30,* 1081–1094.

Symonds, C. P., & Russell, W. R. (1943). Accidental head injuries: Prognosis in service patients. *Lancet,* 7–10.

Tabaddor, K., Mattis, S., & Zazula, T. (1984). Cognitive sequelae and recovery course after moderate and severe head injury. *Neurosurgery, 14,* 701–708.

Teasdale, G., & Jennett, B. (1974). Assessment of coma and impaired consciousness: A practical scale. *Lancet,* 81–83.

Thompson, R. N., Sherer, M., Yablon, S. A., Kennedy, R., & Nick, T. G. (2002). Persistent delirium and outcome following TBI. *Journal of the International Neuropsychological Society, 8,* 219.

Thurman, D., & Guerrero, J. (1999). Trends in hospitalization associated with traumatic brain injury. *Journal of the American Medical Association, 282,* 954–957.

Thurman, D. J., Alverson, C., Browne, D., Dunn, D. A., Guerrero, J., Johnson, R., et al. (1999). *Traumatic brain injury in the United States: A report to Congress.* Atlanta, GA: Centers for Disease Control and Prevention.

Thurman, D. J., Alverson, C., Dunn, K. A., Guerrero, J., & Sniezek, J. E. (1999). Traumatic brain injury in the United States: A public health perspective. *Journal of Head Trauma Rehabilitation, 14,* 602–615.

Traumatic Brain Injury Model Systems National Data Center. (1999). *Traumatic Brain Injury Model Systems national database syllabus.* West Orange, NJ: TBI Model Systems National Data Center.

Trudel, T. M., Tryon, W. W., & Purdum, C. M. (1998). Awareness of disability and long-term outcome after traumatic brain injury. *Rehabilitation Psychology, 53,* 267–281.

van Zomeren, A. H., & Deelman, B. G. (1978). Long-term recovery of visual reaction time after closed head injury. *Journal of Neurology, Neurosurgery, and Psychiatry, 41,* 452–457.

Vespa, P. M., Boscardin, W. J., Hovda, D. A., McArthur, D. L., Nuwer, M. R., Martin, N. A., et al. (2002). Early and persistent impaired percent alpha variability on continuous electroencephalography monitoring as predictive of poor outcome after traumatic brain injury. *Journal of Neurosurgery, 97,* 84–92.

Voogt, R. D. (1996). Quality of life: An aspect of life care planning and long-term care. *NeuroRehabilitation, 7,* 95–117.

Wardlaw, J. M., Easton, V. J., & Statham, P. (2002). Which CT features help predict outcome after head injury? *Journal of Neurology, Neurosurgery, and Psychiatry, 72,* 188–192.

Weed, R. O. (1996). Life care planning and earning capacity analysis for brain injured clients involved in personal injury litigation utilizing the RAPEL method. *NeuroRehabilitation, 7,* 119–135.

Whitmore, M. (1996). Utilization of the life care plan in personal injury litigation: Case evaluation and funding design in the catastrophic needs case. *NeuroRehabilitation*, *7*, 151–156.

Whyte, J., Cifu, D., Dikmen, S., & Temkin, N. (2001). Prediction of functional outcomes after traumatic brain injury: A comparison of two measures of duration of unconsciousness. *Archives of Physical Medicine and Rehabilitation*, *82*, 1355–1359.

Willer, B., Ottenbacher, K. J., & Coad, M. L. (1994). The Community Integration Questionnaire: A comparative examination. *American Journal of Physical Medicine and Rehabilitation*, *73*, 103–111.

Willer, B., Rosenthal, M., Kreutzer, J. S., Gordon, W. A., & Rempel, R. (1993). Assessment of community integration following rehabilitation for traumatic brain injury. *Journal of Head Trauma Rehabilitation*, *8*, 75–87.

Williams, D. H., Levin, H. S., & Eisenberg, H. M. (1990). Mild head injury classification. *Neurosurgery*, *27*, 422–428.

Yablon, S. A. (1996). Posttraumatic seizures. In L. J. Horn & N. D. Zasler (Eds.), *Medical rehabilitation of traumatic brain injury* (pp. 363–394). Philadelphia: Hanley and Belfus.

Yu, E. J., Yablon, S. A., Ivanhoe, C., & Boake, C. (1995). Posttraumatic hydrocephalus: Incidence and outcome following screening of consecutive admissions. *Archives of Physical Medicine and Rehabilitation*, *76*, 1041.

Zhang, J., Jiang, J., Zhong, T., Yu, M., & Zhu, C. (2001). Outcome of 2,284 cases with acute traumatic brain injury. *Chinese Journal of Traumatology*, *4*, 152–155.

Zuckerman, C., & Wollner, D. (1999). End of life care and decision making: How far we have come, how far we have to go. *Hospice Journal*, *14*, 85–107.

9

Neurotoxic Injury

KAREN I. BOLLA

This chapter focuses on the determination of neurotoxic injury subsequent to possible exposure to specific neurotoxicants. A neurotoxin is a chemical or substance that is harmful or fatal to the central nervous system of biological organisms when introduced in certain quantities or doses (Loomis & Hayes, 1996). It is important to remember that even the most innocuous substance can have harmful effects if introduced into the body in high enough doses. For example, even water can be toxic if ingested in large enough quantities. Also, a chemical can be harmful or have adverse effects that are species specific. That is, a chemical that is lethal to an insect may be harmless to a human.

The associations between neurological symptoms and exposure to some specific chemicals are still controversial. Although the literature continues to debate whether low-level chronic exposure results in neurotoxic insult, it is generally accepted that higher levels of exposure can result in neurocognitive sequelae. Even with higher levels of exposure, the association between exposure and central nervous system effects may be reported by some studies; other studies fail to find a similar relationship. A prime example of this is the relationship between solvent exposure and toxic encephalopathy.

Both the scientific and lay communities accept that exposure to solvents causes chronic painter's syndrome or solvent encephalopathy. This well-known syndrome is characterized by headache, fatigue, difficulty concentrating, poor memory, depressed mood, sleep disturbance, decreased libido, and irritability. In fact, in 1985, a World Health Organization working group on the chronic effects of organic solvents on the central nervous system categorized the neurobehavioral effects associated with solvent exposure. These categories were based on the severity of symptoms, and categories are presented in Table 9-1 (Cranmer & Goldberg, 1986).

Painter's syndrome originated in 1979 when Arlein-Soborg, Bruhn, Gyldensted, and Melgaard (1979) from Denmark reported a brain syndrome that they termed chronic painter's syndrome. This report was based on the study of 70 house painters who had an average of 24 years of job-related exposure to solvents and who were referred for medical evaluation for suspected organic solvent intoxication or dementia. Following the release of this report, governments in the Scandinavian countries began to compensate workers for cognitive and psychiatric disabilities determined to be work related.

Although its impact was enormous, this initial description of chronic solvent encephalopathy did not include a control group, made no attempt to control for background variables such as level of education or intelligence, and based its conclusions solely on clinical judgments about the subjective complaints of patients seeking medical treatment. For the most part, reports of neurobehavioral difficulties in workers exposed to solvents are of questionable validity because many of the studies published in the scientific literature contain methodological limitations. Inconsistencies in the literature can be attributed to differences in the populations studied (control and exposed groups) with respect to premorbid level of cognitive and psychiatric functioning, age of the sample, and severity of the exposure (i.e., intensity and duration).

Two critical reviews of the literature (Cranmer & Goldberg, 1986; World Health Organization, 1985) concluded that at least 10 years of exposure are

TABLE 9-1. Categories of the Types of Solvent Encephalopathy

Type I	Subjective nonspecific encephalopathy symptoms only
Type IIa	Sustained personality and mood change; negative neurobehavioral findings; unclear if symptoms are reversible
Type IIb	Impairment of intellectual function documented by objective neurobehavioral test results and possible mild neurological signs; after removal from exposure, symptoms should remain stable or improve, not become worse
Type III	Dementia with neurological signs, neurobehavioral deficits, and possible neuroradiological findings (e.g., frontal lobe atrophy); related to repeated severe exposure (i.e., paint huffers); may be irreversible, but generally does not progress

Note. From Cranmer and Goldberg (1986).

necessary to produce an increased risk of neurobehavioral sequelae from solvent exposure. A number of methodologically sound studies found statistically significant dose-related associations between exposure to solvents and decrements in neurobehavioral test scores, although the magnitude of the effects suggests that they are probably not clinically significant (Bleecker, Bolla, Agnew, Schwartz, & Ford, 1991; Bolla, Schwartz, Agnew, Ford, & Bleecker, 1990; Bolla et al., 1995; Cherry, Hutchins, Pace, & Waldron, 1985; Gade, Mortensen, & Bruhn, 1988; Maizlish, Fine, Albers, Whitehead, & Langolf, 1987; Triebig et al., 1988). It therefore appears that, although 10 years or more of exposure may increase an individual's risk of developing neurobehavioral symptoms, few significant adverse effects may ever actually develop.

This finding emphasizes that if an individual was exposed to a neurotoxicant, the exposure would have had to be of significant intensity and duration to cause symptoms. If there is no evidence of exposure, no relationship can be established between symptoms and exposure to toxicants. Also, if an individual was exposed to sufficiently elevated levels of neurotoxicants, they should have acute symptoms, such as headaches, dizziness, and fatigue, prior to developing chronic symptoms, such as neurocognitive deficits.

As with any diagnostic process, the ability to make a differential diagnosis among neurotoxicant exposure, neurological disease, psychiatric disturbance, or malingering (see chapter 4, this volume) is based on the combined evidence taken from the industrial hygiene data; occupational, medical, social, and academic histories; the physical and neurological examinations; biological monitoring; nerve conduction studies; electroencephalography (EEGs); computed tomography/magnetic resonance imaging (CT/MRI); and the neuropsychological evaluation.

It is therefore essential that patients with potential neurotoxic exposure are evaluated by an interdisciplinary team of health care professionals with expertise in neurotoxicology. Ideally, this "dream team" should be comprised of a neuropsychologist, a neurologist, an occupational medicine physician/internist, an industrial hygienist, and individuals from other medical specialties as necessary (i.e., pulmonologist).

Whereas some health effects, such as pulmonary distress and gastrointestinal symptoms, are noticed immediately by the affected individual, neurocognitive effects may go unrecognized while the individual is acutely ill. Acute, high-level exposure to a toxicant often results in clearly identifiable signs (e.g., delirium, seizures, flulike symptoms, or unconsciousness), but the residual effects, involving alterations in cognition, mood, and personality, are usually quite subtle. The most common clinical presentation is one of poor concentration, short-term memory loss, depressed mood, anxiety, restlessness, loss of interest in work and hobbies, decreased libido, irritability, headaches, weakness, sleep disturbances ranging from insomnia to somnambulism, and symptoms consistent

TABLE 9-2. Symptoms Associated With Heavy Metal Exposure

METAL	ASSOCIATED SYMPTOMS	NEUROLOGICAL FINDINGS	NEUROCOGNITIVE FINDINGS
Aluminum	Respiratory dysfunction	Cognitive decline; halting speech; ataxia	Personality change; fatigue; memory; attention/executive function
Arsenic			
Acute	GI distress; respiratory distress; cardiac distress; elevated temperature; Mee's lines	Headache; nervousness; vertigo; paralysis; seizures; myelopathy; hyperreflexia; neuropathy	Verbal memory; drowsiness; confusion; stupor; organic psychosis resembling paranoid schizophrenia; delirium; agitation; emotional lability
Chronic	Abdominal pain; dermatitis; increased risk of cancer	Headaches; fatigue; restlessness; vertigo; cognitive decline; visual changes or optic neuropathy; seizures; painful sensorimotor peripheral neuropathy	Verbal memory; drowsiness; confusion; stupor; organic psychosis resembling paranoid schizophrenia; delirium; agitation; emotional lability
Lead			
Acute			
Children	Respiratory distress; flulike symptoms	Lethargy; cognitive decline; gait disorder; ataxia; seizures	Lethargy; hyperactivity
Adults	Gastrointestinal distress; miscarriages; joint pain; flulike symptoms	Fatigue; delirium; seizures	Delirium
Chronic			
Children	Changes in auditory threshold; behavioral problems; cognitive decline; learning disabilities; attention-deficit/hyperactivity disorder (ADHD)	Learning disorders	Intelligence; reaction time; perceptual motor performance; memory; reading; spelling; auditory processing; attention
Adults	Miscarriage/stillbirth; arthralgia; anemia; hypertension; gout; renal effects; decreased sperm count	Scoptic visual effects; depression; irritability; sleep disturbance; decline in libido; cognition (learning and memory); fasciculations; paresthesias; sensorimotor polyneuropathy; changes	Depression; apathy; confusion; fatigue; tension; restlessness; anger; visual intelligence; visuomotor; general intelligence; memory; psychomotor speed; rate of learning; attention; visuocon-

Manganese	Anorexia; manganese pneumonia	Headaches; apathy; fatigue; depression; hyperexcitability; dysarthria; psychotic behavior; tremor; gait disorders; microphagia; manganism	Sleepiness; asthenia; anorexia; impaired speech; insomnia; hallucinations; mental excitement; aggression; mania; dementia; frontal lobe dysfunction; emotional lability; manganism; judgment; memory
Mercury Inorganic Acute	Bronchial irritation; chills; gingivitis; gastrointestinal distress; bloody diarrhea; brownish mouth lesions; metallic breath; respiratory distress; renal failure	Weakness; irritability; delirium; psychosis	Confusion
Chronic	Salivary gland swelling; excessive salivation; gingivitis; renal dysfunction	Shyness; fatigue; weakness; personality changes; hyperirritability; insomnia; depression; cognitive decline; visual disturbance; intentional tremor; parkinsonism; seizures; painful paresthesias; peripheral polyneuropathy (sensorimotor axonopathy)	Irritability; avoidant behavior; overly sensitive interpersonal behavior; shyness; depression; lassitude; fatigue; agitation; visuospatial; visual memory; reaction time; learning
Organic	Primarily affects the nervous system	Cognitive decline; neurasthenia; paresthesias; ataxia; restricted visual fields; cortical blindness; peripheral polyneuropathy; intention tremor; motor neuron disease (like amyotrophic lateral sclerosis)	

Note. From Bolla and Cadet (2003); Bolla and Roca (1994).

with peripheral neuropathy. Because this constellation of symptoms is nonspecific and could be related to a host of neurological as well as psychiatric etiologies, determining if these symptoms are a result of neurotoxic injury can be extraordinarily challenging.

CATEGORIES OF TOXINS LEADING TO REFERRAL FOR EVALUATION

The main categories of chemicals associated with central nervous system (CNS) injury are the heavy metals (e.g., lead, mercury), solvents (e.g., mixed solvents, toluene), pesticides (organophosphates), and gases (e.g., carbon monoxide). In addition, work has shown that very heavy doses of drugs of abuse (e.g., alcohol, cocaine, MDMA [Ecstasy], marijuana, methamphetamine) are also associated with lower scores on neuropsychological measures (Bolla, Brown, Eldreth, Tate, & Cadet, 2002; Bolla, Cadet, & London, 1998; Bolla, Funderburk, & Cadet, 2000; Bolla & Ricaurte, 1998; Bolla, Rothman, & Cadet, 1999) and abnormalities in brain activity (Bolla et al., 2003) and brain density (Matochik, London, Eldreth, Cadet, & Bolla, 2003) when measured using neuroimaging methods.

So-called toxic mold in homes, schools, and office buildings has been a prominent topic in the news and is increasingly becoming the basis for litigation. A statement published by the American College of Occupational and Environmental Health Medicine (2002) concluded that there is no scientific evidence linking human health effects, which include neurocognitive effects, to inhaled mycotoxins (a secondary metabolite of mold) in the home, school, or office environment. However, research on the possible neurocognitive sequelae of mold exposure is still needed as there are currently no available scientifically rigorous studies.

An in-depth discussion of the physical, cognitive, and neuropsychiatric symptoms associated with significant exposure to specific neurotoxicants and drugs of abuse is beyond the scope of this chapter, but several reviews are available (Bolla & Cadet, 1999, 2003; Bolla & Roca, 1994; Goetz, 1985; Hartman, 1995; Rosenstock & Cullen, 1994). However, Tables 9-2 to 9-4 summarize the main categories of identified neurotoxicants and the physical and cognitive difficulties generally associated with significant exposure to these substances (Bolla & Cadet, 1999, 2003; Bolla & Roca, 1994). Table 9-5 presents symptoms associated with drugs of abuse (Bolla & Cadet, 2003).

Neurotoxicant–symptom relationships summarized in the tables were extracted from a review of numerous epidemiological studies of effects of various neurotoxicants on the nervous system. Caution must be used because, as with any brain injury, there is large individual variability in the development of symptoms and therefore not all symptoms will be present in a single individual.

Also readily apparent in these tables is that the symptoms resulting from significant exposure to a specific neurotoxicant are quite generic. For example, several neurotoxicants can produce memory, perceptuomotor, and emotional symptoms.

In summary, individuals with known significant neurotoxicant exposures have reported cognitive, physical, and affective changes. With acute, high-level exposure, the physical symptoms appear to be immediate, prominent, and primary. Other primary symptoms may include confusion and mood alterations. Conversely, with chronic low-level exposure, mood and cognitive changes appear to be the primary symptoms. Individuals exposed to neurotoxicants have reported difficulties in the areas of concentration and short-term memory. These individuals also complain of disorientation, depression, irritability, fatigue and sleep disturbances, decreased libido, headaches, and weakness (Bolla & Cadet, 1999, 2003; Goetz, 1985).

Once health effects have been detected, it can be problematic to relate these in a causal fashion to a specific neurotoxicant exposure. The diagnosis of neurotoxicant-related damage is generally one of exclusion. Therefore, other causes of central and peripheral nervous system dysfunction must be ruled out, and a history of significant exposure must be substantiated.

PRINCIPLES OF NEUROTOXICOLOGY

In behavioral neurotoxicology, the ability to make accurate causal inferences about possible exposure and the presence of adverse neurological symptoms relies on how well the available data comply with the principles of neurotoxicology. These include the presence of a dose–response relationship, the biological plausibility of symptoms, and the occurrence of symptoms soon after an exposure.

Of paramount importance is the presence of a *dose–response relationship*. This encompasses the idea that, as the degree of exposure increases (intensity/ concentration or duration), the symptoms (physical, cognitive, and psychological) should also become more severe. That is, there should be a direct relationship between the dose of a chemical agent and the response obtained. Therefore, if a patient reports exposure to a chemical in a well-ventilated area for a short duration of time and claims subsequent severe neurocognitive difficulties, then the symptoms are out of proportion to the level of exposure.

Another principle of neurotoxicology relates to *biological plausibility*. For example, if all of the animal studies show that an extremely high level of exposure to a specific chemical does not produce any health effects in animals, then there would be little reason to suspect that health effects would be produced in humans at a lower level. Another prime example is the waxing and waning of specific symptoms with solvent exposure. Acute significant exposure to solvents

TABLE 9-3. Symptoms Associated With Organic Solvent Exposure

ORGANIC SOLVENTS	ASSOCIATED SYMPTOMS	NEUROLOGICAL FINDINGS	NEUROCOGNITIVE FINDINGS
Mixtures	Irritant effects; contact dermatitis	Headaches; fatigue; irritability; depression; sleep difficulties; cognitive decline; decreased olfaction; peripheral neuropathy; myopathy	Executive functions; eye–hand coordination/manual dexterity; visuoconstruction; odor identification
Carbon disulfide	Pulmonary and dermal irritants; cardiac effects; toxic threshold lowered in alcoholism; diabetes mellitus; renal and hepatic diseases	Headaches; irritability; cognitive decline; psychosis; delirium; hearing loss; loss of corneal reflex; Parkinsonism; peripheral polyneuropathy	Psychosis; depression; personality change; insomnia; eye–hand coordination; motor speed; emotionality; energy level; psychomotor performance; reaction time; vigilance; visuomotor functions, construction; retarded speech
Carbon tetrachloride	Gastrointestinal distress; hiccups; liver and kidney damage; toxic threshold lowered in alcoholism; obesity; diabetes; liver and kidney disease	Intoxication; headaches; vertigo: delirium; seizures; Parkinsonism; optic atrophy; visual difficulties	Lethargy; confusion
Ethylene glycol	Renal effects; cardiopulmonary effects	Restlessness; agitation; seizures; absent corneal reflexes; coma	Fatigue; personality changes; depression

Substance			
Methyl alcohol (methanol)	Gastrointestinal distress	Headache; weakness; incoordination; delirium; hallucinations; visual loss; stupor; seizures; Parkinsonism; death	Personality changes; depression
Methyl-N-butyl ketone (MBK)	Euphoria	Weight loss; sensorimotor polyneuropathy	
N-Hexane	Euphoria	Headaches; poor appetite; mild euphoria; peripheral polyneuropathy	Headaches; depression; euphoria
Toluene (methyl benzene) — Acute exposure	Pulmonary effects; cardiac effects	Euphoria; fatigue; ataxia; dizziness; tremor; cognitive decline; seizures; delirium	Excitation at lower or shorter concentrations; depression at higher concentrations; fatigue; confusion; anxiety; reaction time; concentration
Chronic exposure: huffing		Olfaction; optic atrophy; hearing loss; peripheral neuropathy (in cases with associated N-hexane exposure); alcohol intolerance	Exhilaration; euphoria; disinhibition; Performance IQ: memory; motor control; dementia; attention; visuospatial function; apathy; flattened affect
Trichlorethylene (TCE)	Cardiopulmonary effects; toxic threshold reduced with alcohol	Headaches; insomnia; fatigue; anxiety; trigeminal nerve damage; neuro-ophthalmological findings; alcohol intolerance; cognitive decline; hearing loss; peripheral neuropathy	Headaches; dizziness; fatigue; diplopia; alcohol intolerance; neurasthenia; anxiety; lability; insomnia; concentration; manual dexterity; visuospatial accuracy; reaction time; memory

Note. From Bolla and Cadet (2003); Bolla and Roca (1994).

TABLE 9-4. Symptoms Associated With Exposure to Miscellaneous Neurotoxins

NEUROTOXIN	ASSOCIATED SYMPTOMS	NEUROLOGICAL FINDINGS	NEUROCOGNITIVE FINDINGS
Carbon monoxide	None	Headache; irritability; dizziness; cognitive decline; impaired vision; blindness; deafness; seizures; Parkinsonism; coma	"Apathetic masklike facial expression"; dementia; amnesia; disorientation; irritability; cognitive efficiency and flexibility; verbal and visual memory; spatial deficits
Organophosphates	Gastrointestinal distress; excessive sweating and salivation; hypothermia; liver dysfunction	Headache; fatigue; dizziness; decreased consciousness; sleep disturbance; cognitive decline; blurred vision; absent papillary response; muscular fasciculations; tremor; organophosphate-induced delayed polyneuropathy (OPIDP)	Confusion; fatigue; headache; vigilance; concentration; information processing; depression; anxiety; irritability; memory and learning; visuoconstruction; tension; restlessness; anxiety; apprehension

Note. From Bolla and Cadet (2003); Bolla and Roca (1994).

almost always results in headaches, which then resolve once removed from the source of exposure. Therefore, the characteristic pattern of solvent-induced headaches is that they develop after the individual arrives at work in the morning and resolve after they leave work, on the weekends, and when away on vacations. Biological plausibility is absent if the patient claims that his or her headaches are related to solvent exposure and reports that these headaches last all day and night, 7 days a week, and never remit.

In general, except for carbon monoxide (CO) exposure and organophosphate (i.e., pesticide and nerve agent exposure) exposures, symptoms will occur acutely at the time of high-level exposure. Once the source of the exposure is eliminated, these symptoms will begin to remit or at least remain constant over time. The *proximity to exposure* principle posits that symptoms will not increase after removal from exposure and do not develop after a delayed time interval. As mentioned, the only two known chemicals for which symptoms may worsen following significant exposure are in cases of CO and organophosphate exposure (Parkinson et al., 2002; Senanayake & Johnson, 1982).

TABLE 9-5. Symptoms Associated With Drugs of Abuse

DRUG	NEUROLOGICAL SYMPTOMS	NEUROCOGNITIVE FINDINGS
Alcohol	Peripheral neuropathy	Memory; executive function; visuospatial function
Amphetamine	Meth-induced psychosis; hyper-activity; euphoria; headaches; confusion; vasculitis; strokes	Verbal memory; executive function; attention
Cocaine	Vasoconstriction; stroke	Executive function; visuoperception; psychomotor speed; manual dexterity
MDMA (Ecstasy)	Psychiatric disturbance; sleep disturbance; pupillary dilation; tremors; possible seizures; strokes	Visual and verbal memory; executive function
Marijuana	Vasoconstriction	Memory; executive function; psychomotor speed; manual dexterity
Opiates	Peripheral neuropathy	Memory; executive function

Note. From Bolla and Cadet (2003).

EXPOSURE ASSESSMENT

Establishing Exposure

Are the patient's symptom complaints caused by exposure to a neurotoxic substance? This is the primary referral question addressed to the neuropsychologist in the context of toxic tort litigation. To answer this question with any degree of certainty, it must first be established that an individual has been exposed to a neurotoxicant and if the exposure to the neurotoxicant was sufficient to cause CNS injury. Without empirical evidence documenting an exposure, it is difficult to address the question of causality. In the context of forensic neuropsychology, the inability to establish a strong association between an exposure and neurological effects will not be useful to a plaintiff. On the other hand, the defense can use this absence of empirical exposure data to its advantage. Therefore, it is paramount to establish if an exposure can be documented early in the evaluation process, preferably prior to the initial interview with the patient.

In general, both plaintiff and defense attorneys will already possess or have access to industrial hygiene data. Industrial hygienists collect air, water, soil, and environmental samples in homes, schools, office buildings, and industrial sites. These samples are analyzed by sophisticated analytical chemistry methods (e.g., mass spectroscopy) to ascertain the composition of chemicals in the samples and if the concentrations of the identified chemicals are above the acceptable threshold limit values (TLVs) set by the American Conference of Governmental Industrial Hygienists (2001). The TLVs refer to airborne concentrations of substances in conditions that nearly all workers may be exposed on a daily basis. The TLVs are intended to be used only as guidelines in the practice of industrial hygiene in the control of potential workplace health hazards. The TLVs cannot be used as absolute values above which someone will develop adverse health effects because of the wide variation in individual susceptibility.

In addition to industrial hygiene sampling, other sources documenting exposure-level information can be utilized. For example, in cases of CO poisoning, the fire department will often have records of CO levels in the dwelling where the person was exposed. In addition, emergency room records will contain laboratory data on carboxyhemoglobin levels; if elevated, these will provide evidence that a significant exposure occurred. Because carboxyhemoglobin levels are elevated in smokers, smoking status must be considered when interpreting this information. In a nonsmoker, carboxyhemoglobin levels higher than 8–10% are considered elevated, greater than 50% life threatening; and greater than 70–75% usually fatal (Goetz, 1985). However, for CO exposure, carboxyhemoglobin levels will drop rapidly once the person is removed from the source of exposure. Therefore, it is important to gain knowledge about the time period elapsed between the suspected exposure and the person's treatment in the emergency room, including the time of the blood draw for carboxyhemoglobin levels. This explains why documentation of a significant exposure is of utmost importance and is the first step in determining if CNS symptoms are related to the exposure.

Furthermore, if air samples of CO are higher than the TLV of 50 ppm, then a case for a CO exposure can be made. If, however, the dwelling has been ventilated and the carboxyhemoglobin levels are taken a few hours or days after the maximum exposure, then there will be few industrial hygiene or biological data to support significant CO exposure even if significant exposure has occurred. Without data to verify an exposure, it is difficult to determine the intensity of current and past exposure or even if an individual has been exposed to a toxic chemical. However, knowledge of the toxokinetics of the neurotoxicant is required to interpret this type of information. If there is no empirical evidence of an exposure, it will generally be difficult to relate neurological symptoms to a neurotoxic origin.

Establishing Sufficient Exposure

Often, patients will complain of residual neurocognitive effects following exposure to an unknown chemical, usually one with a strong, unpleasant odor. One such substance is tar used in roofing and highway repair. Many individuals report becoming ill when exposed to tar and claim neurocognitive sequelae as a result of this exposure. However, there is no scientific evidence showing that tar is a neurotoxicant. These odorous chemical irritants may produce allergy-type symptoms (i.e., runny eyes and nose, congestion), but do not cause permanent brain injury. There are an unlimited number of chemical substances encountered in everyday life for which there is no evidence of neurotoxicity.

Once it has been established that an exposure to a potentially neurotoxic chemical has occurred, it then needs to be determined if the exposure was of sufficient duration or intensity to produce neurological injury. To accomplish this task, a biological measurement (a biomarker) of exposure is required. Unfortunately, with the exception of the heavy metals, biomarkers for many neurotoxicants are either difficult to obtain or nonexistent. For example, solvents are difficult to measure because of their rapid metabolism and clearance. N-Hexane, an aliphatic hydrocarbon, has a half-life in fat tissue of about 64 hours. Therefore, N-hexane and other organic solvents are not cumulative chemicals, which means that only recent exposure (i.e., end of work shift) can be evaluated by a biological marker. Even if a patient had elevated levels of N-hexane at one time, the levels would not be elevated after only a few days with no exposure. Cases of solvent exposure can be akin to cases of mild traumatic brain injury with respect to the paucity of empirical data linking neurological injury to an adverse event.

History

Because there is often no definitive evidence (i.e., biomarkers, industrial hygiene data) to make causal inferences about negative neurological effects of a neurotoxic exposure, in-depth histories must be obtained. These histories should include information within the medical, occupational, environmental, social, academic, and psychiatric domains to allow ruling out factors accounting for symptoms and test performance other than the alleged exposure.

Medical history

A detailed medical history is essential to determine if there are alternative explanations for the patient's symptom complaints. Patients should be asked specific questions about previous neurological problems, including head injury, the presence of migraines, sleep disorders, substance use (especially alcohol use), previous learning disabilities (i.e., if they were ever held back a grade in school), symptoms of attention-deficit disorder with and without hyperactivity, or symptoms compatible with carpal tunnel syndrome, which can be confused with symptoms of neurotoxicant-associated polyneuropathy. It is particularly important to review the patient's medical records. It is informative if the patient complains of a long series of severe medical complaints that they believe are caused by neurotoxicant exposure, but there is no history that the patient ever sought medical attention for these symptoms or if they saw physicians for other concerns and did not mention the alleged symptoms.

Occupational and environmental history

We must rely on the occupational and environmental history to determine if there was sufficient exposure to a neurotoxicant to produce neurological effects. An in-depth history relating to a person's occupational setting and specifics of the duties required by the job must be obtained not only from the patient, but also from other sources. Questions that must be addressed are aimed at assessing the work environment in which the potential exposure occurred. Refer to the work of Kilbourne and Weiner (1990) for an occupational history questionnaire.

Does the person work in an industry with potential exposure to a neurotoxicant? Does the person have a job that places him or her close to an exposure? Because the routes of absorption of neurotoxicants are inhalation, ingestion, and dermal absorption, does the individual have a significant exposure that is biologically plausible? For example, although someone lives in a house with lead paint, if the paint is in good shape (i.e., not peeling) and is not disturbed, then there is no potential source of significant exposure. Did the person come in contact with a neurotoxicant? Does the employer enforce safety standards? Is there medical monitoring (i.e., routine testing for elevated lead levels)? If the company does not medically monitor or enforce safety standards, it may not be because of negligence, it may be because the work environment has been determined to be safe. Has the patient experienced symptoms while at work? Have coworkers complained of similar symptoms?

It is also important to determine if individuals claiming neurotoxic exposure are disgruntled workers who have unstable work histories. How many jobs has the patient had? What kind of work performance evaluations has the individual received? Does the patient show unexplained poor job performance evaluations and excessive absenteeism from work long before a claim for exposure is made?

Environmental sources of exposure must also be explored because these may be responsible for the exposure, rather than the work site. What is the person's living situation? Do they live in an old or relatively new home? Do they live in the country or the city? What is the source of water? If water comes from a well, the well may be contaminated. Do they live in old housing in the city that could be contaminated with lead paint? Is the paint in poor repair, and if so, have they tried to remove the lead paint? Does the patient garden? Gardening may be associated with exposure to excessive amounts of pesticides. Has their home been treated with pesticides lately? What are the individual's hobbies? Patients can become ill from high exposure in poorly ventilated areas to paint thinners used in refinishing antique furniture, become lead exposed from lead solder used in making stained glass, and may be exposed to heavy metals from glazes if they make ceramics.

Social, academic, and psychiatric history

Social history is important to gain a feel for psychological stability. Individuals claiming exposure to neurotoxicants may have a long history of antisocial personality disorder, somatoform disorder, major depressive disorder, or childhood traumas. Therefore, it is important to obtain information about the number of marriages, past and current treatments for psychiatric illness, and if there were any instances of physical or sexual childhood trauma. In particular, history of childhood physical or sexual trauma is associated with increased risk for somatization disorder in adulthood (see chapter 10, this volume; Morrison, 1989).

It is also important to ascertain whether there has been a change in neurological status. School records, if available, can provide critical information about premorbid level of functioning (especially national standardized test results). For example, it is not uncommon for a patient to claim to be having difficulty in mathematics or reading as a result of potential exposure. However, very poor grades in these subjects as well as poor scores on a national standardized test compared to a national sample would indicate that the individual has always had trouble in these areas.

The Evaluation

Historically, neuropsychological techniques have consisted of oral and written tests administered by a trained examiner on a one-to-one basis. A number of computerized test batteries have also been developed (i.e., the World Health Organization Neurobehavioral Test Battery and the Neurobehavioral Evaluation System-NES-2; Baker, Letz, & Fidler, 1985) specifically for the evaluation of neurocognitive sequelae of neurotoxicant exposure.

Advantages and disadvantages exist for both interviewer-administered and computer-administered tests (Kane & Kay, 1992). For interviewer-administered tests, the advantages include human interaction and encouragement by the examiner, the ability to determine problem-solving strategies by actually observing the individual perform the tests, and the ability to administer tasks requiring verbal presentation and verbal responses. For example, verbal memory cannot be adequately assessed by a computer without sophisticated computer hardware. The disadvantages of interviewer-administered tests include standardization of administration between different testers and between testing sessions. In epidemiological investigations, interviewer-administered tests are more labor intensive and require a large study team to administer the tests.

Computerized testing offers excellent standardization in administering and scoring. Furthermore, in epidemiological studies, multiple work stations and computers can be set up to test groups of workers simultaneously. However, extensive normative populations may not be available for computer-administered tests, which is not the case for interviewer-administered tests. The normative values for interviewer-administered tests cannot be used to compare the results of written tests adapted for the computer because the performance demands of the tasks change even though the tests appear to be similar (Kane & Kay, 1992).

A thorough assessment includes tests that assess the cognitive domains of intelligence, language, verbal and visual learning and memory, perception, motor/tactile skills, attention, psychomotor speed, executive function, and personality (Lezak, 1995; Spreen & Strauss, 1998). The cognitive areas most often reported to be adversely affected by neurotoxicants are manual dexterity, psychomotor speed, verbal and visual memory and learning, attention, and executive functions (refer to Tables 9-2 to 9-5).

Verbal intelligence can be assessed using the Verbal subtests from the Wechsler Adult Intelligence Scale, Third Edition (WAIS-III) (Wechsler, 1997). For brevity of testing, the Vocabulary subtest can be used alone to obtain a good estimate of verbal intelligence because it correlates highly with the Full-Scale IQ score.

Although there are many standardized tests to evaluate language and aphasia, such as the Western Aphasia Battery (Kertesz, 1980) and the Boston Diagnostic Aphasia Examination (Goodglass, Kaplan, & Barresi, 2000), extensive evaluation of language functioning in suspected cases of neurotoxic exposure is unnecessary because most neurotoxins do not selectively impair language. Therefore, deficits in language (i.e., paraphasias) suggest an alternative etiology for symptoms. The significant aspects of language can be quickly assessed by confrontational naming, repetition of words and phrases, spontaneous writing of a sentence, writing a sentence to dictation, and rating verbal expression.

At low levels, neurotoxins affect new learning and recent memory, and they do not affect remote memory. If gaps exist in the individual's early memories, then a neurotoxic etiology is unlikely. Remote memory can be assessed by asking about significant early life events (wedding or occupational details or historical events).

Difficulty with anterograde memory (ability to learn new information) is one of the characteristics of neurotoxic exposure (Bleecker et al., 1991; Bolla et al., 1995; Schwartz et al., 1993, 2000; Stewart et al., 1999). Therefore, it is important to evaluate this cognitive domain thoroughly with procedures such as the California Verbal Learning Test II (CVLT-II) (Delis, Kramer, Kaplan, & Ober, 2000) and the Rey Auditory Verbal Learning Test (RAVLT) (Rey, 1964). Close inspection of performance patterns on the RAVLT or the CVLT-II in individuals with neurotoxic exposure show a learning effect over the trials, but at a lower rate than expected. Performance on the RAVLT (trials 1–5) also declines as years of exposure to lead increase (Bolla et al., 1995). These tests also allow examination for signs of malingering. For example, the person may be embellishing symptoms if they recall a word consistently on the free recall learning trials, but then fail to recognize it on the Recognition subtest (Binder, Kelly, Villanueva, & Winslow, 2003; Wiggins & Brandt, 1988; Bernard, 1990).

Visual memory can also be assessed with tests such as the Symbol Digit Paired Associate Learning (Kapur & Butters, 1977) task or the Rey-Osterrieth Complex Figure (Osterrieth, 1944).

Sustained attention and executive/motor skills have been reported to be affected by neurotoxic exposure as well. Two tests sensitive in detecting not only neurotoxic exposure, but also any type of CNS damage are the Digit-Symbol Substitution Test from the WAIS-III and the Trail Making Test (Trails A and B) from the Halstead Reitan Neuropsychological Test Battery (Reitan & Davison, 1974). The Wisconsin Card Sorting Test and the Category Test are also sensitive to deficits in executive function and reasoning (Lezak, 1995). The Stroop Test and Consonant Trigrams are measures of divided attention as well as executive functions (Lezak, 1995).

Simple Visual Reaction Time is another test that has been shown to be affected by neurotoxins (Balbus, Stewart, Bolla, & Schwartz, 1997). Reaction time can be measured by using either a reaction-time device or a computer. Stimuli are randomly presented so that the presentation of the next stimulus cannot be anticipated. When this task is given over 44 or more trials, an index of vigilance, sustained attention, and response variability can be determined. In addition to examining the mean or median reaction, the standard deviation has been shown to be especially sensitive for measuring variability in rate of response that appears to be strongly affected by lead exposure (Balbus et al., 1997).

Manual dexterity and coordination have been shown to deteriorate with exposure to various neurotoxins, especially to a combination of organic and inorganic lead (Bolla et al., 1995; Schwartz et al., 1993, 2000, 2001; Stewart et al., 1999). The Purdue Pegboard (Agnew, Bolla-Wilson, Kawas, & Bleecker, 1988; Purdue Research Foundation, 1948) and the Grooved Pegboard (Klove, 1963) are measures of fine motor speed and dexterity. The Finger Oscillation Task (Finger Tapping) (Reitan & Davison, 1974) is a measure of dexterity/simple motor speed. Brain damage from most neurotoxins is diffuse, and significantly faster scores on one hand compared to the other (greater than 10% difference) may suggest a lateralized dysfunction and would therefore be incongruent with a diagnosis of a neurotoxic exposure. Although epidemiological studies find that nondominant hand performance may be more sensitive to lead exposure, the effect is small (Bolla et al., 1995; Schwartz et al., 2001; Stewart et al., 1999).

Not only is it important to use tests that have been shown to be sensitive to detecting subtle neurocognitive effects from exposures, but tests sensitive enough to show a dose–response association are favorable. Significant dose-related associations (increased exposure, poorer performance) between quantitative measures of exposure to a mixture of organic and inorganic lead or only to inorganic lead (duration of exposure, peak tibia bone lead, current blood lead) have been reported for the RAVLT, Serial Digit Learning test, Rey Complex Figure Delayed, Trails A and B, Stroop, Block Design, Purdue Pegboard, and Finger Tapping (Bolla et al., 1995; Schwartz et al., 2000; Stewart et al., 1999). Likewise, increased lifetime weighted-average exposure to a mixture of solvents was associated with decreased performance on the Digit Symbol substitution, Serial Digit learning, Reaction time, Trails A and B, and bilateral finger tapping (Bleecker et al., 1991).

Establishing evidence of dose-related associations on the neuropsychological assessment helps rule out nonneurological psychiatric factors and malingering. Systematically evaluating for malingering must be included in every evaluation of a potential case of neurotoxic exposure. Refer to chapter 4 on malingering for guidelines.

Interpretation of Findings

Adequate normative values for reference

Speculation about the cause of poor performance on a neurobehavioral test must be made with caution. To determine if a score falls outside the normal range, adequate norms must be used for comparison. For example, intellectual ability can predict test performance for verbal, perceptual, executive function, and psychomotor speed tasks (Larrabee, 2000), but few norms are currently available for individuals with low or high levels of intellectual functioning. Comparing the test results of an individual with lower intellectual ability with normative values based on a more intelligent group could lead to the erroneous conclusion of CNS injury when none exists.

This is especially problematic in behavioral neurotoxicology because there are few norms available for unskilled laborers (i.e., blue-collar workers), many of whom never finished high school. Conversely, performance decrements in highly intelligent people may be missed because even their diminished performance may still meet or exceed the upper limits of a normative group representing a more average level of intellectual functioning. In addition, cognitive performance is also influenced by age and sex. Therefore, to ensure an accurate diagnosis, the clinician must use norms that have been adjusted to include the effects of modifying variables such as education, intelligence, age, and sex.

Base rates

When attempting to determine if a patient's cognitive complaints are consistent with those that have been reported with exposure to neurotoxicants, the base rate of the complaint in the general population must be considered. For example, in a study of 40- to 90-year-old community-dwelling healthy individuals, 83% complained of difficulty remembering names, 60% complained that they misplaced items, and 53% complained of word-finding problems (Bolla, Lindgren, Bonaccorsy, & Bleecker, 1991). These base rates increase moderately when associated with head injury of toxic exposure, but increase dramatically once someone enters the legal arena to become a personal injury claimant (Dunn, Lees-Haley, Brown, Williams, & English, 1995; Lees-Haley & Brown, 1993).

Table 9-6 is taken from the work of Dunn et al. (1995) and shows the frequency of symptom complaints in samples of controls, head-injured or toxic-injured individuals, and personal injury claimants. Therefore, it is paramount to remember that just because a patient complains of a specific symptom and that symptom has been reported with exposure to a specific neurotoxicant, this does not mean that the individual was exposed to a chemical that permanently injured the nervous system.

It is important to note that neurobehavioral tests can have high sensitivity but low specificity, meaning that they can be very effective in detecting deficits, but less effective in identifying the causes of those deficits (see chapter 1, this volume, on scientific approach). It is important to determine if cognitive decrements are related to neurotoxicant exposure or to another CNS, medical, or neuropsychiatric disorder. Alterations in performance can be related to age, sex, educational level, native intelligence, cultural differences, cultural deprivation, motivation, involvement in litigation, frustration, fatigue, emotional problems like anxiety and depression, and personality characteristics.

Consequently, although some individual tests are sensitive, they are of little value when attempting to delineate the precise etiology of a person's deficits. The neuropsychological evaluation cannot be used in isolation to make a diagnosis, but rather must be used in combination with medical, social, school, and occupational histories. Although patients may report recent onset of cognitive difficulties, review of school records and prior employment evaluations might indicate long-standing problems (i.e., subnormal intelligence or learning disability).

Furthermore, long-term or heavy alcohol use (Bondi, Drake, & Grant, 1998; Parsons, 1998), heavy cocaine use (Bolla et al., 1999), heavy MDMA use (Bolla et al., 1998), or even very heavy marijuana use (Bolla et al., 2003) may produce a number of cognitive deficits. Medical conditions such as diabetes can cause symptoms of peripheral neuropathy as well as cognitive deficits (Bruce et al., 2003). Other medical conditions to consider in the differential diagnosis are past history of head injury, hypertension, thyroid disease, and renal or hepatic disorders. Depression or anxiety can also produce decrements in neuropsychological test performance. These decrements are usually observed in the areas of attention, learning and memory, processing speed, and psychomotor speed. Because similar cognitive domains are affected by both neurotoxicants and alterations in

TABLE 9-6. Base Rates of Complaints (Symptom Frequency)

SYMPTOM	MEDICAL CONTROLS ($N = 113$)	HEAD INJURED/TOXIC ($N = 68$)	PERSONAL INJURY ($N = 156$)
Anxiety	41	56	87
Trouble sleeping	30	40	81
Headaches	50	57	77
Depression	27	41	76
Tension	24	40	74
Concentration problems	21	34	71
Fatigue	37	56	71
Difficulty concentrating	18	32	69
Impatience	33	41	64
Irritability	27	31	63
Restlessness	16	37	63
Confusion	5	18	58
Feeling disorganized	20	32	58
Thinking clearly	11	27	57
Neck pain[a]	31	40	56
Loss of interest	13	15	51
Easily distracted	15	24	49
Loss of efficiency	10	13	49
Loss of temper	11	19	49
Attention problems	10	25	48
Word finding	12	24	46
Feeling partially disabled	4	16	44
Weakness	6	15	44
Dizziness	21	28	41
Nausea	20	32	39
Sexual problems	8	18	39
Shoulder pain[a]	14	24	38
Slowed thinking	5	16	38
Blurred vision	18	32	37
Rapid heartbeat	15	19	37
Poor judgment	4	16	35
Recent memory problems	5	18	35
Chest pressure	13	13	34
Trouble hearing	12	28	34
Numbness	5	21	34
Painful tingling	5	16	34
Visual problems	7	21	34
Trouble reading	1	6	33
Fear of noncancer illness	6	19	33
Trouble walking	4	6	32
Trembling	5	15	31
Feeling totally disabled	3	3	30
Bumping into things	14	13	30

TABLE 9-6. *Continued*

SYMPTOM	MEDICAL CONTROLS (N = 113)	HEAD INJURED/TOXIC (N = 68)	PERSONAL INJURY (N = 156)
Diarrhea[a]	26	47	28
Perspiring for no reason	5	13	26
Loss of common sense	4	6	24
Marital problems	9	12	24
Fine-motor coordination	2	4	20
Long-term memory problems	0	7	18
Speech problems	2	6	17
Slurred speech	1	6	15
Elbow pain[a]	8	22	14
Impotence	4	2	14
Not knowing where I am	0	4	12
Mean number of symptoms	9	14	25

Note. Adapted from Dunn et al. (1995). Copyright, 1995, John Wiley & Sons, Inc. This material is used by permission of John Wiley & Sons, Inc.

[a]The symptom is a distractor.

mood, it can be difficult to determine the relative contribution of each to decrements in neuropsychological test performance. More specifically, such symptomatology could be related to neurotoxic exposure, to the patient's emotional state, to the patient's personality characteristics, or to some combination of the three.

To determine the etiology of complaints, patterns of performance and inconsistencies during testing (such as superior performance on harder tasks with poor performance on easier ones or lower-than-chance performance on all of the tasks) must be examined carefully. Repeat testing will also assist in this area because test performance should remain relatively static over the course of several days. If significant alterations in test scores are indicated, an affective or motivational disturbance is the likely culprit. If test performance declines without reexposure, then a progressive disease or secondary psychological reaction to the exposure is suspect (Bolla & Rignani, 1997).

Emotional reactions to a perceived exposure may be as important as, or even more important than, the direct physiological effects of the chemicals, especially when considering etiology and persistence of symptoms. Figures 9-1 and 9-2 illustrate the complex relationships between exposure and neurological sequelae (Bolla, 1996). The fear associated with suspected exposures can be stressful enough to cause significant mental disorders such as somatoform disorders, anxiety disorders, adjustment disorders, and typical and atypical posttraumatic stress disorders.

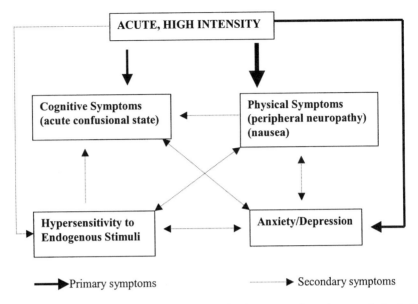

FIGURE 9-1. Schematic representation of the development and persistence of physical, cognitive, and affective symptoms following acute, high-intensity, chemical exposure. Solid lines are primary symptoms and dotted lines are secondary symptoms (Bolla, 2000).

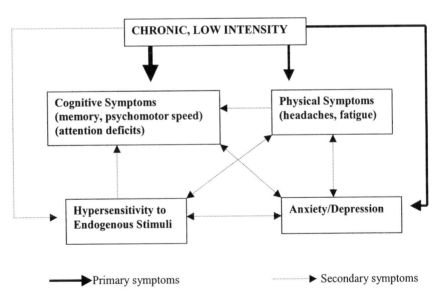

FIGURE 9-2. Schematic representation of the development and persistence of physical, cognitive, and affective symptoms following persistent, low-intensity, chemical exposure. Solid lines are primary symptoms and dotted lines are secondary symptoms (Bolla, 2000).

In addition, specific inherent personality characteristics may predispose an individual to develop physical, cognitive, and psychological symptoms (Bolla-Wilson, Wilson, & Bleecker, 1988; Kellner, 1985; Mechanic, 1972). Clinical observation suggests that more perfectionistic and anxious individuals may be hypersensitive to endogenous stimuli. Expectations by susceptible individuals that exposure to chemicals has adversely affected their health may result in enhanced awareness of normal bodily sensations. This normal physiological activity may then be erroneously attributed to neurotoxic-related abnormal physical, cognitive, and affective symptoms. The degree to which an individual is hypersensitive to endogenous stimuli (normal bodily sensations) may determine the duration and intensity of symptoms. Those psychological mechanisms have been observed in toxic exposure, as well as in persistent postconcussion syndrome (Bolla-Wilson et al., 1988; Mittenberg, DiGuilio, Perrin, & Bass, 1992).

The neuropsychological evaluation provides unique information on the functional integrity of the CNS. As with any diagnostic process, the ability to make a differential diagnosis between neurotoxicant exposure, neurological disease, medical illness, or neuropsychiatric disturbance is based on the combined evidence taken from the medical, occupational, social, and academic histories; physical and neurological exams; biological monitoring; EEG; CT/MRI; and the neuropsychological evaluation.

Central nervous system effects are best discovered with neuropsychological assessment. However, interpretation of decrements in performance on these tests is often erroneous if made by individuals who lack specific expertise in neurobehavioral toxicology. This is illustrated nicely by the N-hexane example presented in this chapter. If the clinician is not knowledgeable about the specific symptoms associated with specific neurotoxic agents, the clinician may conclude that a mild deficit in verbal memory (without having the patient examined for peripheral neuropathy) was caused by exposure to N-hexane when this conclusion would not be biologically plausible.

The neurological examination, EEG, CT scan, and MRI scans are generally not helpful in making a specific diagnosis of toxic encephalopathy, but are helpful in ruling out other causes of the patient's symptoms. In contrast, nerve conduction studies are useful in detecting peripheral neuropathies often associated with exposure to specific chemicals.

For example, the predominant neurological feature of N-hexane exposure is peripheral neuropathy, not cognitive disturbance. Symmetrical sensory dysfunction in the hands and feet is the usual presenting complaint. Weakness in the lower extremities is also a common symptom. Decreased response to pin, vibration, and thermal stimulation is found on examination. The clinician should become suspicious if no symptoms of peripheral neuropathy were ever reported to any doctor by the patient, and the patient is only claiming cognitive problems. If there are no acute effects, it would be highly unlikely to have chronic effects.

After discontinuation of exposure, both CNS and peripheral nervous system effects can recover. When evaluating patients who present with symptoms of a possible neurotoxicant exposure, it is irresponsible to attribute their symptoms routinely to the presence of a neuropsychiatric disorder. It is equally irresponsible to attribute neurotoxic-like symptoms to neurotoxicant exposure without rigorously exploring other etiologies. If other causes for the symptoms are not considered, then many treatable conditions will remain unidentified and untreated.

REFERENCES

Agnew, J., Bolla-Wilson, K., Kawas, C., & Bleecker, M. L. (1988). Purdue Pegboard age and sex norms for ages forty and older. *Developmental Neuropsychology, 4*, 29–35.

American College of Occupational and Environmental Health Medicine. (2002). *Adverse human health effects associated with molds in the indoor environment.* Arlington Heights, IL: American College of Occupational and Environmental Medicine.

American Conference of Governmental Industrial Hygienists. (2001). *Threshold limit values for chemical substances and physical agents and biological exposure indices.* Cincinnati, OH: Author.

Arlien-Soborg, P., Bruhn, P., Gyldensted, C., & Melgaard, B. (1979). Chronic painter's syndrome. Chronic toxic encephalopathy in house painters. *Acta Neurologica Scandinavica, 60*, 149–156.

Baker, E. L., Letz, R. E., & Fidler, A. (1985). A computer administered neurobehavioral evaluation system for occupational and environmental epidemiology. *Journal of Occupational Medicine, 27*, 206–212.

Balbus, J. M., Stewart, W., Bolla, K. I., & Schwartz, B. S. (1997). Simple visual reaction time in organolead manufacturing workers: A comparison of different methods of modeling lead exposure and reaction time. *American Journal of Industrial Medicine, 32*, 544–549.

Bernard, L. C. (1990). Prospects for faking believable memory deficits on neuropsychological tests and the use of incentives in simulation research. *Journal of Clinical and Experimental Neuropsychology, 12*, 715–728.

Binder, L. M., Kelly, M. P., Villanueva, M. R., & Winslow, M. M. (2003). Motivation and neuropsychological test performance following mild head injury. *Journal of Clinical and Experimental Neuropsychology, 25*, 420–430.

Bleecker, M. L., Bolla, K. I., Agnew, J., Schwartz, B. S., & Ford, D. P. (1991). Dose-related subclinical neurobehavioral effects of chronic exposure to low levels of organic solvents. *American Journal of Industrial Medicine, 19*, 715–728.

Bolla, K. (2000). Use of neuropsychological testing in idiopathic environmental intolerance. In P. J. Sparks (Ed.), *State of the art reviews in occupational medicine: Idiopathic environmental illness* (pp. 617–646). Philadelphia: Hanley and Belfus.

Bolla, K., Brown, K., Eldreth, D., Tate, K., & Cadet, J.-L. (2002). Dose-related neurocognitive effects of marijuana use. *Neurology, 59*, 1337–1343.

Bolla, K., & Cadet, J.-L. (1999). Exogenous acquired metabolic disorders of the nervous system: Toxins and illicit drugs. In C. Goetz & E. J. Pappert (Eds.), *Textbook of clinical neurology.* Chicago: Saunders.

Bolla, K., Eldreth, D., London, E. D., Kiehl, K. A., Mouratidis, M., Contoreggi, C., Matochik, J., et al. (2003). Orbitofrontal cortex dysfunction in abstinent cocaine abusers performing a decision-making task. *NeuroImage, 19,* 1085–1094.

Bolla, K., & Roca, R. (1994). The neuropsychiatric sequella of exposure to neurotoxic compounds. In M. L. Bleecker (Ed.), *Occupational neurology and clinical neurotoxicology* (pp. 133–160). Baltimore: Williams and Wilkins.

Bolla, K. I. (1996). Neuropsychological evaluation for detecting alterations in the central nervous system after chemical exposure. *Regulatory Toxicology and Pharmacology, 24,* S48–S51.

Bolla, K. I., & Cadet, J.-L. (2003). Exogenous acquired metabolic disorders of the nervous system: Toxins and illicit drugs. In C. Goetz & E. J. Pappert (Eds.), *Textbook of clinical neurology* (2nd ed., pp. 839–871). Chicago: Saunders.

Bolla, K. I., Cadet, J.-L., & London, E. D. (1998). The neuropsychiatry of chronic cocaine use. *Journal of Neuropsychology and Clinical Neurosciences, 10,* 280–289.

Bolla, K. I., Funderburk, F. R., & Cadet, J.-L. (2000). Differential effects of cocaine and cocaine + alcohol on neurocognitive performance. *Neurology, 54,* 2285–2292.

Bolla, K. I., & Ricaurte, G. (1998). Memory impairment in abstinent MDMA ("ecstasy") users. *Neurology, 51,* 1532–1537.

Bolla, K. I., & Rignani, J. (1997). Clinical course of neuropsychological functioning after chronic exposure to organic and inorganic lead. *Archives of Clinical Neuropsychology, 12,* 123–131.

Bolla, K. I., Lindgren, K. N., Bonaccorsy, C., & Bleecker, M. L. (1991). Memory complaints in the elderly—fact or fiction? *Archives of Neurology, 48,* 61–64.

Bolla, K. I., Rothman, R. B., & Cadet, J.-L. (1999). Dose-related neurobehavioral effects of chronic cocaine use. *Journal of Neuropsychiatry and Clinical Neurosciences, 11,* 361–369.

Bolla, K. I., Schwartz, B. S., Agnew, J., Ford, P., & Bleecker, M. L. (1990). Subclinical neuropsychiatric effects of chronic low level solvent exposure in U.S. paint manufacturers. *Journal of Occupational Medicine, 32,* 671–677.

Bolla, K. I., Schwartz, B. S., Stewart, W., Rignani, J., Agnew, J., & Ford, D. P. (1995). A comparison of neurobehavioral function in workers exposed to a mixture of organic and inorganic lead and in workers exposed to solvents. *American Journal of Industrial Medicine, 27,* 231–246.

Bolla-Wilson, K., Wilson, R. J., & Bleecker, M. L. (1988). Conditioning of physical symptoms after neurotoxic exposure. *Journal of Occupational Medicine, 30,* 684–686.

Bondi, M. W., Drake, A. I., & Grant, I. (1998). Verbal learning and memory in alcohol abusers and polysubstance abusers with concurrent alcohol abuse. *Journal of the International Neuropsychological Society, 4,* 319–328.

Bruce, D. G., Casey, G. P., Grange, V., Clarnette, R. C., Almeida, O. P., Foster, J. K., et al. (2003). Cognitive impairment, physical disability, and depressive symptoms in older diabetic patients: The Fremantle cognition in diabetes study. *Diabetes Research and Clinical Practice, 61,* 59–67.

Cherry, N., Hutchins, H., Pace, T., & Waldron, H. A. (1985). Neurobehavioral effects of repeated occupational exposure to toluene and paint solvents. *British Journal of Industrial Medicine, 41,* 291–300.

Cranmer, J. M., & Goldberg, L. (1986). Human aspects of solvent neurobehavioral effects: Report of the workshop session on clinical and epidemiological topics. *Neurotoxicology, 7,* 57–62.

Delis, D. C., Kramer, J. H., Kaplan, E., & Ober, B. A. (2000). *California Verbal Learning Test* (2nd ed.). San Antonio, TX: Psychological Corporation.

Dunn, J. T., Lees-Haley, P. R., Brown, R. S., Williams, C. W., & English, L. T. (1995). Neurotoxic complaint base rates of personal injury claimants: Implications for neuropsychological assessment. *Journal of Clinical Psychology, 51,* 577–584.

Gade, A., Mortensen, E. L., & Bruhn, P. (1988). Chronic painters "syndrome." A reanalysis of psychological test data in a group of diagnosed cases, based on comparisons with matched controls. *Acta Neurologica Scandinavica, 77,* 293–306.

Goetz, C. G. (1985). *Neurotoxins in clinical practice.* New York: Medical and Scientific Books, Spectrum.

Goodglass, H., Kaplan, E., & Barresi, B. (2000). *The Boston Diagnostic Aphasia Examination.* San Antonio, TX: Psychological Corporation.

Hartman, D. E. (1995). *Neuropsychological toxicology: Identification and assessment of human neurotoxic syndromes* (2nd ed.) New York: Kluwer Academic/Plenum.

Kane, R. L., & Kay, G. G. (1992). Computerized assessment in neuropsychology: A review of tests and test batteries. *Neuropsychology Review, 3,* 1–117.

Kapur, N., & Butters, N. (1977). An analysis of the visuoperceptual deficits in alcoholics. *Journal of the Study of Alcohol, 38,* 2025–2055.

Kellner, R. (1985). Functional somatic symptoms and hypochondriasis: A survey of empirical studies. *Archives of General Psychiatry, 42,* 821–833.

Kertesz, A. (1980). *Western Aphasia Battery.* London, Ontario, Canada: University of Ontario.

Kilbourne, E. W., & Weiner, J. (1990). Occupational and environmental medicine: The internist's role. *Annals of Internal Medicine, 113,* 974–982.

Klove, H. (1963). Clinical neuropsychology. In F. M. Forster (Ed.), *The medical clinics of North America* (pp. 1647–1658). New York: Saunders.

Larrabee, G. J. (2000). Association between IQ and neuropsychological test performance: Commentary on Tremont, Hoffman, Scott and Adams (1998). *Clinical Neuropsychology, 14,* 139–145.

Lees-Haley, P. R., & Brown, R. S. (1993). Neuropsychological complaint base rates of 170 personal injury claimants. *Archives of Clinical Neuropsychology, 8,* 203–209.

Lezak, M. D. (1995). *Neuropsychological assessment* (3rd ed.). New York: Oxford University Press.

Loomis, T. A., & Hayes, A. W. (1996). *Loomis's essentials of toxicology* (4th ed.). San Diego, CA: Academic Press.

Maizlish, N. A., Fine, L. J., Albers, J. W., Whitehead, L., & Langolf, G. D. (1987). A neurological evaluation of workers exposed to mixtures of organic solvents. *British Journal of Industrial Medicine, 44,* 14–25.

Matochik, J. A., London, E. D., Eldreth, D. A., Cadet, J.-L., & Bolla, K. I. (2003). Frontal cortical tissue composition in abstinent cocaine abusers: A magnetic resonance imaging study. *NeuroImage, 19,* 1095–1102.

Mechanic, D. (1972). Social psychologic factors affecting the presentation of bodily complaints. *New England Journal of Medicine, 286,* 1132–1139.

Mittenberg, W., DiGuilio, D. V., Perrin, S., & Bass, A. E. (1992). Symptoms following mild head injury: Expectation as etiology. *Journal of Neurology, Neurosurgery, and Psychiatry, 55,* 200–204.

Morrison, J. (1989). Childhood sexual histories of women with somatization disorder. *American Journal of Psychiatry, 146,* 239–241.

Osterrieth, P. A. (1944). Le test de copie d'une figure complex: Contribution a l'etude de la perception et de la memoire. *Archives de Psychologie, 30,* 286–356.

Parkinson, R. B., Hopkins, R. O., Cleavinger, H. B., Weaver, L. K., Victoroff, J., Foley, J. F., et al. (2002). White matter hyperintensities and neuropsychological outcome following carbon monoxide poisoning. *Neurology, 58*, 1525–1532.

Parsons, O. A. (1998). Neurocognitive deficits in alcoholics and social drinkers: A continuum? *Alcoholism: Clinical and Experimental Research, 22*, 954–961.

Purdue Research Foundation. (1948). *Examiner's manual for the Purdue Pegboard.* Chicago: Science Research Associates.

Reitan, R. M., & Davison, L. A. (1974). *Clinical neuropsychology: Current status and applications.* New York: Hemisphere.

Rey, A. (1964). *L'examen clinique en psychologie.* Paris: Presses Universitaires de France.

Rosenstock, L., & Cullen, M. R. (1994). *Textbook of clinical, occupational and environmental medicine.* Philadelphia: Saunders.

Schwartz, B. S., Bolla, K. I., Stewart, W., Ford, D. P., Agnew, J., & Frumkin, H. (1993). Decrements in neurobehavioral performance associated with mixed exposure to organic and inorganic lead. *American Journal of Epidemiology, 137*, 1006–1021.

Schwartz, B. S., Lee, B. K., Lee, G. S., Stewart, W. F., Lee, S. S., Hwang, K. Y., et al. (2001). Associations of blood lead, dimercaptosuccinic acid-chelatable lead, and tibia lead with neurobehavioral test scores in South Korean lead workers. *American Journal of Epidemiology, 153*, 453–464.

Schwartz, B. S., Stewart, W., Bolla, K. I., Simon, D., Banden-Roche, K., Gordon, B., et al. (2000). Past adult lead exposure is associated with longitudinal decline in neurobehavioral function. *Neurology, 55*, 1144–1150.

Senanayake, N., & Johnson, M. K. (1982). Acute polyneuropathy after poisoning by a new organophosphate insecticide. *New England Journal of Medicine, 306*, 155–157.

Spreen, O., & Strauss, E. (1998). *A compendium of neuropsychological tests* (2nd ed.). New York: Oxford.

Stewart, W., Schwartz, B. S., Simon, D., Bolla, K. I., Todd, A. C., & Links, J. (1999). The relation between neurobehavioral function and tibial and chelatable lead levels in 543 former organolead manufacturing workers. *Neurology, 52*, 610–617.

Triebig, G., Claus, D., Csuzda, I., Druschky, K.-F., Holler, P., Kinzel, W., et al. (1988). Cross-sectional epidemiologic study on neurotoxicity of solvents in paints and lacquers. *International Archives of Occupational and Environmental Health, 60*, 233–241.

Wechsler, D. (1997). *Wechsler Adult Intelligence Scale Third Edition: Administration and scoring manual* (3rd ed.) San Antonio, TX: Psychological Corporation.

Wiggins, E. C., & Brandt, J. (1988). The detection of simulated amnesia. *Law and Human Behavior, 12*, 57–78.

World Health Organization. (1985). *Chronic effects of organic solvents on the central nervous system and diagnostic criteria. Environmental Health Services: Document 5.* Copenhagen, Denmark: Author.

10

Forensic Assessment of Medically Unexplained Symptoms

LAURENCE M. BINDER

Disorders of medically unexplained symptoms without clearly demonstrated pathophysiological origin are characterized more by disability, symptoms, and suffering than by objective medical findings and pathology (Labarge & McCaffrey, 2000). Illnesses including fibromyalgia (Bohr, 1996; Grace, Nielson, Hopkins, & Berg, 1999); chronic fatigue syndrome (CFS; Abbey & Garfinkel, 1991; Buchwald & Garrity, 1994; DeLuca, Johnson, Ellis, & Natelson, 1997; DiPino & Kane, 1996; Fukuda et al., 1994); multiple chemical sensitivities (MCS; Black, 2000; Bolla, 2000; Sparks, 2000); and toxic mold syndrome and sick building syndrome (Burge, 2001; Hardin, Kelman, & Saxon, 2003; M. Hodgson, 2000; Kuhn & Ghannoum, 2003; Reijula & Tuomi, 2003; Robbins, Swenson, Neally, Gots, & Kelman, 2000) usually are of unknown origin and have been referred to as functional somatic syndromes (Barsky & Borus, 1999). This review discusses neuropsychological assessment of medically unexplained symptoms. I do not attempt to provide comprehensive reviews of the above disorders. Instead I focus on certain largely medically unexplained disorders that either are commonly encountered in the practice of forensic clinical neuropsychology in adults or are particular exemplars of functional somatic syndromes. Portions of this chapter were based on previous work (Binder & Campbell, 2004). This chapter is organized in terms of the common assessment issues associated with these disorders.

Forensic neuropsychologists encounter these disorders in two ways. First, persons seeking disability from private insurers or from government entitlement programs often claim one or more of these conditions as an explanation of their inability to work. Second, these disorders are common and may be seen concurrent with other potentially compensable problems, such as alleged toxic encephalopathy (chapter 9, this volume) or traumatic brain injury (chapters 7 and 8, this volume).

ALTERNATIVE EXPLANATIONS FOR SYMPTOMS

Reports of headaches, memory loss, irritability, dizziness, and other physical, cognitive, and emotional complaints are nonspecific. These symptoms are not diagnostic of mild traumatic brain injury, toxic encephalopathy, or other forms of brain dysfunction (Fox, Lees-Haley, Earnest, & Dolezal-Wood, 1995). Negative emotions are more strongly predictive of subjective cognitive symptoms than are objective cognitive problems (Larrabee & Levin, 1986; Seidenberg, Haltiner, Taylor, Hermann, & Wyler 1994; Williams, Little, Scates, & Blockman, 1987). For example, we found that scores on a subjective scale of cognitive impairment were more strongly related to scores on the Beck Depression and Anxiety Inventories than to objective cognitive performance in veterans with illnesses related to the Persian Gulf War (Binder et al., 1999). Patients with fibromyalgia and CFS also have cognitive complaints more severe than their objective deficits (Grace et al., 1999; Tiersky, Johnson, Lange, Natelson, & DeLuca, 1997). In short, cognitive complaints are often an index of emotional distress—emotional distress communicated in a different language from the complaints typically associated with depression and anxiety.

Normal control subjects frequently complained of classic symptoms of traumatic brain injury (TBI) such as memory loss, irritability, headaches, and dizziness (Gouvier, Uddo-Crane, & Brown, 1988). Postconcussive syndrome (PCS) symptoms were at least partly attributable to stress and did not distinguish between those with TBI and control subjects (Gouvier, Cubic, Jones, Brantly, & Cutlip, 1992; Novack, Daniel, & Long, 1984). Among college student controls, many symptoms were as common among controls as among TBI patients (Gouvier et al., 1988). In the Gouvier et al. study, symptoms had the following normative frequencies: memory loss, 20%; loss of interest, 36%; temper problems, 37%; fatigue, 28%. The relatives of the same college student participants also observed high rates of "PCS-like symptoms" in the control group, an observation that suggests that reports of significant others may provide misleading information after suspected mild TBI (Gouvier et al., 1988).

Litigation is associated with neurological complaints despite the absence of any neurological history. Patients in litigation who claim psychological and physical damage and who did not have neuropsychological histories or claims reported the following symptoms on a questionnaire: concentration problems, 78%; confusion, 59%; memory loss, 53%; dizziness, 44%; and word-finding problems, 34% (Lees-Haley & Brown, 1993).

Pseudoneurological symptoms are complaints such as dizziness, memory loss, or weakness of a limb that are not correlated with any objective neurological findings. Pseudoneurological complaints are increased by stressors and can continue chronically (Cardena & Spiegel, 1993; Escobar, Canino, Rubio-Stipec, & Bravo, 1992). One week after the San Francisco earthquake of 1989, 30% of exposed persons complained of dizziness, and 71% complained of concentration difficulty (Cardena & Spiegel, 1993). One year after a flood, there were more pseudoneurological symptoms in persons exposed to the flood than in nonexposed persons (Escobar et al., 1992). Unspecified neurological symptoms were more common in firefighters with posttraumatic stress disorder (PTSD) than in those without this disorder (McFarlane, Atchison, Rafalowicz, & Papay, 1994).

There is evidence that symptoms simply are misattributed to certain events such as head trauma when the symptoms actually are explained by other events or are preexisting. Mittenberg and colleagues introduced the notion of "expectation as etiology" in connection with symptoms after mild TBI, showing that nonpatient controls were able to predict symptoms reported by patients (Mittenberg, DiGuilio, Perrin, & Bass, 1992) and later showing that simple reassurance and education significantly reduced symptoms (Mittenberg, Tremont, Zielinski, Fichera, & Rayls, 1996). Symptomatic patients after mild TBI reported fewer premorbid symptoms than did normal controls (Gunstad & Suhr, 2001; Mittenberg et al., 1992). The same observation was made of people in litigation (Lees-Haley, Williams, & English, 1996). These data suggest that some patients are poor historians and minimize the reports of premorbid problems.

The hypothesis that PCS complaints were unrelated to suspected mild TBI was indirectly tested by comparing patients with mild TBI and more severely head-injured patients on the Minnesota Multiphasic Personality Inventory (MMPI) and the number of PCS complaints (Novack et al., 1984). Patients with mild TBI were nearly twice as likely as the more severely injured to have elevations on the MMPI Hypochondriasis and Hysteria scales. The number of postconcussive symptoms was more strongly associated with elevations of these two MMPI scales than with neuropsychological data. Novack et al. suggested that the number of postconcussive symptoms was an index of emotional adjustment. Leininger, Kreutzer, and Hill (1991) also found an inverse relationship between acute severity of head injury and MMPI abnormality.

ALTERNATIVE EXPLANATIONS FOR COGNITIVE DEFICITS

Like cognitive complaints, cognitive deficits also are not specific to neurological disease or injury. Objective neuropsychological deficits are common in a host of psychiatric disorders. Cognitive deficits occur in affective disorders (reviewed in Burt, Zembar, & Niederehe, 1995; Cassens, Wolfe, & Zola, 1990; Goodwin & Jamison, 1990; Johnson & Magaro, 1987; McAllister, 1981). Patients with depression, particularly inpatients, may have difficulties with attention, abstract thinking, memory, manual dexterity, visuospatial skills (Burt et al., 1995; Cassens et al., 1990), and intellectual decline (Sackeim et al., 1992).

Patients with pseudoneurological symptoms perform poorly on neuropsychological tests. These findings are summarized in detail in a separate section.

GENERAL CHARACTERISTICS OF DISORDERS WITH MEDICALLY UNEXPLAINED SYMPTOMS

Barsky and Borus (1999) described many characteristics of these conditions. The amount of disability contrasts markedly with the degree of measured physical limitations and examination and laboratory abnormalities. Some patients with these conditions tend to view themselves as severely disabled (Hadler, 1999; Moss-Morris, Petrie, & Weinman, 1995; Wolfe et al., 1997), and they often apply for disability payments (Van der Werf, Prins, Jongen, van der Meer, & Bleijenberg, 2000; Wolfe et al., 1997). The degree of disability often is in contrast to the degree of disability reported by patients with demonstrable medical pathology, for example, patients with heart disease, amputations, cancer, or rheumatoid arthritis. According to Barsky and Borus, the fact that subjective distress so often exceeds objective medical findings suggests that symptom magnification is a primary feature of these disorders.

Ford (1997) described similar characteristics in what he labeled "fashionable illnesses." Fashionable illnesses are characterized by vague, subjective, multisystem complaints, a lack of objective laboratory findings, quasi-scientific explanations, overlap of one fashionable diagnosis with another, symptoms consistent with depression or anxiety or both, and denial of psychosocial distress or attribution of it to the illness. According to Ford, fashionable diagnoses represent a heterogeneous collection of physical diseases, somatization, and anxiety or depression.

Patients with medically unexplained symptoms obtain knowledge and beliefs about their conditions from a variety of sources. Often, these patients express skepticism with mainstream medicine (Staudenmayer, 2001). This rejection of mainstream medical thinking is unsurprising because many recognized experts believe that these conditions are of either disputed origin or surrogates for psychological disorders (Abbey & Garfinkel, 1991; Albers & Berent, 2000; Barsky & Borus, 1999; Black, 2000; Bohr, 1996; J. H. Ferguson, 1997; Gabriel et al., 1994; Hadler, 1997; Hennekens et al., 1996; Hyams, Wignall, & Roswell, 1996; Katon & Walker, 1993; Kroenke & Price, 1993; Sanchez-Guerrero, Schur, Sergent, & Liang, 1994; Simon, Katon, & Sparks, 1990; Staudenmayer, 2001;

Walker, Keegan, Gardner, Sullivan, Katon, et al., 1997; Youngjohn, Spector, & Mapou, 1997). As noted by Ford (1997), patients with these disorders reject psychological explanations for their symptoms, preferring biomedical and somatic explanations (Butler, Chalder, & Wessely, 2001; Nimnuan, Hotopf, & Wessely, 2001). Therefore, they seek out health care professionals who share their belief system and who are likely to recommend alternative medical treatment or explanations (Black, 1996; Nimnuan et al., 2001). The general tendency of physicians to provide medical explanations (Nimnuan, Hotopf, & Wessely, 2000) and the proliferation of alternative medicine explanations for symptoms help patients avoid treatment by physicians who interpret somatic symptoms as stress related in origin. Patients often have educated and diagnosed themselves through self-help groups, books and pamphlets, and the Internet (Wessely, 1997), and unexplained illnesses are more likely in adults whose parents suffered from serious illnesses (Hotopf, Mayou, Wadsworth, & Wessely, 1999).

Many of these disorders have overlapping symptoms, reducing the reliability and validity of their diagnoses (Deary, 1999; Wessely, Nimuan, & Sharpe, 1997), and they may not be distinct entities. The same patient could receive a diagnosis of fibromyalgia from a rheumatologist, a diagnosis of CFS from an internist, and a diagnosis of MCS from a clinician interested in that disorder (Buchwald & Garrity, 1994). The complaints of fatigue and joint pain are common to CFS, fibromyalgia, illness related to silicone breast implants, and illnesses related to the Persian Gulf War of 1991.

Not only do the symptoms of these illnesses overlap, but also many of the symptoms are common in healthy samples. Clearly, purportedly "neurological" symptoms such as headaches, fatigue, memory loss, and dizziness occur commonly in the general population (R. J. Ferguson, Mittenberg, Barone, & Schneider, 1999; Gouvier et al., 1988; Kroenke & Price, 1993; Sawchyn, Brulot, & Strauss, 2000). Healthy control participants reported the following frequencies of neurological symptoms: fatigue, 33%; headaches, 58%; forgetfulness, 58%; and poor concentration, 35% (Paniak et al., 2002). Pain also is commonly experienced. In one large survey, joint pains (37%), back pain (32%), headaches (25%), chest pain (25%), arm or leg pain (24%), and abdominal pain (24%) were reported by community dwellers (Kroenke & Price, 1993).

The oft-replicated finding that these symptoms are common in various control samples implies that people who view themselves as able-bodied usually do not find these symptoms to be disabling or pay undue attention to them. Although people with disorders that are medically unexplained may experience some of these symptoms to a more extreme degree than people who consider themselves healthy, clinical observation suggests that some of them also seem to view common symptoms as signs of a serious illness, and some believe their outcome will be bad (Sharpe, Chalder, Palmer, & Wessely, 1997).

Shorter (1992) provided a historical view of illnesses of mysterious origin. He maintained that historical eras and cultures shaped the symptoms of illnesses. The culture surrounding the individual considers some symptoms legitimate, that is, the product of organic disease, and other symptoms illegitimate. The individual is pressured to produce symptoms that are considered legitimate. Different symptoms are considered socially acceptable in different eras. As symptom legitimacy changes over time, people respond by producing different symptoms. Paralysis, for example, no longer is accepted in the mainstream North American culture. In recent years, pain and fatigue have been accepted by our culture. Shorter posited that CFS and fibromyalgia represent contemporary prototypes of culturally induced illnesses.

Shorter (1992) also argued that medical authority has declined, and the influence of the media on popular opinions regarding illness has increased. The media, always searching for new and sensational stories, promotes some illnesses. Rather than depending solely on medical authority for information, support groups also are viewed as sources of information. Shorter noted that advocacy groups were responsible for the name change from CFS to chronic immune dysfunction syndrome, despite the lack of evidence of immune dysfunction in this illness (Wessely, 1997).

According to Shorter (1992), the increasing degree of social isolation may play a role in culturally induced illnesses. He noted that people were less likely to receive consensual validation and feedback regarding the unimportance of common symptoms such as fatigue and headache. In the absence of sensible social input about normal symptoms, people may worry excessively about their significance. Medical care providers with scientifically unsupported explanations also are sources of beliefs about illnesses, and they may be iatrogenic causes of symptom production and maintenance (Black, 2000).

In contrast to many of these arguments, E. Ferguson and Cassaday (2001–2002) hypothesized that these conditions are caused by a complex interaction of biological, psychological, and environmental influences. They emphasized the role of the immune system and its responsiveness to psychological factors. Stressors can weaken the immune system. E. Ferguson and Cassaday suggested that some of these illnesses could be caused by what they called a "bio-associative" mechanism or what psychologists refer to as Pavlovian or classical conditioning. An illness initially caused by a pathogen could be associated with a trigger such as an odor. Later, the illness could be triggered by another odor. In this explanation, the unconditioned stimulus is the pathogen, and the conditioned stimulus is the odor. This theory has received empirical support in the case of MCS (Van den Bergh et al., 2001).

Illnesses with medically unexplained symptoms may be multiply determined (Ford, 1997). For example, a small percentage of veterans with Gulf War illnesses suffered from leishmaniasis, a parasitic disease. Another small group were affected by uranium radiation (McDiarmid et al., 2000). Some Gulf War veterans have diagnoses of CFS or fibromyalgia. There may be multiple etiologies for CFS, both pathophysiological and psychiatric (Afari & Buchwald, 2003).

PSEUDONEUROLOGICAL ILLNESS

Pseudoneurological symptoms are complaints such as dizziness, numbness, weakness, and memory loss that are not associated with objective evidence of neurological disease. Research in this area is useful in the understanding of all medically unexplained symptoms.

Many years ago, evidence of bona fide neurological disease sometimes could not be found using the existing diagnostic tools, potentially making diagnosis of pseudoneurological disease problematic. Slater's (1965) longitudinal study showed that many patients in his era diagnosed with hysteria ultimately were proven to have genuine neurological disease. After the advent of more advanced neurodiagnostic tools, there were unsuccessful efforts to replicate Slater's work. In one study, 56 patients with diagnoses of conversion disorder were followed an average of 4.5 years. Only 2 patients later developed an organic deficit that might have been related to the original episode of illness (Couprie, Wijdicks, Rooijmans, & van Gijn, 1995). Others have reported similar findings (Crimlisk et al., 1998; Kent, Tomasson, & Coryell, 1995; Mace & Trimble, 1996). In contrast to the primitive workups of Slater's era, these studies showed that the majority of patients diagnosed by neurological evaluation as suffering from pseudoneurological illness have not been misdiagnosed.

Despite the absence of neurological disease, patients with pseudoneurological complaints often have measurable neuropsychological deficits. In the first of these studies (Matthews, Shaw, & Klove, 1966), neurological and pseudoneurological patients were compared on the Halstead-Reitan Battery and the Wechsler Adult Intelligence Scale (WAIS). Statistical comparisons yielded significant differences on 17 of 26 variables. However, Matthews et al. stated:

> In spite of the relatively high levels of statistical significance obtained by many of the comparison variables, the use of any single one of them to classify individuals remains a doubtful procedure. Useful cutoff points for the comparison variables could not be established. (p. 250)

More recent neuropsychological investigations of pseudoneurological patients often have studied patients with nonepileptic seizures and consistently have documented poor performance. In these studies, patients were diagnosed with either epileptic or nonepileptic seizures after intensive electroencephalographic (EEG) video telemetry monitoring. Criteria for classification were described in detail in these studies.

The first of these studies (Wilkus, Dodrill, & Thompson, 1984) used a structured test battery with cutoff scores previously established in the same population. The test battery did not show any significant differences between the groups with epileptic and nonepileptic seizures. The epileptic group performed abnormally on an average of 46% of the tests, and the nonepileptic seizure patients produced abnormal scores on an average of 51% of the tests, a nonsignificant difference.

A similar study found no significant differences between patients with epileptic and nonepileptic seizures on 16 neuropsychological measures (Brown, Levin, Ramsay, Katz, & Duchowny, 1991). Based on a qualitative analysis of test data, Brown et al. concluded that the nonepileptic patients had inconsistent abnormalities characteristic of nonneurological conditions.

In another investigation, Binder, Kindermann, Heaton, and Salinsky (1998) compared control participants with epileptic and nonepileptic seizure patients. The two patient groups with seizures performed similarly and demonstrated significant impairment compared with the control group; for example, the nonepileptic seizure patients had a mean WAIS-R (Wechsler Adult Intelligence Scale–Revised) Full Scale IQ of 92.0, a mean score 9.9 points lower than the control group. The difference between the two groups on Trail Making Part B was 31.0 seconds. The mean for the nonepileptic seizure group on Logical Memory I of the Wechsler Memory Scale–Revised was at the 31st percentile, with no data available on this measure from the control group.

Nonepileptic seizure patients performed more poorly than epileptic seizure patients on the Portland Digit Recognition Test (PDRT), a measure of motivation to remember (Binder, Salinksy & Smith, 1994) but they generally did not perform in the range typically associated with malingering on this measure. The PDRT findings in the nonepileptic group (Binder et al., 1994) were consistent with earlier qualitative observations judged by the authors to imply inconsistent effort (Brown et al., 1991). In a mixed group of pseudoneurological cases, 54% were misclassified as brain damaged based on the Generalized Neuropsychological Deficit Scale of the Halstead-Reitan Battery, 34% were misclassified based on the Halstead Impairment Index, and 22% were misclassified using the Average Impairment Rating (Sherer & Adams, 1993).

In addition to measurable neuropsychological impairment, there is significant disability associated with pseudoneurological conditions. Many nonepileptic seizure patients never work again (Barry et al., 1998). The cause of nonepileptic seizures usually is psychiatric. Hence, the cause of disability associated with nonepileptic seizures also is psychiatric.

Investigators have studied the relationships among mild head injury, seizure type, and the opportunity for financial compensation. Epileptic seizures were not commonly found after mild head injury in an epidemiological study, and they were more common after moderate and especially severe head injury (Annegers, Hauser, Coan, & Rocca, 1998). The prevailing opinion is that traumatic seizures of epileptic origin can be caused by cortical contusions. These contusions can be consistent with a head injury defined as mild solely by Glasgow Coma Scale criteria, however, a head injury with a Glasgow score of 13–15 and a contusion is often classified as a complicated mild head injury. If there is no evidence of contusions from acute neuroimaging and if the head injury was trivial with little or no loss of consciousness and little or no posttraumatic amnesia, postinjury seizures usually will be of nonepileptic origin. Nonepileptic seizures, in contrast with epileptic seizures, commonly follow mild head injuries that offer the opportunity for financial compensation (Westbrook, Devinsky, & Geocadin, 1998).

Diagnosis of seizures is within the domain of neurology, particularly the subspecialty of epileptology. Intensive EEG monitoring remains the gold standard method of diagnosis of seizure type. Neuropsychological assessment can aid in the evaluation of postinjury seizures by identifying which patients fit the psychological profile of nonepileptic seizure patients or are likely to be diagnosed as nonepileptic with appropriate diagnostic tools. Persons with neuropsychological correlates of nonepileptic seizures are candidates for intensive EEG monitoring where definitive diagnoses are made.

The MMPI-2 is the best single predictor for the purpose of identifying patients who fit the psychological profile of nonepileptic seizures. According to a review of studies (Dodrill, Wilkus, & Batzel, 1993), in settings with high base rates of nonepileptic seizures, the MMPI-2 is about 70% accurate in predicting the differential of epileptic or nonepileptic seizures as diagnosed by neurology through intensive EEG monitoring. Conversion V profiles and scores on HS or HY above 79 are associated with nonepileptic seizures. Epileptic seizure groups score about 10 points lower on HS and HY than nonepileptic groups (Dodrill et al., 1993). In adult settings, seizure onset generally is more recent in nonepileptic than epileptic seizures. Chronicity of seizures and routine EEGs were combined with the MMPI-2 to yield 86% accuracy in predicting seizure diagnosis with approximately equal accuracy for both types of seizures (Storzbach, Binder, Salinsky, Campbell, & Mueller, 2000).

FIBROMYALGIA

Fibromyalgia is characterized by widespread joint pain, insomnia (Bohr, 1996), and nonrestorative sleep. The diagnosis of fibromyalgia is based on the trigger point exam. In response to 4 kg of finger pressure applied by the examiner, the patient must report pain in at least 11 of 18 trigger points, and the sites with pain must be located both above and below the waist. These criteria have proved problematic (Bohr, 1996; Hadler, 1997) for two reasons. First, it is difficult for a clinician to consistently apply 4 kg of pressure; second, it is not likely that patients will reliably report the experience of pain, an inherently subjective event. Consequently, the illness can be viewed as entirely subjective (Hadler, 1997).

The etiology of fibromyalgia is unknown. It is believed by some investigators that there are neuroendocrine abnormalities associated with fibromyalgia, and that the illness is caused by abnormal sensory processing (Bennett, 1999). However, emotional problems also are associated with neuroendocrine disorders (Barlow, 2000), and it is not clear that there are neuroendocrine abnormalities in fibromyalgia specific to that condition. Some investigators have reported reduced cerebral blood flow in the subcortical and brain stem regions in patients with fibromyalgia (Kwiatet et al., 2000), but similar findings are nonspecific and occur in psychiatric patients (Hakala et al., 2002; Lange, Wang, DeLuca, & Natelson, 1998). Posterior fossa decompression has been used as neurosurgical treatment of fibromyalgia based solely on the rationale of overlapping symptoms with Chiari Type I malformation, but this practice is controversial (Nash, Cheng, Meyer, & Remler, 2002).

There are some well-established facts regarding fibromyalgia. It is far more frequent in females than in males (Wolfe et al., 1995). Persons with fibromyalgia frequently seek disability (Wolfe, Ross, Anderson, Russell, & Hebert, 1997). The condition sometimes is associated with mild neuropsychological deficits (Hart, Martelli, & Zasler, 2000). The fibromyalgia group performed within the normal range on all cognitive measures, although there were some differences between fibromyalgia patients and controls (Grace et al., 1999). Subjective memory complaints were disproportionate to the objective cognitive deficits (Grace et al., 1999). Other investigators found that more than a third of the fibromyalgia patients who either were seeking disability payments or who already were receiving them scored below the cutoffs on measures of motivation to remember (Gervais et al., 2001).

Fibromyalgia patients are more likely than control subjects to have a history of psychiatric problems, including mood and anxiety disorders and more medically unexplained physical symptoms across several organ systems (Walker, Keegan, Gardner, Sullivan, Katon, et al., 1997). Fibromyalgia patients had more evidence of abuse and trauma in both childhood and adulthood, compared with patients with rheumatoid arthritis (Walker, Keegan, Gardner, Sullivan, Bernstein, et al., 1997).

CHRONIC FATIGUE SYNDROME

Diagnostic criteria for CFS in the United States include chronic disabling fatigue and at least four of eight other features, including muscle ache, joint pain, subjective cognitive problems, sore throat, new headache, nonrestorative sleep, postexertion malaise, and swollen lymph glands (Fukuda et al., 1994). These symptoms are similar to those associated with fibromyalgia. Although some symptoms of chronic fatigue are similar to the symptoms of depression, the emotional aspects of depression, such as sadness, anhedonia, and low self-esteem, often seem absent in CFS (Jason et al., 1997). Afari and Buchwald (2003) reviewed CFS. Like fibromyalgia and MCS, it is more prevalent in females than males (Jason et al., 1999).

Neuropsychological impairment has been reported for patients diagnosed with CFS (DiPino & Kane, 1996; Tiersky, Johnson, Lange, Natelson, & Deluca, 1997). A review concluded that intellect and complex problem-solving abilities were preserved, but that CFS patients suffered from a deficit in complex information processing (Tiersky et al., 1997). Clearly, subjective ratings of cognitive impairment are more pronounced than objective neuropsychological findings (Tiersky et al., 1997). There is mixed evidence of motivational problems on neuropsychological testing in patients with CFS. A deficit was found on a forced-choice measure of motivation to remember in a clinical sample (Van der Werf et al., 2000), but not on a similar measure in a research sample who did not consider themselves disabled (Binder et al., 2001).

Chronic fatigue syndrome often is associated with a history of anxiety and affective disorders (Katon, Buchwald, Simon, Russo, & Mease, 1991), but cognitive deficits were found in another study despite the elimination of patients from the sample who reported a history of psychiatric illness (DeLuca et al., 1997). People with CFS were more likely to demonstrate objective cognitive deficits after exercise than controls (LaManca et al., 1998).

Several investigators have studied regional cerebral blood flow in CFS, typically with single photon emitted computerized tomography (SPECT). Early studies suggested that the illness was associated in reductions in cerebral blood flow (Ichise et al., 1992; Schwartz et al., 1994). Subsequent studies parallel results previously reviewed for fibromyalgia: Either there are no abnormalities in CFS (Fischler et al., 1996; Lewis et al., 2001), or the abnormalities are nonspecific and similar to those found in psychiatric groups (Lange et al., 1998). A fluorine-deoxyglucose positron emission tomography (PET) study suggested that hypometabolism in the brain stem was found only in CFS and not in depression (Tirelli et al., 1998), but a study using the same technique found no differences between a group with CFS and a group with somatization disorder (Hakala et al., 2002).

The unclear etiology of CFS has been reviewed (Afari & Buchwald, 2003; Tiersky et al., 1997). Various hypotheses have been advanced, including viral, limbic system, and immune system explanations, all lacking basic scientific support. There is no evidence of a specific viral etiological agent. In some quarters, CFS is viewed as the equivalent of a psychiatric condition. According to this view, patients with CFS are engaging in illness behavior and have normal complaints (Barsky & Borus, 1999).

Wessely and colleagues (Sharpe et al., 1997) have adopted a complex view of the etiology of CFS, emphasizing the distinction among factors that may have predisposed patients to develop the illness, such as lifestyle, work stress, and personality; factors that may have triggered the illness, such as viral infection or life events; and factors that may have perpetuated the illness, such as cerebral dysfunction, sleep disorder, depression, inconsistent activity, and misunderstanding of the illness and fear of making it worse. In a related hypothesis, the illness could be caused by psychological stress or by a quiescent viral infection reactivated by stress (Glaser & Kiecolt-Glaser, 1998).

It also is hypothesized that the low levels of natural killer cells in the immune system explain the illness (Whiteside & Friberg, 1998), although the relationship between low-level immune system activation and CFS symptoms is unclear (Afari & Buchwald, 2003; Wessely, 1997). More controversial is the posterior fossa decompression surgery that also has been performed on fibromyalgia patients (Nash et al., 2002). Others have observed that CFS may be heterogeneous with several infectious and other types of etiologies (Afari & Buchwald, 2003).

MULTIPLE CHEMICAL SENSITIVITIES

The term *multiple chemical sensitivities* (MCS) has been discarded by some authorities (Sparks, 2000) for several reasons, including the fact that there is no conclusive pathophysiological evidence that people with the diagnosis are abnormally sensitive to specific chemicals (Dalton & Hummel, 2000) because the relationship between symptoms and exposures is unproven (but see Dalton, 1999) and because MCS is not a clinically defined disease with generally accepted underlying pathophysiological mechanisms or validated criteria for diagnosis.

As discussed by Sparks (2000), the term *idiopathic environmental intolerance* has been proposed as a replacement. Although MCS is the term commonly employed by many clinicians, the condition has other labels, including chemical intolerance, environmental illness, and total allergy syndrome.

MCS was reviewed comprehensively in an edited volume (Sparks, 2000), and Labarge and McCaffrey (2000) and Staudenmeyer (2001) have provided reviews from neuropsychological and psychological perspectives. The illness is characterized by symptoms in multiple organ systems in reaction to a variety of low levels of chemically unrelated common odors at doses that do not cause symptoms in the general population. The substances causing discomfort in people with MCS are irritants rather than neurointoxicants (Bolla, 2000). The MCS may follow the perception of exposure to harmful chemical substances, as opposed to actual exposure to toxic levels of harmful chemicals, such as occurred in the Persian Gulf War (Reid et al., 2001).

Symptoms of MCS often include fatigue, confusion, dizziness, gastrointestinal, musculoskeletal, and respiratory problems. These symptoms may last for
days or weeks. Patients with MCS believe they are sensitive to certain odors,
and they attempt to avoid common odors such as perfume, gasoline, and other
petroleum products, new carpets, and ordinary household cleansers. Some people with MCS go as far as attempting to avoid close contact with recently
printed matter because of perceived sensitivity to ink. Food allergies are common in this population. The avoidance of so many common substances leads to
disability in many cases. Many patients with MCS also are diagnosed with CFS
and fibromyalgia (Bell, Baldwin, & Schwartz, 1998; Buchwald & Garrity, 1994;
Sparks, 2000) because the symptoms overlap among these disorders.

This clinical entity is controversial, indeed. The clinical ecological approach
views the illness as organic and caused by chemical exposure and recommends
costly lifestyle changes and other interventions. Mainstream medicine has been
particularly critical of the clinical ecological approach (American Academy of
Allergy and Immunology, 1986; American College of Physicians, 1989). Laboratory provocation in patients diagnosed with MCS with the chemicals identified
as incitants yielded extremely low sensitivity and specificity values, data strongly
suggesting that the diagnosis of MCS has no validity (Staudenmayer, Selner, &
Buhr, 1993). Consistent with these results, objective medical findings usually
do not exist (Labarge & McCaffery, 2000). Experimental data provided no evidence that people with MCS are any more sensitive to odors than control subjects (Dalton & Hummel, 2000; Doty, Deems, Frye, Pelberg, & Shapiro, 1988).

A model of MCS involving neurohormonal sensitization of olfactory–limbic
circuits has been proposed (Bell et al., 1998). According to this model, some
individuals can be sensitized by low doses of chemicals that may not have been
troublesome to them in the past. In this model, amplification of responses is
hypothesized to occur in the limbic system, including the mesolimbic dopaminergic (reward) pathway. Subsequent activation of sensitized pathways is purported to lead to impaired function of behavioral, immune, and other systems.
Bell and colleagues have further proposed that the association between early
sexual abuse and MCS exists because sexual abuse sensitizes the limbic system
pathways (Bell, Baldwin, Fernandez, & Schwartz, 1999).

The possible relationship of MCS and classical conditioning has been investigated (Van den Bergh et al., 2001). These authors showed that limited pairings
of a conditioned stimulus of a noxious odor and an unconditioned stimulus of
air rich in carbon dioxide led to the conditioning of both somatic symptoms and
altered respiratory responses in humans in reaction to just the conditioned stimulus of the odor. Importantly, conscious awareness of the relationship between
the odor and the symptoms induced by carbon dioxide was not necessary for
the effects to occur. Symptomatic reactions generalized not only to new, noxious
odors but also to situations in which participants imagined situations in which

the symptoms had occurred. There were individual differences in the effect in that participants who had higher scores on a measure of negative affectivity (neuroticism) or who suffered from nonorganic illnesses had more learned symptoms and more easily generalized the illness response to new odors. Extinction was demonstrated with sufficient exposure to just the conditioned stimulus.

Experimental work on the interaction of health expectancy and the pleasantness of odors also shows a psychological influence on symptomatology (Dalton, 1999). Participants exposed to a solventlike, alcohol scent (butanol), a wintergreen scent, and a balsam scent reported more symptoms when they were warned of solvent exposure than when they were told they would be exposed to a natural extract with a relaxing effect. The odors and self-reported chemical intolerance also had significant effects on symptoms. There are a variety of cognitive influences related to sensory and somatic responses to chemical stimulation (Dalton & Hummel, 2000).

The few available neuropsychological studies of MCS showed little or no evidence of neurocognitive impairment in controlled investigations (Bolla, 2000; Labarge & McCaffrey, 2000). Bolla emphasized the lack of specificity of neuropsychological testing in persons with symptoms of MCS because of the lack of a biological marker of MCS and the absence of evidence of neurocognitive problems among people with MCS symptoms, including cognitive tests thought to be especially sensitive to limbic system dysfunction (Brown-DeGagne & McGlone, 1999). As is true in fibromyalgia and CFS, MCS often is associated with various psychiatric illnesses (Black, 2000; Staudenmayer, 2001).

TOXIC MOLD AND SICK BUILDING SYNDROME

A guideline of the American College of Occupational and Environmental Medicine (Hardin et al., 2003) summarized the state of knowledge regarding toxic mold and human health. Some fungi produce beneficial metabolites known as mycotoxins that can be converted into antibiotics such as penicillin and cyclosporine. *Mold* is the commonplace term for multicellular fungi that grow in a mat. The growth of molds in indoor environments has been cited as the explanation for a variety of nonspecific symptoms. Exposure to fungi and molds is unavoidable unless draconian isolation measures are utilized. Fungi are ubiquitous in all environments and are essential for the decomposition of organic material. Many species of fungi live on the surface of the human body.

Fungi can harm human health through allergy, infection, and toxicity. Allergic responses occur in roughly 5% of the population and usually are experienced as allergic asthma or rhinitis, the latter commonly known as hay fever. Uncommon allergy syndromes include allergic bronchopulmonary aspergillosis and allergic fungal sinusitis. Ingestion of foods with sufficient quantity of certain molds can cause illnesses known as mycotoxicoses. Superficial fungal infections such as *Tinea pedia*, commonly known as athlete's foot, and *Tinea cruris*, commonly known as jock itch, are common in humans.

Of much greater concern are infections in persons who are immunocompromised, including patients on immunosuppressant medications and persons with AIDS and severe diabetes. Previously healthy persons are subject to rare, serious fungal infections caused by fungi including *Cryptococcus* and *Histoplasma* or to hypersensitivity pneumonitis, an exaggerated immune system response after inhalation of large quantities of protein such as fungal proteins. "Organic dust toxic syndrome" has been described after inhalation exposure of agricultural workers to spoiled grain products. These illnesses are associated with thick clouds of dust and not with musty odor from wood with dry rot.

Mycotoxins are not significantly volatile; they do not off-gas into the environment or pass through solid substances such as walls. The musty odor associated with mold is not caused by mycotoxins.

Sick building syndrome is a poorly defined set of symptoms attributed to occupancy of an allegedly contaminated building. Usually, no specific cause is found for the complaints. In some cases, a mycotoxin-producing mold, *Stachybotrys chartarum*, is identified in the building, but generally there is no scientific evidence of a causal relationship between indoor air exposure to *Stachybotrys chartarum* and human illnesses. Hardin et al. (2003) concluded that fungi rarely are significant human pathogens, except through ingestion of contaminated foods, and that current scientific evidence does not support the proposition that human health has been adversely affected by inhaled mycotoxins. Similar views have been expressed by others (Burge, 2001; Kuhn & Ghannoum, 2003; Robbins et al., 2000).

M. Hodgson (2000) suggested that sick building syndrome could be caused by problems associated with humidification and ventilation systems. He also noted that individuals varied in their susceptibility to the two most common building-related problems: mucosal problems in either the nasal passages or eyes. In the only neuropsychological study related to sick building or toxic mold syndrome of which I am aware, there were no difference between exposed persons and controls (M. F. Hodgson et al., 1998). At the present time, there is no credible scientific evidence that toxic mold, buildings, or *Stachybotrys* cause encephalopathy.

A theory of the etiology of medically unexplained conditions such as building-related illnesses, MCS, CFS, and fibromyalgia has been proposed (E. Ferguson & Cassaday, 2001–2002). These medically unexplained symptoms can be explained more parsimoniously as a single symptom cluster than as a set of separate illnesses such as Persian Gulf War illnesses or CFS. The reason these syndromes are persistent is that a "bioassociative mechanism" is established initially through a biological basis (proinflamatory cytokines) as a result of physiological challenges that produce a nonspecific sickness response then associated through the mechanism of classical conditioning with sensory factors such as unpleasant smells like diesel fuel. Cytokine-induced immune system activation temporarily produces memory impairment (Reichenberg et al., 2001).

PSYCHOLOGICAL STRESS AND DISEASE

Human and infrahuman studies indicated that stressors can cause pathological changes in functioning in the immune and endocrine systems and disease (McEwen, 2002). Individuals differ in their biological susceptibility to stressors, possibly because of psychological traits (Kirschbaum et al., 1995). Animal models have shown that early stressors cause chronic alterations in hypothalamic-pituitary-adrenal axis function, chronically negative emotions, and easily elicited alarm reactions in juvenile monkeys, changes that persist into adulthood (Barlow, 2000). In veterans of World War II, the stress of combat experience was associated with an increased risk of physical decline and death (Elder, Shanahan, & Clipp, 1997).

In humans, depression is associated with large changes in immune system functioning, for example, lower natural killer cell activity and change in white blood cell counts (Herbert & Cohen, 1993). Suppression of immune system function persists in persons with past history of PTSD but with no current psychiatric disorder (Kawamura, Kim, & Asukai, 2001). PTSD among Vietnam veterans was associated with self-reported diagnoses of circulatory, digestive, musculoskeletal, nervous system, respiratory, and infectious diseases. In the same study, PTSD was not related to self-reported medical diagnoses of sexually transmitted diseases, cancers, genitourinary, or skin diseases (Boscarino, 1997).

A neuroanatomical model of panic (Gorman, Kent, Sullivan, & Coplan, 2000) was based on animal studies of conditioned fear because of the behavioral and physiological similarities between panic and conditioned fear. Gorman et al. described a fear network with the amygdala interacting with the hippocampus and prefrontal cortex. The amygdala receives the sensation of a conditioned stimulus and coordinates autonomic, sympathetic, and behavioral responses to the conditioned stimulus. Projections from the amygdala to the periaquadactal gray causes postural freezing. The fear network could be inappropriately activated if bodily cues were processed defectively. As noted, early stressors also cause changes in neuroendocrine functioning in the hypothalamic-pituitary-adrenal axis.

Davidson (2000) reviewed further relationships among emotions, psychopathology, and neurophysiology. People have baseline electrophysiological differences that are stable and that predict individual differences in reactivity to emotionally eliciting events. Davidson characterized these differences as forming a neurophysiological vulnerability to the elicitation of both positive and negative emotions. The intensity of negative affect is related to these neurophysiological differences as well as to the immune system functioning and activity of the autonomic nervous system. In infrahuman subjects, early environmental manipulations led to differences in reactivity and brain circuitry (Barlow, 2000; Davidson, 2000).

Severe stressors and PTSD are associated with cognitive abnormalities and structural brain changes in humans. Excess levels of glucocorticoids secreted during stress may contribute to neuronal death and atrophy in the hippocampus in PTSD and major depression (Lee, Ogle, & Sapolsky, 2002; Sapolsky, 2000). Learning and memory were impaired in rape victims with PTSD (Jenkins, Langlais, Delis, & Cohen, 1998). In part, cognitive deficits associated with combat PTSD were associated with premorbid intellect, but controlling for intellect did not eliminate the differences in cognitive functioning between veterans with PTSD and appropriate controls (Vasterling, Brailey, Constans, Borges, & Sutker, 1997). Memory and attention deficits have been associated with diagnoses of PTSD (Bremner et al., 1993; Vasterling, Brailey, Constans, & Sutker, 1998). Hippocampal size was associated with diagnoses of PTSD and depression (Bremner et al., 1995). Neuroimaging findings associated with PTSD have been reviewed (Grossman, Buchsman, & Yehuda, 2002).

Exposure to trauma is associated with the development of medically unexplained physical symptoms, PTSD, depression, and substance abuse (Beckham et al., 1998; Schnurr & Spiro, 1999; Stein, Walker, Hazen, & Forde, 1997). As noted, trauma exposure in those who survive natural disasters is associated with pseudoneurological symptoms (Cardena & Spiegel, 1993; Escobar et al., 1992). Somatization symptoms are associated with both PTSD (Andreski, Chilcoat, & Breslau, 1998) and panic disorder (Katon et al., 1991). Somatization also is associated with a history of childhood sexual abuse (Morrison, 1989). Physical and sexual abuse and other types of trauma also are associated with nonepileptic seizures (Alper, Devinsky, Perrine, Vazquez, & Luciano, 1993; Rosenberg, Rosenberg, Williamson, & Wolford, 2000) and diagnoses of fibromyalgia (Walker, Keegan, Gardner, Sullivan, Bernstein, et al., 1997). A persistent lack of cortisol in traumatized or chronically stressed individuals may increase the risk for medically unexplained symptoms (Heim, Ehlert, & Hellhammer, 2000).

THREATS TO THE ACCURACY OF THE HISTORY
PROVIDED BY THE EXAMINEE

Neuropsychological assessment requires differential diagnosis (Binder, 1997). The patient may be symptomatic because of depression or other psychiatric problems, pseudoneurological problems, developmental learning disabilities, medical illness unrelated to the injury, malingering (chapter 4, this volume), or chronic pain disorder. It is erroneous to attribute symptoms automatically to a TBI (chapters 7 and 8, this volume), alleged neurotoxic exposure (chapter 9, this volume), or other events without performing a differential diagnosis. To make an accurate differential diagnosis, it is essential to obtain accurate historical information. The purpose of this section is to discuss the barriers to obtaining an accurate history and some other confounds in the interpretation of assessment results as well as the possible impact on health of some forms of inaccurate self-disclosure.

Accuracy of Self-Disclosure and Impact on Health

In this section, literature is reviewed to show that the level of accuracy of people who are providing their medical and psychiatric histories or in reporting current psychological distress is less than may generally be assumed by health care professionals. People often are inaccurate in reporting easily defined medical events (Harlow & Linet, 1989). For example, acute medical illnesses and the use of sick leave were not accurately reported a relatively short time later (Rogler, Malgady, & Tryon, 1992). Recall of acute illnesses occurred in only 42% of cases only a month later, and recall of medical events was 70% accurate after 1 month, but only 26% accurate 9–12 months later (Rogler et al., 1992).

People also often are inaccurate reporters of events of potential psychological significance, and these events often are underreported. For example, a longitudinal study found that participants at age 18 years often had recollections discrepant from more contemporaneous data, including reports by their mothers, of family conflict at various ages, earlier self-reports of hyperactivity, and earlier self-reports of depression (Henry, Moffit, Caspi, Langley, & Silva, 1994). A 30-year follow-up of former child guidance clinic patients, using methodology similar to that of Henry et al., examined interview agreement with events previously recorded (Robins et al., 1985). Agreement ranged from low to high, depending on the event. For example, after 30 years, 91% correctly recalled not always living with their parents, but only 47% were cognizant of their family receiving welfare assistance, and only 56% remembered living with relatives.

Traumatic events sometimes are underreported or otherwise distorted. Adults who were sexually abused or otherwise traumatized during childhood or early in adulthood, according to records contemporaneous with the reported abuse, often failed to report this history when directly asked many years later (Widom & Morris, 1997). A longitudinal study of Persian Gulf War veterans found that participants were, in general, more likely to report specific traumatic events 2 years after their return from the Persian Gulf than 1 month after their return (Southwick, Morgan, Nicolaou, & Charney, 1997). These authors felt that exaggeration was the most likely reason for the increase in self-reported exposure to traumatic events, and that this increase over time was associated with psychological distress. A competing hypothesis not ruled out by the authors was that the initial reports minimized meaningful events that later, after reflection, were more fully recalled.

Although Southwick et al. (1997) reported that combat veterans increased their reported exposure to wartime stressors as their psychological distress increased, it generally is true that mental health history is minimized rather than exaggerated (Simon & VonKorff, 1995). In one study, depression was studied by structured interview, and a year later in follow-up the subjects completed a self-report instrument measuring depression (Coyne, Thompson, & Racioppo, 2001). There was no significant overlap between the initial structured interview and self-report after a year, a finding the authors found "disheartening" (Coyne et al., 2001, p. 167). Premorbid somatic and mental symptoms often associated with PCS also were minimized in a longitudinal study of athletes, some of whom sustained concussions while participating in intercollegiate athletics (R. J. Ferguson et al., 1999). R. J. Ferguson et al., who characterized this observation as the "good old days" phenomenon, replicated some of the findings of other researchers (Hilsabeck, Gouvier, & Bolter, 1998; Mittenberg et al., 1992).

Not only is past mental health and medical history incorrectly reported, on the average, in a minimizing direction, but also current mental health problems sometimes are denied. In one investigation, volunteer participants completed self-report ratings of psychiatric symptoms and were rated by an expert on mental health through use of the Early Memory Test (Shedler, Mayman, & Manis, 1993). This test was blindly scored by the expert based on qualitative factors such as self-representation, affective tone, coherence of narrative, and presence of internal contradictions. Some participants were classified as reporting *illusory mental health* because they were abnormal on the Early Memory Test and normal on self-report (Shedler et al., 1993).

Cognitive-behavioral theorists have provided partial explanation for the phenomenon of illusory mental health. Anxiety is conceptualized as comprising three loosely coupled response systems of overt behavior, verbal report, and physiological activation (Lang & Cuthbert, 1984). People often experience stressors physiologically or respond behaviorally without reporting or experiencing a cognitive component of the anxiety; they feel anxious, but are unable to verbalize what is making them anxious (Barlow, 2000).

Lying and Exaggeration

The preceding section discussed inaccurate reporting of mental health and medical history without respect to the intentionality of the inaccurate reporting. This section considers lying, the intentional distortion of information, and exaggeration of history. Mental health experts generally are not permitted to testify in court regarding the credibility of people they have examined, an issue that is determined only by the trier of fact. Despite this evidentiary restriction, experts may choose how much weight to give to reports by examinees regarding preinjury and postinjury history, including educational and occupational attainments, medical history, symptoms, and limitations. An expert should give less weight to improbable statements by an examinee, and statements that cannot be verified are less probable if they are given by a person who is known to have been inaccurate or deceptive about other aspects of personal history. Therefore, attention should be paid to inconsistencies and misstatements, some of which could be lies.

Some people, usually males, exaggerate athletic or military exploits. Some well-publicized incidents of resumé padding by public figures provide examples. An Oregon congressman, Wes Cooley, lost his seat in the 1990s after it was discovered that his claim of military service in the Korean War was false. Cooley also made false claims about motorcycle racing success. A manager of the Toronto Blue Jays baseball team was fired after falsely claiming combat experience in Vietnam, and a University of Notre Dame football head coach was terminated when it was discovered that he exaggerated his football playing experience and education.

Patients also occasionally exaggerate past experiences. A woman undergoing intensive EEG monitoring for diagnosis of medically intractable seizures reported onset of the seizures while serving in an intelligence unit in Vietnam when her jeep struck a land mine, overturning her jeep and causing a cerebral concussion. She was applying for veterans' benefits for an alleged disability. Her service record indicated that she had not served in Vietnam, and the EEG monitoring led to a diagnosis of nonepileptic seizures.

A book has been written about exaggeration of Vietnam War combat exploits (Burkett & Whitley, 1998). One examinee made grandiose claims about his baseball playing prowess despite an obvious physical deformity to his throwing arm that he reported occurred in an accident during adolescence. Another examinee with cerebral palsy reported that he had been a high school football star.

Level of education is related to premorbid and postinjury neuropsychological performance. Whenever possible, self-reported educational attainment should be checked in forensic cases. If transcripts are not available, they should be requested. If one cannot obtain a transcript, most colleges (Johnson-Greene & Binder, 1995) and some high schools will verify by telephone attendance and attainment of degrees and diplomas. One nonforensic patient reported that he had received a degree from the Illinois Institute of Technology. A phone call to this college revealed no record of his attendance. When gently confronted about why he would have made a false report, he replied, "Because it's a good school." The same patient with cerebral palsy who reported that he was a football star also claimed that he had graduated from college. The university in question had no record of his attendance. Grades obtained in high school are exaggerated in forensic cases after mild head trauma (Greiffenstein, Baker, &

Johnson-Greene, 2002). Although determining if this exaggeration is deliberate usually is difficult, the Greiffenstein et al. data underscore the need to review school records rather than rely on self-report.

Medical history sometimes is underreported to such an extreme that it must be questioned if the underreporting is deliberate. A woman with chronic pain had not received any treatment for an alleged injury at work until 20 days had elapsed, when she made a single emergency department visit and then received no additional treatment for another 5 months. Her work-related disability began 7 months after her alleged injury. Her degree of disability was disproportionate to the degree of injury and the medical findings. She failed to provide details to multiple examiners about two separate, similar, financially compensable injuries within the past 10 years.

Psychotherapy notes of treatment prior to a mild head injury, when they are available, sometimes reveal many more sessions of treatment and much more serious psychopathology than reported by the examinee. Such distortions may be deliberate attempts to maximize the financial recovery from litigation, but they also could result from a general tendency to distort past episodes of emotional problems (Coyne et al., 2001).

IMPACT OF DISTORTION OF MEDICAL HISTORY

Data suggest that people who deny psychological problems, that is, people whose psychological defenses do not allow them to recognize their problems, are at risk for medical illnesses because their defenses are associated with increased autonomic reactivity. Shedler et al. (1993) found that participants classified in the illusory mental health group showed greater coronary maximal and mean reactivity than participants in either the subjectively distressed or genuinely healthy groups. Furthermore, in the group with illusory mental health, the lower the self-rating of psychological problems, the greater the coronary reactivity.

There is limited experimental evidence that people with medically unexplained disorders also can be classified as experiencing illusory mental health. In one study, fibromyalgia patients were experimentally presented with emotionally provocative images. These patients reacted more physiologically while acknowledging less affective change than control subjects (Brosschot & Aarsse, 2001). In this study, the fibromyalgia patients were both highly anxious and highly defensive and tended to attribute their physiological responses to somatic rather than psychological causes.

In a series of studies, Pennebaker and colleagues showed that inhibition of thoughts and emotions was associated with increased autonomic nervous system activity in the short term and that inhibition of emotions in the long term served as a cumulative stressor that increased the probability of psychosomatic disease.

Their data also indicated that not discussing an emotional trauma was a harmful form of inhibition. Adults who reported in a questionnaire that they had been subjected to childhood trauma or who suffered recent trauma were more likely to have suffered health problems within the past year (Pennebaker & Susman, 1988). Another survey examined the health effects of a recent, sudden death of a spouse. The more respondents talked about the death of a spouse, the fewer health problems they suffered in the following year. However, the more they simply ruminated about the death without talking about it, the more health problems they suffered (Pennebaker & Susman, 1988). Undergraduates who had the opportunity to write about past emotional trauma experienced a significant drop in visits to the student health center, even when compared with students who wrote about the facts of the trauma without writing about the associated emotions (Smyth, 1998).

In a similar study of the effect of trauma writing, sexual offenders incarcerated for treatment decreased health care visits after a trauma writing exercise (Richards, Beal, Seagal, & Pennebaker, 2000). Writing about emotions led to a beneficial effect in short-term measures of immune system functioning, including circulating total lymphocytes and CD4 (helper) T-lymphocyte levels. Thought suppression was harmful for short-term immune system functioning as measured by CD3 T-lymphocyte levels (Petrie, Booth, & Pennebaker, 1998). Difficulty expressing feelings was associated with increased somatic complaints (Kirmayer & Robbins, 1993).

Studies summarized in the preceding sections demonstrated that people tend to underreport past events, including stressors, episodes of medical and mental problems, and treatment for those problems. Traumatic events, whether encountered during childhood or during adulthood, can cause serious medical and mental health problems directly. These events also can mediate effects that lead to social disruptions and somatic or psychological problems. The medical and mental effects of trauma can be reduced through disclosure and emotional processing. However, disclosure and emotional processing frequently do not occur. In the next section, the implications of these findings for the assessment of medically unexplained disorders are discussed.

ASSESSMENT OF MEDICALLY UNEXPLAINED SYMPTOMS

Conversion disorder in the form of nonepileptic seizures is an excellent model of a pseudoneurological condition often associated with inaccurate self-report of psychiatric symptoms and history. Intensive EEG monitoring and neuroimaging data rule out or make unlikely a diagnosis of epilepsy or other neurological explanations for the seizures. Data reviewed in this chapter indicated that patients with nonepileptic seizures generally have neuropsychological abnormalities.

There are two observations about patients with nonepileptic seizures relevant to the present discussion. First, even after careful evaluation, the majority of these patients do not receive any psychiatric diagnosis other than conversion disorder (Alper, Devinsky, Perrine, Vazquez, & Luciano, 1995). This observation is extraordinary. Despite high levels of disability, despite frequently having a poor prognosis (Ettinger, Devinsky, Weisbrot, Ramakrishna, & Goyal, 1999), and despite the truly bizarre nature of their symptoms, many of these patients neither demonstrate nor report any psychopathology other than their seizures. The extreme nature of the symptom of nonepileptic seizures surely indicates additional underlying psychopathology, but this psychopathology often cannot be detected because it is not acknowledged. Anecdotal evidence shows that some of these patients deny existing, clearcut psychiatric history, including hospitalizations and suicide attempts.

Second, consistent with the fact that some of these patients receive a psychiatric diagnosis only of conversion disorder, the mean MMPI-2 profiles of this population show a Conversion V (Binder et al. 1994; Brown et al. 1991; Wilkus et al. 1984). The highest MMPI-2 elevations, by a wide margin, are on scales Hs and Hy. The mean profiles show much milder elevations on scales measuring symptoms of depression and anxiety. The conventional interpretation of a MMPI-2 Conversion V profile (Greene, 2000) is that the person uses physical symptoms as a form of psychological defense against the experience of psychological complaints and against facing the source of psychological distress. Graham (1990) described this profile as indicating persons who:

present themselves as normal, responsible, and without fault. . . . They prefer medical explanations for their symptoms, and they lack insight into psychological factors underlying their problems . . . they do not show appropriate concern about their symptoms and problems. (p. 90)

It is likely that the lessons of nonepileptic seizure patients with conversion disorders apply, at least in some cases, to other types of medically unexplained disorders. Some studies of people with fibromyalgia, CFS, and other similar conditions show an increased rate of psychiatric problems, especially anxiety and mood disorders, prior to the onset of their illness (Black, 2000; Walker, Keegan, Gardner, Sullivan, Katon, et al., 1997). However, many people with these conditions do not report either mental health treatment or significant episodes of psychiatric disorder prior to the onset of their illnesses, and they do not necessarily report unusual psychological traumas during childhood or adulthood (Staudenmayer, 1996). There also is evidence that people with these disorders both overreact to stressors and deny their anxiety (Brosschot & Aarsse, 2001); that is, they lack insight into their current psychological experience.

It is hypothesized that denial and lack of insight about past and present psychological stressors and current problems occurs commonly in people with medically unexplained disorders (Staudenmayer, 1996). What may be true about people with these conditions is that what they do not know, or what they do not tell the health care professional who is taking the history, is the very thing that might be hurting them. This hypothesis is consistent with the evidence reviewed here and is testable through large-scale, longitudinal investigations.

For example, the cohort of participants followed up for recollections of childhood sexual or physical abuse whose childhood records documented the abuse (Widom & Morris, 1997) or other social upheavals (Henry et al., 1994) could be assessed for relatively common conditions such as fibromyalgia and chronic fatigue. It is hypothesized that participants subjected to childhood traumas will suffer a higher lifetime prevalence of medically unexplained disorders, especially if they do not disclose the childhood traumatic events that were reported earlier. The psychological or psychophysiological pathogen may be less severe than a history of childhood sexual or physical abuse, for example, a neurophysiological predisposition toward intolerance of ordinary stressors, a trait that can be measured (Barlow, 2000; Davidson, 2000).

IMPLICATIONS FOR FORENSIC PRACTICE

Mental health professionals, including neuropsychologists, can perform the most accurate assessment when they have access to mental health and medical records from the past (Coyne et al., 2001). Denial of past mental illness may not be accurate. Moreover, the life events that may have been most damaging to the mental health of the patient under examination may be the very events not reported to the clinician, despite careful inquiry. Records sometimes reveal that the same stressful life events that were denied to the current examiner were acknowledged to previous examiners. Anecdotal evidence suggests that childhood traumatic events sometimes are initially denied and later acknowledged to the same clinician. Asking about a history of psychological traumas in multiple ways or waiting until the examinee is more at ease may increase the probability that the patient will provide accurate information.

Studies reviewed here also have implications specifically for neuropsychological practice. Many people with these disorders have mild neuropsychological abnormalities (Binder et al., 2001; DiPino & Kane, 1996; Grace et al. 1999; Hart et al., 2000; Tiersky et al., 1997) that do not necessarily signify the presence of neurological disease, at least not the way neurological disease currently is defined. Evidence reviewed here clearly indicates that brain chemistry can be altered by psychological traumas. There also is some support for the hypothesis that brain structures may be altered by psychological traumas. These findings blur the distinctions between "organic" and "psychiatric" illnesses.

Cognitive abnormalities are nonspecific. Their presence does not necessarily signify the presence of neurological disease or injury (Bolla, 2000). Cognitive abnormalities may be caused by the considerable natural variability in human performance (Heaton, Grant, & Matthews, 1991), by developmental learning disabilities (O'Donnell, Kurtz, & Ramanaiah, 1983; Selz & Reitan, 1979), or by attention deficit disorder (Fischer, Barkley, Edelbrock, & Smallish, 1990). Neuropsychological impairments also are associated with certain personality disorders, depression, substance abuse, and other psychiatric disorders (Goldman, 1983; Johnson & Magaro, 1987; Judd & Ruff, 1993; McAllister, 1981; O'Leary, Brouwers, Gardner, & Cowdry, 1991).

Assuming that cognitive abnormalities resulted from a valid examination of mental abilities, the neuropsychologist can assist the patient in various ways, such as documenting the findings, measuring the extent of the cognitive problem, suggesting means of coping with the deficits, and recommending and implementing therapy. However, when evaluating patients with medically unexplained disorders such as fibromyalgia or CFS, it should not be assumed that the presence of cognitive abnormalities signifies the presence of a traditionally defined neurological disease affecting the brain.

A history of medically unexplained symptoms or illness provides an explanation for mild cognitive deficits that may be more compelling than a potentially compensable condition such as mild head injury or alleged toxic exposure. The cognitive deficits in information-processing speed, attention, and memory associated with illnesses such as chronic fatigue and fibromyalgia are strikingly similar to the deficits that some authors ascribe to late PCS (chapter 7, this volume) and neurotoxicity (chapter 9, this volume).

Sensible treatment recommendations can be made despite some uncertainty about the possibly multifactorial etiology of these conditions. Cognitive-behavioral therapy combined with graded exercise has been effective for fibromyalgia (Burckhardt, 2002) and CFS (Afari & Buchwald, 2003; Friedberg & Jason, 2001). It also is recommended for MCS (Staudenmayer, 1996), and its value in Gulf War illnesses is under investigation. Clearly, negative expectancies play a role for many people with these ill-defined conditions (Dalton, 1999; Moss-Morris et al., 1995). The classically conditioned responses of MCS are subject to extinction, that is, repeated presentation of the odor without illness (Van den Bergh et al., 2001).

The presence of a medically unexplained disorder, coupled with subjective cognitive complaints, provides a rationale for a neuropsychological evaluation. The evaluation should include an in-depth psychological assessment. The not-always-attainable goal of such an assessment is to provide a psychological explanation for the physical symptoms and to determine which treatment might be helpful. Among the psychological assessment questions that should be answered, whenever possible, are the following: Is a mood disorder present? Is an anxiety disorder present? Has there been sufficient emotional trauma to cause PTSD or posttraumatic stress symptoms? Is there secondary gain or illness behavior in the form of financial incentives or social/familial attention? If one of these conditions is identified, how should it be treated? Psychological problems in the absence of clear physical disease or injury are often the most parsimonious explanations for neuropsychological symptoms.

NOTE

Portions of this chapter were published in "Medically Unexplained Symptoms and Neuropsychological Assessment," by L. M. Binder and K. A. Campbell, 2004, *Journal of Clinical and Experimental Neuropsychology*, *26*(3), 369–392; web site: http://www.psypress.co.uk/journals.asp and are reproduced here with permission.

REFERENCES

Abbey, S. E., & Garfinkel, P. E. (1991). Neurasthenia and chronic fatigue syndrome: The role of culture in the making of a diagnosis. *American Journal of Psychiatry, 148*, 1638–1646.

Afari, N., & Buchwald, D. (2003). Chronic fatigue syndrome: A review. *American Journal of Psychiatry, 160*, 221–236.

Albers, J. W., & Berent, S. (2000). Controversies in neurotoxicology. Current status. *Neurologic Clinics, 18*, 741–763.

Alper, K., Devinsky, O., Perrine, K., Vazquez, B., & Luciano, D. (1993). Nonepileptic seizures and childhood sexual and physical abuse. *Neurology, 43*, 1950–1953.

Alper, K., Devinsky, O., Perrine, K., Vazquez, B., & Luciano, D. (1995). Psychiatric classification of nonconversion nonepileptic seizures. *Archives of Neurology 52*, 199–201.

American Academy of Allergy and Immunology. (1986). Position statement; clinical ecology. *Journal of Allergy and Clinical Immunology, 78*, 269–271.

American College of Physicians. (1989). Clinical ecology. *Annals of Internal Medicine, 111*, 168–178.

Andreski, P., Chilcoat, H., & Breslau, N. (1998). Post-traumatic stress disorder and somatization symptoms: a prospective study. *Psychiatry Research, 79*, 131–138.

Annegers, J. F., Hauser, W. A., Coan, S. P., & Rocca, W. A. (1998). A population-based study of seizures after traumatic brain injuries. *New England Journal of Medicine, 338*, 20–24.

Barlow, D. H. (2000). Unraveling the mysteries of anxiety and its disorders from the perspective of emotion theory. *American Psychologist, 55*, 1247–1263.

Barry, E., Krumholz, A., Bergey, G. K., Chatha, H., Alemayehu, S., & Grattan, L. (1998). Nonepileptic posttraumatic seizures. *Epilepsia, 39*, 427–431.

Barsky, A. J., & Borus, J. F. (1999). Functional somatic syndromes. *Annals of Internal Medicine, 130*, 910–921.

Beckham, J., Moore, S., Feldman, M., Hertzberg, M., Kirby, A., & Fairbank, J. A., (1998). Health status, somatization and severity of posttraumatic stress disorder in Vietnam combat veterans with posttraumatic stress disorder. *American Journal of Psychiatry, 155*, 1565–1569.

Bell, I. R., Baldwin, C. M., Fernandez, M., & Schwartz, G. E. R. (1999). Neural sensitization model for multiple chemical sensitivity: Overview of theory and empirical evidence. *Toxicology and Industrial Health, 15*, 295–304.

Bell, I. R., Baldwin, C. M., & Schwartz, G. E. (1998). Illness from low-level environmental chemicals: Relevance to chronic fatigue syndrome and fibromyalgia. *American Journal of Medicine*, *105*(Supp. 3A), 74S–82S.

Bennett, R. M. (1999). Emerging concepts in the neurobiology of chronic pain: Evidence of abnormal sensory processing in fibromyalgia. *Mayo Clinical Proceedings*, *74*, 385–398.

Binder, L. M. (1997). A review of mild head trauma. Part II: Clinical implications. *Journal of Clinical and Experimental Neuropsychology*, *19*, 432–457.

Binder, L. M., & Campbell, K. A. (2004). Medically unexplained symptoms and neuropsychological assessment. *Journal of Clinical and Experimental Neuropsychology*, *26*, 369–392.

Binder, L. M., Kindermann, S. S., Heaton, R. K., & Salinsky, M. C. (1998). Neuropsychologic impairment in patients with nonepileptic seizures. *Archives of Clinical Neuropsychology*, *13*, 513–522.

Binder, L. M., Salinsky, M. C., & Smith, S. P. (1994). Psychological correlates of psychogenic seizures. *Journal of Clinical and Experimental Neuropsychology*, *16*, 524–530.

Binder, L. M., Storzbach, D., Campbell, K. A., Rohlman, D. S., Anger, W. K., & members of the Portland Environmental Hazards Research Center. (2001). Neurobehavioral deficits associated with chronic fatigue syndrome in veterans with Gulf War unexplained illnesses. *Journal of the International Neuropsychological Society*, *7*, 835–839.

Black, D. W. (1996). Iatrogenic (physician-induced) hypochondriasis: Four patient examples of "chemical sensitivity." *Psychosomatics*, *37*, 390–393.

Black, D. W. (2000). The relationship of mental disorders and idiopathic environmental intolerance. *Occupational Medicine: State of the Art Reviews*, *15*, 557–570.

Bohr, T. (1996). Problems with myofascial pain syndrome and fibromyalgia syndrome. *Neurology*, *45*, 593–597.

Bolla, K. I. (2000). Use of neuropsychological testing in idiopathic environmental testing. *Occupational Medicine: State of the Art Reviews*, *15*, 617–624.

Boscarino, J. A. (1997). Diseases among men 20 years after exposure to severe stress: Implications for clinical research and medical care. *Psychosomatic Medicine*, *59*, 605–614.

Bremner, J. D., Randall, P., Scott, T. M., Bronen, R. A., Seibyl, J. P., Southwick, S. M., et al. (1995). MRI-based measurement of hippocampal volume in patients with combat-related posttraumatic stress disorder. *American Journal of Psychiatry*, *152*, 973–981.

Bremner, J. D., Scott, T. M., Delaney, R. C., Southwick, S. M., Mason, J. W., Johnson, D. R., et al. (1993). Deficits in short-term memory in posttraumatic stress disorder. *American Journal of Psychiatry*, *150*, 1015–1019.

Brosschot, J. F., & Aarsse, H. R. (2001). Restricted emotional processing and somatic attribution in fibromyalgia. *International Journal of Psychiatric Medicine*, *31*, 127–146.

Brown, M. C., Levin, B. E., Ramsay, R. E., Katz, D. A., & Duchowny, M. S. (1991). Characteristics of patients with nonepileptic seizures. *Journal of Epilepsy*, *4*, 225–229.

Brown-DeGagne, A., & McGlone, J. (1999). Multiple chemical sensitivity: A test of the olfactory-limbic model. *Journal of Occupational and Environmental Medicine*, *41*, 366–377.

Buchwald, D., & Garrity, D. (1994). Comparison of patients with chronic fatigue syndrome, fibromyalgia, and multiple chemical sensitivities. *Archives of Internal Medicine*, *154*, 2049–2053.

Burckhardt, C. S. (2002). Nonpharmacologic management strategies in fibromyalgia. *Rheumatologic Diseases Clinics of North America*, *28*, 291–304.

Burge, H. A. (2001). Fungi: Toxic killers or unavoidable nuisances? *Annals of Allergy, Asthma, and Immunology*, *87*(6, Suppl. 3), 52–56.

Burkett, B. G., & Whitley, G. (1998). *Stolen valor: How the Vietnam generation was robbed of its heroes and its history*. Dallas, TX: Verity Press.

Burt, D. B., Zembar, M. J., & Niederehe, G. (1995). Depression and memory impairment: A meta-analysis of the association, its pattern, and specificity. *Psychological Bulletin*, *117*, 285–305.

Butler, J. A., Chalder, T., & Wessely, S. (2001). Causal attributions for somatic sensations in patients with chronic fatigue syndrome and their partners. *Psychological Medicine*, *31*, 97–105.

Cardena, E., & Spiegel, D. (1993). Dissociative reactions to the San Francisco Bay area earthquake of 1989. *American Journal of Psychiatry*, *150*, 474–478.

Cassens, G., Wolfe, L., & Zola, M. (1990). The neuropsychology of depressions. *Journal of Neuropsychiatry and Clinical Neurosciences*, *2*, 202–213.

Couprie, W., Wijdicks, E. F., Rooijmans, H. G., & van Gijn, J. (1995). Outcome in conversion disorder: A follow up study. *Journal of Neurology, Neurosurgery, and Psychiatry*, *58*, 750–752.

Coyne, J. C., Thompson, R., & Racioppo, M. W. (2001). Validity and efficiency of screening for history of depression by self-report. *Psychological Assessment*, *13*, 163–170.

Crimlisk, H. L., Bhatia, K., Cope, H., David, A., Marsden, C. D., & Ron, M. A. (1998). Slater revisited: 6 year follow-up study of patients with medically unexplained motor symptoms. *British Journal of Medicine*, *316*, 582–586.

Dalton, P. (1999). Cognitive influences on health symptoms from acute chemical exposure. *Health Psychology*, *18*, 579–590.

Dalton, P., & Hummel, T. (2000). Chemosensory function and response in idiopathic environmental intolerance. *Occupational Medicine: State of the Art Reviews*, *15*, 539–556.

Davidson, R. J. (2000). Affective style, psychopathology, and resilience: Brain mechanisms and plasticity. *American Psychologist*, *55*, 1196–1214.

Deary, I. J. (1999). A taxonomy of medically unexplained symptoms. *Journal of Psychosomatic Research*, *47*, 51–59.

DeLuca, J., Johnson, S. K., Ellis, S. P., & Natelson, B. H. (1997). Cognitive functioning is impaired in patients with chronic fatigue syndrome devoid of psychiatric disease. *Journal of Neurology, Neurosurgery, and Psychiatry*, *62*, 151–155.

DiPino, R. K., & Kane, R. L. (1996). Neurocognitive functioning in chronic fatigue syndrome. *Neuropsychology Review*, *6*, 47–60.

Dodrill, C. B., Wilkus, R. J., & Batzel, L. W. (1993). The MMPI as a diagnostic tool in non-epileptic seizures. In A. J. Rowan & J. R. Gates (Eds.), *Non-epileptic seizures* (pp. 211–219). Boston: Butterworth-Heinemann.

Doty, R. L., Deems, D. A., Frye, R. E., Pelberg, R., & Shapiro, A. (1988). Olfactory sensitivity, nasal resistance, and autonomic function in patients with multiple chemical sensitivities. *Archives of Otolaryngology and Head and Neck Surgery*, *114*, 1422–1427.

Elder, G. H., Shanahan, M. J., & Clipp, E. C. (1997). Linking combat and physical health: The legacy of World War II in men's lives. *American Journal of Psychiatry*, *154*, 330–336.

Escobar, J. I., Canino, G., Rubio-Stipec, M., & Bravo, M. (1992). Somatic symptoms after a natural disaster: A prospective study. *American Journal of Psychiatry*, *149*, 965–967.

Ettinger, A. B., Devinsky, O., Weisbrot, D. M., Ramakrishna, R. K., & Goyal, A. (1999). A comprehensive profile of clinical, psychiatric, and psychosocial characteristics of patients with psychogenic nonepileptic seizures. *Epilepsia*, *40*, 1292–1298.

Ferguson, E., & Cassaday, H. J. (2001–2002). Theoretical accounts of Gulf War Syndrome: From environmental toxins to psychneuroimmunology and neurodegeneration. *Behavioral Neurology*, *13*, 133–147.

Ferguson, J. H. (1997). Silicone breast implants and neurologic disorders. Report of the Practice Committee of the American Academy of Neurology. *Neurology*, *48*, 1504–1507.

Ferguson, R. J., Mittenberg, W., Barone, D. F., & Schneider, B. (1999). Postconcussion syndrome following sports-related head injury: Expectation as etiology. *Neuropsychology*, *13*, 582–589.

Fischer, M., Barkley, R. A., Edelbrock, C. S., & Smallish, L. (1990). The adolescent outcome of hyperactive children diagnosed by research criteria: II. Academic, attentional, and neuropsychological status. *Journal of Consulting and Clinical Psychology*, *58*, 580–588.

Fischler, B., D'Haenen, H., Cluydts, R., Michiels, V., Demets, K., Bossuyt, A., et al. (1996). Comparison of 99m Tc HMPAO SPECT scan between chronic fatigue syndrome, major depression and healthy controls: An exploratory study of clinical correlates of regional cerebral blood flow. *Neuropsychobiology*, *34*, 175–183.

Ford, C. V. (1997). Somatization and fashionable diagnoses: Illness as a way of life. *Scandinavian Journal of Work and Environmental Health*, *23*(Suppl. 3), 7–16.

Fox, D. D., Lees-Haley, P. R., Earnest, K., & Dolezal-Wood, S. (1995). Base rates of post-concussive symptoms in health maintenance organization patients and controls. *Neuropsychology*, *9*, 606–611.

Friedberg, F., & Jason, L. A. (2001). Chronic fatigue syndrome and fibromyalgia: Clinical assessment and treatment. *Journal of Clinical Psychology*, *57*, 433–455.

Fukuda, K., Straus, S. E., Hickie, I., Sharpe, M. C., Dobbins, J. G., Komaroff, A., et al. (1994). The chronic fatigue syndrome: A comprehensive approach to its definition and study. *Annals of Internal Medicine*, *121*, 953–959.

Gabriel, S. E., O'Fallon, W. M., Kurland, L. T., Beard, C. M., Woods, J. E., & Melton, L. J. (1994). Risk of connective-tissue diseases and other disorders after breast implantation. *The New England Journal of Medicine*, *330*, 1697–1749.

Gervais, R. O., Russell, A. S., Green, P., Allen L. M., Ferrari, R., & Pieschl, S. D. (2001). Effort testing in patients with fibromyalgia and disability incentives. *Journal of Rheumatology*, *28*, 1892–1899.

Glaser, R., & Kiecolt-Glaser, J. K. (1998). Stress-associated immune modulation: Relevance to viral infections and chronic fatigue syndrome. *American Journal of Medicine*, *105*(Suppl. 3A), 35S–42S.

Goldman, M. S. (1983). Cognitive impairment in chronic alcoholics: Some cause for optimism. *American Psychologist*, *38*, 1045–1054.

Goodwin, F., & Jamison, K. (1990). *Manic depressive illness*. New York: Oxford University Press.

Gorman, J. M., Kent, J. M., Sullivan, G. M., & Coplan, J. D. (2000). Neuroanatomical hypothesis of panic disorder, revised. *American Journal of Psychiatry*, *157*, 493–505.

Gouvier, W. D., Cubic, B., Jones, G., Brantley, P., & Cutlip, Q. (1992). Postconcussion symptoms and daily stress in normal and head-injured college populations. *Archives of Clinical Neuropsychology, 7,* 193–211.

Gouvier, W. D., Uddo-Crane, M., & Brown, L. M. (1988). Base rates of post-concussional symptoms. *Archives of Clinical Neuropsychology, 3,* 273–278.

Grace, G. M., Nielson, W. R., Hopkins, M., & Berg, M. A. (1999). Concentration and memory deficits in patients with fibromyalgia syndrome. *Journal of Clinical and Experimental Neuropsychology, 21,* 477–487.

Graham, J. R. (1990). *MMPI-2. Assessing personality and psychopathology.* New York: Oxford University Press.

Greene, R. L. (2000). *The MMPI-2. An interpretive manual* (2nd ed.). Boston: Allyn and Bacon.

Greiffenstein, M. F., Baker, W. J., & Johnson-Greene, D. (2002). Actual versus self-reported scholastic achievement of litigating postconcussion and severe closed head injury claimants. *Psychological Assessment, 14,* 202–208.

Grossman, R., Buchsbaum, M. S., & Yehuda, R. (2002). Neuroimaging studies in post-traumatic stress disorder. *Psychiatric Clinics of North America, 25,* 317–340.

Gunstad, J., & Suhr, J. A. (2001). "Expectation as etiology" versus "the good old days": Postconcussion syndrome symptom reporting in athletes, headache sufferers, and depressed individuals. *Journal of the International Neuropsychological Society, 7,* 323–333.

Hadler, N. M. (1997). Fibromyalgia: La maladie est morte. Vive le malade! *Journal of Rheumatology, 24,* 1250–1251.

Hadler, N. M. (1999). *Occupational musculoskeletal disorders* (2nd ed.). Philadelphia: Lippincott Williams and Wilkins.

Hakala, M., Karlsson, H., Ruotsalainen, U., Koponen, S., Bergman, J., Stenman, H., et al. (2002). Severe somatization in women is associated with altered cerebral glucose metabolism. *Psychological Medicine, 32,* 1379–1385.

Hardin, B. D., Kelman, B. J., & Saxon, A. (2003). Adverse human health effects associated with molds in the indoor environment. *Journal of Occupational and Environmental Medicine, 45,* 470–478.

Harlow, S. D., & Linet, M. S. (1989). Agreement between questionnaire data and medical records. The evidence for accuracy of recall. *American Journal of Epidemiology, 129,* 233–248.

Hart, R. P., Martelli, M. F., & Zasler, N. D. (2000). Chronic pain and neuropsychological functioning. *Neuropsychology Review, 20,* 131–149.

Heaton, R. K., Grant, I., & Matthews, C. G. (1991). *Comprehensive norms for an expanded Halstead-Reitan Battery.* Odessa, FL: Psychological Assessment Resources.

Heim, C., Ehlert, U., & Hellhammer, D. H. (2000). The potential role of hypocortisolism in the pathophysiology of stress-related bodily disorders. *Psychoneuroendocrinology, 25,* 1–35.

Hennekens, C. H., Lee, I. M., Cook, N. R., Hebert, P. R., Karlson, E. W., LaMotte, F., et al. (1996). Self-reported breast implants and connective-tissue diseases in female health professionals: A retrospective cohort study. *Journal of the American Medical Association, 275,* 616–621.

Henry, B., Moffit, T. E., Caspi, A., Langley, J., & Silva, P. A. (1994). On the "Rememberance of Things Past"; a longitudinal evaluation of the retrospective method. *Psychological Assessment, 6,* 92–101.

Herbert, T. B., & Cohen, S. (1993). Depression and immunity: A meta-analytic review. *Psychological Bulletin, 113,* 472–486.

Hilsabeck, R. C., Gouvier, W. D., & Bolter, J. F. (1998). Reconstructive memory bias in recall of neuropsychological symptomatology. *Journal of Clinical and Experimental Neuropsychology*, *20*, 328–338.

Hodgson, M. (2000). Sick building syndrome. *Occupational Medicine*: *State of the Art Reviews*, *15*, 617–624.

Hodgson, M. F., Morey, P., Leung, W., Morrow, L., Miler, D., Jarvis, B. B., et al. (1998). Building-associated pulmonary disease from exposure to *Stachybotrys chartarum* and *Aspergillus versicolor*. *Journal of Occupational and Environmental Medicine*, *40*, 241–248.

Hotopf, M., Mayou, R., Wadsworth, M., & Wessely, S. (1999). Childhood risk factors for adults with medically unexplained symptoms: Results from a national birth cohort study. *American Journal of Psychiatry*, *156*, 1796–1800.

Hyams, K. C., Wignall, F. S., & Roswell, R. (1996). War syndromes and their evaluation: From the U.S. Civil War to the Persian Gulf War. *Annals of Internal Medicine*, *125*, 398–405.

Ichise, M., Salit, I. E., Abbey, S. E., Chung, D. G., Gray, B., Kirsh, J. C., et al. (1992). Assessment of regional cerebral perfusion by 99Tcm-HMPAO SPECT in chronic fatigue syndrome. *Nuclear Medicine Communications*, *13*, 767–772.

Jason, L. A., Richman, J. A., Friedberg, F., Wagner, L., Taylor, R., et al. (1997). Politics, science, and the emergence of a new disease: The case of chronic fatigue syndrome. *American Psychologist*, *52*, 973–983.

Jason, L. A., Richman, J. A., Rademaker, A. W., Jordan, K. M., Pliooplys, A. V., Taylor, R. R., et al. (1999). A community-based study of chronic fatigue syndrome. *Archives of Internal Medicine*, *159*, 2129–2137.

Jenkins, M. A., Langlais, P. J., Delis, D., & Cohen, R. (1998). Learning and memory in rape victims with posttraumatic stress disorder. *American Journal of Psychiatry*, *155*, 278–279.

Johnson, M. H., & Magaro, P. A. (1987). Effects of mood and severity on memory processes in depression and mania. *Psychological Bulletin*, *101*, 28–40.

Johnson-Greene, D., & Binder, L. M. (1995). Evaluation of an efficient method for verifying higher education credentials. *Archives of Clinical Neuropsychology*, *10*, 251–253.

Judd, P. H., & Ruff, R. M. (1993). Neuropsychological dysfunction in borderline personality disorder. *Journal of Personality Disorders*, *7*, 275–284.

Katon, W. J., Buchwald, D. S., Simon, G. E., Russo, J. E., & Mease, P. J. (1991). Psychiatric illness in patients with chronic fatigue and those with rheumatoid arthritis. *Journal of General Internal Medicine*, *6*, 277–285.

Katon, W., & Walker, E. A. (1993). The relationship of chronic fatigue to psychiatric illness in community, primary care and tertiary care samples. In G. R. Bock & J. Whelan (Eds.), *Chronic fatigue syndrome* (pp. 193–211). Chichester, U.K.: Wiley.

Kawamura, N., Kim, Y., & Asukai, N. (2001). Suppression of cellular immunity in men with a past history of posttraumatic stress disorder. *American Journal of Psychiatry*, *158*, 484–486.

Kent, D. A., Tomasson, K., & Coryell, W. (1995). Course and outcome of conversion and somatization disorders: A four-year follow-up. *Psychosomatics*, *36*, 138–144.

Kirmayer, L. J., & Robbins, J. M. (1993). Cognitive and social correlates of the Toronto Alexithymia Scale. *Psychosomatics*, *34*, 41–52.

Kirschbaum, C., Prussner, J. C., Stone, A. A., Federenko, I., Gaab, J., Lintz, D., et al. (199). Persistent high cortisol responses to repeated psychological stress in a subpopulation of healthy men. *Psychosomatic Medicine*, *57*, 468–474.

Kroenke, K., & Price, R. K. (1993). Symptoms in the community. Prevalence, classification, and psychiatric comorbidity. *Archives of Internal Medicine, 153,* 2474–2480.

Kuhn, D. M., & Ghannoum, M. A. (2003). Indoor mold, toxigenic fungi, and *Stachybotrys chartarum*: Infectious disease perspective. *Clinical Microbiology Review, 16,* 144–172.

Kwiatek, R., Barnden, L., Tedman, R., Jarrett, R., Chew, J., Rowe, C., et al. (2000). Regional cerebral blood flow in fibromyalgia: Single-photon-emission computed tomography evidence of reduction in the pontine tegmentum and thalami. *Arthritis and Rheumatology, 43,* 2823–2833.

Labarge, A. S., & McCaffrey, R. J. (2000). Multiple chemical sensitivity: A review of the theoretical and research literature. *Neuropsychology Review, 10,* 183–211.

LaManca, J. J., Sisto, S. A., DeLuca, J., Johnson, S. K., Lange, G., Pareja, J., et al. (1998). Influence of exhaustive treadmill exercise on cognitive functioning in chronic fatigue syndrome. *American Journal of Medicine, 105,* 59S–65S.

Lang, P. J., & Cuthbert, B. N. (1984). Affective information processing and the assessment of anxiety. *Journal of Behavior Assessment, 6,* 369–395.

Lange, G., Wang, S., DeLuca, J., & Natelson, B. H. (1998). Neuroimaging in chronic fatigue syndrome. *American Journal of Medicine, 105*(Suppl. 3A), 50S–53S.

Larrabee, G. J., & Levin, H. S. (1986). Memory self-ratings and objective test performance in a normal elderly sample. *Journal of Clinical and Experimental Neuropsychology, 8,* 275–284.

Lee, A. L., Ogle, W. O., & Sapolsky, R. M. (2002). Stress and depression: Possible links to neuron death in the hippocampus. *Bipolar Disorders, 4,* 117–128.

Lees-Haley, P. R., & Brown, R. S. (1993). Neuropsychological complaint base rates of 170 personal injury claimants. *Archives of Clinical Neuropsychology, 8,* 203–209.

Lees-Haley, P. R., Williams, C. W., & English, L. T. (1996). Response bias in self-reported history of plaintiffs compared with nonlitigating patients. *Psychological Reports, 79,* 811–818.

Leininger, B. E., Kreutzer, J. S., & Hill, M. R. (1991). Comparison of minor and severe head injury: Emotional sequelae using the MMPI. *Brain Injury, 5,* 199–205.

Lewis, D. H., Mayberg, H. S., Fischer, M. E., Goldberg, J., Ashton, S., Graham, M. M., et al. (2001). Monozygotic twins discordant for chronic fatigue syndrome: Regional cerebral blood flow SPECT. *Radiology, 219,* 766–773.

Mace, C. J., & Trimble, M. R. (1996). Ten-year prognosis of conversion disorder. *British Journal of Psychiatry, 169,* 282–288.

Matthews, C. G., Shaw, D. J., & Klove, H. (1966). Psychological test performance in neurologic and "pseudo-neurologic" subjects. *Cortex, 2,* 244–253.

McAllister, T. W. (1981). Cognitive functioning in the affective disorders. *Comprehensive Psychiatry, 22,* 572–586.

McDiarmid, M. A., Keoghm, J. P., Hooper, F. J., McPhaul, K., Squibb, K., Kane, R., et al. (2000). Health effects of depleted uranium on exposed Gulf War veterans. *Environmental Research, 82,* 168–180.

McEwen, B. (2002). *The end of stress as we know it.* Washington, DC: Joseph Henry Press.

McFarlane, A. C., Atchison, M., Rafalowicz, E., & Papay, P. (1994). Physical symptoms in post-traumatic stress disorder. *Journal of Psychosomatic Research, 38,* 715–726.

Mittenberg, W., DiGuilio, D. V., Perrin, S., & Bass, A. E. (1992). Symptoms following mild head injury: Expectation as aetiology. *Journal of Neurology, Neurosurgery, and Psychiatry, 55,* 200–204.

Mittenberg, W., Tremont, G., Zielinski, R. E., Fichera, S., & Rayls, K. R. (1996). Cognitive-behavioral prevention of postconcussion syndrome. *Archives of Clinical Neuropsychology, 11*, 139–145.

Morrison, J. (1989). Childhood sexual histories of women with somatization disorder. *American Journal of Psychiatry, 146*, 239–241.

Moss-Morris, R., Petrie, K. J., & Weinman, J. (1995). The impact of catastrophic beliefs on functioning in chronic fatigue syndrome. *Journal of Psychosomatic Research, 39*, 31–37.

Nash, F., Cheng, J. S., Meyer, G. A., & Remler, B. F. (2002). Chiari type I malformation: Overview of diagnosis and treatment. *Western Medical Journal, 101*, 35–40.

Nimnuan, C., Hotopf, M., & Wessely, S. (2000). Medically unexplained symptoms: How often and why are they missed? *Quarterly Journal of Medicine, 93*, 21–28.

Nimnuan, C., Hotopf, M., & Wessely, S. (2001). Medically unexplained symptoms: An epidemiological study in seven specialties. *Journal of Psychosomatic Research, 51*, 361–367.

Novack, T. A., Daniel, M. S., & Long, D. J. (1984). Factors related to emotional adjustment following head injury. *International Journal of Clinical Neuropsychology, 6*, 139–142.

O'Donnell, J. P., Kurtz, J., & Ramanaiah, N. V. (1983). Neuropsychological test findings for normal, learning-disabled, and brain-damaged young adults. *Journal of Consulting and Clinical Psychology, 51*, 726–729.

O'Leary, K. M., Brouwers, P., Gardner, D. L., & Cowdry, R. W. (1991). Neuropsychological testing of patients with borderline personality disorder. *American Journal of Psychiatry, 148*, 106–111.

Paniak, C., Reynolds, S., Phillips, K., Toller-Lobe, G., Melnyk, A., & Nagy, J. (2002). Patient complaints within 1 month of mild traumatic brain injury: A controlled study. *Archives of Clinical Neuropsychology, 17*, 319–334.

Pennebaker, J. W., & Susman, J. R. (1988). Disclosure of traumas and psychosomatic processes. *Social Science in Medicine, 26*, 327–332.

Petrie, K. J., Booth, R. J., & Pennebaker, J. W. (1998). The immunological effects of thought suppression. *Journal of Personality and Social Psychology, 75*, 1264–1272.

Reichenberg, A., Yirmiya, R., Schuld, A., Kraus, T., Haack, M., Morag, A., et al. (2001). Cytokine-associated emotional and cognitive disturbances in humans. *Archives of General Psychiatry, 58*, 445–452.

Reid, S., Hotopf, M., Hull, L., Ismail, K., Unwin, C., & Wessely, S. (2001). Multiple chemical sensitivity and chronic fatigue syndrome in British Gulf War veterans. *American Journal of Epidemiology, 153*, 604–609.

Reijula, K., & Tuomi, T. (2003). Mycotoxins of aspergilli: Exposure and health effects. *Frontiers of Bioscience, 8*, 3232–3235.

Richards, J. M., Beal, W. E., Seagal, J. D., & Pennebaker, J. W. (2000). Effects of disclosure of traumatic events on illness behavior among psychiatric prison inmates. *Journal of Abnormal Psychology, 109*, 156–160.

Robbins, C. A., Swenson, L. J., Neally, M. L., Gots, R. E., & Kelman, B. J. (2000). Health effects of mycotoxins in indoor air: A critical review. *Applied Occupational and Environmental Hygiene, 15*, 773–784.

Robins, L. N., Schoenberg, S. P., Holmes, S. J., Ratcliff, K. S., Benham, A., & Works, J. (1985). Early home environment and retrospective recall: Test for concordance between siblings with and without psychiatric disorders. *American Journal of Orthopsychiatry, 55*, 27–41.

Rogler, L. H., Malgady, R. G., & Tryon, W. W. (1992). Issues of memory in the Diagnostic Interview Schedule. *Journal of Nervous and Mental Disease, 180*, 215–222.

Rosenberg, H. J., Rosenberg, S. D., Williamson, P. D., & Wolford, G. L. (2000). A comparative study of trauma and posttraumatic stress disorder prevalence in epilepsy patients and psychogenic nonepileptic seizure patients. *Epilepsia, 47,* 447–452.

Sackeim, H. A., Freeman, J., McElhiney, M., Coleman, E., Prudic, J., & Devanand, D. P. (1992). Effects of major depression on estimates of intelligence. *Journal of Clinical and Experimental Neuropsychology, 14,* 268–288.

Sanchez-Guerrero, J., Schur, P. H., Sergent, J. S., & Liang, M. H. (1994). Silicone breast implants and rheumatic disease: Clinical, immunologic, and epidemiologic studies. *Arthritis and Rheumatism, 37,* 158–168.

Sapolsky, R. M. (2000). Glucocorticoids and hippocampal atrophy in neuropsychiatric disorders. *Archives of General Psychiatry, 57,* 925–935.

Sawchyn, J. M., Brulot, M. M., & Strauss, E. (2000). Note on the use of the Postconcussion Syndrome Checklist. *Archives of Clinical Neuropsychology, 15,* 1–8.

Schnurr, P. P., & Spiro, A. A., III. (1999). Combat exposure, PTSD symptoms and health behaviors as predictors of physical health in older veterans. *Journal of Nervous and Mental Disease, 187,* 353–359.

Schwartz, R. B., Garada, B. M., Komaroff, A. L., Tice, H. M., Gleit, M., Jolexa, F. A., et al. (1994). Detection of intracranial abnormalities in patients with chronic fatigue syndrome: Comparison of MR imaging and SPECT. *American Journal of Roentgenology, 162,* 935–941.

Seidenberg, M., Haltiner, A., Taylor, M. A., Hermann, B. B., & Wyler, A. (1994). Development and validation of a Multiple Ability Self-Report Questionnaire. *Journal of Clinical and Experimental Neuropsychology, 16,* 93–104.

Selz, M., & Reitan, R. M. (1979). Neuropsychological test performance of normal, learning disabled, and brain damaged older children. *Journal of Nervous and Mental Disease, 167,* 298–302.

Sharpe, M., Chalder, T., Palmer, I., & Wessely, S. (1997). Chronic fatigue syndrome. A practical guide to assessment and management. *General Hospital Psychiatry, 19,* 185–199.

Shedler, J., Mayman, M., & Manis, M. (1993). The illusion of mental health. *American Psychologist, 48,* 1117–1131.

Sherer, M., & Adams, R. L. (1993). Cross-validation of Reitan and Wolfson's Neuropsychological Deficit Scales. *Archives of Clinical Neuropsychology, 8,* 429–436.

Shorter, E. (1992). *From paralysis to fatigue. A history of psychosomatic illness in the modern era.* New York: The Free Press.

Simon, G. E., Katon, W. J., & Sparks, P. J. (1990). Allergic to life: Psychological factors in environmental illness. *American Journal of Psychiatry, 147,* 901–906.

Simon, G. E., & VonKorff, M. (1995). Recall of psychiatric history in cross-sectional surveys: Implications for epidemiologic research. *Epidemiologic Reviews, 17,* 221–227.

Slater, E. (1965). Diagnosis of "hysteria." *British Medical Journal, 1,* 1395–1399.

Smyth, J. M. (1998). Written emotional expression: Effect sizes, outcome, types, and moderating variables. *Journal of Consulting and Clinical Psychology, 66,* 174–184.

Southwick, S. M., Morgan, C. A., Nicolaou, A. L., & Charney, D. S. (1997). Consistency of memory for combat-related traumatic events in veterans of Operation Desert Storm. *American Journal of Psychiatry, 154,* 173–177.

Sparks, P. J. (2000). Idiopathic environmental intolerances: Overview. *Occupational Medicine: State of the Art Reviews, 15,* 497–510.

Staudenmayer, H. (1996). Clinical consequences of the EI/MCS "diagnosis": Two paths. *Regulatory Toxicology and Pharmacology, 1*(Part 2), S96–S110.

Staudenmayer, H. (2001). Idiopathic environmental intolerances (IEI): Myth and reality. *Toxicology Letters, 120,* 333–342.

Standenmayer, H., Selner, J. C., & Buhr, M. P. (1993). Double-blind provocation chamber challenges in 20 patients presenting with "multiple chemical sensitivity." *Regulatory Toxicology and Pharmacology, 18,* 44–53.

Stein, M., Walker, J., Hazen, A., & Forde, D. (1997). Full and partial posttraumatic stress disorder: Findings for a community survey. *American Journal of Psychiatry, 154,* 1114–1119.

Storzbach, D., Binder, L. M., Salinsky, M. C., Campbell, B. R., & Mueller, R. M. (2000). Improved prediction of nonepileptic seizures using combined MMPI and EEG measures. *Epilepsia, 41,* 332–337.

Tiersky, L. A., Johnson, S. K., Lange, G., Natelson, B. H., & DeLuca, J. (1997). Neuropsychology of chronic fatigue syndrome: A critical review. *Journal of Clinical and Experimental Neuropsychology, 19,* 560–586.

Tirelli, U., Chierichetti, G., Tavio, M., Simonelli, C., Bianchin, G., Zanco, P., et al. (1998). Brain positron emission tomography (PET) in chronic fatigue syndrome: Preliminary data. *American Journal of Medicine, 105*(Suppl. 3A), 54S–58S.

Van den Bergh, O., Devriese, S., Winters, W., Veulemans, H., Nemery, B., Eelen, P., et al. (2001). Acquiring symptoms in response to odors: A learning perspective on multiple chemical sensitivity. *Annals of the New York Academy of Sciences, 933,* 278–290.

Van der Werf, S. P., Prins, J. B., Jongen, P. H. J., van der Meer, J. W. M., & Bleijenberg, G. (2000). Abnormal neuropsychological findings are not necessarily a sign of cerebral impairment: A matched comparison between chronic fatigue syndrome and multiple sclerosis. *Neuropsychiatry, Neuropsychology, and Behavioral Neurology, 13,* 199–203.

Vasterling, J. J., Brailey, K., Constans, J. I., Borges, A., & Sutker, P. (1997). Assessment of intellectual resources in Gulf War veterans: Relationship to PTSD. *Assessment, 4,* 51–59.

Vasterling, J. J., Brailey, K., Constans, J. I., & Sutker, P. B. (1998). Attention and memory dysfunction in posttraumatic stress disorder. *Neuropsychology, 12,* 125–133.

Walker, E. A., Keegan, D., Gardner, G., Sullivan, M., Bernstein, D., & Katon, W. J. (1997). Psychosocial factors in fibromyalgia compared with rheumatoid arthritis: II. Sexual, physical, and emotional abuse and neglect. *Psychosomatic Medicine, 59,* 572–577.

Walker, E. A., Keegan, D., Gardner, G., Sullivan, M., Katon, W. J., & Bernstein, D. (1997). Psychosocial factors in fibromyalgia compared with rheumatoid arthritis: I. Psychiatric diagnoses and functional disability. *Psychosomatic Medicine, 59,* 565–571.

Wessely, S. (1997). Chronic fatigue syndrome: A 20th century illness? *Scandinavian Journal of Work and Environmental Health, 23*(Suppl. 3), 17–34.

Wessely, S., Nimnuan, C., & Sharpe, M. (1997). Functional somatic syndromes: One or many? *Lancet, 354,* 936–939.

Westbrook, L. E., Devinsky, O., & Geocadin, R. (1998). Nonepileptic seizures after head injury. *Epilepsia, 39,* 978–982.

Whiteside, T. L., & Friberg, D. (1998). Natural killer cells and natural killer cell activity in chronic fatigue syndrome. *American Journal of Medicine, 105*(Suppl. 3A), 27S–34S.

Widom, C. S., & Morris, S. (1997). Accuracy of adult recollections of childhood victimization: Part 2. Childhood sexual abuse. *Psychological Assessment, 9,* 34–46.

Wilkus, R. J., Dodrill, C. B., & Thompson, P. M. (1984). Intensive EEG monitoring and psychological studies of patients with pseudoepileptic seizures. *Epilepsia, 25,* 100–107.

Williams, J. M., Little, M. M., Scates, S., & Blockman, N. (1987). Memory complaints and abilities among depressed older adults. *Journal of Consulting and Clinical Psychology, 55,* 595–598.

Wolfe, F., Anderson, J., Harkness, D., Bennett, R. M., Caro, X. J., Goldenberg, D. L., et al. (1997). Work and disability status of persons with fibromyalgia. *Journal of Rheumatology, 24,* 1171–1178.

Wolfe, F., Ross, K., Anderson, J., Russell, I. J., & Hebert, L. (1995). The prevalence and characteristics of fibromyalgia in the general population. *Arthritis and Rheumatism, 38,* 19–28.

Youngjohn, J. R., Spector, J., & Mapou, R. L. (1997). Neuropsychological findings in silicone breast-implant complainants: Brain damage, somatization, or compensation neuroses? *The Clinical Neuropsychologist, 11,* 132–141.

11

Assessing Civil Competencies in Older Adults With Dementia: Consent Capacity, Financial Capacity, and Testamentary Capacity

DANIEL C. MARSON
KATINA HEBERT

Impairment of competency, or decision-making capacity (Appelbaum & Gutheil, 1991), is an inevitable consequence of the dementias of Alzheimer's disease (AD) and Parkinson's disease (PD) (Dymek, Atchison, Harrell, & Marson, 2001; D. C. Marson, Ingram, Cody, & Harrell, 1995; D. C. Marson, Schmitt, Ingram, & Harrell, 1994). As capacities for memory, judgment, reasoning, and planning erode, AD patients eventually lose decision-making capacity in every sphere of life. Specific competencies that are lost include the capacity to make medical decisions (D. C. Marson, Ingram, et al., 1995; D. C. Marson, McInturff, Hawkins, Bartolucci, & Harrell, 1997); to consent to research (Kim, Caine, Currier, Leibovici, & Ryan, 2001); to manage financial affairs (D. Marson, 2001b; D. Marson, Sawrie, et al., 2000); to execute a will (Spar & Garb, 1992; Walsh, Brown, Kaye, & Grigsby, 1997); to drive (Drachman, Swearer, & Group, 1993; Hunt et al., 1997); to manage medications (Barberger-Gateau, Dartigues, & Letenneur, 1993); to live independently; and ultimately to handle even the most basic activities of daily life. Patients with PD and dementia have demonstrated deficits in medical decision-making capacity (Dymek et al., 2001; D. Marson & Dymek, in press) and are likely to be impaired in other higher-order capacities such as financial management skills. Loss of competency in dementia has crucially important consequences for patients and their families, for health care and legal professionals, and for society as a whole (D. C. Marson et al., 1994).

Considerable progress has been made in understanding the pathogenesis, pathophysiology, and neurocognitive changes that occur in AD (Butters, Salmon, & Butters, 1994; Cummings & Benson, 1992; Cummings, Vinters, Cole, & Khachaturian, 1998) and in PD with dementia (Emre, 2003; Mahler & Cummings, 1990; Woods & Troster, 2003). In contrast, we still know relatively little about functional impairment in AD and related dementias and in cognitive aging. In particular, we do not understand well the phenomenon of loss of competency. Although a number of conceptual studies of competency exist (Marson & Ingram, 1996), only recently have actual empirical studies of competency loss in dementia and other neurocognitive and medical disorders appeared (Grisso & Appelbaum, 1995a, 1995b; Janofsky, McCarthy, & Folstein, 1992; D. Marson, Sawrie, et al., 2000; D. C. Marson, Ingram, et al., 1995). These empirical studies of competency represent a new and exciting field of clinical and ethical research (D. Marson & Ingram, 1996).

This chapter presents conceptual and clinical approaches to assessing civil competencies in cognitively impaired patients with AD and PD. We begin by outlining basic theoretical concepts that provide a general context for understanding competency assessment and research. We then focus on conceptual and empirical aspects of three specific civil competencies: medical decision-making capacity (treatment consent capacity), financial capacity (FC), and testamentary capacity (capacity to execute a will). In the area of treatment consent, we consider a cognitive model of consent capacity and then review psychometric and neuropsychological studies of this competency in patients with AD and with PD with dementia. In the area of FC, we present a clinically based conceptual model and then review recent psychometric studies of this competency in patients with AD and mild cognitive impairment (MCI). In the area of testamentary capacity, we present the legal elements of this capacity, and then discuss the need for conceptual and empirical research regarding this important civil competency. A preliminary cognitive neuropsychological model of testamentary capacity is proposed, and a prototype assessment instrument is described. We conclude the section by describing two approaches to clinical assessment of testamentary capacity: contemporaneous and retrospective.

Finally, in a chapter epilogue, we note strengths and limitations of competency research in older adults with dementias like AD and PD and suggest directions for future research in the field.

CONCEPTUAL ISSUES IN COMPETENCY ASSESSMENT

Competency is an elusive and often misunderstood medical-legal construct (D. Marson & Briggs, 2001). Sound clinical assessment and empirical research in the area of competency requires identification and clarification of terminology and basic concepts (D. C. Marson et al., 1994). In this section, we highlight a number of key points and principles.

What Is "Competency"?

Competency concerns an individual's legal capacity to make certain decisions and to perform certain acts (Appelbaum & Gutheil, 1991). In our society, the law presumes that adults have the capacity to exercise choices and make decisions for themselves until proven otherwise (Appelbaum & Roth, 1981). However, neurological and psychiatric illnesses may impair the ability to make such decisions in a rational manner. In addition, some individuals with developmental or acquired disabilities in childhood will never, even as adults, possess the capacities necessary to make such decisions. In these circumstances, the state, through exercise of its protective *parens patriae* power, may deem these persons incompetent and appoint substitute decision makers (Kapp, 1992). Accordingly, competency may be usefully defined as "a threshold requirement for an individual to retain the power to make decisions for themselves" (Appelbaum & Gutheil, 1991, p. 218). Because a finding of incompetency may entail a significant deprivation of rights and autonomy, competency evaluations and determinations are serious matters (Appelbaum & Gutheil, 1991; D. C. Marson et al., 1994).

Capacity Versus Competency

The terms *capacity* and *competency* are often used interchangeably (D. Marson & Briggs, 2001). However, although related, the terms are actually also distinct concepts (Kapp, 1992). Capacity denotes a clinical status as judged by a health care professional, whereas competency denotes a legal status as determined by a legal professional (i.e., a judge). A capacity evaluation involves a clinical assessment and judgment based on a patient's history, presentation, and test performance. A judge may consider such clinical capacity findings as part of his or her competency decision-making process, but will also consider other sources of authority, such as statutes, case law precedent, and principles of equity and justice. It is important and useful to be mindful of the capacity/competency distinction in approaching competency issues, even when for reasons of convenience the terms are often used interchangeably (D. Marson & Briggs, 2001).

Multiple Competencies: Competency to Do What?

The term competency is often used in an undifferentiated way to describe a variety of capacities (D. C. Marson et al., 1994). Competency, however, is not a unitary concept or construct: There is not simply "one" competency. The normal adult has distinct and multiple competencies, including the capacity to make a will, to drive, to consent to medical treatment, to manage financial affairs, and ultimately, to manage all of his or her personal affairs. Each capacity involves a distinct combination of functional abilities and skills that sets it apart from other competencies (Grisso, 1986). For example, the cognitive and physical capacities requisite for driving are arguably quite distinct from those for making a will (D. Marson & Briggs, 2001). In addition, each competency tends to operate in a context specific to itself (Grisso, 1986). For example, the capacity to consent to treatment almost always arises in a medical setting. The reality of multiple competencies indicates that the operative question should not be "Is he or she competent?" but rather, "Is he/she competent to do X in Y context?" (D. C. Marson et al., 1994).

Specific Versus General Competency

One useful distinction for analyzing different competencies is that of "specific" versus "general" competency (Appelbaum & Gutheil, 1991). *General competency* is defined as the capacity to manage "all one's affairs in an adequate manner" (Appelbaum & Gutheil, 1991, p. 219) and is the focus of most state statutes in the United States governing guardianship. *Specific competency*, in contrast, concerns the capacity to perform a specific act or set of specific actions (Appelbaum & Gutheil, 1991). As suggested, there are many specific competencies recognized by the law (D. Marson, 2001a), including the capacity to manage financial affairs, make a will, be a parent (adoption and custody), stand trial, and consent to medical treatment. In our experience, each specific competency must be approached and analyzed discretely because each has distinct functional abilities underlying it.

Limited Competency

Because competency determination by its nature results in a categorical assignment (e.g., competent vs. incompetent), in the past competency outcomes were treated as dichotomous, "all-or-nothing" propositions (Appelbaum & Gutheil, 1991). *Limited competency* refers to the fact that, within a general or specific competency, an individual may have the capacity to perform some actions, but not others. For example, a mildly demented patient with AD may no longer be able to handle more complex investment and financial decisions, but might still be able to write checks and handle small daily sums of money (D. Marson, 2001a; D. Marson & Briggs, 2001). Such an individual could be characterized, therefore, as having limited competency to manage his or her financial affairs. The legal system has recognized the importance of limited competency through its use of limited guardianships and conservatorships.

Intermittent Competency and Restoration of Competency

It is important to realize that competency status may change over time (D. Marson, 2001a; D. Marson & Briggs, 2001). For example, fluctuations in chronic psychiatric illness may periodically compromise an individual's capacity to give consent to medication or to manage his or her personal affairs. The competency of a patient with dementia, in contrast, is usually more stable over time. In situations of intermittent competency, periodic reevaluations are indicated. In some cases, the underlying neurological or psychiatric condition compromising an individual's competency may resolve, resulting in the individual regaining decision-making abilities. In such cases, legal competency may be restorable through a formal court hearing and decision.

Dementia Diagnosis Does Not Constitute Incompetency

A diagnosis of dementia or other neurological/psychiatric disorder is not synonymous with incompetency (D. Marson, 2001a; D. Marson & Briggs, 2001). A patient who meets the NINCDS-ADRDA (National Institute of Neurological and Communication Disorders and Stroke-Alzheimer's Disease and Related Disorders Association) criteria for probable AD (McKhann et al., 1984) may nonetheless be competent to consent to medical treatment or research or perform other activities such as driving or managing financial affairs. A determination of competency should always involve a "functional" analysis: Does the person possess the skills and abilities integral to performing a specific act in its context? Dementia diagnosis is certainly a relevant factor in evaluating competency. However, because diagnosis conveys no specific functional information, it cannot by itself be dispositive of the competency question (D. C. Marson et al., 1994).

Neuropsychological Impairment Does Not Constitute Incompetency

For similar reasons, neuropsychological and mental status test measures cannot decide issues of capacity to consent (D. Marson, 2001a; D. Marson & Briggs, 2001). Such test results are important for diagnosing AD and for measuring level of cognitive impairment, and they certainly are relevant to a competency evaluation. However, again, they cannot by themselves be dispositive of the competency issue (Grisso, 1986; High, 1992). As noted by Grisso, decision makers must go further and "present the logic that links these clinical observations [ie., test results] to the capacities with which the law is concerned" (Grisso, 1986, p. 8). For example, neuropsychological impairments in attention, auditory verbal comprehension, and abstractive capacity become relevant to a competency determination only when they are meaningfully related to competency-specific functional impairments—for example, the inability to express a treatment preference or to explain the treatment choice rationally (D. C. Marson, Chatterjee, Ingram, & Harrell, 1996; D. C. Marson, Cody, Ingram, & Harrell, 1995; D. C. Marson, Hawkins, McInturff, & Harrell, 1997).

CAPACITY TO CONSENT TO MEDICAL TREATMENT

In this section, we discuss conceptual and empirical aspects of the capacity to consent to medical treatment (treatment consent capacity). This competency is a fundamental aspect of personal autonomy because it concerns intimate decisions regarding the care of a person's body and mind (D. Marson & Briggs, 2001). Consent capacity refers to a patient's cognitive and emotional capacity to accept a proposed treatment, to refuse treatment, or to select among treatment alternatives (Grisso, 1986; Tepper & Elwork, 1984). In the United States, consent capacity is the cornerstone of the medical-legal doctrine of informed consent, which requires that a valid consent to treatment be informed, voluntary, and competent (Kapp, 1992; D. C. Marson, Ingram, et al., 1995). From a functional standpoint, consent capacity may be viewed as an "advanced activity of daily life" (ADL, activity of daily living) (Wolinsky & Johnson, 1991) and important aspect of functional health and independent living skills in both younger and older adults.

As a competency, consent capacity is distinctive for several reasons: (a) it arises in a medical and not a legal setting; (b) it generally involves a physician, psychologist, or other health care professional and not a legal professional, as decision maker; and (c) these judgments are rarely subject to judicial review (Grisso, 1986). As discussed in this chapter, clinicians are not deciding competency in a formal legal sense. However, their decisions can have the same effect as a courtroom determination insofar as the patient loses decision-making power (Appelbaum & Gutheil, 1991).

As discussed in the section on psychometric studies, consent capacity becomes increasingly impaired in dementia and more specifically in AD as the disease progresses (D. C. Marson, Ingram, et al., 1995). As cognitive skills such as memory, reasoning, judgment, and planning decline, patients lose the ability to encode and process medical information and to make coherent treatment decisions. Because it is often unclear at what point cognitive decline translates into loss of competency, the question of whether a dementia patient is competent to consent to treatment is of considerable interest to health care providers (Farnsworth, 1990; D. C. Marson et al., 1994; Sherlock, 1984).

Cognitive Model for Consent Capacity

Consent capacity may be conceptualized as consisting of three core cognitive tasks: comprehension and encoding of treatment information; information processing and internally arriving at a treatment decision; and communication of the treatment decision to a clinical professional (Alexander, 1988; D. Marson, 2001a; D. Marson & Briggs, 2001; D. C. Marson & Harrell, 1999). These core cognitive tasks occur in a specific context: a patient's dialogue with a physician, psychologist, or other health care professional about a medical condition and potential treatments (D. C. Marson, Ingram, et al., 1995). The comprehension/encoding task involves oral and written comprehension, and encoding, of novel and often complex medical information presented verbally to the patient by the treating clinician. The information processing/decision-making task involves the patient processing (at different levels, depending on the complexity of the information and treatment options) the consent and other information presented, integrating this information with established declarative and episodic knowledge (including personal values and risk preferences), rationally weighing this information, and arriving internally at a treatment decision. The decision communication task involves the patient communicating his or her treatment decision to the clinician in some understandable form (e.g., oral, written, or gestural expression of consent/nonconsent).

This model affords a basis for understanding the cognitive structure of consent capacity decisions and also loss of competency in neurodegenerative disorders (D. Marson, 2001a; D. Marson & Briggs, 2001). For example, short-term memory ability is relevant to consent capacity because impaired learning and short-term recall will limit the amount of encoded medical information available for further processing. Similarly, receptive language measures are relevant to capacity to consent because of their sensitivity to reduced comprehension of treatment related information. Conceptualization and executive function measures are important to consent capacity because of their relevance to organized processing of treatment information. Measures of judgment and reasoning are equally important as they make possible a patient's rational weighing of all this information and his or her internal determination of a treatment choice. Measures of expressive language (e.g., semantic memory), in turn, may be important because of their relevance to effective communication of the treatment choice in the patient–clinician dialogue. In this regard, it should be noted that treatment consent capacity is a highly verbally mediated competency (the only pragmatic arguably is the signature on the form), and thus verbal measures are likely to load highly on it (D. C. Marson & Harrell, 1999).

Psychometric Assessment of Consent Capacity

A number of investigators have developed instruments for assessment of consent capacity in different patient populations (Edelstein, Nygren, Northrop, Staats, & Pool, 1993; Grisso & Appelbaum, 1991, 1995b; Grisso, Appelbaum, Mulvey, & Fletcher, 1995; Janofsky et al., 1992; D. Marson, Earnst, Jamil, Bartolucci,

& Harrell, 2000; D. C. Marson, Ingram, et al., 1995; Marson, McInturff, et al., 1997). Our group has developed an instrument for empirically assessing the capacity of patients with dementia to consent to medical treatment under different legal standards (Capacity to Consent to Treatment Instrument, CCTI) (D. C. Marson, Ingram, et al., 1995).

Specifically, we developed two specialized clinical vignettes (A, neoplasm, and B, cardiac) designed to test competency under five distinct standards of consent capacity. Each vignette presented a hypothetical medical problem and symptoms and two treatment alternatives with associated risks and benefits. The medical content of each vignette was reviewed by a neurologist with expertise with the elderly and dementia. The vignettes, which are presented orally and in writing to subjects in an uninterrupted disclosure format (Grisso & Appelbaum, 1991), were written at a fifth- to sixth-grade reading level (Flesch, 1974), with low syntactic complexity and a moderate information load. The administration format for each vignette approximates an informed consent dialogue and requires the subject to consider two different treatment options with associated risks and benefits.

Administration involves subjects simultaneously reading and listening to an oral presentation of the vignette information. Subjects then answer questions designed to test consent capacity under five different legal thresholds or standards. These standards or thresholds have been drawn from case law and the psychiatric literature (Appelbaum & Grisso, 1988; Roth, Meisel, & Lidz, 1977). In order of increasing difficulty for patients with AD-type dementia (D. C. Marson, Ingram, et al., 1995), they are as follows:

S1: Capacity simply to "evidence" a treatment choice

S3: Capacity to "appreciate" the consequences of a treatment choice

S4: Capacity to reason about treatment/provide "rational reasons" for a treatment choice

S5: Capacity to "understand" the treatment situation and treatment choices

The above standards represent different thresholds for evaluating capacity to consent (D. C. Marson et al., 1994). For example, S1 (evidencing a choice) requires nothing more for competency than a subject's communication of a treatment choice. S3 (appreciating consequences) is of moderate difficulty and requires patients to appreciate how a treatment choice will affect them personally. S4 (rational reasons) bases competency on a subject's capacity to supply rational reasons for the treatment choice. S5 is a comprehension standard and requires a patient to demonstrate conceptual and factual knowledge concerning the medical condition, symptoms, and treatment choices and their respective risks/benefits.

It should be noted that these four standards can be readily applied to other competencies to consent, such as capacity to consent to research, and to decisional capacity generally.

In addition to these four standards, there is an additional consent-related ability described as making the "reasonable" treatment choice (when the alternative is manifestly unreasonable) (Roth et al., 1977). This ability, which we reference as [S2], emphasizes outcome rather than the mere fact of a decision or how it has been reached. The patient who fails to make a decision that is roughly congruent with the decision that a reasonable person in like circumstances would make is viewed as incompetent. The [S2] ability is not an accepted legal standard for judging consent capacity because of concerns about arbitrariness in determining what constitutes a "reasonable choice" (Tepper & Elwork, 1984). Accordingly, [S2] is referenced in brackets to distinguish it from the other four established abilities. However, [S2] remains useful as a means of understanding treatment preferences of patients with neurocognitive disorders (Dymek et al., 2001).

The CCTI has a detailed and well-operationalized scoring system for each vignette standard. In prior work with AD patients, three trained raters achieved high interrater reliability for standards with both interval scales ($r > .83$, $p < .0001$) (S3–S5) and categorical scales (>96% agreement) (S1, [S2]) (D. C. Marson, Ingram, et al., 1995). The CCTI scoring system permits evaluation of both a subject's competency performance and a competency status on each standard. By *competency performance*, we refer to the quantitative score that a subject achieves on a particular standard as determined by the CCTI scoring system. By *competency status*, we refer to the categorical outcome (capable, marginally capable, or incapable) of a subject on a standard based on use of psychometric cutoff scores derived from normal control performance (D. C. Marson, Ingram, et al., 1995).

Consent Capacity in Patients With Alzheimer's Disease

Capacity performance and outcomes

The CCTI has been used to investigate empirically loss of competency in patients with AD ($n = 29$) and older controls ($n = 15$). Using Mini-Mental State Examination (MMSE) scores (Folstein, Folstein, & McHugh, 1975), AD subjects were divided into groups of mild dementia (MMSE > 20) ($n = 15$) and moderate dementia (MMSE > 10 and <20) ($n = 14$). Performance on the five standards was compared across groups.

As shown in Table 11-1, the CCTI discriminated the performance of the normal control, mild AD, and moderate AD subgroups on three of the five standards. Although the three groups performed equivalently on minimal standards requiring merely a treatment choice (S1) or the reasonable treatment

TABLE 11-1. Performance on Capacity to Consent to Treatment Instrument (CCTI) Capacity Standards by Group

	N	LS1 0–4	[LS2][a] 0–1	LS3 0–10	LS4 0–12	LS5 0–70
Older controls	15	4.0 (0.0)	.93	8.7[b] (1.2)	10.3[c,]* (3.8)	58.3* (6.6)
Mild AD	15	3.9 (0.4)	1.00	7.1 (2.0)	6.1[d] (3.4)	27.3[d] (9.6)
Moderate AD	14	3.6 (0.9)	.79	5.9 (2.7)	2.3 (2.4)	17.9 (10.6)

Note. Adapted from D. C. Marson, Ingram, et al. (1995). Copyright 1995 American Medical Association. Reprinted by permission. AD, Alzheimer's disease.
[a]No group differences emerged on [LS2] ($\chi^2 = 4.2$, $p = .12$).
[b]Normal mean differs significantly from moderate AD mean ($p < .001$).
[c]Normal mean differs significantly from mild AD mean ($p < .01$).
[d]Mild AD mean differs significantly from moderate AD mean ($p < .01$).
*$p < .0001$.

choice [S2], patients with mild AD performed significantly below controls on more difficult standards requiring rational reasons (S4) and understanding treatment information (S5). Patients with moderate AD performed significantly below controls on appreciation of consequences (S3), rational reasons (S4), and understanding treatment (S5) and significantly below patients with mild AD on S4 and S5 (D. C. Marson, Ingram, et al., 1995).

In addition to capacity performance, the outcome status of AD patients on the standards was experimentally classified (capable, marginally capable, incapable) using psychometric cutoff scores referenced to control group performance on each standard. As shown in Table 11-2, assignment of capacity status resulted in a consistent pattern of compromise (marginally capable and incapable outcomes) among AD patients that related to both dementia stage and stringency of standard. Mild AD patients demonstrated substantial compromise on S4 (53%) and S5 (100%), the two most stringent and clinically relevant CCTI standards. Patients with moderate AD demonstrated significant compromise on the three more complex and clinically relevant standards S3 (64%), S4 (93%), and S5 (100%)). The results raised the concern that, depending on circumstances (such as the complexity of intervention, the level of treatment risk, and the standard to be applied), many patients with mild AD as well as a majority of patients with moderate AD may lack consent capacity (D. Marson & Briggs, 2001; D. C. Marson, Ingram, et al., 1995).

Cognitive predictors of consent capacity

In addition to providing a standardized basis for evaluating competency performance and outcome, instruments like the CCTI also provide a psychometric criterion for investigating neurocognitive changes associated with loss of con-

TABLE 11-2. Experimental Outcomes by Capacity to Consent to Treatment
Instrument (CCTI) Capacity Standard and Group

STANDARD/GROUP	CAPABLE	MARGINALLY CAPABLE	INCAPABLE
S1 evidencing choice			
Controls	15 (100%)	0 (0%)	0 (0%)
Mild AD	13 (87%)	2 (13%)	0 (0%)
Moderate AD	11 (79%)	1 (7%)	2 (14%)
[S2] reasonable choice			
Controls	14 (93%)		1 (7%)
Mild AD	15 (100%)		0 (0%)
Moderate AD	11 (79%)		3 (21%)
S3 appreciate consequences			
Controls	14 (93%)	1 (7%)	0 (0%)
Mild AD	10 (67%)	2 (14%)	3 (20%)
Moderate AD	5 (36%)	2 (14%)	7 (50%)
S4 reasoning			
Controls	14 (93%)	1 (7%)	0 (0%)
Mild AD	7 (47%)	5 (33%)	3 (20%)
Moderate AD	1 (7%)	3 (22%)	10 (71%)
S5 understand treatment			
Controls	15 (100%)	0 (0%)	0 (0%)
Mild AD	0 (0%)	1 (7%)	14 (93%)
Moderate AD	0 (0%)	0 (0%)	14 (100%)

Note. Adapted from D. C. Marson, Ingram, et al. (1995). Copyright 1995, American Medical
Association. Control $N = 15$; mild AD $N = 15$; moderate AD $N = 14$). AD, Alzheimer's disease.

sent capacity in neurocognitive disorders such as AD. We used the CCTI and a
neuropsychological test battery sensitive to dementia in the above subject sample to identify cognitive predictors of declining competency performance in AD
patients under the four standards (D. C. Marson et al., 1996; D. C. Marson,
Cody, et al., 1995). Table 11-3 presents stepwise multiple regression results for
the combined AD group for these standards.

Findings from these psychometric studies suggested that multiple cognitive
functions are associated with loss of consent capacity in patients with AD, as
measured by the CCTI standards (D. C. Marson et al., 1996; D. C. Marson,
Cody, et al., 1995). Deficits in conceptualization, semantic memory, and probably verbal recall appear to be associated with the significantly impaired capacity
of patients with both mild and moderate AD to understand a treatment situation
and choices (S5). Deficits in simple executive dysfunction (word fluency) appear linked to the impaired capacity of patients with both mild and moderate

TABLE 11-3. Multivariate Cognitive Predictors of Capacity Performance in the Alzheimer's Disease Group ($N = 29$)

S1 (EVIDENCING CHOICE)		S3 (APPRECIATING CONSEQUENCES)		S4 (REASONING)		S5 (UNDERSTANDING TREATMENT)	
R^2	p	R^2	p	R^2	p	R^2	p
SAC .44	.0001	CFL 58	.0001	DRS IP .36	.0008	DRS CON	.70	.0001
						BNT	.11	.001

Note. Adapted from Marson et al. (1996). Copyright 1996, American Academy of Neurology. Reprinted by permission. No measures achieved univariate or multivariate significance for the control group. CFL, Controlled Oral Word Asssociation Test (Benton & Hamsher, 1978); BNT, Boston Naming Test; CFL, Controlled Oral Word Fluency (Kaplan, Goodglass, & Weintraub, 1983); DRS CON, Dementia Rating Scale Conceptualization subscale (Mattis, 1976); DRS IP, Dementia Rating Scale Initiation/Perseveration subscale (Mattis, 1976); SAC, Simple Auditory Comprehension Screen (Eisenson, 1954).

AD to provide rational reasons for a treatment choice (S4) and to the impaired capacity of patients with moderate AD to identify the consequences of a treatment choice (S3). Finally, receptive aphasia and semantic memory loss (severe dysnomia) may be associated with the impaired ability of patients with advanced AD to evidence a simple treatment choice (S1). The results offer insight into the relationship between different legal thresholds of competency and the progressive cognitive changes characteristic of AD and represent an initial step toward a neurological model of competency (D. C. Marson et al., 1996; D. C. Marson, Cody, et al., 1995).

Consent Capacity in Patients With Parkinson's Disease and Dementia

Over the past decade, most competency research involving older adult populations has focused on AD (Kim et al., 2001; D. Marson, Earnst, et al., 2000; D. C. Marson, Ingram, et al., 1995; D. C. Marson, McInturff, et al., 1997; D. C. Marson et al., 1994). Relatively little attention had been given to consent capacity in patients with PD and its dementia syndrome. PD is one of the most prevalent and disabling of neurological disorders (Jacobs, Stern, & Mayeux, 1997); over time, patients become extremely incapacitated by their progressive motor and cognitive impairments (D. Marson & Dymek, in press). Impairment of medical decision-making capacity in PD and its dementia syndrome is likely to differ in important ways from that in AD because these two dementias have differing neuropathology and neurological substrates and cognitive, psychiatric, and motor features (Mahler & Cummings, 1990; Stern, Richards, Sano, & Mayeux, 1993). The prominence of motor dysfunction in PD has tended to obscure the contributions of cognitive change and dementia to patients' functional decline. In this regard, consent capacity is a competency that is particularly suitable for study in PD because it is primarily a verbally based construct (D. Marson & Dymek, in press).

Capacity performance and outcomes in patients
with Parkinson's disease and dementia

Twenty patients aged 60 years and older with idiopathic PD and cognitive impairment were recruited from the Movement Disorders Clinic at the University of Alabama at Birmingham (Dymek et al., 2001). Inclusion criteria for the PD group were (a) a positive diagnosis by a neurologist with expertise in movement disorders of idiopathic PD based on symptomatology, neurological examination, disease development, and positive response to antiparkinsonian medication; (b) patient- or caregiver-reported complaints of cognitive impairment in the PD patient; and (c) psychometric evidence of cognitive impairment, as measured by a Dementia Rating Scale (DRS) Total Score (Mattis, 1976) of 130 and below. All PD patients were taking antiparkinsonian medications.

Although a formal dementia diagnosis using *Diagnostic and Statistical Manual of Mental Disorders* (*DSM*) criteria (American Psychiatric Association, 1994) was not used in the study, most if not all of the PD patients were demented, as reported by the participating neurologist (Dr. Atchison, coauthor of the original study) and as reflected by the DRS Total Score mean of 117 (14.5 *SD*) (Dymek et al., 2001) (Table 11-4). Thus, the PD patient group in this study probably closely approximated how a formally diagnosed group of patients with Parkinson's disease dementia syndrome (PDDS) would perform. Accordingly, we reference the PD group as PDDS to reflect its probable dementia status.

As reflected in Table 11-4, the control and PDDS patients groups did not differ in years of education (Dymek et al., 2001). The PDDS group was older than the control group. The mean DRS Total Score of the PDDS group fell significantly below that of controls and reflected an overall mild level of dementia. The mean DRS Total Score of the older control group was indicative of normal cognitive function (Dymek et al., 2001).

The PDDS group performed significantly below the control group ($p < .05$) on all four core CCTI consent abilities: evidencing a choice, appreciating consequences, reasoning about treatment (rational reasons), and understanding treatment (S1, S3–S5) (Dymek et al., 2001; D. Marson & Dymek, in press). The patients with PDDS performed equivalently with controls only on the experimental consent ability of reasonable choice ([S2]) (Dymek et al., 2001).

Capacity status of patients with PDDS on the standards was classified (capable, marginally capable, incapable) using psychometric cutoff scores referenced to control group performance (D. C. Marson, Ingram, et al., 1995) (Table 11-5).

TABLE 11-4. Group Comparisons on Demographic, Dementia Screen, and Capacity to Consent to Treatment Instrument (CCTI) Consent Standard Variables

VARIABLE	OLDER CONTROLS ($N = 20$)		PDDS PATIENTS ($N = 20$)		F	p
	MEAN (*SD*)	RANGE	MEAN (*SD*)	RANGE		
Age	68.1 (5.8)	(60–79)	75.0 (7.5)	(63–86)	10.4	.003
Education	14.8 (2.3)	(9–18)	14.3 (3.1)	(9–20)	0.34	.56
DRS total score	141.2 (3.1)	(138–144)	117.3 (14.5)	(72–129)	51.8	.0001
S1 Evidencing choice	4.0 (0.0)	(4)	3.6 (0.8)	(1–4)	5.9	.020
[S2] reasonable choice	0.95 (0.2)	(0–1)	0.95 (0.2)	(0–1)	—	—
S3 appreciate consequences	8.9 (1.2)	(6–10)	7.5 (2.5)	(1–10)	5.7	.022
S4 reasoning about treatment	10.9 (3.7)	(6–21)	5.1 (3.2)	(1–11)	27.9	.000
S5 understanding treatment	59.0 (6.0)	(51–68)	36.8 (13.0)	(1–60)	47.8	.000

Note. Adapted from Dymek et al. (2001). Copyright 2001, AAN Enterprises Inc. Reprinted by permission. DRS, Dementia Rating Scale; PDDS, Parkinson's disease dementia syndrome.

Similar to patients with AD (see AD sections), patients with PD demonstrated a pattern of capacity compromise (defined as the combination of marginally capable and incapable outcomes) that related to stringency of the standard: [S2], 5%; S1, 30%; S3, 45%; S4, 55%; and S5, 80%.

Patients with PDDS demonstrated significant deficits across all four core CCTI capacity standards. The PDDS group demonstrated a trend toward poorer performance on the standards as their difficulty increased, with impairment greatest for the most complex and clinically challenging standards of reasoning and understanding. Similarly, capacity outcomes of the PDDS patients reflected a pattern of increasing compromise (marginally capable and incapable outcomes) across these four standards, ranging from 30% compromise on evidencing a choice (S1) to 80% compromise on understanding treatment (S5). Similar to findings in studies with patients with AD (D. C. Marson, Ingram, et al., 1995), it appears that these four standards may be hierarchical in difficulty for PDDS patients, with standards tapping reasoning (S4) and medical treatment information comprehension (S5) the most difficult and requiring a level of information retention and processing that may be beyond the capacity of many patients with PDDS.

TABLE 11-5. Experimental Capacity Outcomes by Capacity to Consent
to Treatment Instrument (CCTI) Standard and Patient Group

	CAPABLE	MARGINALLY CAPABLE	INCAPABLE
S1 evidencing choice			
Controls	20 (100%)	0 (0%)	0 (0%)
PDDS patients	14 (70%)	5 (25%)	1 (5%)
[S2] reasonable choice			
Controls	19 (95%)	—	1 (5%)
PDDS patients	19 (95%)	—	1 (5%)
S3 appreciate consequences			
Controls	17 (85%)	3 (15%)	0 (0%)
PDDS patients	11 (55%)	5 (25%)	4 (20%)
S4 reasoning about treatment			
Controls	20 (100%)	0 (0%)	0 (0%)
PDDS patients	9 (45%)	10 (50%)	1 (5%)
S5 understanding treatment			
Controls	20 (100%)	0 (0%)	0 (0%)
PDDS patients	4 (20%)	3 (15%)	13 (65%)

Note. From Dymek et al. (2001). Copyright 2001, AAN Enterprises Inc. Reprinted
by permission. Capable: For S3–S5, scores falling at or above 1.5 *SD* below the
control group mean on the S; for S1, a score of 4; for [S2], a score of 1. Marginally
capable: For S3–S5, scores falling between 1.5 and 2.5 *SD* below the control group
mean on the S; for S1, a score of 3; no marginally capable outcomes are possible
on [S2]. Incapable: For S3–S5, scores falling below 2.5 or more *SD* below the
control group mean on the S; for S1, a score of 0–2; for [S2], a score of 0.

*Cognitive predictors of consent capacity in Parkinson's disease
patients with dementia*

We were interested in identifying cognitive predictors of PDDS patient performance and outcome on the CCTI capacity standards. Tables 11-6 and 11-7
present the four strongest univariate correlates and the multivariate predictor of
PDDS patient performance and capacity outcome on three of the standards. No
neuropsychological measures correlated significantly ($p < .05$) with S3 or [S2]
on the univariate level (Dymek et al., 2001), and thus these two standards were
excluded from subsequent multivariate analyses, and no predictor models are
reflected in the two tables (Dymek et al., 2001).

The neuropsychological findings suggested that declines in executive functions, and to a lesser extent memory, are key neurocognitive changes associated
with competency loss in patients with PD (Dymek et al., 2001; D. Marson &
Dymek, in press). Executive dysfunction was closely associated with PDDS
patient performance on S5 (understanding treatment) and S4 (reasoning about

TABLE 11-6. Neuropsychological Predictors of Capacity Standard Performance for Parkinson's Disease Dementia Syndrome Patients ($n = 20$)

STANDARD VARIABLE(S)	PREDICTOR	UNIVARIATE CORRELATION		STEPWISE REGRESSION	
		r	p	$cumR^2$	p
S1 evidencing	DRS Memory	.73	.000	.55	.000[a]
choice	WAIS-R Comprehension	.67	.002		
	DRS Attention	.58	.008		
	EXIT 25	−.53	.02		
S4 rational	EXIT 25	−.67	.002	.45	.002[a]
reasons	Trails B	−.60	.005		
	DRS Attention	.58	.008		
	WMS-LM II	.48	.04		
S5 understanding	EXIT 25	−.75	.000	.56	.000[a]
treatment	DRS Memory	.71	.000	.68	.000[b]
	WAIS-R Comprehension	.70	.001		
	WMS-R LM II	.65	.002		

Note. From Dymek et al. (2001). Copyright 2001, AAN Enterprises Inc. Reprinted by permission. See text for definition of abbreviations

[a]Step 1.
[b]Step 2.

TABLE 11-7. Neuropsychological Predictors of Experimental Capacity Standard Outcomes in the PDDS Group

STANDARD	PREDICTOR VARIABLE(S)	CLASSIFICATION ACCURACY RATE,[a] %
S1 evidencing choice	DRS Memory	70
	DRS Memory/WAIS-R Comprehension	100
S4 rational reasons	EXIT 25	90
	EXIT 25/Trails B	95
S5 understanding treatment	EXIT 25	90
	EXIT 25/DRS Memory	95

Note. From Dymek et al. (2001). Copyright 2001, AAN Enterprises Inc. Reprinted by permission. See text for definitions of abbreviations.

[a]Percentage of capacity outcomes on each standard that were accurately classified by the respective neuropsychological predictor variable(s). As there are three outcomes (capable, marginally capable, incapable), a chance classification rate would be 33%.

treatment). Specifically, simple measures of executive function (EXIT 25) (Royall, Mahurin, & Gray, 1992) and memory (DRS Memory) (Mattis, 1976) predicted S5 performance, together accounting for 68% of score variance. Using the EXIT 25, nonparametric discriminant function analysis showed a very high classification rate of S5 competency outcomes (90%), which increased to 95% when both the EXIT 25 and DRS Memory were used. The EXIT 25 is a bedside test of simple executive abilities, including verbal and spatial fluency, inhibition, primitive reflexes, and set flexibility (Royall et al., 1992). DRS Memory is a composite measure of memory, consisting of short-term verbal recall items, orientation items, and verbal and visual recognition items (Mattis, 1976). Thus, basic executive and to a lesser extent memory functions appear to mediate the capacity of patients with PDDS to comprehend a treatment situation and choices. This finding was consistent with the task demands of S5, which require conceptual organization as well as recall of factually complex material (Dymek et al., 2001; Dymek, Marson, & Harrell, 1999).

Executive dysfunction was also closely associated with PDDS patient performance on S4 (reasoning). Again, the EXIT 25 was the key predictor of S4 performance, accounting for 45% of score variance. Using the EXIT 25, nonparametric discriminant function analysis showed a very high classification rate of S4 competency outcomes (90%), which increased to 95% when using both EXIT 25 and Trails B (Reitan, 1958). Trails B is a measure of visuomotor sequencing and set flexibility that is strongly associated with executive ability (Reitan, 1958). Thus, basic executive functions also appear to mediate the capacity of patients with PDDS to provide rational reasons for a choice of medical treatment. This finding was consistent with the task demands of S4, which require a subject to integrate information regarding two treatment choices and their risk/benefit profiles and to provide logical reasons (pro and con) for his or her treatment choice.

Simple memory and comprehension/judgment abilities were associated with PDDS patient performance on S1. As discussed, S1 is a minimal standard requiring only communication of a treatment choice. DRS Memory emerged as the only multivariate predictor of PDDS patients' S1 scores ($R^2 = .55$, $p = .000$), and it correctly classified 70% of patient competency outcomes. When DRS Memory was coupled with Wechsler Adult Intelligence Scale–Revised (WAIS-R) Comprehension, they together correctly classified 100% of S1 competency outcomes. These findings suggest that simple memory and comprehension/judgment deficits underlie the declining capacity of patients with PD simply to communicate a treatment choice (S1).

The available neuropsychological findings from this study are consistent with prior literature proposing a strong association between the frontal-subcortical disconnection syndrome of PD and executive dysfunction (Mahurin, Feher, Nance, Levy, & Pirozzolo, 1993; White, Au, Durso, & Moss, 1992). The most problematic CCTI standards were the reasoning and comprehension standards (S4 and S5), which are cognitively most complex (Dymek et al., 1999; D. C. Marson, Ingram, et al., 1995). Previous research has shown that patients with PD perform well on simple cognitive tasks, but as the task complexity increases, performance deteriorates, likely a result of impaired higher-order executive control of cognitive processes (Girotti et al., 1986; Gotham, Brown, & Marsden, 1988). The findings are also consistent with research on patients with frontal lobe dementia and significant executive dysfunction who show impaired decision-making capacity despite intact language, memory, perception, and absence of apraxia and agnosia (Schindler, Rachmandi, Matthews, & Podell, 1995). Thus, the findings of the present study point to important relationships in PD among cognitive impairment, executive dysfunction, and competency loss (Dymek et al., 2001; D. Marson & Dymek, in press).

CAPACITY TO MANAGE FINANCIAL AFFAIRS

Background

In this section, we discuss conceptual and empirical aspects of a second and very different civil competency: capacity to manage financial affairs (FC). Financial capacity comprises a broad range of conceptual, pragmatic, and judgment abilities critical to the independent functioning of adults in our society (D. Marson & Briggs, 2001; D. Marson, Sawrie, et al., 2000). As such, it differs in many respects from medical decision-making capacity, which is almost exclusively a verbally mediated capacity.

Epidemiological studies in the elderly have suggested that FC is an "advanced" ADL (Wolinsky & Johnson, 1991). The advanced ADLs are mediated by higher cognitive function and can be distinguished from "household" ADLs (e.g., meal preparation, shopping, housework) and "basic" ADLs (e.g., bathing, dressing, walking) (Wolinsky & Johnson, 1991). Financial capacity comprises a complex set of abilities, ranging from basic skills of identifying and counting coins/currency, to conducting cash transactions, to managing a checkbook and bank statement, to higher-level abilities of making investment decisions. As might be expected, such abilities can vary enormously across individuals, depending on a person's socioeconomic status, occupational attainment, and overall financial experience (D. Marson, 2001b; D. Marson & Briggs, 2001; D. Marson, Sawrie, et al., 2000). Along with medical decision making, driving, and mobility, FC is a vital aspect of individual autonomy in our society.

Loss of FC has a number of important consequences for dementia patients and families and important implications for health care and legal professionals (D. Marson, 2001b; D. Marson & Briggs, 2001; D. Marson, Sawrie, et al., 2000). First, loss of FC can have economic and household consequences. People suffering from dementia, such as AD, often have difficulties paying their bills and carrying out basic financial tasks (Overman & Stoudemire, 1988). They are continually at risk for making decisions that endanger assets needed for their own long-term care or intended for testamentary distribution to family members. Second, there are also important psychological consequences to FC loss. Much like loss of the car keys, loss of control over personal funds implicates a core aspect of personal independence in our society and can lead to depression and other significant psychological consequences (Moye, 1996). Third, loss of FC has clinical significance to health care professionals. Impairments in higher-order financial skills and judgment are often early functional changes demonstrated by dementia patients (D. Marson, Sawrie, et al., 2000) and some patients with MCI (Griffith et al., 2003). As discussed in the section on psychometric studies, research has demonstrated that patients suffering from mild AD demonstrate significant impairments in most financial activities and in many specific financial abilities (D. Marson, Sawrie, et al., 2000).

Fourth, declining FC is closely linked to legal issues of elder abuse (D. Marson, Sawrie, et al., 2000). Financial exploitation is an all-too-common form of elder abuse commonly associated with victims' diminished or impaired mental capacities (Nerenberg, 1996). There are daily media accounts of older adults victimized in consumer fraud and other scams (Bryant, 1996; Walton, 2002). Older adults can also be more covert victims of undue influence exercised by family members, professionals, and third parties (D. Marson, Huthwaite, & Hebert, 2004; Spar & Garb, 1992).

Finally, loss of FC can trigger important legal issues of guardianship and conservatorship (Grisso, 1986; D. Marson, Sawrie, et al., 2000). Disproportionately high numbers of older adults are subjects each year of conservatorship proceedings because of the high incidence of dementias and other mental and medical illnesses affecting financial competency in this age group (Grisso, 1986). These legal proceedings involve significant time and expense for families (D. Marson & Briggs, 2001).

Conceptual Model of Financial Capacity

Despite its clear relationship to everyday living and independence, there has been a surprising lack of conceptual and empirical study of FC. We present here a conceptual model of FC in older adults (D. Marson, Sawrie, et al., 2000; D. Marson & Zebley, 2001). This model has been the basis for instrument development and for ongoing studies of FC in AD and other clinical populations.

Because FC represents a broad continuum of activities and specific skills, it may be best conceptualized as a series of domains of activity that each have specific clinical relevance (D. Marson & Briggs, 2001; D. Marson, Sawrie, et al., 2000). Examples of these domains include handling basic monetary skills, carrying out cash transactions, managing a checkbook, and managing a bank statement. This domain-based approach is clinically oriented and is consistent with the presumed multidimensionality of FC and its variability across individuals. It is also consistent with the legal doctrine of limited financial competency adopted within most state legal jurisdictions, which recognizes that an individual may be competent to carry out some financial activities and not others (Grisso, 1986; D. Marson & Briggs, 2001; D. Marson, Sawrie, et al., 2000).

In addition to domains of activity, our model identifies specific financial abilities or tasks (D. Marson, 2001b; D. Marson, Sawrie, et al., 2000). Tasks reflect more basic financial skills that comprise domain-level capacities. For example, the domain of financial conceptual knowledge might draw on specific abilities such as understanding simple concepts like a loan or savings and pragmatically applying such concepts in everyday life (e.g., selecting interest rates, identifying a medical deductible, and making simple tax computations). The domain of financial judgment might consist of tasks related to detection/awareness of financial fraud or of making informed investment choices. Therefore, tasks represent abilities that constitute broader, clinically relevant domains of financial activity. We have defined tasks as simple or complex, depending on the level of cognitive resources they appear to require (D. Marson, 2001b; D. Marson, Sawrie, et al., 2000).

Our model also includes FC at the global level (Griffith et al., 2003; D. Marson & Zebley, 2001). Competency is ultimately an overall categorical judgment or classification made by a clinician or legal professional. Thus, the conceptual model of FC currently has three levels (Griffith et al., 2003): (a) specific financial abilities or tasks, each of which is relevant to a particular domain of financial activity; (b) general domains of financial activity, which are clinically relevant to the independent functioning of community-dwelling older adults; and (c) overall FC, which reflects a global measure of capacity based on the summation of domain- and task-level performance. Our conceptual model of FC currently comprises 9 domains, 18 tasks, and 2 global levels. It is presented in Table 11-8.

Psychometric Study of Financial Capacity in Alzheimer's Disease

In addition to the limited conceptual understanding of FC, until recently there have been few empirical studies (D. Marson & Briggs, 2001; D. Marson, Sawrie, et al., 2000). The Financial Capacity Instrument (FCI) is a psychometric instrument designed by our group to assess performance of older adults at the task, domain, and global levels of the conceptual model. The original FCI (FCI-6) assessed 6 domains and 14 tasks (Marson, Sawrie, et al., 2000) (the global level was introduced in later versions of the FCI as described in the section on FC in patients with MCI below).

TABLE 11-8. Revised Conceptual Model of Financial Capacity: Nine Domains and Eighteen Tasks

	TASK DESCRIPTION	TASK DIFFICULTY
Domain 1, Basic Monetary Skills		
Task 1a, naming coins/currency	Identify specific coins and currency	Simple
Task 1b, coin/currency relationships	Indicate relative monetary values of coins/currency	Simple
Task 1c, counting coins/currency	Accurately count groups of coins and currency	Simple
Domain 2, Financial Conceptual Knowledge		
Task 2a, define financial concepts	Define a variety of simple financial concepts	Complex
Task 2b, apply financial concepts	Practical application/computation using concepts	Complex
Domain 3, Cash Transactions		
Task 3a, one-item grocery purchase	Enter into simulated one-item transaction; verify change	Simple
Task 3b, three-item grocery purchase	Enter into simulated three-item transaction; verify change	Complex
Task 3c, change/vending machine	Obtain change for vending machine use; verify change	Complex
Task 3d, tipping	Understand tipping convention; calculate/identify tips	Complex
Domain 4, Checkbook Management		
Task 4a, understand checkbook	Identify and explain parts of check and check register	Simple
Task 4b, use checkbook/register	Enter into simulated transaction; pay by check	Complex

354

Domain 5, Bank Statement Management		
Task 5a, understand bank statement	Identify and explain parts of a bank statement	Complex
Task 5b, use bank statement	Identify specific transactions on bank statement	Complex
Domain 6, Financial Judgment		
Task 6a, detect mail fraud risk	Detect and explain risks in mail fraud solicitation	Simple
Task 6c, detect telephone fraud risk	Detect and explain risks in telephone fraud solicitation	Simple
Domain 7, Bill Payment		
Task 7a, understand bills	Explain meaning and purpose of bills	Simple
Task 7b, prioritize bills	Identify overdue utility bill	Simple
Task 7c, prepare bills for mailing	Prepare simulated bills, checks, envelopes for mailing	Complex
Domain 8, knowledge of assets/estate	Indicate/verify asset ownership, estate arrangements	Simple
Domain 9, investment decision making	Understand options; determine returns; make decision	Complex
Global 1, sum of Domains 1–7	Overall functioning across tasks and domains	Complex
Global 2, sum of Domains 1–8	Overall functioning across tasks and domains	Complex

Note. From Griffith et al. (2003). Copyright 2003, American Academy of Neurology. Reprinted by permission.

In an initial study, a sample of 23 older controls and 53 patients with AD (30 with mild dementia and 23 with moderate dementia) were administered the FCI-6 (Marson, Sawrie, et al., 2000). As shown in Table 11-9, we found that patients with mild AD performed equivalently with control subjects on Domain 1 (basic monetary skills), but significantly below controls on the other five domains. Patients with moderate AD performed significantly below controls and patients with mild AD on all domains. On the FCI tasks, patients with mild AD performed equivalently with controls on simple tasks such as naming coins/currency, counting coins/currency, understanding parts of a checkbook, and detecting risk of mail fraud. Those with mild AD performed significantly below controls on more complex tasks such as defining and applying financial concepts, obtaining change for vending machine use, using a checkbook, understanding and using a bank statement, and making an investment decision. Patients with moderate AD performed significantly below controls and patients with mild AD on all tasks (Marson & Briggs, 2001; Marson, Sawrie, et al., 2000).

Using a cut-score method derived from control performance (Marson & Briggs, 2001; Marson, Sawrie, et al., 2000), we translated the quantitative performance of the patients with AD into capacity outcomes (capable, marginally capable, incapable) on the domains. Table 11-10 presents capacity outcomes for the mild and moderate AD subgroups on the FCI-6 domains. In the context of a prototype instrument and small control sample, these outcomes should be interpreted cautiously. However, patients with mild AD demonstrated an interesting pattern of capacity loss across the domains. Although approximately 50% of patients with mild AD were found capable on Domains 1, 2, and 3, less than 30% were found capable on Domains 4 and 5 (checkbook management, bank statement management), and less than 15% were found capable on Domain 6 (financial judgment). These findings suggested that the FCI domains may form a hierarchy of difficulty for patients with mild AD. Moderate AD patients, in contrast, demonstrated very high rates of incapable outcomes on all FCI domains (range 90–100%). The relationship of the AD patients' dementia level to their capacity outcomes was statistically robust for all domains (Table 11-10) (Marson, Sawrie et al., 2000).

The findings from this initial study represented the first empirical effort to investigate loss of FC in patients with AD (Marson & Briggs, 2001). The findings suggested that, early in AD, there is significant impairment of FC. Patients with mild AD appeared to experience deficits in complex financial abilities (tasks) and some level of impairment in almost all financial activities (domains). Patients with moderate AD appeared to experience loss of both simple and complex financial abilities and severe impairment across all financial activities. Based on these initial findings, we proposed two preliminary clinical guidelines

TABLE 11-9. Financial Capacity Instrument 6 (FCI-6) Domain and Task Performance by Group

	SCORE RANGE	CONTROLS (n = 23)		MILD AD (n = 30)		MODERATE AD (n = 20)	
Domain 1, basic monetary skills	0–79	77.9[a]	(1.9)	75.5[c]	(3.5)	57.9	(16.3)
Task 1a, naming coins/ currency	0–30	30.0[a]	(0.0)	30.0[c]	(0.0)	26.7	(4.7)
Task 1b, coin/currency relationships	0–37	36.0[a]	(1.8)	34.0[c]	(3.0)	22.7	(9.2)
Task 1c, counting coins/ currency	0–12	11.9[a]	(0.3)	11.5[c]	(0.8)	8.6	(3.8)
Domain 2, financial concepts	0–41	35.5[a, b]	(2.7)	29.6[c]	(5.4)	19.1	(6.3)
Task 2a, defining concepts	0–16	13.0[a, b]	(1.9)	9.7[c]	(2.9)	7.1	(2.7)
Task 2b, applying concepts	0–25	22.5[a, b]	(1.4)	19.9[c]	(3.6)	12.0	(4.6)
Domain 3, cash transactions	0–48	46.2[a, b]	(2.7)	38.6[c]	(8.5)	22.2	(10.1)
Task 3a, one-item purchase	0–16	15.3[a]	(2.5)	14.4[c]	(3.2)	8.6	(4.9)
Task 3b, three-item purchase	0–16	15.2[a, b]	(1.3)	10.7[c]	(5.0)	4.6	(3.3)
Task 3c, change/vending machine	0–16	15.7[a, b]	(0.6)	13.6[c]	(2.8)	9.0	(4.1)
Domain 4, checkbook/register	0–62	60.2[a, b]	(2.1)	50.7[c]	(8.0)	33.3	(16.1)
Task 4a, understanding checkbook	0–32	30.7[a]	(1.5)	27.9[c]	(3.1)	20.6	(7.6)
Task 4b, using checkbook	0–30	29.5[a, b]	(1.5)	22.8[c]	(6.1)	12.2	(9.1)
Domain 5, bank statement	0–40	37.4[a, b]	(2.2)	28.6[c]	(7.6)	14.9	(7.2)
Task 5a, understanding bank statement	0–22	19.7[a, b]	(2.1)	15.0[c]	(4.1)	8.0	(3.6)
Task 5b, using bank statement	0–18	17.7[a, b]	(0.9)	13.6[c]	(4.3)	6.9	(4.1)
Domain 6, financial judgment	0–37	30.0[a, b]	(3.0)	20.8[c]	(5.4)	10.7	(5.1)
Task 6a, detecting fraud risk	0–10	8.6[a]	(2.0)	7.8[c]	(2.2)	6.9	(2.8)
Task 6b, investment decision	0–27	21.4[a, b]	(2.1)	13.0[c]	(4.4)	5.3	(3.5)

Note. From D. Marson, Sawrie, et al. (2000). Copyright 2000, American Medical Association. Reprinted by permission. AD, Alzheimer's disease.

[a]Normal control mean differs from moderate AD mean using least significant difference post hoc test ($p < .01$).

[b]Normal control mean differs from mild AD mean ($p < .01$).

[c]Mild AD mean differs from moderate AD mean ($p < .01$).

TABLE 11-10. Capacity Outcomes on Financial Capacity Instrument 6 (FCI-6) Domains Across Alzheimer's Disease (AD) Patient Subgroups

	CAPABLE		MARGINALLY CAPABLE		INCAPABLE		p^*
Domain 1, basic monetary skills							.0002
Mild AD patients	53%	(16/30)	17%	(5/30)	30%	(9/30)	
Moderate AD patients	10%	(2/20)	0%	(0/20)	90%	(18/20)	
Domain 2, financial concepts							.002
Mild AD patients	47%	(14/30)	13%	(4/30)	40%	(12/30)	
Moderate AD patients	5%	(1/20)	5%	(1/20)	90%	(18/20)	
Domain 3, cash transactions							.0002
Mild AD patients	47%	(14/30)	10%	(3/30)	43%	(13/30)	
Moderate AD patients	0%	(0/20)	0%	(0/20)	100%	(20/20)	
Domain 4, checkbook/register							.02
Mild AD patients	27%	(8/30)	13%	(4/30)	60%	(18/30)	
Moderate AD patients	0%	(0/20)	5%	(1/20)	95%	(19/20)	
Domain 5, bank statement							.003
Mild AD patients	27%	(8/30)	16%	(5/30)	57%	(17/30)	
Moderate AD Patients	0%	(0/20)	0%	(0/20)	100%	(20/20)	
Domain 6, financial judgment							.007
Mild AD patients	13%	(4/30)	37%	(11/30)	50%	(15/30)	
Moderate AD patients	0%	(0/18)	6%	(1/18)	94%	(17/18)	

Note. From D. Marson, Sawrie, et al. (2000). Copyright 2000, American Medical Association. Reprinted by permission.
*Significance of difference in capacity outcomes across dementia stage (mild vs. moderate AD) using chi square.

for assessment of FC in patients with mild and moderate AD (Marson, Sawrie, et al., 2000):

(1) Mild AD patients are at significant risk for impairment in most financial activities, in particular complex activities like checkbook and bank statement management. Areas of preserved autonomous financial activity should be carefully evaluated and monitored. (2) Moderate AD patients are at great risk for loss of all financial activities. Although each AD patient must be considered individually, it is likely that most moderate AD patients will be unable to manage their financial affairs. (p. 883)

Psychometric Study of Financial Capacity in Mild Cognitive Impairment

In a subsequent study, our group also examined FC in patients with MCI (Griffith et al., 2003). There is increasing evidence to support the existence of a preclinical phase in the development of AD (Collie & Maruff, 2000; Grady et al., 1988; Morris et al., 1993). The term MCI denotes a transitional phase between normal cognitive aging and dementia (Morris et al., 2001; Petersen et al., 2001). Diagnostic criteria for MCI remain controversial (Ritchie, Artero, & Touchon, 2001), and there may be different MCI subtypes (Petersen et al., 2001). *Amnestic MCI*, a prodromal condition involving memory loss and progressing over time to AD, is the most common and best-characterized form. Diagnostic criteria for amnestic MCI include (a) subjective complaints of memory loss, preferably confirmed by an informant; (b) objective impairment on memory testing compared to age and educational norms; (c) normal performance overall on general cognitive tests; and (d) generally preserved activities of daily living (Petersen et al., 2001).

The criteria requirement that patients with MCI not show any functional change has been challenged. There is emerging evidence that individuals with MCI do experience changes in everyday function prior to dementia diagnosis (Daly et al., 2000; Morris, 2002; Ritchie, Artero, & Touchon, 2001; Touchon & Ritchie, 1999). Such empirical findings make sense conceptually because MCI appears to be a dynamic transitional period throughout which cumulative cognitive and functional change presumably occur. Thus, although an individual at "entry" into MCI may have only focal memory impairment and little or no ADL impairment, the same individual at MCI "departure" (conversion to early AD) will have cognitive impairments beyond memory and notable declines in ADLs. A flexible approach to the diagnostic criteria appears increasingly indicated as it is often difficult on presentation to determine where on the MCI continuum an individual patient may be (Griffith et al., 2003).

To investigate functional change in MCI, our group believed that a cognitively complex IADL (instrumental activity of daily living) like FC would be a good place to focus. In addition, we also believed that using a standardized and normed psychometric measure like the FCI might reveal more subtle performance changes in the MCI group that might otherwise go undetected by conventional IADL rating forms.

As reflected in Table 11-11, the FCI-9 was administered to groups of older controls, patients with amnestic MCI, and patients with mild AD (Griffith et al., 2003). The groups were well matched on demographic variables of education, gender, race, and socioeconomic status (Griffith et al., 2003). At the domain level, using $p < .01$ for overall group effect, controls performed significantly better than mild AD subjects on all domains with the exception of Domain 6 (financial judgment) and Domain 8 (knowledge of assets/estate). Controls performed significantly better than the MCI group on Domains 2 (financial concepts), 5 (bank statement management), and 7 (bill payment). In turn, the MCI group performed significantly better than patients with mild AD, $p < .05$, on

TABLE 11-11. Comparisons of Group Performance on the Financial Capacity Instrument (FCI)

	SCORE RANGE	CONTROLS (n = 21) X (SD)	MCI PATIENTS (n = 21) X (SD)	AD PATIENTS (n = 22) X (SD)	P (TWO TAILED)	POST HOC $p < .05$
Domain 1, basic monetary skills	0–48	45.2 (3.5)	44.3 (3.7)	41.0 (6.3)	.011	C M > A
Naming coins/currency	0–8	7.9 (0.3)	7.8 (0.4)	7.6 (0.7)	.050	C > A
Coins/currency relationships	0–28	24.9 (3.4)	24.8 (3.5)	22.0 (5.5)	.044	—
Counting coins/money	0–12	12.0 (0.2)	11.7 (0.5)	11.5 (1.2)	.119	—
Domain 2, financial concepts	0–40	36.9 (3.2)	33.1 (4.7)	27.6 (7.5)	.001	C > M > A
Understanding concepts	0–15	13.8 (1.2)	12.9 (1.8)	11.2 (2.6)	.001	C M > A
Applying concepts	0–25	23.1 (2.4)	20.2 (3.6)	16.4 (5.3)	.001	C > M > A
Domain 3, cash transactions	0–30	27.0 (3.4)	24.8 (3.6)	20.6 (5.9)	.001	C M > A
One-item transaction	0–6	6.0 (0.0)	5.8 (0.6)	5.5 (1.1)	.044	C > A
Multiitem transaction	0–7	6.1 (1.9)	5.7 (1.8)	4.5 (2.4)	.037	C > A
Vending machine	0–9	8.6 (0.9)	8.0 (1.4)	5.6 (1.9)	.001	C M > A
Tipping	0–8	6.3 (1.7)	5.4 (1.5)	5.1 (2.1)	.068	—
Domain 4, checkbook management	0–54	53.2 (1.5)	50.6 (2.9)	42.9 (8.0)	.001	C M > A
Understanding checkbook	0–24	23.5 (0.8)	22.8 (1.5)	21.2 (2.5)	.001	C M > A
Using checkbook	0–30	29.6 (1.4)	27.9 (2.2)	21.7 (6.0)	.001	C M > A

	Range	Control M (SD)	MCI M (SD)	AD M (SD)	p	
Domain 5, bank statement management	0–38	35.2 (2.7)	29.9 (5.6)	23.3 (8.3)	.001	C > M > A
Understanding bank statement	0–18	16.2 (1.6)	13.4 (2.7)	10.6 (3.9)	.001	C > M > A
Using bank statement	0–20	19.1 (1.5)	16.5 (4.0)	12.7 (4.9)	.001	C > M > A
Domain 6, financial judgment	0–26	25.6 (1.2)	23.2 (3.7)	23.5 (3.5)	.029	C > M A
Mail fraud	0–8	8.0 (0.0)	7.3 (1.3)	7.1 (1.6)	.045	C > A
Telephone fraud	0–18	17.6 (1.2)	15.9 (3.0)	16.4 (2.3)	.051	—
Domain 7, bill payment	0–46	43.7 (3.3)	38.4 (6.2)	28.3 (9.6)	.001	C > M > A
Understanding bills	0–6	5.9 (0.4)	5.1 (1.2)	4.7 (1.6)	.006	C > M A
Identifying/prioritizing bills	0–13	12.6 (0.6)	12.3 (1.1)	10.9 (1.7)	.001	C M > A
Preparing bills for mailing	0–27	25.1 (3.3)	20.4 (6.1)	12.7 (8.4)	.001	C > M > A
Domain 8, assets and estate arrangements[a]	0–20	18.1 (1.6)	17.4 (2.6)	16.2 (2.8)	.068	—
Domain 9, investment decision making[b]	0–17	13.9 (2.9)	12.4 (2.3)	9.2 (3.5)	.001	C M > A
FCI total score (Domains 1–7)	0–282	266.8 (13.2)	243.8 (21.7)	207.2 (38.0)	.001	C > M > A
FCI total score (Domains 1–8)	0–302	282.1 (14.1)	264.0 (17.8)	223.8 (39.9)	.001	C M > A

Note. Adapted from Griffith et al. (2003). Copyright 2003, American Academy of Neurology. Reprinted by permission. AD, Alzheimer's disease; MCI, mild cognitive impairment. C > A, control mean is greater than AD mean; C > M > A, control mean is greater than MCI and AD means, and MCI mean is greater than AD mean; C > MA, control mean is greater than MCI and AD means; CM > A, control and MCI means are greater than AD mean.

[a]Control = 15, MCI = 13, AD = 21.
[b]Control = 21, MCI = 19, AD = 18.

Domains 1 (basic monetary skills), 2, 3 (cash transactions), 4 (checkbook management), 5, 7, and 9 (investment decision making). There were no domains on which the MCI group performed better than controls.

At the task level, controls performed significantly better than those in the mild AD group on most tasks, with the exception of simple tasks of basic monetary skills and cash transactions (Griffith et al., 2003). Controls performed significantly better than the MCI group on tasks of applying financial concepts, understanding and using a bank statement, understanding bills, and preparing bills for mailing. The MCI group in turn performed significantly better than the mild AD group on tasks of understanding and applying financial concepts, using a vending machine, understanding and using a checkbook, understanding and using a bank statement, prioritizing bills, and preparing bills for mailing, There were no tasks on which the MCI group performed better than controls.

For overall FC (Domains 1–7), control participants performed significantly better than MCI and AD participants, and MCI participants performed significantly better than AD participants. On an experimental measure of overall FC that included knowledge of assets and estate arrangements (Domains 1–8), smaller samples of control and MCI subjects performed significantly better than AD patients ($p < .001$), but did not differ significantly from each other.

This study represents one of the first published reports of psychometric evidence for higher-order functional decline and capacity loss in MCI (Griffith et al., 2003). Using a direct assessment approach, we found that patients with amnestic MCI demonstrated significant, albeit mild, declines on some (but not all) financial abilities compared to age, education, gender, and racially matched normal controls. MCI patients showed a decline in overall FC (Domains 1-7) of 1.74 *SD* units compared to control subjects (Table 11-11). These results strongly suggested that decline in financial abilities is an aspect of functional change in MCI (Griffith et al., 2003).

Summary of Financial Capacity Research

In summary, these two studies supported the value of the conceptual model and the FCI as new approaches for assessing FC in patients with neurodegenerative disease. The FCI represents a potential advance in functional assessment in dementia (Moye, 2003). It is specific to the construct of FC and is based on a model conceptualizing FC as a series of discrete spheres of activity (domains) linked to independent community function. The FCI operationalizes domains with actual tests of specific financial abilities (tasks) that are objective and behaviorally anchored. It also provides global estimates of FC useful to clinicians. Finally, the FCI has demonstrated initial construct validity by discriminating the financial performance and capacity outcomes of controls, patients with mild AD, and patients with moderate AD (Marson, Sawrie, et al., 2000) and the performance of controls, amnestic MCI patients, and mild AD patients (Griffith et al., 2003).

TESTAMENTARY CAPACITY

Background

In this section, we discuss conceptual and clinical aspects of a third civil competency: capacity to make a will (testamentary capacity). The freedom to choose how one's property and other possessions will be disposed of following death—known as the right of *testation*—is a fundamental right under Anglo-American law (Frolik, 2001; D. Marson et al., 2004). A key requirement of the law of testation is that a testator (person making the will) have *testamentary capacity* or *competency*: "that measure of mental ability which is recognized in law as sufficient for the making of a will" (Black, 1968, p. 1644). If testamentary capacity is lacking at the time of execution of the will, the will is invalid and void in effect (Perr, 1981). The legal requirement of testamentary capacity exists across all state jurisdictions.

To make a valid will, the law also requires that the testator be free from *undue influence* by another individual who may profit from a new will or a legal amendment of an existing will (codicil) (Spar, Hankin, & Stodden, 1995). Thus, a validly executed will may be voided by the court if the court deems that the volition of the testator was in effect supplanted by an individual exercising undue influence over him or her. The doctrine of undue influence, which also exists across state jurisdictions, is analytically distinct from testamentary capacity insofar as it applies in cases in which the testator possesses testamentary capacity (Frolik, 2001). Nonetheless, in the case of a will contest, these two legal issues often co-occur and intertwine.

Anglo-American law has strongly supported testation over intestacy (Frolik, 2001; D. Marson et al., 2004). Public policy and legal precedent have clearly favored allowing individuals to choose how their property will be distributed after death rather than leaving such decisions to state laws governing intestacy. However, despite the legal system's tendency to favor the rights of the testator, cases challenging the validity of wills and specifically the testamentary capacity or independent volition of testators are common and in fact appear to be increasing in number (Nedd, 1998). This increase in will contest litigation reflects a number of factors, particularly our aging society and increasing numbers of older adults with neurological, psychiatric, and medical impairments that adversely affect their mental capacities (D. Marson et al., 2004). Other factors include the breakdown of the nuclear family and increase in blended families with conflicting agendas and the enormous transfer of wealth currently ongoing between the World War II and baby boomer generations (Nedd, 1998).

Legal Elements of Testamentary Capacity

The current legal requirements for testamentary capacity in the United States vary to some degree from state to state, but in many states (although not all), four specific criteria or elements are recognized. A testator must (a) understand the nature of the testamentary act (i.e., know what a will is); (b) understand and recollect the nature and situation of his or her property; (c) have knowledge of the persons who are the natural objects of his or her bounty; and (d) know the manner in which the disposition of the property is to occur (D. Marson et al., 2004; Spar & Garb, 1992).

The way in which these elements are weighed by courts in determining the validity of a will varies across states (Frolik, 2001; Spar et al., 1995). Some states require that the testator meet only one of the criteria for a will to be valid; others require that the testator understand a will and demonstrate memory of all property and potential heirs and hold this information in mind while developing a plan for disposition of assets (Spar & Garb, 1992; Walsh et al., 1997).

In addition to the four elements mentioned, many states also require that the testator at the time the will is executed not exhibit delusions or hallucinations that result in a will that excludes or favors potential heirs based on false beliefs or is uncharacteristic of the testator's preferences in the absence of delusions and hallucinations (Spar & Garb, 1992; Walsh et al., 1997). However, a will may be ruled valid if delusions and hallucinations are discrete, unassociated with the testator's property and potential heirs, or have seemingly little or no impact on the testator's plan for the disposition of assets (D. Marson et al., 2004; Walsh et al., 1997).

Undue Influence and Testamentary Capacity

As mentioned, undue influence is a legal issue not only related to, but also distinct from, testamentary capacity. In situations of undue influence, the testator is at least marginally competent, but is subjected to direct or indirect coercion that subverts his or her volition and thus the validity of the will. The resulting will reflects the preferences of the coercing party rather than the testator, benefits the coercing party over other potential heirs, and is inconsistent with what the testator's wishes would be in the absence of this influence (Haldipur & Ward, 1996). Indicators of undue influence include the active participation of the coercing party in attaining a will or controlling the testamentary act, the role of the coercing party as an advisor or confidant to the testator and his or her use of this relationship to influence the way in which the testator disposed of his or her assets, and provisions within the will that are inconsistent with prior or subsequent expressions of the testator's intent in executing a will (Frolik, 2001; D. Marson et al., 2004).

Chronic physical and mental illness as well as memory loss and cognitive dysfunction associated with dementia often increase the dependency of older adults on others, thereby increasing their susceptibility to undue influence (Haldipur & Ward, 1996). Susceptibility to undue influence is not restricted to individuals who require assistance in their general care and decision making. As such, a will may also be ruled invalid by the courts even in the absence of medical or mental illness if other indicators of undue influence are present (Walsh et al., 1997).

Conceptual Basis of Testamentary Capacity

Currently, there is little or no published research investigating the conceptual or empirical bases of testamentary capacity (D. Marson et al., 2004). In part, this reflects the still-early developmental stage of the field of capacity assessment generally. With the exception of treatment consent capacity, for which there is now a reasonable body of research (Appelbaum & Grisso, 1995; Grisso & Appelbaum, 1995b; Grisso et al., 1995; Kim et al., 2001; D. C. Marson, Ingram, et al., 1995), relatively little conceptual and empirical research has been conducted thus far regarding other important civil competencies, such as FC (D. Marson, 2001b; D. Marson, Sawrie, et al., 2000).

However, this point notwithstanding, the area of testamentary capacity has been neglected. Although (as discussed below) there is literature providing general clinical guidelines and tips for assessment of testamentary capacity, there is currently no body of harder research that can inform and advance the field. Specifically, we have identified no cognitive or neuropsychological models, direct assessment instruments, or published empirical research in the psychological literature regarding either testamentary capacity or undue influence. Given the prevalence and importance of inheritance by will, this represents a key knowledge gap in neuropsychological forensic science as it relates to civil competencies and the elderly.

Some initial ideas for development of a cognitive conceptual model of testamentary capacity can be found in the legal and psychological literature. Walsh and colleagues, in conjunction with the American Bar Association, identified several factors required for the determination of testamentary capacity as defined in medical terms (Walsh et al., 1997). These are "functional autonomy, working memory, orientation, attention, and calculation" (§2.08, pp. 2–20 to 2–21). Likewise, research on medical decision making and FC found correlations between these civil competencies and performance on neuropsychological measures of conceptualization, calculation, semantic memory, verbal recall, and executive function, particularly word fluency (D. Marson, Sawrie, Stalvey, McInturff, & Harrell, 1998; D. C. Marson et al., 1996; D. C. Marson, Cody, et al., 1995).

However, there are no data in literature that specifically correlate performance on neuropsychological measures with testamentary capacity. Neuropsychological testing is useful in measuring specific cognitive skills, but can only indirectly measure the specific functional elements for executing a will. As such, further research is needed to identify the neuropsychological functions most strongly associated with each element of testamentary capacity and to develop a strong theoretical model of testamentary capacity that takes into consideration both legal and medical perspectives.

Thus, a starting point for addressing this theoretical gap would be to develop a cognitive (neuro)psychological model for the legal elements of testamentary capacity. Our capacity research group has begun work in this area and offers the following preliminary discussion concerning hypothesized cognitive components for each the four legal elements of testamentary capacity (D. Marson et al., 2004). These are outlined next.

1. *Cognitive Functions Related to Understanding the Nature of a Will.* This element requires a testator to understand the purposes and consequences of a will, and to express these verbally or in some other adequate form to an attorney or judge. Possible cognitive functions involved may include semantic memory regarding terms such as death, property and inheritance, verbal abstraction and comprehension abilities, and sufficient language abilities to express the testator's understanding. Recognition items may assist a testator with expressive language problems. A reply of "Yes" or "No" to an attorney's queries regarding the nature of a will is unlikely to be satisfactory in this regard as such responses do not clearly support the testator's independent understanding of the element. Similarly, a testator's signature on a legal document by itself does not demonstrate understanding because a signature is an automatic procedural behavior not dependent on higher-level cognition (Greiffenstein, 1996).

2. *Cognitive Functions Related to Knowing the Nature and Extent of Property.* The second legal element of testamentary capacity requires that the testator remember the nature and extent of his or her property to be disposed. As reported in this section, some states differ in their interpretation of this (Walsh et al., 1997, §2.04 Variation in Requirements, pp. 2–13). Possible cognitive functions involved here would include semantic memory concerning assets and ownership, historical memory and short-term memory enabling recall of long-term and more recently acquired assets and property, and comprehension of the value attached to different assets and property. If the testator has recently purchased new possessions prior to his or her execution of a will, then impairment in short-term memory (the hallmark sign of early AD) can significantly impact his or her recall of these items. Testators also must be able to form working estimates of value for key pieces of property that reasonably approximate their true value; it is likely that executive function abilities play a role here.

3. *Cognitive Functions Related to Knowing the Objects of One's Bounty.* This legal element requires that the testator be cognizant of those individuals who represent his or her natural heirs or other heirs who can place a reasonable

claim on the estate. Historical and short-term episodic personal memory of these individuals, and of the nature of their relationships with the testator, would appear to be prominent cognitive abilities associated with this element. As dementias like AD progress, testators may be increasingly unable to recall family members and acquaintances, leading ultimately to failure to recognize these individuals in photographs or even when presenting in person.

4. *Cognitive Functions Related to a Plan for Distribution of Assets.* This final legal element of testamentary capacity requires that the testator be able to express a basic plan for distributing his or her assets to his or her intended heirs. Insofar as this element integrates the first three elements in a supraordinate fashion, the proposed cognitive basis for this element arguably represents an integration of the cognitive abilities underlying the other three elements. Accordingly, higher-order executive function abilities are implied as the testator must demonstrate a projective understanding of how future dispositions of specific property to specific heirs will occur.

The preliminary cognitive psychological model of testamentary capacity proposed here represents a first step toward model building in this area. Such a model would require empirical verification in an older adult sample through use of a relevant testamentary capacity instrument and neuropsychological test measures. However, as suggested, there is currently a lack of psychological assessment instruments specific to this domain of forensic practice (but in the legal sphere, refer to the Legal Capacity Questionnaire (Walsh et al., 1997, §1.10, pp. 1–17 to 1–22). As testamentary capacity matures as an area of civil competency practice and research, it is anticipated that conceptually based assessment instruments will emerge.

Prototype Assessment Instrument for Testamentary Capacity

As discussed, no standardized psychological measures of testamentary capacity currently are available. A psychometric instrument currently in development by our research group is the Testamentary Capacity Instrument (TCI; Marson & Hebert, 2004). The TCI is a structured, psychometric measure for assessing and differentiating the testamentary capacity of cognitively intact versus cognitively impaired older adults.

The TCI measures capacity according to the four legal elements of testamentary capacity discussed in the preceding section. Performance on each element is based on the individual's ability to recall or recollect information pertinent to the execution of a will. The degree to which memory for relevant information is required by law varies (Walsh et al., 1997). For this reason, each of the four elements is measured using free recall, multiple-choice, and forced-choice items. An individual who may not be able to recall information pertinent to a legal element freely may still be able to identify this information accurately in a

recognition or forced-choice (yes/no or true/false) format. All items are administered verbally and in writing and are scored according to a quantitated scoring
system. The scoring system in turn supports three judgment outcomes for testamentary capacity: capable, marginally capable, and incapable. In this regard, the
TCI outcomes are similar (although not identical) to those for the Legal Capacity Questionnaire (see preceding section).

The TCI also has separate sections that support guided questioning regarding
the potential occurrence of lucid intervals, the presence of delusions/hallucina-
tions impacting testamentary capacity, and the testator's susceptibility to undue
influence.

Although if necessary the TCI is designed to be a stand-alone assessment, its
administration to an older adult testator should ideally co-occur with a comprehensive neuropsychological evaluation. The latter cognitive and emotional test
data will provide an important overall context for the evaluation and can help
inform specific testamentary capacity findings as well as the clinician's overall
judgment of capacity.

Standardized assessment of testamentary capacity involves certain methodological challenges that require attention (D. Marson et al., 2004). Unlike
knowledge of a will, information concerning a testator's assets/property, his or
her natural heirs, and his or her plan of distribution is individual specific and
not as readily amenable to standardized inquiry across patients/clients. Accordingly, it is very important to obtain accurate information regarding the testator's
property and heirs from reliable collateral sources to evaluate and verify the
testator's responses to questions tapping these three legal elements. Thus, the
TCI explicitly seeks collateral information for all four legal elements.

However, collateral sources sometimes may have limited or inaccurate information regarding the testator's assets or relationships with potential heirs. In
addition, collateral sources may have potential conflicts of interest insofar as
they are often also prospective heirs of the testator. Such conflicts of interest
may thus bias responses of collateral sources to inquiries regarding the testator's
assets and heirs, as well as regarding the testator's general cognitive function,
psychiatric health, and quality of relationships with other prospective heirs.
These issues obviously require application of clinical judgment by the examiner
in selecting collateral sources and using the TCI and related instruments.

Clinical Assessments of Testamentary Capacity

Current mental health practice in cases of testamentary capacity can be divided
into two major areas: clinical interviews of living testators and family members
contemporaneous with a will execution (Spar & Garb, 1992) and retrospective
analyses of testamentary capacity and undue influence in cases involving a now-

deceased or incompetent testator (Greiffenstein, 1996; D. Marson et al., 2004). In each of these areas, current practice patterns vary quite widely in approach and quality, in large part because of uneven conceptual understanding among many practitioners of capacity assessment generally (D. Marson, 2001a; D. C. Marson & Harrell, 1996) and of the legal requirements of testamentary capacity and undue influence specifically.

Contemporaneous assessment of testmentary capacity

In certain circumstances, an attorney or a judge, or a family member, may request that a mental health professional assess the capacity of a living testator prior to his or her execution of a will. Two common scenarios underlie such a referral. The attorney or judge may have concerns about the testamentary capacity of the proposed testator and therefore will seek clinical expertise and input on the issue before proceeding further. Alternatively, in cases of ongoing or anticipated family conflict, the foresighted attorney may seek to preempt a future will contest by having a client undergo a capacity assessment prior to will execution.

Spar and colleagues have written on the topic of contemporaneous clinical assessment of testamentary capacity and undue influence (Spar & Garb, 1992; Spar et al., 1995). Their clinical interview guidelines for testamentary capacity published in 1992 continue to represent a key contribution to forensic practice in this area. The key aspects of the interview are to "assess the legal elements of testamentary capacity, identify any features of the testator's personality and mental status that could affect susceptibility to undue influence, and determine the nature, extent, and general functional consequences of mental illness, if any" (pp. 171–172). The authors highlighted the importance of conducting the clinical interview close to the moment the testamentary document is executed. Interviews conducted close to the time of testamentary document execution are more likely to be influential in court than those conducted at more distant time periods. This consideration is important as courts generally place great emphasis on the testator's mental functioning at the time in question and recognize that individuals' mental functioning can vary at different time points (*Allen v. Sconyers*, 1995).

A second and perhaps more difficult challenge for the clinical examiner is to obtain as much information as possible about the testator's possessions and names and relationships of potential heirs to the testators (D. Marson et al., 2004). This can be a difficult task when the testator's informants are limited to family members who serve to profit from the examiner's testimony. An objective source of information regarding a testator's potential heirs and possessions is strongly recommended, but may not always be practical. A private interview with only the testator is recommended to limit outside influences. A videotaped recording of the interview with the testator may prove beneficial for illustrating the lack of outside influences; however, this should first be discussed with the testator's attorneys.

Retrospective assessment of testamentary capacity

Although direct, contemporaneous evaluations of testamentary capacity are desirable and useful, they probably do not represent the majority of forensic evaluations in this area (D. Marson et al., 2004). More often than not, neuropsychologists and other mental health professionals are called on by attorneys for or against the will/estate, by the probate court, or by interested family members to examine indirect evidence and render retrospective opinions regarding testamentary capacity and, if applicable, regarding undue influence. Retrospective evaluations of testamentary capacity arise after the death (or sometimes the incompetency) of a testator when heirs or other interested parties contest a will on grounds that the decedent lacked testamentary capacity at the time of will execution. Although recognized by courts, no clear rules for conducting such evaluations have been established (Spar & Garb, 1992).

The process of retrospective evaluation has sometimes been described as a "neuropsychological autopsy" (Greiffenstein, 1996), and neuropsychological methods and knowledge can be particularly useful for these purposes (D. Marson, 2002). Greiffenstein has proposed several steps for determining testamentary capacity retrospectively (Greiffenstein, 1996). First, the clinician should consider whether the legal issue at hand pertains to testamentary capacity, undue influence, or both. Next, the date of the legal transaction should be identified because this date will help determine the relevance of contemporaneous mental status and medical and lay testimony evidence. This is typically the date in which the will was signed. The clinician must also identify the type of neurological or psychiatric disorder that the testator had and determine which, if any, cognitive abilities were impacted. This is done by gathering evidence of normal and abnormal cognitive and emotional behavior occurring as close as possible to the date of will execution.

There are a number of information sources that can assist a clinician in making an indirect assessment of testamentary capacity (Spar & Garb, 1992). These include the testator's business records, checkbook and other financial documents, and personal documents such as family films, videos, notebooks, and diaries. Medical records yield particularly useful information, including mental status and neuropsychological testing, diagnosis, level of impairment, and behavioral observations. Clinicians may also find it beneficial to interview the testator's family, friends, business associates, and other involved professionals (i.e., physician, attorney, accountant, notary public, etc.) regarding the testator's cognitive and functional abilities during the time that the will was executed.

Neuropsychologists may also seek to rely on information collected from dementia staging instruments, such as the Clinical Dementia Rating scale and the
Global Deterioration Scale (Morris, 1993; Reisberg, Ferris, deLeon, & Crook,
1982). In cases of Alzheimer's type dementia, these scales permit the clinician
to assess dementia stage retrospectively based on the contemporaneous mental
status and behavioral evidence in the record. For example, a clinician may determine from such evidence that a patient with AD was functioning at Global
Deterioration Scale Stage 6. Such individuals may occasionally forget the name
of the spouse on whom they are entirely dependent for survival, are largely
unaware of all recent events and experiences in their lives, and have very
sketchy knowledge of their past lives (Reisberg et al., 1982). Such specific
staging information will be very useful to a clinician seeking to determine
whether an individual during this time had testamentary capacity or another type
of legal capacity. Thus, dementia stage in turn becomes an evidentiary source
that clinicians and probate courts can both use in making retrospective capacity
determinations.

Ultimately, the clinician must assemble all of the information described here
and make judgments and offer testimony as to whether the testator had testamentary capacity or was subject to undue influence at the prior relevant time
points. In some cases, it may not be possible to render such judgments if there
is insufficient evidence of the testator's cognitive, emotional, and functional
abilities contemporaneous with the prior will execution.

SUMMARY

In this chapter, we examined conceptual, empirical, and clinical aspects of competency loss in dementia by focusing on three specific civil competencies: treatment consent capacity, FC, and testamentary capacity. It should be apparent that
our group has used AD, and to a lesser extent PD with dementia, as the clinical
context for understanding loss of competency. By virtue of its relentless progressive nature, AD is perhaps the most useful prism with which to begin to understand relationships between abnormal cognition and loss of decisional capacity.
At the same time, it must be acknowledged that some of the reported study
results may be quite specific to the AD or PD context and may not always
necessarily generalize well to other dementias (Dymek et al., 2001) or to normal
aging. For this reason, it is very important to understand how cognitive changes
in other neurodegenerative diseases such as Huntington's disease, amyotrophic
lateral sclerosis, or multiple sclerosis, acquired disorders such as severe traumatic brain injury or cerebrovascular accident, and dementing processes such as
vascular dementia may also affect different competencies (Dymek et al., 2001;
Marson & Dymek, in press). In addition, normal age-related cognitive changes

may affect higher-order functional capacities like consent capacity and FC (Diehl, Willis, & Schaie, 1995; Park, 1992; Willis, 1996). Little is known about whether and to what extent such normative age-related changes may affect the competency of nondemented older adults. Thus, studies using different age cohorts of normal adults, as well as patient groups with neurodegenerative diseases and dementias other than AD and PD, are necessary to expand our understanding of competency in dementia and in normal aging.

ACKNOWLEDGMENT

The work in this chapter was supported in part by an Alzheimer's Disease Center Core grant (National Institutes of Health [NIH], NIA 1 P30 AG10163) (L. Harrell, primary investigator) and an Alzheimer's Disease Research Center grant (NIH, NIA 1P50 AG16582) (L. Harrell, primary investigator) from the National Institute on Aging; a grant from the National Institute of Mental Health (NIH, NIMH 1 R01 MH55427); and grants from the Alzheimer's Association (IIRG 93-051 and PRG-91-122) (D. Marson, primary investigator) and the Alzheimer's Disease Cooperative Study (NIH, NIA AG 10483-12) (L. Thal, primary investigator).

REFERENCES

Alexander, M. (1988). Clinical determination of mental competence. *Archives of Neurology*, *45*, 23–26.

Allen v. Sconyers, So.2d (Vol. 669, p. 113): Alabama (1995).

American Psychiatric Association. (1994). *Diagnostic and statistical manual of mental disorders* (4th ed.). Washington, DC: American Psychiatric Association.

Appelbaum, P., & Grisso, T. (1988). Assessing patients' capacities to consent to treatment. *New England Journal of Medicine, 319*, 1635–1638.

Appelbaum, P., & Grisso, T. (1995). The MacArthur Treatment Competence Study. I: Mental illness and competence to consent to treatment. *Law and Human Behavior, 19*, 105–126.

Appelbaum, P., & Gutheil, T. (1991). *Clinical handbook of psychiatry and the law* (2nd ed.). Baltimore: Williams and Wilkins.

Appelbaum, P., & Roth, L. (1981). Clinical issues in the assessment of competence. *American Journal of Psychiatry, 138*, 1462–1467.

Barberger-Gateau, P., Dartigues, J., & Letenneur, L. (1993). Four Instrumental Activities of Daily Life score as predictor of 1-year incident dementia. *Age and Aging, 22*, 457–463.

Benton, A., & Hamsher, K. (1978). *Multilingual aphasia examination*. Iowa City, IA: University of Iowa.

Black, H. (1968). *Black's Law Dictionary* (4th ed.). St. Paul, MN: West.

Bryant, W. (1996, March 3). Woman out $5,300 in two cons. *Birmingham News*, p. A15.

Butters, M., Salmon, D., & Butters, N. (1994). Neuropsychological assessment of dementia. In M. Storandt & G. VandenBos (Eds.), *Neuropsychological assessment of demen-*

tia and depression in older adults: A clinician's guide (pp. 33–59). Washington, DC: American Psychological Association.

Collie, A., & Maruff, P. (2000). The neuropsychology of preclinical Alzheimer's disease and mild cognitive impairment. *Neuroscience and Biobehavioral Reviews, 24,* 365–374.

Cummings, J., & Benson, D. (1992). *Dementia: A clinical approach.* Stoneham, MA: Butterworth.

Cummings, J., Vinters, H., Cole, G., & Khachaturian, Z. (1998). Alzheimer's disease: Etiologies, pathophysiology, cognitive reserve, and treatment opportunities. *Neurology, 51*(Suppl. 1), S2–S17.

Daly, E., Zaitchik, D., Copeland, M., Schmahmann, J., Gunther, J., & Albert, M. (2000). Predicting conversion to Alzheimer disease using standardized clinical information. *Archives of Neurology, 57,* 675–680.

Diehl, M., Willis, S., & Schaie, K. (1995). Everyday problem solving in older adults: Observational assessment and cognitive correlates. *Psychology and Aging, 10,* 478–491.

Drachman, D., Swearer, J., & Group, C. S. (1993). Driving and Alzheimer's disease: The risk of crashes. *Neurology, 43,* 2448–2456.

Dymek, M., Atchison, P., Harrell, L., & Marson, D. (2001). Competency to consent to treatment in cognitively impaired patients with Parkinson's disease. *Neurology, 56,* 17–24.

Dymek, M. P., Marson, D. C., & Harrell, L. (1999). Factor structure of capacity to consent to medical treatment in patients with Alzheimer's disease: An exploratory study. *Journal of Forensic Neuropsychology, 1,* 27–48.

Edelstein, B., Nygren, M., Northrop, L., Staats, N., & Pool, D. (1993, August). *Assessment of capacity to make medical and financial decisions.* Paper presented at the 101st Annual Convention of the American Psychological Association, Toronto, Ontario, Canada.

Eisenson, J. (1954). *Examining for aphasia.* New York: Psychological Corporation.

Emre, M. (2003). What causes mental dysfunction in Parkinson's disease? *Movement Disorders, 18*(Suppl. 6), S63–S71.

Farnsworth, M. (1990). Competency evaluations in a general hospital. *Psychosomatics, 31,* 60–66.

Flesch, R. (1974). *The art of readable writing.* New York: Harper and Row.

Folstein, M., Folstein, S., & McHugh, P. (1975). Mini-Mental State: A practical guide for grading the cognitive state of the patient for the physician. *Journal of Psychiatry Research, 12,* 189–198.

Frolik, L. (2001). The strange interplay of testamentary capacity and the doctrine of undue influence: Are we protecting older testators or overriding individual preferences? *International Journal of Law and Psychiatry, 24,* 253–266.

Girotti, G., Grassi, M., Carella, F., Soliveri, P., Musicco, M., Lamperti, E., et al. (1986). Possible involvement in attention processes in Parkinson's disease. In M. Yahr & K. Bergmann (Eds.), *Advances in neurology* (pp. 425–429). New York: Raven Press.

Gotham, A., Brown, R., & Marsden, C. (1988). "Frontal" cognitive functions in patients with Parkinson's disease "on" and "off" levodopa. *Brain, 111,* 199–231.

Grady, C., Haxby, J., Horowitz, M., Sundaram, M., Berg, E., Schapiro, M., et al. (1988). Longitudinal study of the early neuropsychological and cerebral metabolic changes in dementia of the Alzheimer's type. *Journal of Clinical and Experimental Neuropsychology, 10,* 576–596.

Greiffenstein, M. (1996). The neuropsychological autopsy. *Michigan Bar Journal*, *75*(5), 424–425.

Griffith, H., Belue, K., Sicola, A., Krzywanski, S., Zamrini, E., Harrell, L., et al. (2003). Impaired financial abilities in mild cognitive impairment: A direct assessment approach. *Neurology*, *60*, 449–457.

Grisso, T. (1986). *Evaluating competencies: Forensic assessments and instruments*. New York: Plenum Press.

Grisso, T., & Appelbaum, P. (1991). Mentally ill and non-mentally ill patients' abilities to understand informed consent disclosure for medication. *Law and Human Behavior*, *15*, 377–388.

Grisso, T., & Appelbaum, P. (1995a). A comparison of standards for assessing patients' capacities to make treatment decisions. *American Journal of Psychiatry*, *19*, 149–166.

Grisso, T., & Appelbaum, P. (1995b). The MacArthur Treatment Competence Study. III: Abilities of patients to consent to psychiatric and medical treatments. *Law and Human Behavior*, *19*, 149–169.

Grisso, T., Appelbaum, P., Mulvey, E., & Fletcher, K. (1995). The MacArthur Treatment Competence Study. II: Measures of abilities related to competence to consent to treatment. *Law and Human Behavior*, *19*, 127–148.

Haldipur, C., & Ward, M. (1996). Competence and other legal issues. In M. Hersen & V. Van Hasselt (Eds.), *Psychological treatment of older adults: An introductory text* (pp. 103–125). New York: Plenum Press.

High, D. (1992). Research with Alzheimer's disease subjects: Informed consent and proxy decision-making. *Journal of the American Geriatric Society*, *40*, 950–957.

Hunt, L., Murphy, C., Carr, D., Duchek, J., Buckles, V., & Morris, J. (1997). Reliability of the Washington University Road Test: A performance-based assessment for drivers with dementia of the Alzheimer type. *Archives of Neurology*, *54*, 707–712.

Jacobs, D., Stern, Y., & Mayeux, R. (1997). Dementia in Parkinson's disease, Huntington's disease, and other degenerative conditions. In T. Feinberg & M. Farah (Eds.), *Behavioral neurology and neuropsychology* (pp. 579–587). New York: McGraw-Hill.

Janofsky, J., McCarthy, R., & Folstein, M. (1992). The Hopkins Competency Assessment Test: A brief method for evaluating patients' capacity to give informed consent. *Hospital and Community Psychiatry*, *43*, 132–136.

Kaplan, E., Goodglass, H., & Weintraub, S. (1983). *Boston Naming Test*. Philadelphia: Lea and Febiger.

Kapp, M. (1992). *Geriatrics and the law: Patient rights and professional responsibilities*. New York: Springer.

Kim, S., Caine, E., Currier, G., Leibovici, A., & Ryan, M. (2001). Assessing the competence of persons with Alzheimer's disease in providing informed consent for participation in research. *American Journal of Psychiatry*, *158*, 712–717.

Mahler, M., & Cummings, J. (1990). Alzheimer disease and the dementia of Parkinson disease: Comparative investigations. *Alzheimer Disease and Associated Disorders*, *4*(3), 133–149.

Mahurin, R., Feher, E., Nance, M., Levy, J., & Pirozzolo, F. (1993). Cognition in Parkinson's disease and related disorders. In R. Parks, R. Zec, & R. Wilson (Eds.), *Neuropsychology of Alzheimer's disease and other dementias* (pp. 247–268). New York: Oxford University Press.

Marson, D. (2001a). Loss of competency in Alzheimer's disease: Conceptual and psychometric approaches. *International Journal of Law and Psychiatry*, *8*, 109–119.

Marson, D. (2001b). Loss of financial capacity in dementia: Conceptual and empirical approaches. *Aging, Neuropsychology and Cognition, 8,* 164–181.

Marson, D. (2002, October). *CME Workshop: Assessment of civil competencies in the elderly: Theory, research, and clinical case studies.* Paper presented at the 22nd Annual Conference of the National Academy of Neuropsychology, Miami, Florida.

Marson, D., & Briggs, S. (2001). Assessing competency in Alzheimer's disease: Treatment consent capacity and financial capacity. In S. Gauthier & J. L. Cummings (Eds.), *Alzheimer's disease and related disorders annual 2001* (pp. 165–192). London: Dunitz.

Marson, D., & Dymek, M. (in press). Competency in patients with Parkinson's disease and dementia. *Ethics, Law, and Aging.*

Marson, D., Earnst, K., Jamil, F., Bartolucci, A., & Harrell, L. (2000). Consistency of physicians' legal standard and personal judgments of competency in patients with Alzheimer's disease. *Journal of the American Geriatrics Society, 48,* 911–918.

Marson, D., & Hebert, K. (2004). Assessment of testamentary capacity in older adults: A conceptual model and prototype instrument. Manuscript in preparation.

Marson, D., Huthwaite, J., & Hebert, K. (2004). Testamentary capacity and undue influence in the elderly: A jurisprudent therapy perspective. *Law and Psychology Review, 28,* 71–96.

Marson, D., & Ingram, K. (1996). Competency to consent to treatment: A growing field of research. *Journal of Ethics, Law, and Aging, 2,* 59–63.

Marson, D., Sawrie, S., Snyder, S., McInturff, B., Stalvey, T., Boothe, A., et al. (2000). Assessing financial capacity in patients with Alzheimer's disease: A conceptual model and prototype instrument. *Archives of Neurology, 57,* 877–884.

Marson, D., Sawrie, S., Stalvey, T., McInturff, B., & Harrell, L. (1998, February). *Neuropsychological correlates of declining financial capacity in patients with Alzheimer's disease.* Platform presentation at the 26th Annual Meeting of the International Neuropsychological Society, Honolulu, HA. [Abstract published in *Journal of the International Neuropsychological Society, 4,* 37 (1998).]

Marson, D., & Zebley, L. (2001). The other side of the retirement years: Cognitive decline, dementia, and loss of financial capacity. *Journal of Retirement Planning, 4*(1), 30–39.

Marson, D. C., Chatterjee, A., Ingram, K. K., & Harrell, L. E. (1996). Toward a neurologic model of competency: Cognitive predictors of capacity to consent in Alzheimer's disease using three different legal standards. *Neurology, 46,* 666–672.

Marson, D. C., Cody, H. A., Ingram, K. K., & Harrell, L. E. (1995). Neuropsychologic predictors of competency in Alzheimer's disease using a rational reasons legal standard. *Archives of Neurology, 52,* 955–959.

Marson, D. C., & Harrell, L. E. (1996). Decision making capacity: In reply. *Archives of Neurology, 53,* 589–590.

Marson, D. C., & Harrell, L. E. (1999). Neurocognitive models that predict physician judgments of capacity to consent in patients with mild Alzheimer's disease. In D. Park, R. Morrell, & K. Shifrin (Eds.), *Medical information processing and aging* (pp. 109–126). New York: Erlbaum.

Marson, D. C., Hawkins, L., McInturff, B., & Harrell, L. E. (1997). Cognitive models that predict physician judgments of capacity to consent in mild Alzheimer's disease. *Journal of the American Geriatrics Society, 45,* 458–464.

Marson, D. C., Ingram, K. K., Cody, H. A., & Harrell, L. E. (1995). Assessing the competency of patients with Alzheimer's disease under different legal standards. *Archives of Neurology, 52,* 949–954.

Marson, D. C., McInturff, B., Hawkins, L., Bartolucci, A., & Harrell, L. E. (1997). Consistency of physician judgments of capacity to consent in mild Alzheimer's disease. *Journal of the American Geriatrics Society*, *45*, 453–457.

Marson, D. C., Schmitt, F., Ingram, K. K., & Harrell, L. E. (1994). Determining the competency of Alzheimer's patients to consent to treatment and research. *Alzheimer's Disease and Associated Disorders*, *8*(Suppl. 4), 5–18.

Mattis, S. (1976). Dementia rating scale. In R. Bellack & B. Karasu (Eds.), *Geriatric psychiatry*. New York: Grune & Stratton.

McKhann, G., Drachman, D., Folstein, M., Katzman, R., Price, D., & Stadlan, E. (1984). Clinical diagnosis of Alzheimer's disease: Report of the NINCDS-ADRDA work group under the auspices of the Department of Health and Human Services Task Force on Alzheimer's disease. *Neurology*, *34*, 939–944.

Morris, J. (1993). The Clinical Dementia Rating (CDR): Current version and scoring rules. *Neurology*, *43*, 2412–2414.

Morris, J. (2002). Challenging assumptions about Alzheimer's disease: Mild cognitive impairment and the cholinergic hypothesis. *Annals of Neurology*, *51*(2), 143–144.

Morris, J., Edland, S., Clark, C., Galasko, D., Koss, E., Mohs, R., et al. (1993). The consortium to establish a registry for Alzheimer's disease (CERAD). Part IV. Rates of cognitive change in the longitudinal assessment of probable Alzheimer's disease. *Neurology*, *43*, 2457–2465.

Morris, J., Storandt, M., Miller, J., McKeel, D., Price, J., Rubin, E., et al. (2001). Mild cognitive impairment represents early stage Alzheimer's disease. *Archives of Neurology*, *58*, 397–405.

Moye, J. (1996). Theoretical frameworks for competency in cognitively impaired elderly adults. *Journal of Aging Studies*, *10*, 27–42.

Moye, J. (2003). Guardianship and conservatorship. In T. Grisso (Ed.), *Evaluating competencies: Forensic assessments and instruments* (2nd ed., pp. 309–390). New York: Plenum Press.

Nedd, H. (1998, July 30). Fighting over the care of aging parents: More siblings clashing over money and control. *USA Today*, p. 1A.

Nerenberg, L. (1996). *Financial abuse of the elderly*. Washington, DC: National Center on Elder Abuse.

Overman, W., & Stoudemire, A. (1988). Guidelines for legal and financial counseling of Alzheimer's disease patients and their families. *American Journal of Psychiatry*, *145*, 1495–1500.

Park, D. (1992). Applied cognitive aging research. In F. Craik & T. Salthouse (Eds.), *Handbook of aging and cognition* (pp. 449–493). Hillsdale, NJ: Erlbaum.

Perr, I. (1981). Wills, testamentary capacity and undue influence. *Bulletin of the American Academy of Psychiatry and the Law*, *9*(1), 15–22.

Petersen, R., Doody, R., Kurz, A., Mohs, R., Morris, J., Rabins, P., et al. (2001). Current concepts in mild cognitive impairment. *Archives of Neurology*, *58*, 1985–1992.

Reisberg, B., Ferris, S., deLeon, M., & Crook, T. (1982). The Global Deterioration Scale for assessment of primary degenerative dementia. *American Journal of Psychiatry*, *139*, 1136–1139.

Reitan, R. (1958). Validity of the Trail Making Test as an indication of organic brain damage. *Perceptual and Motor Skills*, *8*, 271–276.

Ritchie, K., Artero, S., & Touchon, J. (2001). Classification criteria for mild cognitive impairment: A population based validation study. *Neurology*, *56*, 37–42.

Roth, L., Meisel, A., & Lidz, C. (1977). Tests of competency to consent to treatment. *American Journal of Psychiatry, 134,* 279–284.

Royall, D., Mahurin, R., & Gray, K. (1992). Bedside assessment of executive cognitive impairment: The Executive Interview. *Journal of the American Geriatrics Society, 40,* 1221–1226.

Schindler, B., Rachmandi, D., Matthews, M., & Podell, K. (1995). Competency and the frontal lobe: The impact of executive dysfunction on decisional capacity. *Psychosomatics, 36,* 400–404.

Sherlock, R. (1984). Competency to consent to medical care: Toward a general view. *General Hospital Psychiatry, 6,* 71–76.

Spar, J., & Garb, A. (1992). Assessing competency to make a will. *American Journal of Psychiatry, 149,* 169–174.

Spar, J., Hankin, M., & Stodden, A. (1995). Assessing mental capacity and susceptibility to undue influence. *Behavioral Sciences and the Law, 13,* 391–403.

Stern, Y., Richards, M., Sano, M., & Mayeux, R. (1993). Comparison of cognitive changes in patients with Alzheimer's disease and Parkinson's disease. *Archives of Neurology, 50,* 1040–1045.

Tepper, A., & Elwork, A. (1984). Competency to consent to treatment as a psychological construct. *Law and Human Behavior, 8,* 205–223.

Touchon, J., & Ritchie, K. (1999). Prodromal cognitive disorder in Alzheimer's disease. *International Journal of Geriatric Psychiatry, 14,* 556–563.

Walsh, A. C., Brown, B. B., Kaye, K., & Grigsby, J. (1997). *Mental capacity: Legal and medical aspects of assessment and treatment* (2nd ed.). Deerfield, IL: Clark, Boardman, and Callaghan.

Walton, V. (2002, February 2). Con man sentenced to 20 years. *Birmingham News,* pp. 11A–12A.

White, R., Au, R., Durso, R., & Moss, M. (1992). Neuropsychological function in Parkinson's disease. In R. White (Ed.), *Clinical syndromes in adult neuropsychology: The practitioner's handbook.* New York: Elsevier Science.

Willis, S. (1996). Everyday cognitive competence in elderly persons: Conceptual issues and empirical findings. *The Gerontologist, 36,* 595–601.

Wolinsky, F., & Johnson, R. (1991). The use of health services by older adults. *Journal of Gerontology: Social Sciences, 46,* 345–357.

Woods, S., & Troster, A. (2003). Prodromal frontal/executive dysfunction predicts incident dementia in Parkinson's disease. *Journal of the International Neuropsychology Society, 9,* 17–25.

12

Criminal Forensic Neuropsychology and Assessment of Competency

ROBERT L. DENNEY

Clinical neuropsychologists provide unique services in a wide variety of settings. Although the idea of forensic neuropsychological practice may bring to mind involvement in personal injury and other civil tort cases, there are a growing number of clinical neuropsychologists providing services to participants in criminal forensic proceedings as well (Giuliano, Barth, Hawk, & Ryan, 1997). This trend is understandable given the apparent higher rates of brain injury among criminal populations (Martell, 1992a). Borum and Grisso (1995) surveyed test use in criminal forensic evaluations and found 46–50% of forensic psychologists indicated they used some type of neuropsychological assessment in their pretrial evaluations. Mittenberg, Patton, Canyock, and Condit (2002) presented the results of a national survey of board certified neuropsychologists regarding the estimated base rates of symptom exaggeration and malingering. The 131 survey respondents indicated they completed a total of 33,531 annual evaluations. Of these evaluations, 34% were considered forensic in nature (19% personal injury, 11% disability/workers' compensation, and 4% criminal litigation. This 4% constituted 1,341 criminally related forensic evaluations per year for just 131 practitioners. One could argue this sample is a unique subset of neuropsychology practitioners; nevertheless, the information reveals the reality that neuropsychology has something to contribute to criminal forensic matters (Denney & Wynkoop, 2000; Martell, 1992b).

Clinical neuropsychology's involvement in the criminal judicial system is understandable because the field has much to contribute when issues of cognition compromising central nervous system pathologies arise. Neuropsychologists can bring to the judicial system their understanding of neuroanatomy, neuropathology and most important, how neuropathological conditions affect thinking skills and decision-making capacity (Bigler & Clement, 1997; Lezak, 1995).

No less important is neuropsychology's ability to identify when unusual behaviors are not caused by neuropathological conditions. The obvious example is feigning of deficits, but nonneuropathological conditions come to play as well, such as psychopathy, other personality disturbances, and general psychiatric concerns. Ruling out neurocognitive deficits in nonneurological conditions is just as important as identifying the presence of potentially disabling neurocognitive concerns. Further, such evaluations can delineate neurocognitive functioning when diagnostic issues other than neuropathology exist, such as developmental and psychiatric conditions.

Criminal courts need clear understanding regarding a defendant's cognitive functioning when there is concern that it may be compromised. It has been long held that the U.S. Constitution requires defendants to have adequate understanding and the ability to aid in their own behalf when facing criminal proceedings affecting their "liberty or life" (*Youtsey v. United States*, 1899).

Under the U.S. Constitution, society can deprive people of their liberty only under two doctrines, *police power* and *parens patriae*. *Parens patriae* refers to the government looking after the citizen's welfare in a parental role. An example includes civil commitment procedures for mental health treatment. Police power is, of course, the criminal justice system. The U.S. Constitution outlines minimal acceptable rights for citizens of the United States under federal and state laws. States can always provide more personal rights than dictated by the U.S. Constitution, but not less.

The aspects of the Constitution most relevant for practitioners interfacing with the criminal justice system are the 5th, 6th, and 14th Amendments. The 5th Amendment includes the right to be free from self-incrimination. The 6th Amendment guarantees the right to counsel and representation. The 14th Amendment establishes that everyone will have equal protection under the law. Last, both the 5th and 14th Amendments declare that no one will lose "life, liberty, or property" without due process of the law.

Constitutional guidelines have tremendous implication for the practice of neuropsychology in criminal areas. For example, due process requires a mentally competent defendant. Aside from mental competency, there are other times during criminal proceedings when courts can benefit from neuropsychological expertise, such as mental state of the defendant at the time of the crime, mitigating issues and treatment needs to consider at the time of sentencing, and prerelease assessment of potential increased dangerousness. Participants in the criminal judicial system can benefit from the input of neuropsychology, but neuropsychologists need to understand the unique aspects of forensic work in the criminal setting and have specialized knowledge and techniques for competent practice (Melton, Petrila, Poythress, & Slobogin, 1997; Sullivan & Denney, 2003).

The goal of this chapter is to provide neuropsychological practitioners with an introductory understanding of issues involved in practicing in the criminal forensic arena in general and the assessment of competency to stand trial in particular. Chapter 13 continues the introduction by focusing on assessment of criminal responsibility, diminished capacity and responsibility, dangerousness assessment, death penalty, and ethical and professional development issues.

CRIMINAL FORENSICS AS A SUBSPECIALTY
OF FORENSIC NEUROPSYCHOLOGY

In the "Petition for the Recognition of Forensic Psychology as a Specialty in Professional Psychology," the American Board of Forensic Psychology and American Psychology–Law Society jointly defined forensic psychology in this manner (Forensic Specialty Council, 2000):

[Forensic psychology is] the professional practice by psychologists within the areas of clinical psychology, counseling psychology, neuropsychology, and school psychology, when they are engaged regularly as experts and represent themselves as such, in an activity primarily intended to provide professional psychological expertise to the judicial system. (p. 6)

Under this definition, forensic neuropsychology could be viewed as a specialty area within clinical neuropsychology. Neuropsychologists can provide expertise to the judicial system in civil as well as criminal areas. In this regard, the application of neuropsychological expertise to criminal forensic matters could be considered a subspecialty of forensic neuropsychology. Although good clinical neuropsychological skill and expertise form the basis of sound practice, forensic neuropsychology, particularly criminal forensic matters, requires understanding of a unique knowledge domain beyond that of sound clinical practice (Denney & Wynkoop, 2000; Martell, 1992b; Sullivan & Denney, 2003).

FORENSIC NEUROPSYCHOLOGY
AS A UNIQUE PRACTICE SETTING

There are striking differences between neuropsychology practice in the general clinical setting and that of the forensic setting, particularly the criminal realm. Goals of the two specialties, by definition, differ greatly. For example, the goal of clinical evaluation is most often alleviation of human suffering and improvement of levels of functioning through evaluation and development of efficient intervention. With the exception of treatment recommendations, the goal of forensic evaluation is most often to determine whether a defendant's psychological problems meet a specific legal standard. These disparate goals create different assumptions, roles, alliances, and methods (Denney & Wynkoop, 2000; Goldstein, 2003; Greenberg & Shuman, 1997; Heilbrun, 2001).

Assumptions

In clinical practice, neuropsychologists assume, for the most part, that patients voluntarily seek help because they want relief from bothersome symptoms. There is often a diagnosable condition that occasions the service, whether the service is assessment or intervention. Certainly, within the neurorehabilitation setting, an alliance is built. The overriding theme is one of collaboration, mutual goals, and belief. Criminal defendants are often not self-referred, or even voluntary, recipients of services. In many instances, they may not have a psychological or neuropsychological complaint. In addition, the possibility of harsh punishment can create tremendous motivation to manipulate the evaluator and judicial system (Rogers, 1997). It is counterproductive to assume defendants have neurocognitive deficits, want help for deficits, or will present themselves in an honest manner within such a harsh and potentially punitive setting. It is no surprise, then, that these differences in assumptions result in different roles for neuropsychologists.

Roles

There are striking differences between the roles of clinical provider and forensic examiner. Heilbrun (2001) outlined differences between the roles of forensic examiner and treatment clinician. As can be seen from Table 12-1, the differences between the two roles reveal themselves in a variety of attitudes and behaviors. The clinical provider maintains a role consistent with helping the patient. Rather than patient–helper, however, the forensic evaluator maintains a more neutral role, a role consistent with being a "seeker of truth" and judicial educator (Greenberg & Shuman, 1997; Saks, 1990). It can often be a difficult role to maintain. The evaluator should realize his or her opinion has the potential to do significant harm, particularly from a standard psychotherapeutic mindset. Potential consequences can be great. Probably the most serious example includes capital cases, for which the evaluator must provide an opinion on competence to be executed. A neuropsychologist who is uncomfortable with the task of being an unbiased seeker of truth should avoid forensic practice.

Alliance

Developing therapeutic alliances with neurorehabilitation patients is required for successful rehabilitation outcomes. Sohlberg and Mateer (2001) went so far as to

TABLE 12-1. Differences Between Treatment and Forensic Roles
for Mental Health Professionals

DIMENSION	THERAPEUTIC	FORENSIC
Purpose	Diagnose and treat symptoms of illness	Assist decision-maker or attorney
Examiner–examinee relationship	Helping role	Objective or quasi-objective stance
Notification of purpose	Implicit assumptions about purpose shared by doctor and patient	Formal and explicit notification
Who is being served	Individual patient	Variable; may be court, attorney, and patient
Nature of standard considered	Medical, psychiatric, neuropsychological	Medical, psychiatric, neuropsychological, and legal
Data sources	Self-report, behavioral observations, medical diagnostic procedures, and neuropsychological testing; occasional corroborative information	Self-report, behavioral observations, medical diagnostic procedures, and neuropsychological testing; nearly always incorporate corroborative and surreptitious observation by others
Response style of examinee	Assumed to be predominantly reliable	Not assumed to be reliable
Clarification of reasoning and limits of knowledge	Optional	Very important
Written report	Brief, conclusory statement common	Lengthy and detailed, documents findings, reasoning, and conclusions
Court testimony	Not expected	Expected

Note. From Heilbrun (2001, p. 9). Copyright 2001 by Kluwer Academic/Plenum Publishing. Adapted with permission.

include it as a basic principle of cognitive rehabilitation. They noted, "Cognitive rehabilitation requires a sound therapeutic alliance among the therapist, client, and family members or care givers" (p. 21). A therapeutic alliance allows the therapist to foster motivation and hopefulness on behalf of the patient (Parenté & Herrmann, 1996). Forensic evaluations are not therapeutic endeavors. As such, the forensic examiner's allegiance is with finding the truth in a thorough, ethical manner.

Relatedly, it must be remembered who is the recipient of these services. In general clinical work, the patient is clearly the recipient. In this manner, the patient is the client. The client role is less clear in forensic endeavors. Forensic examiners must realize the patient is generally not the client. More typically, the recipient of services, particularly evaluative services, is the court (and by extension, the jury) or attorney. Other distinctions between the two roles are presented in Table 12-1.

Lack of therapeutic alliance in forensic evaluation does not, however, eliminate the need to develop rapport with the defendant or to treat him or her with dignity and respect. Rapport fosters self-disclosure and motivation to perform during neuropsychological testing, and appropriate motivation and effort are the bane of neuropsychology (Hom & Denney, 2002). It is possible to maintain a professional and ethical relationship while maintaining the strict boundaries of the forensic evaluation process. The difference in alliance between clinical and forensic evaluations is exemplified in the absence of confidentiality in criminal forensic practice. Issues of confidentiality are addressed in the Ethical and Professional Issues section of chapter 13, this volume.

Methodology

Given the different assumptions, roles, and alliances, it is no surprise competent and ethical forensic evaluation requires somewhat different methodology from that of routine clinical practice. Clinical practice typically incorporates an interview with the patient, and perhaps an informant familiar with the patient, and neuropsychological testing to characterize the patient's difficulties or to arrive at a diagnosis and make treatment recommendations. The entire process is designed to provide assistance to the patient, his or her caregivers, and medical managers in a timely fashion. Forensic assessment requires a broader base of information sources than is typical of clinical practice.

The evaluator must also place more weight on objective test results than subjective complaints, self-report checklists, and behavior during clinical interviews. Systematic assessment of negative response bias and malingering is a necessity in the criminal forensic setting. Surreptitious observation can be invaluable, particularly when signs of poor motivation or symptom exaggeration exist (Denney & Wynkoop, 2000; Wynkoop & Denney, 1999). The evaluator must carry out the evaluation much like a detective would attempt to sleuth out the truth. It can take time to locate and review past medical and educational records and interview others familiar with the defendant.

Nonetheless, this "search for truth" requires the forensic psychologist to gather information from a wide variety of sources aside from the defendant and to consider more critically the defendant's self-report. Along with specialized knowledge domains, the contrast in methodology between clinical and forensic practice is a major difference between specialties. This difference in theoretical basis necessitates a broader model of practice.

Denney and Wynkoop (2000) adapted Mrad's (1996) multiple data source model (MDSM) to the practice of criminal forensic neuropsychology. The model represents a synthesis of various authors in forensic psychology (Grisso, 1988; Melton et al., 1997; Shapiro, 1984, 1991, 1999), particularly related to the assessment of sanity (and other past mental states). The model is represented in Figure 12-1. Although designed to guide the evaluator in tapping all relevant information sources for identifying a defendant's mental state at the time of the offense, it is also helpful as a general model of forensic assessment. The model ensures the evaluator will acquire corroborative information rather than relying on the defendant's self-report and presentation during interviews and testing.

The first two columns represent sources of information (self-report and corroborative), which when combined can lead to an understanding of mental state. Each row represents a different point in time (currently, historically, and a specific time in the past). There should be reasonable consistency between each of the columns and rows. The model is discussed more thoroughly as it relates to sanity in chapter 13, this volume. It can be quite helpful in the assessment of competency as well because it facilitates information acquisition from objective information sources, particularly when dealing with retrospective competency.

The following case exemplifies the need to acquire corroborative information about the defendant's past behavior. It also demonstrates how evaluations for competency can lead to complicated additional judicial inquiries. The case started out as a reasonably simple evaluation for competency to be sentenced, but it quickly evolved into an evaluation of past competency to stand trial and sanity.

"Where's the Video?": A Case of Vital Corroborative Data

A 70-year-old man with diabetes was convicted by a jury of gambling and money laundering. After his conviction, defense acquired a mental health evaluation by a neuropsychiatrist in preparation for diminished capacity arguments during sentencing. The neuropsychiatrist found signs of periventricular white matter changes on magnetic resonance imaging and concluded the man was not competent to be sentenced. The court referred him for inpatient mental health evaluation to address competency to proceed with sentencing.

During this evaluation more than one of his recent attorneys and the defendant's wife (a codefendant also convicted) reported him having terrible debilitation, particularly at the time of the recent trial. The case became quite complicated because new charges were brought against the man for jury tampering and obstruction of justice secondary to allegations he contacted and attempted to manipulate a juror during the recent trial. The judge in charge of the jury tampering/obstruction case requested a mental health evaluation focused on criminal responsibility. Both issues were addressed during the same inpatient evaluation, with reports going to separate courts.

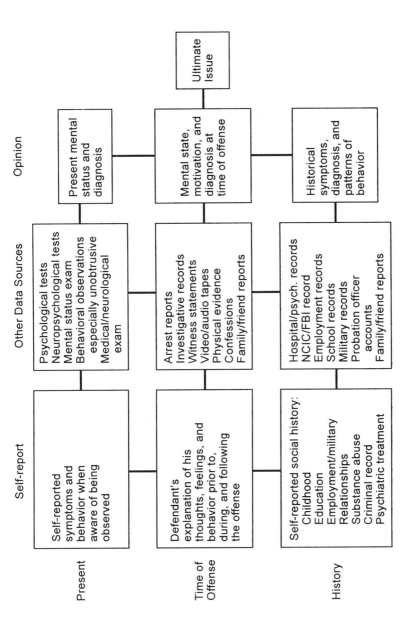

Figure 12-1. Multiple data source model. Reproduced with permission of David Mrad, Ph.D.

Neuropsychological testing revealed only minor bilateral motor slowing. All other results, including measures of attention, concentration, learning, memory, and abstract reasoning, were in the range of average to slightly above average given his age and educational background. Regarding his current functioning, I considered him competent to proceed, but the issue was much more complicated regarding his past mental state.

Regarding the time of the trial, I received a great deal of information from the defense attorney and very little information from prosecution beyond basic investigative material, including the contacted juror statements and the defendant's private investigator's statements. This man assisted the defendant in acquiring personal information about the juror. Available information suggested a combination of uncontrolled insulin-dependent diabetes mellitus, recent subcortical strokes, stress of the trial, and depression resulted in some level of cognitive compromise at the time of the trial. I provided this opinion regarding his appreciation of the wrongfulness of contacting a juror (sanity):

There is evidence of mental illness or defect at the time [of the alleged offense]. . . . Although his judgment was impacted to a degree, he was not so incapacitated by illness as to cause him to not understand what he was doing or what was going on around him. On the contrary, his behavior as outlined in the investigative reports suggested he made comments and acted in a manner consistent with someone who knew their actions were wrong and/or potentially illegal.

As a result of my opining that the defendant had "some amount of incapacity at the time," defense now claimed he was incompetent during past trial and counsel was ineffective by not noticing this fact. The first court then requested a retrospective competency evaluation to determine if he was, in fact, competent to stand trial during the jury trial in which he was convicted on gambling and money laundering.

During this evaluation, striking new information came to light. During the lengthy trial process, the defendant was out of jail on bond and living at his home. In his free time, he was carrying out real estate transactions, and the other businessperson with whom he was interacting described his negotiation and financial analysis skills as "good as always."

More striking yet was the fact he was going through divorce proceedings in a local court during the same week as the criminal trial. When he was not in federal court, he was in divorce court. His divorce attorney was one of the attorneys claiming how impaired he was during the criminal trial. The best part was the fact that this particular divorce court videotaped all its proceedings. On several videotapes, dated the same week and interspersed with court appearances in the criminal trial, the defendant was vigorously questioned by his attorney regarding real estate property lines and property values while pointing out boundaries on a map. He was able to follow rapid-fire questioning and respond quickly. The were no signs of cognitive compromise on these tapes.

Last, and even more astounding, was the acquisition of court transcripts of a postconviction detention hearing at which the defendant's attorney (the very one claiming how incompetent he was during the trial) was arguing before the court that the court should release the defendant on bond because his assistance was needed in preparation for sentencing. The attorney actually made statements to the effect that he expected the defendant to continue working on the case as well as he did during the trial and that his help had been invaluable; he was like having a "paralegal."

All of this new information flew in the face of my previous opinion that he demonstrated some cognitive deficits during the trial. My opinion changed, and I explained in the report how the new information had an impact on my reasoning. The defendant was found by the court to have been competent during the trial. This case demonstrates how easy it is to come to a determination and only later find out vital information had not been received. Solid corroborative information regarding defendant behavior during examination of mental state at the time of the offense is vital in nearly any circumstance, but particularly when there is documented presence of potentially debilitating disease.

This case demonstrates the complexity of neuropsychological assessment in the criminal forensic setting. Using the multiple data source model as a template to ensure information from all relevant areas should increase diagnostic clarity and provide the needed information to address forensic questions competently. Even having the appropriate information, however, will not facilitate the evaluator making a correct formulation about forensic questions if he or she does not understand the correct legal standards relevant to that forensic question. I now turn to one of the most commonly encountered legal issues, criminal competency.

CRIMINAL COMPETENCIES

Competency is broadly considered the capacity to decide or perform certain functions. From a legal perspective, a large portion of the concept of competency includes the cognitive construct of "knowledge." It implies a person's understanding of issues pertaining to participation in a specific legal proceeding (Reisner & Slobogin, 1990). This understanding includes some sense of appreciation for such issues as nature of the procedure, risks, likelihood of success, available alternative options and strategies, and relative advantages/disadvantages of potential courses of action.

The issue of competency can arise during any phase of the criminal judicial process, from the first contact a suspect has with law enforcement to the time of sentencing and even to the point of execution in capital cases. Table 12-2 presents an overview of these points, with brief descriptions (Grisso, 1988).

Threshold to Seek Competency Evaluation

Competency evaluations are the most commonly requested mental health studies in criminal forensics. Defense attorneys typically raise the issue of a defendant's competency to proceed; however, prosecutors and judges (in what is termed *sua sponte*) can raise the issue as well. When defense counsel raises the issue, often it is over the objection of the defendant. This event places the defense attorney in a unique ethical position between fulfilling the wishes of the client and also protecting his or her constitutional right to a fair trial. It also strains the attorney–client relationship (Melton et al., 1997).

Steadman, Monahan, Hartstone, Davis, and Robbins (1982) found that 6,500 defendants were adjudicated not competent to stand trial and committed to public mental institutions for treatment in 1978. They estimated this result came

TABLE 12-2. Specific Competencies in the Criminal Justice Process

COMPETENCY TO	GENERAL ISSUE IN QUESTION
Confess (or to waive rights at pretrial investigations)	Understanding and appreciation of rights to silence and legal counsel when the rights may be waived at the request of law enforcement investigators seeking a self-incriminating statement
Plead guilty	Understanding and appreciation of above and of the right to a jury trial, the right to confront one's accusers, and the consequences of a conviction
Waive right to counsel	Understanding and appreciation of the dangers of self-representation at trial
Stand trial	Ability to assist an attorney in developing and presenting a defense and to understand the nature of the trial and its potential consequences
Be sentenced	Understanding and appreciation of nature of the sentence to be imposed (after trial has resulted in conviction)
Waive further appeal (when facing an execution)	Understanding and appreciation of right for additional appeal and potential consequences of waiving it
Be executed	Understanding and appreciation of nature and purpose of the punishment, and ability to assist counsel in any available appeal

Note. Competency to Stand Trial Evaluations: A Manual for Practice (p. 3), by T. Grisso, 1988, Sarasota, FL: Professional Resource Press. Copyright 1988 by Professional Resource Exchange, Inc. Reprinted with permission. The wording of these definitions does not conform to prevailing legal terminology. The definitions are intended only to convey the general issues raised in each specific competency.

from 25,000 requested competency evaluations. Hoge and colleagues (1997) cited a personal communication from Thomas Grisso regarding information derived from a 50-state survey (Grisso, Cocozza, Steadman, Fisher, & Greer, 1994) in which state forensic directors were asked to estimate the number evaluations of competency to stand trial performed. The total estimate was from 24,000 to 39,000 studies. It is not surprising that so many competency evaluations are done in the United States as the threshold to raise concern over competency is quite low, as revealed by the U.S. Supreme Court in *Pate v. Robinson* (1966) and *Drope v. Missouri* (1975).

Theodore Robinson was found guilty of murder and sentenced to life in prison by the Illinois state court. Although his attorney contended throughout the court proceedings that Robinson was not competent to proceed and was insane at the time of the offense and Robinson's relatives and family friend testified during the trial that he was insane, the trial court never stopped the trial to have him examined for competence. Robinson's history included significant childhood traumatic brain injury, subsequent erratic behavior, and state hospitalization as an adult for psychotic behavior. It was later argued that Robinson "deliberately waived the defense of his competence to stand trial by failing to demand a [competency] hearing as provided by Illinois law" (*Pate v. Robinson*, 1966, p. 821). The U.S. Supreme Court responded, "It was contradictory to argue that a defendant may be incompetent, and yet knowingly or intelligently 'waive' his right to have the court determine his capacity to stand trial" (p. 821). The High Court concluded the trial court's failure to address the competency issue deprived him of his right to a fair trial. The Court went on to conclude that a hearing on competency should occur whenever the evidence raises a "bona fide doubt" as to the defendant's competency.

The U.S. Supreme Court considered this issue further in the interesting case of *Drope v. Missouri* (1975). James Drope was charged with rape. Prior to trial, the defense had a psychiatrist evaluate him; the psychiatrist concluded he needed mental health treatment. The defense requested a delay in the proceedings for the defendant to receive psychiatric treatment, but the trial judge denied the request and proceeded with trial.

During the trial, the defendant's wife (the victim) testified and confirmed his history of "strange behavior." On the second day of the trial, he shot himself in the stomach in an apparent suicide attempt and was hospitalized. The judge denied a request for mistrial and continued the trial even without the defendant's presence, citing his absence as voluntary. The jury found him guilty, and he was sentenced to life in prison. The case eventually came before the U.S. Supreme Court to determine whether the trial court erred in not addressing the competency issue. The Supreme Court concluded there was certainly enough evidence to meet the bona fide doubt standard presented in *Pate*. Trial courts should consider any evidence coming from irrational behavior, demeanor at trial, or any prior medical opinions. Disconcerting information from even one of these sources may trigger an inquiry into the defendant's competency to proceed.

In the time since these two cases were decided, it has become clear that courts will rarely refuse a request for competency evaluation. This very low threshold for referral results in the fact that most defendants referred for competency evaluation are competent to proceed. Consistent with this belief is the finding that an estimated 26% of those competency evaluations mentioned in the Steadman et al. (1982) survey were considered not competent by the court.

Roesch and Golding (1980) reviewed a number of studies reporting rates of incompetency among competency evaluations to range from 1.2% to 77%. Melton and colleagues (1997) suggested "when more rigorous (i.e., more valid) evaluation standards and procedures are applied, the percentage found incompetent is typically less than 10%" (p. 135). This low rate of incompetency occurs for at least two other reasons beyond a low threshold to request evaluation. As it will become apparent, the threshold for competency to stand trial is not very high.

Last, many competency referrals occur for reasons unrelated to mental health concern, such as attorney ignorance, confusion between sanity and competency, as an information-seeking ruse, as a tactical delay, and for strategic planning of the case (Melton et al., 1997; Roesch & Golding, 1978; Rosenberg & McGarry, 1972).

Competency as a U.S. Constitutional Right

The concept of not allowing a mentally "defective" defendant to progress through the criminal judicial system can be traced to at least the middle 1600s in British Common Law (Melton et al., 1997). In 1899, the U.S. Court of Appeals for the 6th Circuit determined it was a violation of the U.S. Constitution's 14th Amendment right to due process to allow a mentally incompetent person to proceed through the criminal judicial process (*Youtsey v. United States*, 1899). The circuit court wrote that it was:

Fundamental that an insane person can neither plead to an arraignment, be subjected to a trial, or, after trial, receive judgment, or after judgment, undergo punishment. . . . It is not "due process of law" to subject an insane person to trial upon an indictment involving liberty or life. (pp. 940–941)

In 1899, the term *insane* was more broadly defined and often referred to lack of competency, as in this passage. *Youtsey* established the constitutionality of adjudicative competency, but it was not until 1960 that the U.S. Supreme Court established a holding on what constituted the difference between competency and incompetency (*Dusky v. United States*, 1960).

In *Dusky*, the U.S. Supreme Court identified the requirement that a person needed a rational as well as factual understanding for competency to stand trial. Milton Dusky was arrested in August 1958 for kidnapping a 15-year-old girl, transporting her from Kansas to Missouri, and raping her. He was referred for mental health evaluation, and a psychiatrist testified Dusky was "unable to properly understand the proceedings against him and unable to adequately assist counsel in his defense" (p. 402) because of severe mental illness. He was found competent, nonetheless, because he was oriented and had some recollection of the events in question. He was then convicted of kidnapping. The U.S. Court of Appeals for the 8th Circuit affirmed the conviction.

The U.S. Supreme Court reviewed the case, overturned the conviction, and remanded it back to the trial court for new competency assessment, indicating the level of competency was not adequate. They wrote, "It is not enough for the district judge to find that the defendant is oriented to time and place and has some recollection of events" (p. 402). Dusky was to receive a new trial if he was found competent under the new standard. The following has been now termed the *"Dusky* standard" (*Dusky v. United States*, 1960):

[The] test must be whether he has sufficient present ability to consult with his lawyer with a reasonable degree of rational understanding—and whether he has a rational as well as factual understanding of the proceedings against him. (p. 402)

The *Dusky* standard spells out the minimal level of competency necessary under the U.S. Constitution for all criminal jurisdictions in the United States. As such, it has been written into statute in one form or other in most jurisdictions in the United States (Favole, 1983). Although wording varies, each jurisdiction addresses these two prongs, factual and rational, at the minimum.

Dusky also made several other key points. Competency is an issue of *current* ability as opposed to mental state at some time in the past (the exception, of course, is an evaluation of retrospective competency, as briefly touched in the above case example). Implied is the need to remain competent for the foreseeable near future, at least as long as the upcoming proceeding.

Occasionally, a defendant's competency will vary from week to week in what amounts to a "moving target." Under these circumstances, providing treatment, reevaluation, and guaranteeing the defendant a fair trial process can be difficult work for the judge.

The term *ability* to consult with his or her lawyer implies capacity to do so rather than desire to do so. It is not unusual for criminal defendants not to want to cooperate with counsel for reasons not rooted in mental illness. The ability to identify the motivation for this lack of cooperation is the task of the forensic evaluator. Further, it is important to keep in mind "ability to assist" counsel does not imply a constitutional right to a "meaningful attorney–client relationship" (*Morris v. Slappy*, 1983).

Last, the standard also includes the phrase *reasonable level of understanding*, rather than a perfect level of understanding; a criminal defendant is not expected to have perfect understanding. Although these small components of the *Dusky* standard are important, the core issue of concern remains the nature of "rational as well as factual understanding."

According to Reisner and Slobogin (1990), factual understanding comprises a person's strict understanding. Examples include a defendant's ability to repeat information provided, paraphrasing that information in their own words, and displaying an ability to put the information into use. The defendant presents rational understanding as involving a rational manipulation of the information. It can be evaluated by observing how information is used in decision making and includes such abilities as judgment, comprehension, good reality testing, rational weighing of risks and benefits, and relevance of facts to the immediate situation. Although there are various descriptions of specific points within this concept of competency for various activities, the general understanding of competency as outlined in *Dusky* is the core aspect of competency for any point in the criminal judicial process.

One issue *Dusky* does not explicitly address is the presence of mental abnormality beyond lack of knowledge. Milton Dusky was considered to have a severe mental illness, so the issue was in the record before the U.S. Supreme Court (Frederick, DeMier, & Towers, 2004). It was simply not listed in the final Court decision.[1] Subsequent case law makes it clear the competency deficiency must be caused by mental abnormality as opposed simply to ignorance. Individuals can be unable to assist in their defense for purely physical reasons, but as it relates to cognitive functioning, some type of diagnosable mental condition is required. Most jurisdictions make this requirement much more clear. An example is the current federal statute (Title 18, U.S.C., Section 4241a). The statute is very reminiscent of *Dusky*, with added emphasis on mental abnormality: "The defendant, as a result of mental disease or defect, is unable to understand the nature and consequences of the proceedings against him or assist properly in his defense."

The current federal standard also highlights another aspect of competency by replacing "consult" with "assist" regarding working with counsel. There is no definitive rule as to how much ability one needs to assist "properly." The amount of assistance necessary to give direction to counsel or rally a defense on one's own behalf likely varies depending on the complexity of the case. In this regard, the standard for competency to proceed implicates the need to evaluate the context and situational demands into which the defendant will likely need to go. Grisso (1986, 1988) provided insight into the need to consider contextual issues in determining competence to proceed.

Competency as a Contextual Issue

Grisso (1988) presented a conceptual framework that emphasized the contextual nature of criminal competency. From this perspective, the likely demands placed on a defendant must be considered before determining whether the defendant can rise to the level of performance required. Although subsequent U.S. Supreme Court case law (*Godinez v. Moran*, 1993) implied otherwise, it is still a valuable exercise in understanding the nature of the interaction between the defendant's capabilities and the likely situational demands. Viewing competency as an adaptive function in this manner makes the process of determining what neurocognitive deficits likely play a role in the defendant's lack of competence and provides guidance in determining prognosis and treatment needs. Grisso presented five areas of analysis relevant for neuropsychologists performing competency evaluations: functional description of specific abilities, causal explanations for deficits in competency abilities, interactive significance of deficits in competency ability, conclusory opinions about legal competency and incompetency, and prescriptive remediation for deficits in competency abilities.

Functional description of specific abilities

The primary objective of a competency evaluation is not foreign to clinical neuropsychology because it deals with describing functional strengths and weaknesses. The difference is in knowing specific legal standards sufficiently to appreciate the relevance of those deficits to the determination of competency.

Causal explanations for deficits in competency abilities

The logical next step is determining the cause of those deficiencies, another task well known by neuropsychologists. The key here is, again, knowing the appropriate legal standard and how that standard is applied. Neuropsychologists are equipped to communicate neuroanatomical and neuropathological bases for deficits presented and to rule out other potential causes of performance (ignorance, situational influences, cultural influences, and malingering). Lack of knowledge pertaining to the law (ignorance) is not grounds for incompetency. The knowledge and reasoning skill deficits must be rooted in diagnosable pathology.

Interactive significance of deficits in competency ability

The neuropsychologist should attempt to place the defendant's strengths and weaknesses into context, that is, how the neurocognitive function interacts with the ecological demands required of him or her given the specific legal situation. Although case law suggests the standard for competency does not change based on the complexity of the case, the level of rational and factual understanding required is not necessarily interpreted in the same manner for every situation.

The demands required of the defendant will vary given the complexity of the case. In this regard, two defendants with the exact same neurocognitive deficits could vary in their competence based on the complexity of the case. More is required from a defendant in a long, multiple-count bank fraud trial than for a single charge of illegal reentry after deportation. Likewise, pleading guilty will press cognitive capacity less than a lengthy trial. Before concluding a defendant's competency, there must be a sense of which demands will be placed on him or her through the particular legal proceedings. This gray aspect of competency determination is an excellent example of why it is important to remember the judge makes the final decision regarding a defendant's competency, not the expert witness.

Conclusory opinions about legal competency and incompetency

Evaluators provide opinions regarding the defendant's competency. The trier of fact (in this instance, the judge) will make the actual legal finding regarding competence. The forensic neuropsychologist's role is simply to provide an expert opinion for the court's consideration. Judges consider other salient facts beyond that provided by the forensic neuropsychologist before making a legal ruling.

Grisso (1986, 1988) made the argument that mental health professionals should refrain from actually providing a definitive opinion on competency. He suggested instead that they limit their opinions to clinical conclusions, particularly in those areas most relevant to competency, and allow the trier of fact to make the final legal decision. The final legal decision before the court is considered the "ultimate issue." In competency hearings, the ultimate issue is whether the defendant is competent to proceed. Providing an opinion on the ultimate issue has been debated, particularly when the expert is providing an opinion before a jury. There is relatively pervasive case law and statute limiting mental health experts from providing ultimate issue opinions on sanity, and in some jurisdictions, there are formal limits on providing ultimate issue opinions on competency as well.

Grisso (1988) pointed out three reasons to refrain from providing ultimate issue opinion testimony in the area of competence. First, psychologists are experts in mental health issues, not law. He argued they are not in a position to know which demands will be placed on a defendant in the course of his or her legal actions. In this regard, clinicians should leave the opinion up to those who are experts in the judicial process. Second, an argument has been made that mental health experts can have too great an influence on the minds of legal decision makers. Although such may be the case in jury trials, it is difficult to fathom that a judge will be unduly swayed to an opinion of even the best-qualified neuropsychologist. Third, Grisso suggested no new information is provided to the judge by mental health professionals giving their opinions on the ultimate issue after a description of the neuro/psychopathology with its functional strengths and weaknesses is made. In some jurisdictions, however, the expert is required to provide an opinion on the ultimate issue regarding competency (Title 18 U.S. Code, Sections 4241 and 4247). The debate on providing ultimate issue opinions on competency will likely continue in academic settings and scholarly writings whether or not it makes any real difference in the court room.

Prescriptive remediation for deficits in competency abilities

If the forensic neuropsychologist believes the defendant is not competent, it is his or her responsibility to provide prognostic considerations and outline remedial options from a clinical perspective, truly the neuropsychologist's element. The clinician can educate the court regarding the nature of the condition, which treatment options are available, and the likely success potential for each. Grisso (1988) pointed out these issues to consider:

- Whether the defendant's deficits are remediable;
- If so, the treatment that is required for remediation;
- How long the remediation is likely to require;
- The local facilities or programs in which the treatment is available; and
- The conditions of restriction represented by each of these facilities. (p. 21)

Depending on the nature of the legal case, courts may have the option to place defendants in community treatment or rehabilitation programs. In many instances, the court has little option but to refer the defendant to forensic hospitals run by state or federal correctional agencies. For example, the federal law dictates that U.S. district judges are to commit incompetent defendants to the custody of the U.S. attorney general for inpatient mental health treatment focused on competency restoration (Title 18, U.S.C., Section 4241d).

Customarily, mental health treatment facilities under the department of corrections have little in the way of neurocognitive remediation capability. It is important to remember the goal of treatment is remediation of deficits sufficient to restore competency. This level of therapeutic outcome is likely lower than that espoused in general clinical rehabilitation. The ultimate goal is the ability to advance successfully through legal proceedings rather than successful independent living and community reentry.

More Detailed Considerations of Competency

Others have attempted to define further the functional capacities that go into competency as formulated in *Dusky*. A previously cited (Grisso, 1986; Melton et al., 1997) example is Florida's 2002 Title XLVII (Criminal Procedure and Corrections), Chapter 916.12 (Mentally Deficient and Mentally Ill Defendants), which spells out the standard of incompetency in this manner, starting with paragraph (2):

(2) The experts shall first determine whether the person is mentally ill and, if so, consider the factors related to the issue of whether the defendant meets the criteria for competence to proceed; that is, whether the defendant has sufficient present ability to consult with counsel with a reasonable degree of rational understanding

and whether the defendant has a rational, as well as factual, understanding of the pending proceedings.

(3) In considering the issue of competence to proceed, the examining experts shall first consider and specifically include in their report the defendant's capacity to:

1. Appreciate the charges or allegations against the defendant;
2. Appreciate the range and nature of possible penalties, if applicable, that may be imposed in the proceedings against the defendant;
3. Understand the adversarial nature of the legal process;
4. Disclose to counsel facts pertinent to the proceedings at issue;
5. Manifest appropriate courtroom behavior; and
6. Testify relevantly; and include in their report any other factor deemed relevant by the experts.

(4) If the experts should find that the defendant is incompetent to proceed, the experts shall report on any recommended treatment for the defendant to attain competence to proceed. In considering the issues relating to treatment, the examining experts shall specifically report on:

1. The mental illness causing the incompetence;
2. The treatment or treatments appropriate for the mental illness of the defendant and an explanation of each of the possible treatment alternatives in order of choices;
3. The availability of acceptable treatment and, if treatment is available in the community, the expert shall so state in the report; and
4. The likelihood of the defendant's attaining competence under the treatment recommended, an assessment of the probable duration of the treatment required to restore competence, and the probability that the defendant will attain competence to proceed in the foreseeable future.

There have been clinician/researchers involved in attempting to operationalize *Dusky* and provide evaluators with specific functional abilities. The Group for the Advancement of Psychiatry (1974) developed a 21-point list of abilities from competency assessment instruments available at the time (Table 12-3). These abilities can assist the evaluator by providing an outline and road map for clinical interviewing. Failure in any one point does not necessarily constitute incompetency, but the points help ensure evaluators identify and consider all relevant issues before coming to conclusions.

In contrast to the detail that came out of criminal competency research at the hands of behavioral scientists is the emphasis on the most *basic* elements of competency presented by judges in case law. *Wieter v. Settle* was an interesting case in the U.S. District Court for the Western District of Missouri in 1961. Although *Wieter v. Settle* is not a jurisdictionally authoritative decision, meaning it does not have much power to control other judicial decisions, it has been presented widely to better enable mental health professionals to understand the very basic aspects of "reasonable understanding" as it relates to mental health competency (Denney & Wynkoop, 2000; Grisso, 1988; Stafford, 2003).

Wieter was arrested and charged with a federal misdemeanor offense after he claimed to have placed a bomb on a commercial airliner traveling from Seattle,

TABLE 12-3. Group for the Advancement of Psychiatry 21-Item List to Assist in the Evaluation of Competency

1. Understand current legal situation.
2. Understand current charges.
3. Understand facts relevant to the case.
4. Understand the legal issues and procedures in the case.
5. Understand legal defenses available in the defendant's behalf.
6. Understand the dispositions, pleas, and penalties possible.
7. Appraise the likely outcomes.
8. Appraise the roles of defense counsel, prosecuting attorney, judge, jury, witnesses, and defendant.
9. Identify and locate witnesses.
10. Relate to defense counsel.
11. Trust and communicate relevantly with counsel.
12. Comprehend instructions and advice.
13. Make decisions after receiving advice.
14. Maintain a collaborative relationship with counsel and help plan legal strategy.
15. Follow testimony for contradictions or errors.
16. Testify relevantly and be cross-examined if necessary.
17. Challenge prosecution witnesses.
18. Tolerate stress at the trial and while awaiting trial.
19. Refrain from irrational and unmanageable behavior during trial.
20. Disclose pertinent facts surrounding the alleged offense.
21. Protect self by using available legal safeguards.

Note. From Group for the Advancement of Psychiatry (Report 89, 1974). Formulated by the Committee on Psychiatry and Law. Reproduced with permission.

Washington, to Los Angeles, California. He was found not competent to stand trial and committed for inpatient mental health treatment. After 18 months, he filed a habeas corpus motion seeking relief from mental health commitment and release because he already spent more time in custody than he would have if convicted of the misdemeanor.

A psychiatrist filed a report indicating Wieter was still not competent because of mental illness. The U.S. District Court reheard the case and disagreed with the psychiatric opinion. In considering the man competent, the court outlined eight minimal abilities required for competency to proceed (Table 12-4). Subsequent case law substantially softened the requirement for memory of the events such that a competent defendant does not necessarily need to recall details of the alleged offense (*Wilson v. United States*, 1968). This issue is addressed further under competency and amnesia.

Competency as Decisional Capacity

Much of the discussion around *Dusky* has to do not only with knowledge, but also with the ability to go through a process. Implied within the concept of

TABLE 12-4. Minimal Ability Requirements for Criminal Competency as Outlined by the U.S. District Court in *Wieter v. Settle* (1961)

1. Mental capacity to appreciate his or her presence in relation to time, place, and things.
2. Elementary mental processes such that he or she apprehends (i.e., seizes and grasps with what mind he or she has) that he or she is in a court of justice, charged with a criminal offense.
3. Apprehends that there is a judge on the bench.
4. Apprehends that there is a prosecutor present who will try to convict him or her of a criminal charge.
5. Apprehends that he or she has a lawyer (self-employed or court-appointed) who will undertake to defend him or her against that charge.
6. Apprehends that he or she will be expected to tell his or her lawyer the circumstances, to the best of his or her mental ability (whether colored or not by mental aberration), the facts surrounding him or her at the time and place where the law violation allegedly occurred.
7. Apprehends that there is, or will be, a jury present to pass on evidence adduced as to his or her guilt or innocence of such charge.
8. He or she has memory sufficient to relate those things in his or her own personal manner.

Note. Adapted for clarity.

competency to proceed is decisional capacity, that is, the idea of capacity to make important legal decisions. Contrasted with decisional capacity is procedural capacity, by which a person can understand the nature and consequences of proceedings. Criminal defendants make many decisions in the process of assisting in their defense, but there are some decisions that have unique standing because they involve waiving rights guaranteed under the U.S. Constitution. Three examples are the right to remain silent, right to counsel, and right to trial. I address each of these in turn.

Competency to confess

The 5th Amendment of the U.S. Constitution guarantees the right to be free from self-incrimination, and the 6th Amendment guarantees the right to counsel. The U.S. Supreme Court affirmed these rights in *Miranda v. Arizona* (1966). As a result of this famous case, the concept has become known as the "right to remain silent." If the suspect waives the right to silence and input from counsel, any statements given can be used against him or her. The Court spelled out the need for any statements given by the suspect to be *voluntary, intelligent,* and *knowing* for them to be admissible in later criminal proceedings.

Although *Miranda* appeared to limit law enforcement deception, later court cases have outlined that:

As long as the person subjected to interrogation appears to understand the right to remain silent and the right to counsel subsequent waiver of those rights will usually be "knowing and intelligent"; other types of misunderstandings or misimpressions are not relevant to the admissibility issue. (Melton et al., 1997, p. 159)

Greater emphasis has been placed on the term, voluntary, in subsequent cases as much of the concern has revolved around what constitutes "coercion."

Coercion was addressed in light of mental health concerns by the U.S. Supreme Court in *Colorado v. Connelly* (1986). Barry Francis Connelly flew from Boston to Denver to confess to the Denver police about a murder committed several months earlier in Colorado. Despite repeated *Miranda* warnings that he need not talk, he insisted on giving self-incriminating details of the murder. Police observed no overt signs of mental illness. Later testimony presented that the defendant was "compelled" to confess by command hallucinations from God.

The U.S. Supreme Court ultimately opined that the "respondent's perception of coercion flowing from the 'voice of God,' however important or significant such a perception may be in other disciplines, is a matter to which the United States Constitution does not speak" (p. 524). There needed to be police activity amounting to "overreaching" to find his confession not voluntary. The Court confirmed that the waiver of *Miranda* rights must be knowing, intelligent, and voluntary. Regardless of the *Colorado v. Connelly* decision's emphasis on police overreaching, both *Miranda* and *Connelly* suggest mental health professionals have a place in evaluating the competency of criminal defendants to confess.

Competency to plead guilty and waive counsel

Post-*Dusky* courts also struggled with the level of competency required to waive the constitutional right to counsel and trial. Both of these rights were addressed and the concepts brought together in *Godinez v. Moran* (1993), which spelled out the current standard in these areas.

In 1966, the U.S. Supreme Court decided *Westbrook v. Arizona*, which questioned whether a general competency hearing addressing *Dusky* language was adequate when the defendant chose to waive right to counsel. Westbrook was initially found competent to stand trial. He then dismissed his attorney and chose to act as his own attorney (termed acting *pro se*). The High Court eventually reviewed the case and sent it back to the trial court, suggesting the need to determine whether the defendant made an "intelligent and competent" waiver of his constitutional right to counsel. This finding suggested a higher standard of competency to act as one's own attorney than that outlined in *Dusky*.

In a non–mental health, but related, case, *Faretta v. California* (1975), the U.S. Supreme Court concluded that competency to waive the right to an attorney is not based on a determination of the defendant's level of legal knowledge. Even though it may be bad judgment, competent defendants can act as their own attorneys regardless of how ignorant they are in the law and criminal procedure.

A discussion on the issue of waiving one's right to trial by pleading guilty needs to start with a non–mental health case. In 1970, the U.S. Supreme Court decided *North Carolina v. Alford*. Alford chose to plead guilty in a capital murder case simply to avoid the possibility of the death penalty. In his statement pleading guilty, he asserted he did not do the crime, but was pleading guilty to avoid the death penalty. The U.S. Supreme Court reviewed the issue based on the question of whether Alford was coerced by the gravity of the situation into waiving his right to a trial. The Court summarized the issue that defendants must *voluntarily, knowingly*, and *understandingly* waive a right to trial. They found Alford had made a "voluntary and intelligent choice among alternatives;" his plea was not compelled merely by the risk of execution.

The *Alford* decision set the stage for the 1973 U.S. Court of Appeals for the 6th Circuit decision in *Sieling v. Eyman*. In this case, the 9th Circuit established what appeared to be a higher standard to waive rights to trial and plead guilty. The court seemed to propose a standard of a "reasoned choice among alternatives" in addition to the general *Dusky* criteria. The U.S. Supreme Court encompassed each of these concerns and appeared to resolve the inconsistencies with their reasoning in *Godinez v. Moran* (1993).

Richard Moran was charged with murdering a bartender and bar patron in August 1984. A few days later, he allegedly murdered his wife and attempted suicide by shooting himself in the abdomen. He survived and was handed over to police in the hospital recovery room. He was found competent to stand trial and initially pleaded not guilty. Two and one half months later, he requested that his defense attorney be discharged, and that he be allowed to plead guilty. The trial court accepted his waiver of counsel and trial once assured that he was not pleading guilty in response to threats or promises, and that he understood the charges and potential consequences facing him.

In 1985, Moran was sentenced to death. In 1987, he filed a petition for post-conviction relief claiming he had not been mentally competent to represent himself. The trial court, Nevada Supreme Court, and U.S. District Court rejected his appeal, but the U.S. Court of Appeals for the 9th Circuit reversed the prior decisions, holding the due process clause of the 14th Amendment required the court to hold a competency inquiry before accepting his decision to discharge counsel and enter a guilty plea. Similar to the reasoning in *Sieling v. Eyman* (1973), the Court required a reasoned-choice-among-alternatives inquiry. The U.S. Supreme Court took up the question of whether the competency standard for pleading guilty or waiving right to counsel was higher than the competency standard for standing trial. They rejected the 9th Circuit's use of reasoned choice and concluded:

We can conceive of no basis for demanding a higher level of competence for those defendants who choose to plead guilty . . . nor do we think that a defendant who waives his right to the assistance of counsel must be more competent than a defendant who does not. (p. 332)

Although the Court specifically indicated the *Dusky* standard was not increased, they made this slight enhancement:

A finding that a defendant is competent to stand trial, however, is not all that is necessary before he may be permitted to plead guilty or waive his right to counsel. In addition to determining that a defendant who seeks to plead guilty or waive counsel is competent, a trial court must satisfy itself that the waiver of his constitutional rights is knowing and voluntary. (p. 333)

Godinez trumped the reasoning presented in *Westbrook* and *Sieling* by establishing that competency to plead guilty or waive counsel requires no higher standard than competency to stand trial. However, the trial court must now specifically place in the record an inquiry into the defendant's thought process to verify it is a "knowing" and "voluntary" decision. *Godinez* recapitulated *Dusky* and spelled out the minimum required standard for decisional capacity.

Burden and Standard of Proof

It is helpful for neuropsychologists to understand how courts make decisions. Evidence is compared to sometimes vague legal standards in a manner remotely analogous to hypothesis testing. As with science, the court starts out with a default assumption. In the example of criminal conviction, defendants are assumed innocent until shown otherwise. Enough evidence must be demonstrated on the record to move the mind of the trier of fact (judge or jury) to a level "beyond reasonable doubt" to find the defendant guilty of the crime. In this example, the prosecution carries the burden of proof, and the standard of proof is beyond reasonable doubt.

There are three major standards of proof: beyond reasonable doubt, clear and convincing, and preponderance of the evidence. Although quite artificial, behavioral scientists can use percentages to communicate better the concept to such legal terms. In this regard, beyond reasonable doubt is most similar to 90% to 95% ($p < .05$), clear and convincing approximates 75%, and preponderance amounts to just slightly better than half (51%; Melton et al., 1997, p. 202). Each of these standards is used during different inquiries in criminal procedure, and there are other standards used by appellate courts when reviewing trial court records. I turn to two criminal competency cases to demonstrate the standard of proof and who holds the burden in competency determinations.

In 1984, Teofilo Medina stole a gun, held up four business establishments, murdered three employees, attempted to rob a fourth, and shot at two passersby. He was apprehended, tried, and convicted of three counts of first-degree murder. Before the trial, defense moved for a hearing on Medina's competency to stand trial. He was found competent, although there was conflicting expert testimony. After the guilty verdict, Medina reinstated a previously withdrawn plea of not guilty by reason of insanity. The jury found him sane, and he was sentenced to death.

On appeal, it was argued his constitutional right to due process was violated by placing the burden of proof on him to establish his incompetence to stand trial. In 1992, the U.S. Supreme Court heard the case and held (a) the California statute requiring that the party asserting incompetency of the defendant to stand trial had the burden of proving incompetence did not violate procedural due process rights of the defendant, and (b) the statute providing for the presumption of competency did not violate procedural due process.

Medina v. California (1992) not only revealed it is constitutional to place the incompetency burden on the defendant, but also revealed that the burden is on *whoever* asserts that the defendant is not competent because defendants are presumed competent to stand trial. The table turns after the court has found a defendant not competent and commits him or her to mental health treatment for restoration of competency. At the end of treatment, the burden is now on whoever asserts the defendant is competent to proceed because it is assumed the defendant remains not competent. The issue of who carries the burden of proof in competency determinations is not particularly critical given the particular standard of proof involved. The importance of this standard of proof was addressed by the U.S. Supreme Court in *Cooper v. Oklahoma* (1996).

In Oklahoma at the time Byron Cooper was charged with murdering an 86-year-old man during the course of a burglary, defendants in criminal prosecutions were assumed competent to stand trial until shown otherwise by clear and convincing evidence. Questions regarding Cooper's competence were raised on five separate occasions before and after the trial. Initially, a pretrial judge relied on a psychologist's opinion that Cooper was not competent and committed him to a state hospital for treatment. After 3 months of treatment, however, the trial court found him competent to proceed. At this point, he was presumed competent until shown by clear and convincing evidence not competent. One week before trial, the lead defense attorney raised the issue of competence, but the judge held to his earlier determination that Cooper was competent.

On the first day of trial, his bizarre behavior led to a further competency hearing. Additional expert testimony was heard suggesting Cooper was incompetent, but there was concern about malingering. The judge held to his earlier determination and pushed on with the trial. Cooper was found guilty. Before sentencing, defense moved for a mistrial and another competency hearing, but the motions were denied. Cooper was sentenced to death. The Oklahoma Court of Criminal Appeals affirmed the decision.

The court of appeals ruling was overturned by a unanimous decision of the U.S. Supreme Court. It was concluded Oklahoma's clear and convincing evidence rule regarding proof of incompetence "offends a principle of justice that is deeply rooted in the traditions and conscience of our people" (p. 362). By holding to a clear and convincing standard, the state runs too great a risk of finding an incompetent defendant competent to proceed and thereby violating his or her due process rights under the 14th Amendment. Although *Medina* provided that it is constitutionally sound to place the burden on defendants, *Cooper* dictated that the standard of proof in determining incompetency can be no more strict than preponderance of the evidence, that is, just enough to tip the scales.

Competency to Refuse an Insanity Defense

As demonstrated in *Faretta v. California* (1975), competent defendants have the right to make decisions that may not be in their best interests or are otherwise demonstrative of poor judgment. Occasionally, it is difficult to tell whether such decisions reflect poor judgment. Such is the case when a mentally ill (but competent) defendant has a very good case for a successful insanity defense, but he or she chooses to forgo that defense. Judge Bazelon of the Court of Appeals for the District of Columbia wrote these words about society's responsibility in this regard (*Whalem v. United States*, 1965):

In the courtroom confrontations between the individual and society the trial judge must uphold this structural foundation by refusing to allow the conviction of an obviously mentally irresponsible defendant, and when there is sufficient question as to a defendant's mental responsibility at the time of the crime, that issue must become part of the case. (pp. 818–819)

In *Whalem* (1965), the appeals court held that the trial court could impose an insanity defense on a competent defendant even against the defendant's desires. That reasoning was reviewed after the *North Carolina v. Alford* (1970) and *Faretta* (1975) decisions in another District of Columbia Circuit Court case, *Frendak v. United States* (1979).

Paula Frendak's coworker, Willard Titlow, was fatally shot on the first floor of their office building. Frendak traveled out of Washington, D.C., on a multistate, multicountry trip before she was apprehended in Abu Dhabi, United Arab Emirates, for not surrendering her passport. She was found to possess a pistol and 45 rounds of ammunition. She was extradited back to the United States and charged with first-degree murder. She underwent multiple competency evaluations and was ultimately found competent. Frendak was convicted.

The trial court then overrode her conviction and found her not guilty by reason of insanity. She appealed partly to reject the insanity plea. The District of Columbia Court of Appeals held that the trial judge may not force an insanity defense on a defendant found competent to stand trial if the defendant *intelligently* and *voluntarily* decided to reject the insanity defense. There were several potentially intelligent rationales for rejecting an insanity defense (*Frendak v. United States*, 1979):

1) A defendant may fear that an insanity acquittal will result in the institution of commitment proceedings which lead to confinement in a mental institution for a period longer than the potential jail sentence.
2) The defendant may object to quality of treatment or the type of confinement to which he or she may be subject in an institution for the mentally ill.
3) A defendant, with good reason, may choose to avoid the stigma of insanity.
4) Other collateral consequences of an insanity acquittal can also follow the defendant throughout life (e.g., the right to vote, serve on a federal jury, or even restrict his or her ability to obtain a drivers license).
5) A defendant also may oppose the imposition of an insanity defense because he or she views the crime as a political or religious protest which a finding of insanity would denigrate. (pp. 376–378)

It is important for a forensic examiner to be aware of these potential reasons for wanting to avoid an insanity defense because the rationale for choosing a defense goes to competency by way of "assisting properly" in one's defense. The evaluator will need to assess the impact of any mental illness on the defendant's ability to make an intelligent and voluntary judgment in this regard.

Competency Assessment Tools

There are a number of CATs available to assist in the assessment of competency to proceed. Some of these tools are simply interview outlines; others are structured interviews and more formalized tests. They all have one characteristic in common, however: They do not determine who is or is not competent to proceed. As with all competent neuropsychological evaluations, such tools aid in clinical determination, but do not replace a thorough integration of all relevant information as part of a multiple data source assessment. Several CATs have limited utility at this point and receive only a brief mention here. I then review the Competency Assessment Instrument (CAI, and its revised version R-CAI), Fitness Interview Test–Revised (FIT-R), Georgia Court Competency Test (GCCT, and its revised version GCCT-MSH), Competency Assessment for Standing Trial for Defendants With Mental Retardation (CAST*MR), and the MacArthur Competency Assessment Tool–Criminal Adjudication (MacCAT-CA) in more detail because these tools appear to have greater utility in criminal forensic neuropsychological evaluations. Special mention is made of a newly published instrument, the Evaluation of Competency to Stand Trial–Revised (ECST-R).

The Competency Screening Test (CST; Laboratory of Community Psychiatry, 1973; Lipsitt, Lelos, & McGarry, 1971) was developed as a brief screening test to aid in deciding who needed more throughout assessment regarding competency to proceed. It was devised by a group of psychiatrists, psychologists, and lawyers with a National Institute of Mental Health grant from the Center for

Studies of Crime and Delinquency. It is a 22-item sentence-completion test. Each of the items is scored 0, 1, or 2 and summed for a total score. Total scores below 21 suggest further competency assessment is warranted. There has been criticism of the CST on conceptual, psychometric, and predictive utility grounds. See Grisso, Borum, Edens, Moye, and Otto (2003) for a more thorough review. The CST may have value as a general screener for agencies, but it appears to have limited utility for neuropsychologists performing competency evaluations.

The Interdisciplinary Fitness Interview (Golding, Roesch, & Schreiber, 1984) was developed as a research tool for Canadian jurisdictions. The semistructured interview format includes items on psychopathology as well as legal issues. The unique aspect of the procedure includes a joint interview of an attorney with a mental health professional. No additional research has come out on the Interdisciplinary Fitness Interview since Grisso's detailed review of it in 1986.

The Computer Assisted Determination of Competency to Proceed (Barnard et al., 1991, 1992) is a computer-administered, 272-item, 18-scale test that addresses social history, psychological functioning, and legal knowledge. Items include yes/no, true/false, and multiple choice formats. It takes over an hour to administer, and the computer produces a narrative report summary. It was designed to provide organized and relevant information directly from the defendant for the clinician to review prior to a face-to-face interview. Preliminary research of the instrument seemed positive, but there were significant concerns about its initial validation. There has been no published research of the instrument since 1992, and there is no published manual (Grisso et al., 2003). In her review of the instrument, Stafford (2003) recommended research use only at this point. See Melton and colleagues (1997) for a more detailed review and discussion.

Competency Assessment Instrument

The CAI (Laboratory of Community Psychiatry, 1973; McGarry, Lelos, & Lipsitt, 1973) was developed alongside the CST. It is a semistructured interview that takes about 45 minutes to administer. It was originally developed with a scoring system based on 5-point Likert ratings of 13 competency-related functions. The functional domains were derived from appellate cases, legal literature, and experience of the multidisciplinary development team (Stafford, 2003). There are no standardized administration rules. Although clinicians are free to formulate their own questions to address each knowledge domain, example questions are provided for each.

The original CAI manual did not specify the order in which the functions should be addressed, and many of the questions required only yes or no answers. It was revised by forensic practitioners working in the Trial Competency Program at Atascadero State Hospital in California on three different occasions over the course of 20 years (Riley, 1998). The order of questions was changed to flow more logically during a competency interview. Questions were also added and reworded in a more open-ended format. An additional domain was added to deal with capacity to cope with stress of incarceration prior to trial. Riley stressed "probing of an area should continue until the examiner is satisfied that as much as is reasonably possible is known about [the domain]" (p. 14). He further pointed out it is not always necessary to ask every question under each dimension as some questions are not appropriate given the charge (e.g., misdemeanor) or current stage of legal proceedings (e.g., questions about trial when the defendant is facing sentencing).

Administration of the CAI remains flexible. A portion of the Revised CAI is shown in Table 12-5.[2] Although the CAI and R-CAI use a scoring system with cutoffs for incompetency, the scoring system is generally used solely for research. The instrument is more commonly used as an interview outline and guide to guarantee important areas are not overlooked during the competency interview process (Denney & Wynkoop, 2000; Stafford, 2003).

The Fitness Interview Test–Revised

The Fitness Interview Test (FIT; Roesch, Webster, & Eaves, 1984) was a Canadian adaptation of the CAI. It included additional items regarding trial procedures and a separate section addressing general defendant mental status. An extensive revision occurred secondary to Canada's 1992 revision of the Criminal Code (Roesch, Zapf, Eaves, & Webster, 1998). Changes in the FIT were substantial (Grisso et al., 2003). The FIT-R retained the structured interview format. It starts with four introductory questions (such as "Do you have a lawyer at this point?") then moves on to 70 questions grouped in 16 headings under the following three major sections (which correspond to the Criminal Code of Canada, Section 2):

Section I: Understanding the Nature or Object of the Proceedings: Factual Knowledge of Criminal Procedure

1. Understanding of Arrest Process
2. Understanding of the Nature and Severity of Current Charges
3. Understanding of the Role of Key Participants
4. Understanding of the Legal Process
5. Understanding of Pleas
6. Understanding of Court Procedure

Section II: Understanding the Possible Consequences of the Proceedings: Appreciation of Personal Involvement in and Importance of the Proceedings

7. Appreciation of the Range and Nature of Possible Penalties
8. Appraisal of Available Legal Defenses
9. Appraisal of Likely Outcome

TABLE 12-5. Portions of the Revised Competency Assessment Instrument (CAI)

1. Understanding of Charge(s):
   What are you charged with?
   Is this a felony or misdemeanor?
   Which is more serious?
   What would anyone have to do to commit the crime of?
2. Appreciation of Penalties:
   If you're found guilty as charged, what are the possible sentences the Judge could give you?
   Where would you serve such a sentence?
   What does probation mean?
   What are some of the conditions a person must follow on probation?
   What happens if a person is found Not Guilty?
   Where do they send people found Not Guilty by Reason of Insanity?
3. Appraisal of Available Defenses:
   What pleas can a person enter in court?
   What does Not Guilty mean?
   Guilty?
   Not Guilty by Reason of Insanity?
4. Appraisal of Functions of Courtroom Participants:
   In the courtroom during a trial, what is the job of
   a. Public Defender?
   b. District Attorney?
   c. Judge
   d. Jury
   e. Defendant
   f. Witnesses
5. Understanding the Court Procedures:
   Do defendants always have to testify in their own cases?
   If you do have to testify, will you have to tell everything that happened?
   If you testify, who asks you questions first?
   Then who can ask you questions?
   What is the district attorney trying to do?
   What is the difference between a court trial and a jury trial?

Note. From Laboratory of Community Psychiatry, Harvard Medical School (1973, p. 1). Originally published by National Institute of Mental Health, Department of Health Education and Welfare Publication No. (ADM) 77-103. Reproduced with permission of Paul D. Lipsitt. Revised by John A. Riley, Ph.D.; reproduced with permission.

Section III: Communicate with Counsel: Ability to Participant in Defense

10. Capacity to Communicate Facts to Lawyer
11. Capacity to Relate to Lawyer
12. Capacity to Plan Legal Strategy
13. Capacity to Engage in Own Defense
14. Capacity to Challenge Prosecution Witnesses
15. Capacity to Testify Relevantly
16. Capacity to Manage Courtroom Behavior (p. 27)

As in the CAI, responses to questions are rated 0, 1, or 2 for adequacy. Scores are summed to achieve performance for each section as well as overall total performance. There are no norms available.

Grisso and colleagues (2003) cited the work of Viljoen, Roesch, and Zapf (in preparation) regarding multidisciplinary interrater reliability. He noted, "Averaged across professions, correlations for most items were in the .80 to .95 range, with a few in the .70s" (with one falling to .67) (p. 105). Section correlations averaged .70, .54, .59 for Sections I, II, and III, respectively. Despite these low numbers, "Average correlation for the overall judgement of fitness was .98" (p. 105).

Although the results are confounded by differences between U.S. and Canadian conceptualizations of competency, a comparison between the FIT-R and the MacArthur Competency Assessment Tool–Criminal Adjudication demonstrated a 76% agreement for 100 male forensic inpatients referred for competency evaluation (Zapf & Roesch, 2001). Grisso and colleagues (2003) recommended factor analysis of the FIT-R to understand further its construct validity. Additional research (Zapf, Roesch, & Viljoen, 2001) suggested the FIT-R has strong negative predictive value as a screening tool. Overall, the FIT-R appears to be a valid and useful tool for assisting neuropsychologists in the assessment of fitness for trial in Canadian jurisdictions.

Georgia Court Competency Test

The Georgia Court Competency Test (GCCT) was developed as an in-house competency screening tool at Central State Hospital, Milledgeville, Georgia, to assess competency to proceed in a relatively rapid manner (Wildman et al., 1980). In its original form, it was comprised of 17 questions designed to address knowledge of courtroom and legal proceedings, current charges and possible penalties, and relationship with an attorney. Johnson and Mullett (1988) modified the instrument and raised the number of items to 21 (now referred to as the GCCT-MSH). Nicholson (1992, cited in Rogers, Grandjean, Tillbrook, Vitacco, & Sewell, 2001) reviewed available reliability studies of the GCCT and concluded the test has moderately high test–retest reliability, high α coefficients, and excellent interscorer reliability.

Early research suggested the GCCT had a stable three-factor structure, termed "general legal knowledge," "courtroom layout," and "specific legal knowledge" (Bagby, Nicholson, Rogers, & Nussbaum, 1992; Nicholson, Briggs, & Robertson, 1988). Rogers, Ustad, Sewell, and Reinhart (1996) and Ustad, Rogers, Sewell, and Guarnaccia (1996) failed to demonstrate this factor structure with confirmatory factor analysis, but exploratory factor analysis with mentally ill jail and forensic hospital samples suggested two factors related to "legal knowledge." Research revealed classification rates of 68% to 78% on the GCCT (Wildman et al., 1980) and 81.8% on the GCCT-MSH (Nicholson, Robertson, Johnson, & Jensen, 1988).

Gothard, Rogers, and Sewell (1995) demonstrated the instrument's susceptibility to malingering and added an eight-item Atypical Presentation scale. In their subsequent analysis, the Atypical Presentation scale demonstrated a 90% classification rate for individuals simulating psychosis.

Although the GCCT-MSH has a become a popular instrument throughout a variety of jurisdictions (Grisso, 1986), it was recently criticized for only representing the factual knowledge prong of the *Dusky* standard (Rogers et al., 2001). The GCCT-MSH is a helpful CAT that only takes about 20 minutes to administer, but clinicians need to remember it remains a screening instrument designed to augment competency assessment.

Competence Assessment for Standing Trial for Defendants
With Mental Retardation

The CAST*MR[3] was developed by Everington and Luckasson (1992) to overcome difficulties inherent in using open-ended questions with mentally retarded defendants. The first 40 items are three alternative multiple choice questions dealing with basic legal concepts and knowledge that would help the defendant assist in his or her defense. The last 10 items are open-ended questions dealing with the specific charges and situation of the defendant. Each of these items are scored as 0, 0.5, or 1 point based on accuracy and detail. Results are totaled for each of the three sections (basic legal concepts, skills to assist defense, and understanding case events) as well as a total score. The procedure takes about 30–40 minutes to administer. Results are then compared with performances (mean and standard deviation) of four groups of criminal defendants: not mentally retarded (MR); MR but not referred for evaluation; MR, referred for pretrial evaluation and considered competent; and MR, referred for pretrial evaluation and considered not competent.

Everington (1990) outlined the development of the CAST*MR. Cronbach's α and Kuder-Richardson 20 coefficients ranged from .93 to .85 for three groups of older adolescents and adults with MR from two states. The 2-week, test–retest Pearson *r*'s were .90 and .89. Subsequent studies using criminal defendants from Wisconsin, Ohio, Maryland, and New Mexico were completed. Ten checks of interrater reliability were done, which resulted in 100% agreement for the multiple choice items and 80% agreement for open-ended questions. Interrater agreement improved to 86.6% with a larger number of comparisons (Everington & Dunn, 1995).

Competent/not competent classification agreement rates with independent forensic examiners varied from 62.9% to 71.43%, similar to hit rates of the GCCT and GCCT-MSH. There is no research on the impact malingering has on the

CAST*MR. Its structure suggests it is an easy instrument on which to feign incompetency. As with other CATs, results need integration into the overall competency evaluation results rather than relying solely on a test score.

MacArthur Competency Assessment Tool–Criminal Adjudication

The MacCAT-CA; Poythress et al., 1999) is a trimmed down, clinical version of the broader research instrument, MacArthur Structured Assessment of Competencies of Criminal Defendants (MacSAC-CD; Otto et al., 1998). The Mac-CAT-CA is a structured interview consisting of 22 items organized under three domains: Understanding, Reasoning, and Appreciation. Four questions under Understanding and Reasoning incorporate a brief vignette about two individuals fighting during a pool game in a bar.

One individual strikes the other with a pool cue and is charged with a crime. The subject taking the MacCAT-CA must assume the mindset of the defendant in the vignette to answer questions under Understanding and Reasoning. Several questions under Understanding incorporate brief training after initially inadequate responses and follow up with additional questioning. Items under Reasoning are of two types. The first requires the test subject to indicate which of two facts are more important for the hypothetical defendant to tell his attorney. The other items require the subject to choose between two alternative pleading options.

Scoring focuses on the reasoning behind the choice. The Appreciation items rely on the test subject's actual legal situation rather than the hypothetical vignette. The subject must compare his or her situation to that of others and decide whether he or she is "more likely," "less likely," or "just as likely" to have various outcomes. Summary scores are obtained for each section (Understanding, Reasoning, and Appreciation). The MacCAT-CA takes about 45 to 60 minutes to administer.

Interrater reliability was determined with 48 protocols from the norming sample (Otto et al., 1998; Poythress et al., 1999). Scale score intraclass correlations were .90 (Understanding), .85 (Reasoning), and .75 (Appreciation). Rogers (2001) pointed out these scores were likely inflated because of hierarchical questions that cue raters. Nevertheless, Rogers et al. (2001) reported results from Rogers and Grandjean (2000) for 14 subjects that produced interrater correlations from .92 to .99. There are no published test–retest correlations. Cronbach's αs were .85 (Understanding), .81 (Reasoning), and .88 (Appreciation) based on the original studies (Otto et al., 1998).

MacCAT-CA norms are based on 283 adjudicated incompetent defendants, 249 mentally ill defendants presumed competent, and 197 randomly selected jail inmates also presumed competent. Subjects came from six states and ranged in age from 18 to 65 years. Of the sample, 90% were male. Approximately half of the sample were non-Hispanic white defendants (Poythress et al., 1999).

Percentile rank scores are provided for each of the scales in the MacCAT-CA manual.

Predictive ability of the MacCAT-CA appears reasonably strong and as good as the CST and GCCT-MSH (Stafford, 2003). Each of the scale scores was correlated with the a priori competency classifications (Understanding, .36; Reasoning, .42; Appreciation, .49). Performance of the incompetent groups was significantly lower than that of the presumed competent groups.

The manual includes scale cutoff scores as well as tables that address sensitivity, specificity, false-negative rate, and positive and negative predictive value for every score of each MacCAT-CA scale (Poythress et al., 1999). Grisso et al. (2003) highlighted the fact that, although the MacCAT-CA authors provided cutoffs, they discouraged users from taking these indicators as signs of competency or incompetency. The MacCAT-CA does not include an index of subject response set, and Rogers, Sewell, Grandjean, and Vitacco (2002) demonstrated the susceptibility of the MacCAT-CA to malingering.

Evaluation of Competency to Stand Trial–Revised

The ECST-R (Rogers, Tillbrook, & Sewell, 2004) represents a promising new endeavor in the assessment of competence to proceed. The ECST-R is a structured interview composed of four main sections with an additional set of "background" questions (Rogers et al., 2001, p. 510). It was developed to measure the two *Dusky* prongs, understanding and ability to assist counsel, from both factual as well as rational perspectives. The Consult With Counsel scale includes 10 questions to assess the attorney–client relationship. The scale also incorporates five criteria: "(i) perceptions of the relationship, (ii) defendant's expectations of the attorney, (iii) defendant's understanding of the attorney's expectations, (iv) resolving disagreements, and (v) special means of communicating with the attorney" (p. 510). The Factual Understanding scale includes 15 questions regarding courtroom participants. The Rational Understanding is comprised of 10 questions that measure the defendant's ability to make rational decisions. In addition, the ECST-R includes an Atypical Presentation scale to assist in identifying feigned incompetency.

Rogers et al. (2001) evaluated the internal and interrater reliabilities of the ECST-R by combining data from previous studies. The α coefficients for the combined data were .72 (Consult With Counsel), .86 (Rational Understanding), .90 (Factual Understanding), and .93 (total score). Interrater reliability correlations were .97 (Consult With Counsel), .99 (Rational Understanding), 1.00 (Factual Understanding), and 1.00 (total score).

In this regard, performance of the ECST-R was commensurate with that for the MacCAT-CA and somewhat better than for the GCCT-MSH. Principle axis factoring of the ECST-R revealed a strong two-factor solution accounting for 43.5% of the variance. This solution produced 21 substantial and unique loadings with only 2 cross loadings. The two factors corresponded to Factual Understanding and Rational Understanding (Ability to Consult With Counsel fell under Rational Understanding). The strength of the ECST-R appears to be its emphasis on rational understanding and its inclusion of an internal validity indicator. Additional research is required to determine the measure's incremental validity in determination of competency to proceed.

Applicability of Competency Assessment Tools to Neuropsychological Evaluation

As competency is a contextual issue, each of the CAT authors cautioned against the use of strict cutoffs and recommended using their instruments to augment the competency evaluation by obtaining standardized information about the defendant's level of understanding and reasoning ability related to legal issues. It is up to the neuropsychologist to bring together each defendant's cognitive strengths and weaknesses as they relate to issues of competency. It is possible a defendant may perform well on any of these competency instruments and yet demonstrate such severe cognitive deficits as to bring their competency into serious question. Likewise, it may very well be possible for a defendant to perform poorly on a CAT for reasons indirectly related to competency.

None of the CATs have been validated with brain-injured or neurological populations. Anecdotally, I have seen brain-injured defendants who have been found competent to proceed have trouble with taking the perspective of the hypothetical defendant during the MacCAT-CA. It is not surprising that individuals with poor mental flexibility would perform poorly on this test. Brain-injured defendants appear to tolerate the GCCT-MSH and CAST*MR more easily.

Regarding the CAST*MR, Stafford (2003) noted, "This instrument contributes legally relevant data and norms to the assessment of mentally retarded *or otherwise cognitively impaired* defendants" (p. 369; emphasis added). Empiricism aside, the CAST*MR does allow comparisons between a brain-injured defendant's performance and that of competent and incompetent individuals with mental retardation. This qualitative comparison can be helpful in evaluating the competence of brain-injured defendants as results can help validate perceptions of the defendant's basic level of knowledge (Denney, 2002).

None of the CATs include measures of cognitive ability beyond legal knowledge and decision-making capacity. The CAST*MR and MacCAT-CA both correlate positively with IQ (Everington & Dunn, 1995; Poythress et al., 1999). Little is known regarding the impact neurocognitive deficits have on competency to proceed. Clearly, there is a role for neurocognitive measures in establishing a criminal defendant's cognitive strengths and weaknesses.

Nestor, Daggett, Haycock, and Price (1999) retrospectively studied the neuropsychological functioning of 181 defendants who underwent inpatient evaluations at Bridgewater State Hospital in Massachusetts for competency to stand trial. The sample consisted of 128 defendants considered competent to proceed and 53 defendants considered not competent to proceed. Subjects were predominantly diagnosed with psychotic and major mood disorders. There were no comparisons of ethnic/racial differences, which substantially limits the study. Also, sample selection bias was a concern. Despite these shortcomings, results suggested competent defendants score higher in areas of psychometric intelligence, attention, memory (particularly verbal), episodic memory (Logical Memory), and verbal and nonverbal social intelligence (Comprehension and Picture Arrangement), but not semantic memory (Vocabulary and Information) or achievement. See Table 12-6 for specific test scores.

TABLE 12-6. Neuropsychological Test Scores for Competent and Not Competent Groups

MEASURE	COMPETENT	NOT COMPETENT	p	EFFECT SIZE
Intelligence				
WAIS-R FIQ	88.25 (15.09)	82.00 (14.44)	<.01	.054
WAIS-R VIQ	88.54 (15.28)	83.06 (15.24)	<.01	.046
WAIS-R PIQ	89.01 (15.50)	82.79 (14.07)	<.01	.043
Memory				
WMS-R GMI	88.12 (19.83)	78.25 (18.62)	<.01	.061
WMS-R VerMI	89.26 (17.40)	80.17 (15.87)	<.01	.070
WMS-R VisMI	92.06 (17.69)	84.64 (20.01)	<.05	.039
Attention/concentration				
WMS-R A/CI	87.58 (19.45)	84.00 (21.09)	ns	
TMT-A sec.	36.70 (17.03)	55.00 (32.19)	<.01	.101
TMT-B sec.	121.29 (92.90)	146.93 (112.74)	ns	
Executive function				
WCST Cat.	3.98 (2.06)	3.19 (2.06)		ns
Academic abilities				
WRAT-R Rd.	81.22 (19.41)	78.88 (23.30)	ns	
WRAT-R Sp.	77.31 (19.14)	76.71 (22.73)	ns	
WRAT-R A.	79.89 (18.48)	75.05 (22.05)	ns	

Note. A, arithmetic; A/CI, Attention/Concentration Index; Cat., Category Test; FIQ, full-scale IQ; GMI, General Memory Index; PIQ, performance IQ; Rd., reading; sec., seconds; Sp., spelling; TMT-A, Trail Making Test-A; TMT-B, Trail Making Test-B; VerMI, Verbal Memory Index; VIQ, Verbal IQ; VisMI, Visual Memory Index; WAIS-R, Wechsler Adult Intelligence Scale–Revised; WCST, Wisconsin Card Sorting Test; WMS-R, Wechsler Memory Scale–Revised; WRAT-R, Wide-Range Achievement Test–Revised. Adapted from "Competence to Stand Trial: A Neuropsychological Inquiry," by P. G. Nestor, D. Daggett, J. Haycock, and M. Price, 1999, *Law and Human Behavior, 23,* pp. 397–412.

These results, and logic, would suggest neuropsychological assessment of competency to stand trial should focus on intelligence, attention and concentration, speed of mental processing, verbal learning and memory, mental flexibility, social reasoning, and decision-making capacity. Such results would also be helpful from a prescriptive perspective. More research on the impact of neurocognitive functioning and competency to proceed needs to occur.

Last, none of these competency instruments have indices of cognitive validity. Only the GCCT-MSH and ECST-R have associated validity indicators, and these are directed toward psychosis. All of the CATs have substantial face validity and appear easy to fake by defendants simply claiming ignorance or lack of cognitive ability. Competency assessment tools are helpful adjunct procedures, but competency evaluations of traumatically brain-injured defendants require a broader neurocognitive evaluation with a battery of tests that include measures of negative response bias specific to neurocognitive functioning.

Amnesia and Competency to Stand Trial

Claimed amnesia for the alleged criminal activity is not unusual (Schacter, 1986). Estimates range from 23% to 65% for homicide (Bradford & Smith, 1979; Guttmacher, 1955; Leitch, 1948; Parwatikar, Holcomb, & Menninger, 1985). Of 100 cases of claimed amnesia, 90% pertained to murder or attempted murder (Hopwood & Snell, 1933). The rates of claimed amnesia appear much lower for nonhomicide crimes. Taylor and Kopelman (1984) found 8% claimed amnesia for 120 cases of nonhomicide violent crimes, and there were no claims of amnesia for 47 nonviolent crimes.

Relevant to legal issues, amnesia has been classified as organic or functional and chronic or limited. Schacter (1986) provided this summary:

In the large majority of criminal cases that involve amnesia, the loss of memory either has a functional origin or concerns only a single critical event. I have found no cases in the literature in which a patient afflicted with chronic organic amnesia has come before the courts on a serious criminal matter that is related to his or her memory disorder. Organic factors may play a role when concussion, alcohol intoxication, or epileptic seizure occurs during a crime, with subsequent limited amnesia for the crime itself, but in these cases memory problems typically do not exist prior to the crime. (p. 287)

It appears the most common form of organic amnesia is limited to specific events and is secondary to alcohol or drug intoxication at the time of the alleged crime. Criminal defendants occasionally experience a neurological disease severe enough to hinder recall of events around the time of the offense or experience a stroke or other neurological event after their arrest, but before trial, that will raise concern about their competency in general and their recollection of allegedly criminal events in particular (Wynkoop & Denney, 1999). It is possible for defendants to experience the neurological trauma at the time of their arrest (e.g., gunshot wounds, head trauma from motor vehicle accidents). In these instances, it is not unreasonable to suspect some loss of memory for events directly preceding arrest, which can include the crime that occasioned the arrest. A defendant's ability to recall events constituting the alleged offense is an important issue and one that speaks to their ability to establish a reasonable defense against criminal prosecution.

Amnesia has the capacity to limit competency to stand trial substantially. For example, the last criteria put forth by the court in *Wieter v. Settle* (1961, Table 4) includes "memory sufficient to relate those things in his/her own personal manner." In 1968, however, the U.S. Court of Appeals for the District of Columbia addressed the issue in an interesting manner in *Wilson v. United States*. Defendant Wilson incurred a traumatic brain injury when his vehicle hit a tree at the conclusion of a high-speed chase. He was unconscious at the scene after having "fractured his skull and ruptured several blood vessels in his brain" (p. 461). He remained unconscious for 3 weeks. Subsequently, he denied recollection of his offenses (five counts of assault with a deadly weapon and robbery). There were no observable mental difficulties beyond his claimed memory loss. He was found competent and convicted. The federal court of appeals concluded that amnesia, in and of itself, did not *necessarily* eliminate competency to stand trial. The court outlined six criteria for determining the impact amnesia has on competency (Table 12-7). Note most of these criteria (3–6) relate to strictly investigative and prosecutory issues. For example, the court made this conclusion regarding the strength of the prosecution's case (*Wilson v. United States*, 1968):

Most important here will be whether the Government's case is such as to negate all reasonable hypotheses of innocence. If there is any substantial possibility that the ac-

TABLE 12-7. Criteria for Impact of Amnesia on Competency

1. The extent to which the amnesia affected the defendant's ability to consult with and assist his lawyer.
2. The extent to which the amnesia affected the defendant's ability to testify in his own behalf.
3. The extent to which the evidence could he extrinsically reconstructed in view of the defendant's amnesia. Such evidence would include evidence relating to the crime itself as well as any reasonably possible alibi.
4. The extent to which the government assisted the defendant and his counsel in that reconstruction.
5. The strength of the prosecution's case.
6. Any other facts and circumstances that would indicate whether or not the defendant had a fair trial.

Note. Issues set forth in *Wilson v. United States* (391 F.2d 460, 1968), pp. 463–464, to aid trial courts in determining whether or not amnesia for the alleged offense substantially impacts the defendant's competency to stand trial.

cused could, but for his amnesia, establish an alibi or other defense, it should be presumed that he would have been able to do so. (p. 464)

Issues relating to the nature of legal cases are explicitly non–mental health.
The extent to which the amnesia affects the defendant's ability to consult with
his or her lawyer and testify in his or her own behalf, however, are clinical
issues. Neuropsychologists have the knowledge and tools to speak directly to
these concerns. Given the issues outlined in *Wilson v. United States*, a trial court
may rule a defendant competent to proceed even with legitimate amnesia. It is
easy to understand why courts are concerned about claimed amnesia and the
possibility of malingering.

Researchers long presented the perspective that a substantial number of amnestic claims for criminal events are feigned (Adatto, 1949; Bradford & Smith,
1979; Hopwood & Snell, 1933; Lynch & Bradford, 1980; O'Connell, 1960;
Parwatikar, Holcomb, & Menninger, 1985; Power, 1977; Price & Terhune,
1919). There have been a variety of methods presented to evaluate legitimacy
of claimed amnesia (see Rubinsky & Brandt, 1986; Schacter, 1986). Symptom
validity testing has been adapted for evaluating the veracity of criminal defendants claiming partial amnesia for the alleged offense as well as total retrograde
amnesia, also including the offense (Denney, 1996; Frederick, Carter, & Powel,
1995; Frederick & Denney, 1998).

Symptom validity testing for remote memory entails creating, from investigative records (including eye witness accounts and prosecutory reconstructions)
and information regarding defendant's life history from collateral informants for
those defendants claiming total retrograde amnesia, two-alternative forced-
choice questions based on information about the alleged criminal activity. Questions can also be developed to assess recollection of well-known facts about
courtroom participants and the criminal law process as these areas can be considered a component of remote memory. Developed questions are presented to
the defendant orally. Only those questions for which the defendant claims no
recollection are kept in the analysis. Results are applied to the binomial theorem
to identify below-chance responding. Significantly worse-than-chance performance provides evidence the defendant actually knew the correct material but
was intentionally choosing the wrong answer to appear impaired. See Denney
(1996) for a thorough description of the process. Although time consuming, the
procedure has demonstrated considerable clinical utility (Denney, 1996; Wynkoop & Denney, 1999) and a sound statistical basis (Frederick & Denney, 1998).

Treatment of the Incompetent Defendant

The courts have authority to commit incompetent defendants for mental health
treatment involuntarily. *Jackson v. Indiana* (1972), a famous and far-reaching
U.S. Supreme Court case, outlined that the length of such commitments must

have a "rational relationship" to the nature of the commitment. In other words, it is not constitutional to hold someone strictly for treatment to restore competency longer than the person would have been held if convicted of the crime. Criminal defendants *can* be held longer if they are considered dangerous to themselves or others as a result of mental illness, however.

Continued commitment for danger to self requires a change from a criminally established commitment to a civil commitment procedure. Most jurisdictions have a process for continued criminal commitment for those defendants considered dangerous to others. For example, in the federal system, 18 U.S.C., § 4246, allows continued commitment of an incompetent defendant who is judicially determined to "presently suffer from a mental disease or defect as a result of which his release would create a substantial risk of bodily injury to another person or serious damage to property of another" but only until a "suitable" (i.e., safe) state placement is found, or the defendant is no longer dangerous because of mental illness. Involuntary commitment for treatment to restore competency to proceed does not necessarily mean treatment with psychiatric medications, however.

In *Riggins v. Nevada* (1992), the U.S. Supreme Court provided vague guidance regarding medicating incompetent defendants over their objections. Although the justices indicated "treatment with antipsychotic medication was medically appropriate and, considering less intrusive alternatives, essential for the sake of [the defendant's] own safety or the safety of others" (p. 135), they did not spell out whether involuntary treatment simply to restore competency was appropriate.

In an earlier decision (*Washington v. Harper*, 1990), the court described a balance between state interests and rights of an incarcerated man by citing "overriding state interest" as adequate authority to force medicate. In a similar vein, courts have found the prosecution of dangerous defendants a reasonable state interest such that forced medication for trial competency was justified (*United States v. Charters*, 1988; *Khiem v. United States*, 1992).

This position appears to be tacitly supported by the U.S. Supreme Court given the fact they refused to review the District of Columbia Circuit Court's decision to allow forced medication of Russell Weston, a clearly violent man,[4] to restore his competency to stand trial in a capital case. The U.S. Supreme Court provided an opinion regarding involuntary medication for competency restoration of a nonviolent defendant during June 2003, but the impact of the *Sell v. United States* decision is still unclear.

Charles Sell, a St. Louis area dentist, was originally charged with insurance fraud, Medicare fraud, and money laundering.[5] He had a history of psychotic mental illness. Dr. Sell was initially found competent to stand trial, but regressed to a more clearly psychotic state. He was then found not competent to stand trial and was committed for mental health treatment to restore his competency

FORENSIC NEUROPSYCHOLOGY

to proceed. It was recommended he receive antipsychotic medication, but he would not consent. Over the course of the next 6 years, the defense argued that he had a right to refuse treatment with antipsychotic medications. The 8th Circuit Court ruled in favor of forcibly medicating him, but stayed the order, pending review by the U.S. Supreme Court. The U.S. Supreme Court vacated the circuit court order and remanded the case back to the district court for further consideration. The High Court concluded that the forcible administration of antipsychotic medication solely to restore competency could be done under certain circumstances.

First, the Court recommended trial courts consider such cases based on *Washington v. Harper* (1990) grounds (i.e., is the person dangerous to self or others grounds). If so, there is no legal concern. If the defendant is not dangerous to self or others, then these four issues must be resolved affirmatively by the trial court in order to justify forced medication: (a) There are *important* government interests; (b) those important government interests will be *significantly furthered* by medication; (c) the medication is *necessary* (i.e., there are no less-intrusive alternatives); and (d) such medicine is *medically appropriate*.

The full impact of the *Sell* decision is not yet completely clear. At this point in the federal jurisdiction, criminal defendants committed to inpatient treatment for purposes of restoration who do not consent to take antipsychotic medication after psychiatric recommendation often undergo an additional hearing (*Sell* hearing) for the referring district court to consider first the issue of dangerousness, then the four points outlined by the U.S. Supreme Court. In this manner, the referring court can authorize forced administration of antipsychotic medication solely for the restoration of competency.

SUMMARY

This chapter introduced the practice of neuropsychology in the criminal forensic arena as a unique practice opportunity. Neuropsychologists are more commonly applying principles of brain–behavior relationships and assessment results to the specific questions of criminal courts. Although neuropsychology has a great deal to offer the courts, practice of neuropsychology in this setting requires different assumptions and different methods of evaluation from that of typical clinical settings. Neuropsychologists must recognize that, in forensic settings, the client is typically not the patient. The evaluator's alliance is with the truth rather than the patient or referral source. As a result of this different conceptual standing, neuropsychologists incorporate slightly different methodology by including corroborative information sources and systematic assessment of negative response bias and malingering.

The chapter covered the mental health case law at it relates to criminal competency and how it applies to various points in criminal proceedings. Particularly, the *Dusky* standard and its conceptual bases were emphasized. Case law related to decisional competency, such as pleading guilty, waiving right to counsel, and refusing an insanity defense, was addressed. The impact of amnesia on competency as well as methods to assess its veracity were covered. Last, treatment issues were addressed as they related to hospitalization and forced treatment for the sole purpose of restoring competency.

Chapter 13 furthers the discussion of neuropsychological practice in the criminal forensic arena by expanding on the multiple data source model and applying it to criminal responsibility evaluations. The history and current standing of the insanity defense are covered. Issues around sentencing are presented, such as diminished capacity and responsibility, dangerous prediction, and death penalty. Last, general ethical and professional development issues are addressed. Neuropsychologists have an opportunity to make substantial contributions to each of these criminal areas if they have the prerequisite knowledge base and understand important legal and ethical issues inherent in criminal forensics.

NOTES

Opinions expressed in this chapter are those of the author and do not necessarily represent the position of the Federal Bureau of Prisons or the U.S. Department of Justice.

1. Frederick, DeMier, and Towers obtained primary source documents related to *Dusky*.
2. Those wishing to obtain the CAI may request the Competency to Stand Trial and Mental Illness Packet from Paul Lipsitt, LL.B., Ph.D., at Student Mental Health Clinic, Boston University, 881 Commonwealth Avenue, West Entrance, Boston, MA 02215. The Revised CAI may be obtained from John Riley, Ph.D., Forensic Services, Atascadero State Hospital, P.O. Box 7001, Atascadero, CA 93423-7001.
3. Ordering information: IDS Publishing, P.O. Box 389, Worthington, OH 43085; phone (614) 885-2323.
4. Weston was charged with a shooting rampage in the U.S. Capital building, which resulted in the deaths of two Capital Police. The facts of the case clearly revealed Weston as the perpetrator.
5. He has subsequently been charged with attempted murder of a federal agent, but the U.S. Supreme Court is making its decision based solely on the facts as if Sell was considered a nondangerous criminal defendant.

REFERENCES

Adatto, C. P. (1949). Observations on criminal patients during narcoanalysis. *Archives of Neurology and Psychiatry, 62,* 82–92.

Bagby, R. M., Nicholson, R. A., Rogers, R., & Nussbaum, D. (1992). Domains of competency to stand trial: A factor analytic study. *Law and Human Behavior, 16,* 491–507.

Barnard, G. W., Nicholson, R., Hankins, G., Raisani, K., Patel, N., Gies, D., et al. (1992). Item metric and scale analysis of a new computer-assisted competency assessment instrument (CADCOMP). *Behavioral Sciences and the Law, 10,* 419–435.

Barnard, G. W., Thompson, J. W., Freeman, W. C., Robbins, L., Gies, D., & Hankins, G. C. (1991). Competency to stand trial: Description and evaluation of a new computer assisted assessment tool (CADCOMP). *Bulletin of the American Academy of Psychiatry and Law, 19,* 367–381.

Bigler, E. D., & Clement, P. F. (1997). *Diagnostic clinical neuropsychology* (3rd ed.). Austin, TX: University of Texas Press.

Borum, R., & Grisso, T. (1995). Psychological test use in criminal forensic evaluations. *Professional Psychology: Research and Practice, 26,* 465–473.

Bradford, J. W., & Smith, S. M. (1979). Amnesia and homicide: The Padola case and a study of 30 cases. *Bulletin of the American Academy of Psychiatry and Law, 7,* 219–231.

Colorado v. Connelly, 107 S.Ct. 515 (1986).

Cooper v. Oklahoma, 517 U.S. 348 (1996).

Denney, R. L. (1996) Symptom validity testing of remote memory in a criminal forensic setting. *Archives of Clinical Neuropsychology, 11,* 589–603.

Denney, R. L. (2002, October). *Neuropsychological assessment in the criminal forensic arena: Competencies, sanity, and ethics.* Presentation given at the 22nd Annual National Academy of Neuropsychology Conference, South Miami Beach, FL.

Denney, R. L., & Wynkoop, T. F. (2000). Clinical neuropsychology in the criminal forensic setting. *Journal of Head Trauma Rehabilitation, 15,* 804–828.

Drope v. Missouri, 420 U.S. 162 (1975).

Dusky v. United States, 362 U.S. 402 (1960).

Everington, C. T. (1990). The Competence Assessment for Standing Trial for Defendants With Mental Retardation (CAST-MR): A validation study. *Criminal Justice and Behavior, 17,* 147–168.

Everington, C. T., & Dunn, C. (1995). A second validation study of the Competence Assessment for Standing Trial for Defendants With Mental Retardation (CAST-MR). *Criminal Justice and Behavior, 22,* 44–59.

Everington, C. T., & Luckasson, R. (1992). *Competence Assessment for Standing Trial for Defendants With Mental Retardation (CAST*MR): Test manual.* Worthington, OH: IDS.

Faretta v. California, 422 U.S. 806 (1975).

Favole, R. J. (1983) Mental disability in the American criminal process: A four issue survey. In J. Monahan & H. Steadman (Eds.), *Mentally disordered offenders: Perspectives from law and social science* (pp. 281–295) New York: Plenum Press.

Forensic Specialty Council. (2000). *Petition for the recognition of forensic psychology as a specialty in professional psychology.* Submitted to the American Psychological Association, Washington, DC.

Frederick, R. I., Carter, M., & Powel, J. (1995). Adapting symptom validity testing to evaluate suspicious complaints of amnesia in medicolegal evaluations. *Bulletin of the American Academy of Psychiatry and the Law, 23,* 231–237.

Frederick, R. I., DeMier, R. L., & Towers, K. (2004). *Assessing competency to stand trial: Foundations in case law.* Sarasota, FL: Professional Resource Press.

Frederick, R. I., & Denney, R. L. (1998). Minding your "ps and qs" when using forced-choice recognition tests. *Clinical Neuropsychologist, 12,* 193–205.

Frendak v. United States, 408 A.2d 364 (1979).

Giuliano, A. J., Barth, J. T., Hawk, G. L., & Ryan, T. V. (1997). The forensic neuropsychologist: Precedents, roles, and problems. In R. J. McCaffrey, A. D. Williams, J. M. Fisher, & L. C. Laing (Eds.), *The practice of forensic neuropsychology: Meeting challenges in the courtroom* (pp. 1–36). New York: Plenum Press.

Godinez v. Moran, 125 L. Ed. 2d, 509 U.S. 389 (1993).

Golding, S., Roesch, R., & Schreiber, J. (1984). Assessment and conceptualization of competency to stand trial: Preliminary data on the Interdisciplinary Fitness Interview. *Law and Human Behavior, 8*, 321–324.

Goldstein, A. M. (2003). Overview of forensic psychology. In I. B. Weiner (Series Ed.) & A. M. Goldstein (Vol. Ed.), *Handbook of psychology, Vol. 11: Forensic psychology* (pp. 3–20). Hoboken, NJ: Wiley.

Gothard, S., Rogers, R., & Sewell, K. W. (1995). Feigning incompetency to stand trial: An investigation of the GCCT. *Law and Human Behavior, 19*, 363–373.

Greenberg, S. A., & Shuman, D. W. (1997). Irreconcilable conflict between therapeutic and forensic roles. *Professional Psychology: Research and Practice, 28*, 50–57.

Grisso, T. (1986). *Evaluating competencies: Forensic assessments and instruments.* New York: Plenum Press.

Grisso, T. (1988). *Competency to stand trial evaluations: A manual for practice.* Sarasota, FL: Professional Resource Exchange.

Grisso, T., Borum, R., Edens, J. F., Moye, J., & Otto, R. K. (2003). *Evaluating competencies: Forensic assessments and instruments* (2nd ed.). New York: Kluwer Academic/Plenum.

Grisso, T., Cocozza, J., Steadman, H. J., Fisher, W., & Greer, A. (1994). The organization of pretrial forensic evaluation services: A national profile. *Law and Human Behavior, 18*, 377–394.

Group for the Advancement of Psychiatry. (1974). *Misuse of psychiatry in the criminal courts: Competency to stand trial.* New York: Committee on Psychiatry and the Law.

Guttmacher, M. S. (1955). *Psychiatry and the law.* New York: Grune and Stratton.

Heilbrun, K. (2001). *Principles of forensic mental health assessment.* New York: Kluwer Academic/Plenum.

Hoge, S. K., Bonnie, R. J., Poythress, N., Monahan, J., Eisenberg, M., & Feucht-Haviar, T. (1997). The MacArthur adjudicative competence study: Development and validation of a research instrument. *Law and Human Behavior, 21*, 141–179.

Hom, J., & Denney, R. L. (2002). Preface. In J. Hom & R. L. Denney (Eds.), *Detection of negative response bias in forensic neuropsychology* (pp. xi–xvi). New York: Haworth Press.

Hopwood, J. S., & Snell, H. K. (1933). Amnesia in relation to crime. *Journal of Mental Science, 79*, 27–41.

Jackson v. Indiana, 406 U.S. 715 (1972).

Johnson, W. G., & Mullett, N. (1988). Georgia Court Competency Test-R. In M. Hersen & A. S. Bellack (Eds.), *Dictionary of behavioral assessment techniques* (p. 234). New York: Pergamon.

Khiem v. United States, 612 A.2d 160 (DC, 1992).

Laboratory of Community Psychiatry, Harvard Medical School. (1973). *Competency to stand trial and mental illness* (DHEW Publication No. ADM77–103). Rockville, MD: Department of Health, Education, and Welfare.

Leitch, A. (1948). Notes on amnesia in crime for the general practitioner. *Medical Press, 219*, 459–463.

Lezak, M. D. (1995). *Neuropsychological assessment* (3rd ed.). New York: Oxford.

Lipsitt, P. D., Lelos, D., & McGarry, A. L. (1971). Competency for trial: A screening instrument. *American Journal of Psychiatry, 128*, 105–109.

Lynch, B. E., & Bradford, J. M. W. (1980). Amnesia: Its detection by psychophysiological measures. *Bulletin of the American Academy of Psychiatry and the Law, 8*, 288–297.

Martell, D. A. (1992a). Estimating the prevalence of organic brain dysfunction in maximum-security forensic psychiatric patients. *Journal of Forensic Science, 37*, 878–893.

Martell, D. A. (1992b). Forensic neuropsychology and the criminal law. *Law and Human Behavior, 16*, 313–336.

McGarry, A. L., Lelos, D., & Lipsitt, P. D. (1973). *Competency to stand trial and mental illness.* Washington, DC: U.S. Government Printing Office.

Medina v. California, 505 U.S. 437 (1992).

Melton, G. B., Petrila, J., Poythress, N. G., & Slobogin, C. (1997). *Psychological evaluations for the courts* (2nd ed.). New York: Guilford Press.

Miranda v. Arizona, 384 U.S. 436 (1966).

Mittenberg, W., Patton, C., Canyock, E. M., & Condit, D. C. (2002). Base rates of malingering and symptom exaggeration. *Journal of Clinical and Experimental Neuropsychology, 24*, 1094–1102.

Morris v. Slappy, 461 U.S. 1 (1983).

Mrad, D. (1996, September). *Criminal responsibility evaluations.* Paper presented at Issues in Forensic Assessment Symposium, Federal Bureau of Prisons, Atlanta, GA.

Nestor, P. G., Daggett, D., Haycock, J., & Price, M. (1999). Competence to stand trial: A neuropsychological inquiry. *Law and Human Behavior, 23*, 397–412.

Nicholson, R. A., Briggs, S. R., & Robertson, H. C. (1988). Instruments for assessing competency to stand trial: How do they work? *Professional Psychology: Research and Practice, 19*, 383–394.

Nicholson, R. A., Robertson, H. C., Johnson, W. G., & Jensen, G. (1988). A comparison of instruments for assessing competency to stand trial. *Law and Human Behavior, 12*, 313–321.

North Carolina v. Alford, 400 U.S. 25 (1970).

O'Connell, B. A. (1960). Amnesia and homicide. *British Journal of Delinquency, 10*, 262–276.

Otto, R., Poythress, N., Edens, J., Nicholson, R., Monahan, J., Bonnie, R., et al. (1998). Psychometric properties of the MacArthur Competence Assessment Tool—Criminal Adjudication. *Psychological Assessment, 10*, 435–443.

Parenté, R., & Herrmann, D. (1996). *Retraining cognition: Techniques and applications.* Gaithersburg, MD: Aspen.

Parwatikar, S. D., Holcomb, W. R., & Menninger, K. A., II. (1985). The detection of malingered amnesia in accused murderers. *Bulletin of the American Academy of Psychiatry and the Law, 13*, 97–103.

Pate v. Robinson, 383 U.S. 375 (1966).

Power, D. J. (1977). Memory, identification and crime. *Medicine, Science, and the Law, 17*, 132–139.

Poythress, N., Nicholson, R., Otto, R., Edens, J., Bonnie, R., Monahan, J., et al. (1999). *The MacArthur Competence Assessment Tool—Criminal Adjudication: Professional manual.* Odessa, FL: Psychological Assessment Resources.

Price, G. E., & Terhune, W. B. (1919). Feigned amnesia as a defense reaction. *Journal of the American Medical Association, 72*, 565–567.

Reisner, R., & Slobogin, C. (1990). *Law and the mental health system* (2nd ed.). St. Paul, MN: West.

Riggins v. Nevada, 504 U.S. 127 (1992).

Riley, J. A. (1998, March) *Introducing the Revised-CAI and assessment of trial competency—Use of the Revised-Competency Assessment Instrument handbook.* Presentation at American Psychology–Law Society Biennial Conference, Redondo Beach, CA.

Roesch, R., & Golding, S. (1978). Legal and judicial interpretation of competency to stand trial. *Criminology, 16,* 420.

Roesch, R., & Golding, S. (1980). *Competency to stand trial.* Urbana-Champaign: University of Illinois Press.

Roesch, R., Webster, C., & Eaves, D. (1984). *The Fitness Interview Test: A method for examining fitness to stand trial.* Toronto, Ontario, Canada: Research Report of the Centre of Criminology, University of Toronto.

Roesch, R., Zapf, P., Eaves, D., & Webster, C. (1998). *Fitness Interview Test* (rev. ed.). Burnaby, British Columbia, Canada: Mental Health, Law and Policy Institute, Simon Fraser University.

Rogers, R. (1997). Introduction. In R. Rogers (Ed.), *Handbook of diagnostic and structured interviewing* (pp. 1–19). New York: Guilford Press.

Rogers, R. (2001). Focused forensic interviews. In R. Rogers (Ed.), *Handbook of diagnostic and structured interviewing* (pp. 296–357). New York: Guilford Press.

Rogers, R., & Grandjean, N. R. (2000, March). *Competency measures and the Dusky Standard: A conceptual mismatch?* Biennial convention of the American Psychology-Law Society, New Orleans, Louisiana.

Rogers, R., Grandjean, N. R., Tillbrook, C. E., Vitacco, M. J., & Sewell, K. W. (2001). Recent interview-based measures of competency to stand trial: A critical review augmented with research data. *Behavioral Sciences and the Law, 19,* 503–518.

Rogers, R., Sewell, K. W., Grandjean, N. R., & Vitacco, M. (2002). The detection of feigned mental disorders on specific competency measures. *Psychological Assessment, 14,* 177–183.

Rogers, R., Tillbrook, C. E., & Sewell, K. W. (2004). *Evaluation of Competency to Stand Trial–Revised.* Lutz, FL: Psychological Assessment Resources, Inc.

Rogers, R., Ustad, K. L., Sewell, K. W., & Reinhart, V. (1996). Dimensions of incompetency: A factor analytic study of the Georgia Court Competency Test. *Behavioral Sciences and the Law, 14,* 323–330.

Rosenberg, A. H., & McGarry, L. (1972). Competency for trial: The making of an expert. *American Journal of Psychiatry, 128,* 1092–1096.

Rubinsky, E. W., & Brandt, J. (1986). Amnesia and criminal law: A clinical overview. *Behavioral Sciences and the Law, 4,* 27–46.

Saks, M. J. (1990). Expert witnesses, nonexpert witnesses, and nonwitness experts. *Law and Human Behavior, 14,* 291–313.

Schacter, D. L. (1986). Amnesia and crime: How much do we really know? *American Psychologist, 41,* 286–295.

Sell v. United States, ____ U.S. ____ (2003).

Shapiro, D. L. (1984). *Psychological evaluation and expert testimony.* New York: van Nostrand Reinhold.

Shapiro, D. L. (1991). *Forensic psychological assessment.* Boston: Allyn and Bacon.

Shapiro, D. L. (1999). *Criminal responsibility evaluations: A manual for practice.* Sarasota, FL: Professional Resource Press.

Sieling v. Eyman, 478 F.2d 211 (1973).

Sohlberg, M. M., & Mateer, C. A. (2001). *Cognitive rehabilitation.* New York: Guilford Press.

Stafford, K. P. (2003). Assessment of competence to stand trial. In I. B. Weiner (Series Ed.) & A. M. Goldstein (Vol. Ed.), *Handbook of psychology, Vol. 11: Forensic psychology* (pp. 359–380). Hoboken, NJ: Wiley.

Steadman, H., Monahan, J., Hartstone, E., Davis, S., & Robbins, P. (1982). Mentally disordered offenders: A national survey of patients and facilities. *Law and Human Behavior, 6*, 31–38.

Sullivan, J. P., & Denney, R. L. (2003). Constitutional and judicial foundations in criminal forensic neuropsychology. *Journal of Forensic Neuropsychology, 3*, 13–44.

Taylor, P. J., & Kopelman, M. D. (1984). Amnesia for criminal offences. *Psychological Medicine, 14*, 581–588.

United States v. Charters, 863 F.2d 302 (4th Cir., 1988).

Ustad, K. L., Rogers, R., Sewell, K. W., & Guarnaccia, C. A. (1996). Restoration of competency to stand trial: Assessment with the GCCT-MSH and the CST. *Law and Human Behavior, 20*, 131–146.

Washington v. Harper, 494 U.S. 210 (1990).

Westbrook v. Arizona, 384 U.S. 150 (1966).

Whalem v. United States, 346 F.2d 812 (DC Cir., 1965).

Wieter v. Settle, 193 F. Supp. 318 (W.D. Mo., 1961).

Wildman, R., Batchelor, E., Thompson, L., Nelson, F., Moore, J., Patterson, M., et al. (1980). *The Georgia Court Competency Test: An attempt to develop a rapid, quantitative measure for fitness for trial.* Unpublished manuscript, Forensic Services Division, Central State Hospital, Milledgeville, GA.

Wilson v. United States, 391 F.2d 460 (DC Cir., 1968).

Wynkoop, T. F., & Denney, R. L. (1999). Exaggeration of neuropsychological deficit in competency to stand trial. *Journal of Forensic Neuropsychology, 1*, 29–53.

Youtsey v. United States, 97 F. 937, 940 (6th Circ. 1899).

Zapf, P. A., & Roesch, R. (2001). A comparison of MacCAT-CA and FIT for making determinations of competency to stand trial. *International Journal of Law and Psychiatry, 24*, 81–92.

Zapf, P. A., Roesch, R., & Viljoen, J. L. (2001). The utility of the Fitness Interview Test for assessing fitness to stand trial. *Canadian Journal of Psychiatry, 46*, 426–432.

13

Criminal Responsibility and Other Criminal Forensic Issues

ROBERT L. DENNEY

In chapter 12, I presented criminal forensic neuropsychology as a subspecialty of forensic psychology. It is a practice area that requires a unique knowledge base. The forensic role requires an appreciation of the significantly different alliance, goals, and methodology. I introduced the multiple data source model (MDSM) of forensic assessment. I described mental health case law regarding competency to proceed and outlined decisional competency as it relates to confessions, pleading guilty, waiving one's right to an attorney, and refusing an insanity defense. The impact of amnesia on competency and treatment to restore competency were also addressed. Each of these areas establishes a foundation to cover the more advanced areas of criminal forensics presented here.

In this chapter, I expand on the forensic assessment model, particularly as it pertains to the assessment of criminal responsibility. I cover the historical antecedents of the insanity defense and its current legal conceptualizations. Sentencing issues, such as diminished capacity and responsibility, prediction of dangerousness, and death penalty, are covered. The chapter ends with general ethical and professional development issues for neuropsychologists entertaining the idea of developing proficiency in criminal forensics.

Part of the unique knowledge base in criminal forensics is the realization that forensic evaluators do not share the same goals as general clinical providers. The client is typically not the patient, and the evaluator's alliance is with the

425

truth as opposed to the patient or referral source. As such, forensic neuropsy-chologists utilize a different methodology that includes extensive use of corrob-orative information and the systematic assessment of negative response bias and malingering. The conceptual difference of this approach is best exemplified, in methodological terms, by the multiple data source model of assessment.

MULTIPLE DATA SOURCE MODEL

The MDSM is presented in Figure 12-1 (see p. 385, this volume). It represents a synthesis of the works of various authors in forensic psychology in general (Grisso, 1988; Melton, Petrila, Poythress, & Slobogin, 1997) and Shapiro's work in criminal responsibility evaluation in particular (1984, 1991, 1999). The primary aspects of this integrated model were first presented by Mrad (1996), adapted and published for use in criminal forensic neuropsychology (Denney & Wynkoop, 2000), and later applied to civil forensic work (McLearen, Pietz, & Denney, 2004).

Figure 12-1 provides an overall picture of how information sources are classi-fied and integrated to form reasonable clinical decisions and adequate support for specific forensic questions, particularly those that involve an opinion about behavior at some point in the past. Most commonly, the past opinion will deal with mental state at the time of a specific crime, but occasionally retrospective competency evaluations occur as well. Using this model better ensures that the evaluator considers relevant information, identifies inconsistencies between data sources, and comes to a reasonable conclusion, whether addressing past mental states or current diagnostic issues.

Figure 12-1 represents a cross-tabulation of information sources (self-report and corroborative information) and points on the time line (currently, the time of the offense, and life history). The three rows represent periods of time. The top row includes information to address current mental functioning. The lower row refers to life history. The middle row focuses on mental state, behavior, and motivation at the time of the alleged offense (or the row can represent any event in the past, such as retrospective study of competency to stand trial, enter a guilty plea, waive right to counsel, understanding *Miranda* warning, and com-petence to confess). The focus on mental state, behavior, and motivation for that time period has been referred to as MSO for mental state (at the time of the) offense (Melton et al., 1997). The left column of self-report covers the defen-dant's perception and recollection, and the middle column focuses on informa-tion derived from sources other than the defendant. Self-report and corroborative information cover each of the three time periods. The third column refers to the clinician's opinion about mental state and likely diagnosis for each period of time.

There should be a general flow of consistency between boxes vertically and horizontally. For example, a defendant's self-reported history in the area of mental health symptoms should be reasonably consistent with their current mental state and MSO given known understanding of the natural course for that particular mental health concern. The age of onset and symptom manifestation should make sense. Likewise, medical records, family reports, and current assessment techniques should be reasonably consistent from past to present. The major consistency check, however, occurs horizontally. Defendant's report of personal history should be consistent with educational records, medical records, family reports, and so on. This consistency acts as a veracity check and cannot be ignored. The ultimate focus after incorporating current and background information is the row dealing with MSO. It deserves special consideration.

Mental State at Offense

Like every other aspect of this model, there should be reasonable consistency between defendant self-report regarding thoughts and actions during and around the time of the offense and that of corroborative sources. It is customary to discuss with the defendant his or her perception of events leading up to the alleged offense, behaviors and motivations during the events, and what happened afterward. Although it is desirable to interview the defendant about such issues, occasionally the defendant's mental illness interferes. The defendant may be unwilling to talk about it or may indicate that his or her attorney directed him or her not to speak of events leading up to the alleged offense. In such cases, coordinating a telephone conversation between the defendant and his or her attorney is often helpful. Federal Rule of Criminal Procedure 12.2(c)(4) provides this protection for federal defendants:

No statement made by a defendant in the course of any examination conducted under this rule (whether conducted with or without the defendant's consent), no testimony by the expert based on the statement, and no other fruits of the statement may be admitted into evidence against the defendant in any criminal proceeding except on an issue regarding mental condition on which the defendant [has either introduced mental health evidence or notice of intent to rely on a mental health defense].

The protection is provided for subjects of court-ordered evaluations, for which questions of the defendant's willingness to cooperate most commonly arise. Relatedly, 12.2(d) allows the court to exclude any expert evidence (even defense evidence) if the defendant does not cooperate with a court-ordered examination. Reminding defense counsel of such rules and allowing the defendant to consult with counsel often resolves the defendant's concern and allows the evaluation to proceed as usual. Occasionally, defendants are quite suspicious of their attorney and will not cooperate because of paranoid ideation. Typically, these instances relate to evaluations for competency to stand trial and are court ordered. The evaluator will need to progress with the evaluation with whatever information becomes available and limit his or her opinions appropriately.

In the federal system, as in most states, intent to rely on an insanity defense requires notification to the court by the defense. In this regard, defendants are generally, ostensibly, cooperative because they have discussed the potential referral for mental health evaluation with counsel before making the request to the judge. An insanity-referred defendant who indicates no desire to use a mental health defense raises a unique concern. Because insanity is an "affirmative" defense, meaning the defense must actively seek it and carries the burden of proof, competent defendants have the right to refrain from a mental health defense. Continuing a mental health evaluation on the issue of sanity is problematic if the defendant does not want a mental health defense.

Under this circumstance, the issue goes more to competence to refuse an insanity defense (see chapter 12). These issues are discussed further under Ethical and Professional Issues. The point here is that, most of the time, defendants are willing to provide their perspective of their functioning at MSO if they are seeking a mental health defense. Occasionally, defendants will be unable to do so because of acute mental illness or significant neurocognitive deficits. Inability to provide self-report information does not necessarily eliminate the ability to determine MSO, but it often limits the opinion to some degree. The amount of limitation depends on the quality of corroborative information at MSO.

Acquisition of corroborative information at MSO is *paramount* in evaluations of sanity and past mental states. In this regard, the middle box under Other Data Sources for MSO is vital under any circumstance and should be viewed as a kingpin of the model. Examples of other data sources dealing with MSO include witness statements, videotape and audiotape recordings (actual observed defendant behavior), family reports, and courtroom transcripts. Each of the surrounding boxes must be rationally consistent with the information from this domain. Synthesizing information from each of the other boxes allows the evaluator to derive a reasoned opinion about the defendant's MSO. Once this is done, the evaluator can consider the ultimate issue, that is, whether the defendant's mental health compromised and altered thinking meets the legal definition in question (e.g., insanity, retrospective competency).

It will become apparent under sections dealing with standards for insanity in this chapter that presence of a mental disease or defect is not enough by itself to conclude lack of criminal responsibility. Making such a judgment simply on presence of mental abnormality, without analyzing defendant's behavior with corroborative information, constitutes what has been referred to as the "forensic leap of faith" (Denney & Wynkoop, 2000; Mrad, 1996). To the right of the opinion about MSO box is the ultimate issue box (Figure 12-1, p. 385, this volume). The separation of this box from the opinion box signifies a distinctly separate analysis that requires comparison of the MSO opinion to the specific legal standard (e.g., insanity) in that criminal jurisdiction. As will become apparent, insanity standards are not uniform across jurisdictions.

CRIMINAL RESPONSIBILITY

A conclusion of criminal responsibility (guilt) for a criminal offense requires proof, beyond reasonable doubt, of two elements, *actus reus* and *mens rea*. *Actus reus* refers to the performance of a prohibited act. *Mens rea* refers to the mental state, literally "guilty mind." Mental health professionals address *mens rea* when they provide opinions on sanity and diminished capacity.

Historical Introduction to Insanity

The concept of evaluating the perpetrator's mental state and culpability is as old as documented history. Mosaic law, written in the 13th century B.C. (e.g., Numbers 35:22), describes situations in which "intention" to murder is translated as "malice aforethought" (Jewish Publication Society, 1982). Suggestions of exculpatory "madness" were apparent in preclassical Greek writing (Robinson, 1996). Greek moral philosophy clearly addressed inner will. With the sixth century Justinian Code, ecclesiastical law influenced secular law by introducing *mens rea* more formally. It became clear that mental illness influenced a defendant's *mens rea*, and courts began wrestling with the definition of insanity.

Early British legal history recognized the unjustness of holding persons responsible for acts stemming from mental aberrations. From 1265 on, legal scholars used terms such as "wild beast," "idiots, madmen, [those who] wholly loseth memory and understanding," and "infant, brute or wild beast" (Melton et al., 1997). Some British courts during the 1700s concentrated more on the focused issues of an individual's understanding between good and evil and right and wrong. In the 1800s, some British jurisdiction broadened insanity by using such volitional concepts as "controlling disease" and "acting power within which cannot be resisted." Finally, in 1843 Daniel M'Naghten was found not guilty by reason of insanity for shooting the British prime minister's personal secretary (*Rex v. M'Naghten*, 1843).

> Ye people of England: exult and be glad,
> for ye're now at the will of the merciless mad . . .
> Thomas Campbell (published in several English papers
> in response to M'Naghten's acquittal, 1843)

Daniel M'Naghten[1] had a persecutory delusional belief that incorporated the Tory Party leader, Prime Minister Robert Peel. He traveled to London to ambush Prime Minister Peel, but inadvertently shot Peel's personal secretary, Edward

Drummond. He was acquitted as insane, and there was immediate outcry in public and Parliament as demonstrated by Thomas Campbell's satire (Moran, 1981). After much debate regarding the nature of sanity, the House of Lords called the judges of the Supreme Court to answer five specific questions. The answers to these questions became the M'Naghten rules. A portion of those rules outlined a strictly right/wrong test for insanity, which has become known as the M'Naghten test. Here is the key portion of that judicial decision:

> To establish a defence on the ground of insanity it must be clearly proved that, at the time of committing of the act, the party accused was labouring under such a defect of reason, from disease of the mind, as not to know the nature and quality of the act he was doing, or, if he did know it, that he did not know he was doing what was wrong. (p. 210)

Insanity in the United States

The M'Naghten right/wrong test for insanity became the standard in the United States as well as England, although it was criticized for its rigidity and sole reliance on cognitive understanding (Melton et al., 1997). This criticism gradually led U.S. jurisdictions to loosen the standard for insanity. The "irresistible impulse" rule was first adopted in Alabama (*Parsons v. State*, 1887) and later by a federal jurisdiction (*Davis v. United States*, 1895). This rule was a straightforward volitional controls standard. As described in *Parsons*, a defendant would be considered not responsible if each of these two conditions were met:

> (1) If, by reason of the duress of . . . mental disease he had so far lost the power to choose between the right and wrong, and to avoid doing the act in question, as that his free agency was at the time destroyed: (2) and if, at the same time, the alleged crime was so connected with such mental disease, in the relation of cause and effect, as to have been the product of it solely. (cited in Melton et al., 1997, p. 191)

In 1954, the District of Columbia Court of Appeals carried on similar language when it adopted a little-known New Hampshire "product test" (*State v. Jones*, 1871), in part secondary to criticisms of rigidity and narrowness of previous standards (*Durham v. United States*, 1954). Also, in response to the growing hope in psychoanalysis as a method of understanding human nature, Judge Bazelon opened the doors to psychiatry in the criminal courts by defining insanity as any action that is a "product of mental disease or defect" (*Durham v. United States*, 1954). This new *Durham* standard was exceptionally broad and had occasionally been referred to as the "but for" test, meaning but for the mental illness, the crime would have never occurred. The *Durham* "product test" was a hopeful experiment in humanizing the criminal law, but difficulties inherent in such a broad and poorly defined test soon appeared.

Several legal decisions over the next 20 years attempted to tighten the product test for insanity by redefining mental disease (*McDonald v. United States*, 1962) and by limiting what mental health professionals could say in front of a jury

(*Washington v. United States*, 1967). By 1972, nearly every federal jurisdiction in the United States adopted the American Law Institute's (ALI's) *Model Penal Code* criteria (1955),[2] which included a two-prong test for insanity involving cognition and volition (*United States v. Brawner*, 1972). Under the ALI standard, a defendant could be found insane if he or she lacked substantial capacity, as a result of mental disease or defect, to appreciate the criminality (or wrongfulness) of his or her acts *or* to conform his or her conduct to the requirements of the law (Table 13-1). Either one, or both, of these prongs must be "substantially" impaired as a result of "mental disease or defect."

In many respects, the ALI standard combined the M'Naghten right/wrong knowledge test with the irresistible impulse test. Nevertheless, there were distinct differences that made the ALI criteria a much more attainable standard. The ALI replaced M'Naghten's rigid term, "did not know" with a more flexible "appreciate" standard. In addition, the M'Naghten standard suggested an "all-or-nothing" criteria with "*did not* know" as opposed to the ALI's "lacked substantial capacity" formulation. Many jurisdictions also chose to adopt the word *wrongfulness* rather than *criminality*. The wrongfulness term references the point that a person can hold a moral appreciation of wrongfulness as opposed to simply appreciating the act was criminal. On the other side of the coin, however, the ALI formulation contained a second "optional" paragraph, termed the *caveat paragraph*, that effectively eliminated repeated criminal acts, in and of themselves (i.e., antisocial personality disorder), as constituting mental disease. The ALI standard was adopted by a majority of jurisdictions in the United States and remains a popular standard today (Melton et al., 1997).

John Hinckley and the Insanity Defense Reform Act

The ALI standard was in place in 1981 when John Hinckley shot President Ronald Reagan, Press Secretary James Brady, and two law enforcement personnel. He was believed to have a delusional disorder by which he believed this act would endear him to a particular Hollywood actress. He was found not guilty

---

TABLE 13-1. Key Elements of the American Law Institute's *Model Penal Code* Standard for Insanity

The ALI proposed a two-prong test, cognition and volition:
  A. Lacks substantial capacity as result of mental disease or defect to:
    1. appreciate criminality (optionally, wrongfulness), or
    2. conform conduct to requirements of the law.
It contained an optional "caveat paragraph":
  B. Repeated criminal behavior does not constitute a mental disease.

Note. Adapted from American Law Institute (1955).

TABLE 13-2. Current Federal Standard (Title 18, U.S.C., § 17)

(a) *Affirmative defense.* It is an affirmative defense to a prosecution under any Federal statute that, at the time of the commission of the acts constituting the offense, the defendant, as a result of a severe mental disease or defect, was unable to appreciate the nature and quality or the wrongfulness of his acts. Mental disease or defect does not otherwise constitute a defense.

(b) *Burden of proof.* The defendant has the burden of proving the defense of insanity by clear and convincing evidence.

by reason of insanity under the volitional prong of the ALI standard. There was an immediate public backlash that resulted in the Insanity Defense Reform Act (IDRA) as part of the broader Crime Control Act, which became law in 1984. This standard is currently in place within the federal jurisdiction and sets the basis for insanity in a majority of state jurisdictions. Title 18, U.S.C., § 17 contains the current federal definition of insanity (Table 13-2).

The federal statute effectively eliminated the volitional prong and required the presence of a "severe" mental disease or defect. It changed the burden of proof to keep it on the defense by a clear and convincing evidence standard rather than automatically switching the burden over to the prosecution by beyond reasonable doubt when the sanity issue is raised (which was the case previously). This change makes insanity an "affirmative defense." It retained the ALI standard's use of "appreciate" rather than the strict M'Naghten knowledge test. The U.S. Congress also added paragraph (b) to Federal Rule of Evidence (FRE) 704, which placed a restriction against mental health professionals providing an opinion in front of a jury on the ultimate issue of whether the defendant is insane or not and, more broadly, whether the defendant could appreciate the wrongfulness of his or her behavior. Although unable to provide that opinion verbally in front of a jury, professionals are directed to provide their opinion in written reports [18, U.S.C., § 4247(c)(4)(B)]. The IDRA also established that once an individual is acquitted by reason of insanity, he or she is committed to the U.S. attorney general for secure hospitalization and is assumed dangerous until evaluated and judicially determined to be otherwise (18, USC, § 4243).

Nature, Quality, and Wrongfulness

The exact meanings of nature, quality, and wrongfulness have been debated. Melton and colleagues (1997) considered these words a two-prong standard of (a) nature and quality and (b) wrongfulness (p. 198). They suggested that individuals who do not meet the first standard will likely not meet the second. Further, nature and quality are often ignored altogether as juries focus on wrongfulness (Goldstein, 1967, cited in Melton et al., 1997). Shapiro (1984, 1991, 1999) described the view that nature and quality have subtle differences. Nature is quite basic, such that, "When the defendant picked up the gun, did he know the object was a gun?" The concept of quality goes more to consequences. A defendant would not appreciate the consequences if he beheaded his sleeping brother thinking it would be funny to see the brother get up and look for his head in the morning. Shapiro and colleagues (Goldstein, Morse, & Shapiro, 2003) considered the terms one basic concept. Experience has shown criminal responsibility concerns that focus on nature and quality are rare as most considerations balance on the defendant's appreciation of wrongfulness.

Is Wrongfulness Moral or Criminal?

The ALI standard included the optional use of the word "wrongfulness" in place of "criminality" (Table 13-1). This option reflected the possibility that a criminal defendant may have appreciated that his or her act was criminal, but because of mental illness, believed it was morally justified. This concept was initially presented in 1915 by Judge Cordozo in New York, who described "misperceptions" as a result of mental disease that could cause a defendant to believe his or her act was morally justified (*People v. Schmidt*, 1915). In 1970, the U.S. Court of Appeals for the 9th Circuit (federal jurisdictions in California, Oregon, Washington, Arizona, Montana, Idaho, Nevada, Alaska, and Hawaii) adopted wrongfulness and gave the example of a delusion leading to belief in moral justification (*Wade v. United States*, 1970). In a similar case, the 9th Circuit reiterated the point that the moral justification must be a result of mental disease (*United States v. Sullivan*, 1976). The 9th Circuit Court went further in 1977 by declaring juries should be instructed that wrongfulness can be interpreted as moral rather than criminal *only* if there are facts in the case that raise this unique distinction (*United States v. Segna*, 1977).

Not only are *Wade*, *Sullivan*, and *Segna* noteworthy for raising the issue of moral wrongfulness in the federal jurisdiction and outlining its use, but also they refer to the ALI standard. In 1988, the U.S. Court of Appeals for the 8th Circuit applied this same clarification and procedure to the post-Hinckley IDRA insanity standard (*United States v. Dubray*, 1988). *Dubray* also clarified the FRE 704(b) limitation of testimony on the ultimate issue of sanity by allowing testimony on motivation, mental state, and diagnosis at the time of the offense. *Dubray* only governs federal jurisdictions in the 8th Circuit (North Dakota, South Dakota, Minnesota, Nebraska, Iowa, Missouri, and Arkansas), but many other jurisdiction throughout the country have adopted this definition of wrongfulness as well.

A case study in wrongfulness

Let us assume a mother[3] of a very young child becomes psychotic with delusions that the only way to save her child from the fires of hell is to drown him. She realized she would be arrested afterward and likely convicted of murder because she understood it is against the law to kill her child. Although realizing this fact, she earnestly believed killing her child was the right thing to do because, in her psychotic state of understanding, it was the *only* possible way for her to truly *save* her child.

In this scenario, the woman appreciated the nature of the act; that is, she realized the act would terminate the life of her child on earth. She also appreciated the quality of the act in that the consequences included her son's death and even the fact she would be arrested and likely convicted. The issue of her appreciation of wrongfulness becomes much more problematic. She clearly appreciated the criminality of her actions as she even voiced her awareness of her arrest and likely conviction. It is reasonable in this instance, given a jurisdiction that interprets wrongfulness as moral rather than strictly criminal, to argue she did not appreciate the moral wrongfulness and was, therefore, insane. Although criminally wrong, she believed it was the morally right thing to do as it was the only way she could save her child from hell.

This scenario highlights the importance of understanding the law in the jurisdiction in which the case is prosecuted. In a strictly criminal jurisdiction, a mental health expert should opine that she was sane. In a jurisdiction in which wrongfulness can mean moral as well as criminal, the expert should raise the issue of her appreciating the moral wrongfulness and opine that she was insane. Not understanding this difference in the law can cause otherwise quite competent and respected mental health experts to come to a wrong conclusion. The importance in evaluating a criminal defendant's sanity is applying our skills in evaluation and diagnosis to the correct standard of law.

Current Status of the Insanity Defense

The federal jurisdictions are uniformly IDRA right or wrong because of statutory authority. As of 1995, about half the states had adopted the federal standard in one form or other, and about 20 states use a version of the ALI criteria (Melton et al., 1997). With only a few exceptions, a forensic evaluator performing sanity evaluations for state jurisdictions will likely be using a form of the ALI or IDRA criteria, which means he or she will evaluate the defendant's understanding of the nature, quality, and wrongfulness of the acts and, possibly, the defendant's capacity to conform his or her conduct to the requirements of the law. New Hampshire still relies on the product test. Idaho, Montana, and Utah have eliminated the insanity defense altogether, although mental health experts can still testify on *mens rea* (Melton et al., 1997).

Some states have adopted a "guilty but mentally ill" (GBMI) provision in addition to an insanity defense as an alternative verdict for juries to consider. This finding would convict a defendant of the crime, but make it clear he or she is mentally ill and in need of treatment. The GBMI provision has been significantly criticized on conceptual grounds and, in most cases, does not appear to ensure mental health treatment for the convicted (Melton et al., 1997).

A surprising finding is that, even with these various formulations, including ALI, IDRA, and abolition of the insanity defense, research suggests no difference between conviction rates or rates of hospitalization (Steadman et al., 1993). Apparently this finding is because every state has a method of hospitalizing mentally ill persons convicted of crimes (Favole, 1983), and individuals acquitted by reason of insanity appear to spend the same amount of time securely hospitalized as they would have been incarcerated if convicted (Steadman et al., 1993).

Insanity and Traumatic Brain Injury

Changing the insanity standard back to a test of appreciation for right and wrong would appear to make it a much more difficult standard to meet for potentially insane defendants, particularly when their "mental disease or defect" is caused by traumatic brain injury (TBI). Contrary to this appearance, however, the overall incidence of insanity pleas and their ultimate success rates seem to have changed little since the reform (Steadman et al., 1993). Also contrary to public perception is the finding that insanity defenses are relatively rare, and successful insanity acquittals are even less common (Silver, Cirincione, & Steadman, 1994; Steadman et al., 1993). National data are available that reveal only 2,542 people were found insane in the entire United States in 1980 (Steadman, Rosenstein, MacAskiel, & Manderschied, 1988). As said by the legal scholar, Michael Perlin, successful insanity acquittals are "rarer than snake bites in Manhattan" (Perlin, 1992).

The incidence of brain injury–related insanity acquittals appears to be even rarer. Steadman and colleagues studied four states regarding insanity pleas, acquittals, and diagnostic characteristics before and after the Hinckley-related reforms (Steadman et al., 1993). They did not specifically identify brain injury as a diagnostic category, but they found 69% of those entering insanity pleas had schizophrenia, another psychosis, or major affective disorder. Nestor and Haycock studied murderers committed to the state hospital (Nester & Haycock, 1997). Of the 13 insanity acquittees referred for neuropsychological evaluation, 12 were considered psychotic at the time of the crime. Melton his colleagues reported the results of six studies that revealed 67% to 97% of insanity acquittees had a significant psychosis, suggesting psychosis is usually required for successful insanity defense (Melton et al., 1997).

There are no studies identifying the rates of a neuropsychological basis for insanity. Available research would suggest the condition would need to rise to the level of psychosis for success, particularly in those jurisdictions without the volitional prong in the insanity standard. Of 456 consecutive referrals for sanity evaluation at the U.S. Medical Center during the early 1990s, only 17 were diagnosed with an organic mental illness, and none were considered insane (Denney & Wynkoop, 2000). Cochrane, Grisso, and Frederick (2001) combined additional cases ($N = 1,170$) from this database to cover a longer period of time and found little support for insanity opinions based on organic disorders.

Denney and Wynkoop (2000) provided the example of an insanity evaluee diagnosed with dementia caused by Alzheimer's disease and considered insane for disorderly conduct and trespassing on U.S. postal property. The defendant had delusions that the U.S. Postal Service was stealing his mail. In this instance, psychosis caused his insanity, and Alzheimer's dementia caused his psychosis.

In many instances, it is apparent that cases are not referred for evaluation because they are not prosecuted when an organic mental illness was severe enough at the time to clearly result in criminal actions (called *pretrial diversion*). Of those that are prosecuted, many are dealt with at the level of competency to stand trial. Given the often static or degenerative nature of neurological conditions, these people are found not competent to stand trial and remain so. Consequently, they never reach a point at which sanity is at issue.

It is apparent that evaluators more often face insanity evaluations when some form of less-obvious organic mental disorder is present and may have had an impact on the defendant's past behavior. It has been presented that, for mild cases without psychosis, it will likely be difficult to support an insanity defense with the current right/wrong standard (Denney & Wynkoop, 2000). Under the ALI standard, such defenses would appear to have a greater chance of success (Melton et al., 1997).

Brain Injury and Insanity: Importance of the Multiple Data Source Model and Not Ignoring Data

The following case example demonstrates the importance of obtaining corroborative information as part of a neuropsychological evaluation on the issue of criminal responsibility. Although it is important to use the MDSM (Figure 12-1, p. 385, this volume) for acquiring information, it is imperative the information is integrated in a manner consistent with the known natural course of TBI. This is the only way to arrive at a reasonable forensic conclusion regarding such complicated issues.

A 28-year-old man was charged with armed bank robbery and referred for evaluation of his sanity. Nine years previously, he was in a serious motor vehicle accident and experienced a possible TBI with potential brief loss of consciousness (medical records were not available). There were no known complications. Two years later, he became a police officer and joined the department's Special Weapons and Tactics team. He won awards on the police force for his excellent work. He started experiencing significant stress secondary to a deathly sick child and overwhelming debt. He was diagnosed with posttraumatic stress disorder (PTSD) and major depression in the community. Nine years after the putative TBI, he robbed a bank.

The defendant was referred for an evaluation regarding his criminal responsibility in light of his history of PTSD and major depression. In seeking other data regarding his mental state at the time of the offense, investigative records revealed that, when he went into the bank, he carried a handgun. He ushered all the bank employees into an office. He acquired access to the walk-in safe. Last, *he asked the employees where the videotape recording device was that videotaped bank robberies.* He then went to the room and confiscated the videotape that had recorded his entrance to the bank. He locked the employees in the office and departed. Throughout the robbery, he demanded employees not look at his face and to turn away from him. Given the entirety of information available using the MDSM, the evaluator provided this opinion:

Although he had been diagnosed prior to the robbery with PTSD and depression, behavior described in the offense suggested he well understood what he was doing and the wrongfulness of his actions. He used a gun to gain control of the bank employees. He carried with him a bag for money. He ordered them not to give him bait money or dye packs. He cautioned them against pulling any alarm. He demanded the video tape from the security camera. He pulled the telephone out of the room in which he left them. He repeatedly told them to not look at him. After leaving the bank, he changed his outward appearance and attempted to flee the area.

The defendant was subsequently evaluated by a neuropsychologist hired by the defense. The neuropsychologist provided this opinion:

He suffers cognitive deterioration from his head injury, with his IQ 40–50% below his memory functions and achievement skills. The weak score on ability to attend and concentrate is consistent with this deterioration. Additionally, in the critical area of thinking abstractly and solve problems in a hypothetical-deductive fashion, as measured by the Category Test, he was in the impaired range. Given these limitations from his 1985 head injury, when stressed, he had little or no reserve to call upon for coping skills. *I do not agree that his reality contact was not substantially impaired at the time of the offense* [emphasis added]. In my opinion, he saw no options and had no choices. He did not act rationally and did not appreciate the consequences of his actions.

This opinion was provided by an expert who had read the previous report and knew of the defendant's actions in the bank. He nonetheless ignored this vital corroborative information about the man's behavior and concluded that not only was his abstract thinking and hypothetical-deductive problem-solving skills impaired, but also his reality contact was impaired. Aside from ignoring important corroborative information from the time of the offense, the evaluator also disregarded the atypical pattern of recovery for brain injury. The defendant had become a decorated police officer and SWAT team member *after* the claimed head injury. Barring some intervening event to the brain, there is no explanation for that course of recovery from brain injury. A comparison of information dealing with past history, current presentation, and time of the alleged offense would have revealed these striking inconsistencies.

Criminal Responsibility Assessment Tools

Rogers (1984) developed the Rogers Criminal Responsibility Assessment Scales (R-CRAS) as a tool to assist in the evaluation of criminal responsibility. It contains 25 scales focused on areas relevant to the ALI standard, with four additional variables related to the GBMI standard and an additional variable for the right/wrong standard (M'Naghten and IDRA). The instrument helps clinicians rate the defendant in several areas: reliability regarding potential malingering; signs indicative of organic mental illness, mental retardation, and mental illness; and whether there were indications of cognitive impairment or loss of behavioral control at the time of the alleged offense. Each of these areas requires a Likert-style rating, which then culminates in a decision tree that produces the clinical opinion: sane, insane, or no opinion. Interrater reliability and concordance between opinions based on R-CRAS rating and court verdicts are both respectable (Melton et al., 1997).

Although the R-CRAS promises increased scientific rigor in the process of sanity evaluations, it has been criticized regarding its method of "quantifying" vague clinician judgments (Melton et al., 1997). See the work of Golding and Roesch (1987), Rogers and Ewing (1992), and Golding, Skeem, Roesch, and Zapf (1999) for discussion of these criticisms. The R-CRAS may prove invaluable as a training tool for evaluators learning to perform criminal responsibility evaluations, but available research suggests the R-CRAS is rarely used in forensic practice (Borum & Grisso, 1995).

DIMINISHED CAPACITY AND RESPONSIBILITY

Diminished capacity is considered a *mens rea* defense. In other words, it refers to a decreased level of culpability because of lesser intent (Clark, 1999). In this regard, first-degree murder, second-degree murder, and manslaughter differ in their level of intent. Without invoking the insanity defense, defendants occasionally bring mental state into play by claiming a decreased level of intent because of such factors as alcohol or drug intoxication, medication use, and neurological conditions (Melton et al., 1997). An extreme example is the automatism defense, by which defendants claim no conscious awareness of their acts. Examples have included crimes committed while sleepwalking, during a seizure, while unaware secondary to head injury or other encephalopathic conditions, and even during dissociative episodes (Barnard, 1998). Although courts have generally allowed testimony to this issue, they have limited its use when the defendant experienced the disability previously and should have taken precautions to prevent a potential criminal event. An example would be a man with a known history of aggression secondary to complex-partial seizure disorder who refuses prophylactic treatment to help avoid seizures (and thereby aggression and assault).

When considering diminished capacity, it must be realized that there are both general and specific intent crimes. Felon in possession of a weapon is an example of a general intent crime. By definition, possessing the weapon carries with it the prerequisite intent as long as the defendant understood, or should have understood, that it was illegal for him or her to possess a weapon. Bank robbery requires specific intent, that is, resolve for a particular act to occur. *Intent* must be differentiated from *motive*. Motive prompts an act, whereas intent "refers only to the state of mind with which the act is done" (West Publishing, 1990, p. 810).

The most common basis for diminished capacity is intoxication (Marlowe, Lambert, & Thompson, 1999). An example would include whether a defendant could form the prerequisite intent to first-degree murder. It may very well be that alcohol intoxication made this level of intent rather unlikely. Under this circumstance, a jury could use a lesser included offense such as second-degree murder or even manslaughter, depending on the facts of the case.

A similar argument can be made for the effects of neurological compromise. An example would include a dentist charged with inappropriate dispensing of narcotics and whose judgment was compromised by early frontal dementia. The compromise may not be so severe as to eliminate intent fully (which should result in an acquittal), but it can allow the jury to apply the law in a fair manner.

A related, and often confused, term is *diminished responsibility*. This term actually refers to mitigating circumstances of the crime that warrant a lesser punishment (Clark, 1999). Such issues are brought before the court at the time of sentencing. Diminished responsibility is particularly relevant in jurisdictions that no longer have the volitional prong in their insanity standard. Individuals with frontal lobe damage often have impulse control problems that potentially impact their ability to refrain from performing certain criminal acts. Deficits in cognitive, emotional, and behavioral controls secondary to neurological compromise are relevant to a defense against many criminal charges, either at trial or at sentencing.

ASSESSING RISK OF DANGEROUSNESS

It is not uncommon for neuropsychologists involved in criminal proceedings to be asked by the court to assess a criminal defendant's propensity for violence if released from custody. The issue of dangerousness is certainly relevant in cases of neurological compromise (Volavka, Martell, & Convit, 1992). Such questions can arise during detention hearings at any phase of the criminal proceedings. Potential for dangerousness is generally always an issue for defendants who are considered not competent to stand trial and unrestorable. In the federal jurisdiction, the presiding court must address the defendant's potential dangerousness to others and significant property of others on release because the charges can be dismissed when a mentally defective defendant is considered unlikely to become competent in the foreseeable future (18, U.S.C., § 4241 and 4241).

Unrestorable incompetent defendants in the federal jurisdiction can be held in a secure hospital indefinitely if they are considered dangerous because of mental defect (18, U.S.C., § 4246). Nearly the same issue arises after a defendant is found insane and hospitalized in a secure facility (18, U.S.C., § 4243). The issue can come up again when a sentenced inmate who is potentially dangerous because of mental disease or defect reaches the end of a sentence because federal statute allows potential extended commitment (18, U.S.C., § 4246). In each of these scenarios, the Federal Bureau of Prisons under authority of the U.S. attorney general has the mandate and challenge to find suitable state placement—a placement that will further ensure public safety. Most states have similar statutory procedures. Consequently, it is common for mental health professionals to provide expert opinions on risk of dangerousness for the deciding court on each of these occasions.

Assessment of risk in the prediction of future dangerousness poses certain ethical dilemmas as it balances the liberty interests of the individual against the safety needs of the community (Grisso & Applebaum, 1992). Given the liberty interests involved, it is imperative neuropsychologists performing this function conform their work to the standard of practice as outlined in current literature. In *Barefoot v. Estelle* (1983), James P. Grigson testified regarding defendant Barefoot's dangerousness without ever meeting the man. Justice Blackmun wrote, "Doctor Grigson testified that whether Barefoot was in society at large or in a prison society there was a '*one hundred percent and absolute*' chance that Barefoot would commit future acts of violence that would constitute a continuing threat to society" (emphasis original; Justice Blackmun, dissent, p. 3408). Although an egregiously overstated conclusion, recent research suggests that mental health professionals can predict violence at a rate significantly better than chance when they include relevant factors in the decision analysis (Monahan, 1992; Monahan & Steadman, 1994; Mossman, 1994).

Factors Known to Increase Risk of Dangerousness

In this section, I focus on factors relevant for the assessment of future risk of violence. There is quite a large body of research on risk assessment in general and specifically on that pertaining to sex offenders. I consider general issues of risk assessment and that which logically pertains to neuropsychology. For a recent review pertaining to risk assessment of sexual predators, see the work of Conroy (2003).

Much of the research regarding violence prediction, and certainly that dealing with sex offenders, have dealt with *static* and *dynamic* prediction variables (Bonta, Law, & Hanson, 1998). Static variables refer to fixed and unchanging facts regarding an individual's life (e.g., number and nature of past violent offenses, demographic characteristics), and dynamic variables can change. These variables are subdivided into *stable* and *acute* dynamic variables. Stable variables have the potential for change (e.g., substance abuse history), and acute variables are clearly situation specific (e.g., intoxication). The bulk of actuarial research on violence prediction focuses on static variables (Conroy, 2003).

The research of Swanson and colleagues suggested that being male, young, of lower socioeconomic status, and an abuser of drugs or alcohol, having a major mental disorder, and particularly having a major mental disorder in combination with substance abuse/dependence are demographic factors that increase risk of violence in the community (Swanson, Holzer, Ganju, & Jono, 1990). Meta-analysis suggests that the strongest predictor of future violence is past violence (Mossman, 1994). Monahan and colleagues (2001) reported results of the MacArthur Violence Risk Assessment Study, the largest study of community violence prediction of its kind (Monahan, 2003). The study included male and female civilly committed patients from several facilities, with follow-up in the community at 20 weeks and 1 year after discharge. They focused on variables believed to relate to potential violence (see Melton et al., 1997, and Monahan, 2003, for a more thorough review).

Rather than just static and dynamic variables, the MacArthur study considered variables in four factors: *dispositional, historical, contextual,* and *clinical.* Dispositional factors included demographic (e.g., age, gender, race), personality (e.g., impulsivity and psychopathy), and cognitive concerns (IQ and neurological impairment). Historical factors included social history (family, work, and education), mental hospitalization history (prior hospitalizations and compliance), and history of crime and violence. Contextual factors included perceived stress, social support systems, and physical aspects of the environment (e.g., presence of weapons). Clinical factors included Axis I diagnosis, symptoms, Axis II diagnosis, level of functioning, and substance abuse.

The MacArthur study (Monahan, 2003; Monahan et al., 2001) revealed some surprises and confirmations regarding violence. Prior violence and criminality were strongly associated with community violence in this group of psychiatric patients. The prevalence rates for men and women were actually about the same, but the nature of the violence was different. Women are more likely to be violent toward family members, but violence from men is more likely to result in serious injury. History of childhood physical abuse, but not sexual abuse, appears associated with postdischarge violence. As in the Swanson et al. (1990) study, presence of substance abuse or dependence in conjunction with mental illness significantly raised potential for violence; however, a diagnosis of a major mental illness was associated with a lower rate of violence compared to personality or adjustment disorders. Also, presence of schizophrenia appeared less associated with violence than depression or bipolar disorder. Delusions and hallucinations were associated with violence less than nondelusional suspiciousness and presence of violent thoughts. Those scoring high in anger during hospitalization were twice as likely to commit violent acts after discharge than those with low anger scores. The nature of the environment also played a role in violence determination, with high-crime neighborhoods more associated with postdischarge violence. There is little indication in the MacArthur study that neurological compromise contributed to an increased likelihood of postdischarge violence. The facts that only a few of these subjects had neurologically related concerns and that brain injury did not appear to be assessed thoroughly clouds the potential contribution that neurological disorder may have on postdischarge violence.

Neurocognitive contributions to risk have been studied less thoroughly. Research with childhood neuropathology implied that early cerebral deficits can predispose future dangerousness, particularly when combined with the environmental factor of an abusive family (Golden, Jackson, Peterson-Rohne, & Gontkovsky, 2002; Lewis, Lovely, Yeager, & Della Femina, 1989; Lewis et al., 1985). It is logical that neuropsychological factors can play a role in the production of violence.

Neuropathology and the Potential for Violence

It is well known that large portions of the brain are involved in inhibition of behavior. Damage to the prefrontal cortex and temporal poles or frontal-subcortical system or diffuse axonal shearing can cause a behavioral disinhibition syndrome, often termed "pseudopsychopathic," that can surface as a combination of jocularity, impulsivity, behavioral dyscontrol, and sexual disinhibition (Benson & Miller, 1997; Mesulam, 2000; Mills, Cassidy, & Katz, 1997). See the work of Damasio and Anderson (2003) for a review of clinical cases that manifested these personality characteristics.

A classic example of this syndrome is found in the case of Phineas Gage, a 19th century railroad foreman who survived an explosion in which an iron tamping bar (about 1 m long, 3 cm wide) was blasted up under his cheekbone and out through the top of his head. His physician described the change in his personality by writing that the "equilibrium . . . between his intellectual faculties and animal propensities seems to have been destroyed" (Harlow, 1868, reprinted in Macmillan, 2000, p. 414). One—possibly augmented—account of Gage described him as "so loudmouthed, boisterous, and profane that eventually 'the police drove him from Boston Common' " (Blackington, 1956, cited in Macmillan, 2000, p. 97).

Many researchers are implicating the prefrontal and frontal lobes in violence and criminal behavior (Best, Williams, & Coccaro, 2002; Brower & Price, 2001; New et al., 2002; Raine, 2002; Raine et al., 1998; Volkow et al., 1995). Correspondingly, decreased executive functioning appears to be associated with an increase in some forms of aggression (Barratt, Stanford, Kent, & Felthous, 1997; Giancola, Moss, Martin, Kirisci, & Tarter, 1996; Paschall & Fishbein, 2002; Villemarette-Pittman, Stanford, & Greve, 2003). Electroencephalogram and evoked potential alterations have been implicated in violence as well (Bars, Heyrend, Simpson, & Munger, 2001; Conklin & Stanford, 2002; Drake, Hietter, & Pakalnis, 1992; Drake, Pakalnis, Brown, & Hietter, 1988; Evans, 1997; Gerstle, Mathias, & Stanford, 1998; Houston & Stanford, 2001; Kiehl, Hare, Liddle, & McDonald, 1999; Mathias & Stanford, 1999; Raine & Venables, 1988; Raine, Venables, & Williams, 1990). There are also lines of research implicating neurochemical alterations and violence (Gregg & Siegel, 2001; Linnoila & Charney, 1999; Miczek, 1987; Siegal & Shaikah, 1992), with a particular emphasis on decreased 5-HT (serotonin) and its treatment with selective serotonin reuptake inhibitors (Coccaro, 1992; Coccaro & Kavoussi, 1997; Coccaro et al., 1989; Dolan, Deakin, Roberts, & Anderson, 2002; Kavoussi, Liu, & Coccaro, 1994; Kent et al., 1988; Linnoila et al., 1983; Shaikah, De Lanerolle, & Siegel, 1997). The research appears to support the proposed two-part classification of violent behavior as either premeditated or impulsive (Barratt, Stanford, Dowdy, Liebman, & Kent, 1999; Frick, 1995; A. B. Heilbrun, Heilbrun, & Heilbrun, 1978; Hubbard et al., 2002; Malone et al., 1998; Pulkkinen, 1996; Scarpa & Raine, 2000; Smithmyer, Hubbard, & Simons, 2000; Vitaro, Gendreau, Tremblay, & Oligny, 1998; Weinshenker & Siegel, 2002).

Among the impulsively aggressive, there appears to be substantial evidence of neurocognitive compromise consistent with previous research regarding executive dysfunction among the violent (Giancola et al., 1996; Mungus, 1988; Stanford, Greve, & Gerstle, 1997). In addition, the impulsively aggressive appear responsive to treatment with antiseizure medications (Barratt, Kent, Bryant, & Felthous, 1991; Barratt, Stanford, Felthous, & Kent, 1997; Stanford et al., 2001).

Houston, Stanford, Villemarette-Pittman, Conklin, and Helfritz (2003) suggested "growing evidence of neurobiological deficits specific to impulsive aggressive behavior (i.e., reduced central serotonergic functioning, executive dysfunction, [and] prefrontal deficits) may serve as markers of an ineffective behavioral control system in these individuals." The nature of the deficits in those with impulsive, reactive aggression, in concert with apparent treatment benefits of antiseizure medication, may even suggest the possibility of neuroregulatory abnormality. Overall, there appears to be enough research implicating a relationship between neurocognitive functioning and aggression, particularly the impulsive type, to indicate neuropsychology has a place in the evaluation of violent criminal defendants (Brower & Price, 2001).

Risk Assessment Tools

Given the generally improved prediction accuracy of actuarial information over clinical judgment, several successful efforts to develop risk assessment tools have occurred (Monahan, 2003).

The Hare Psychopathy Checklist–Revised (PCL-R; Hare, 1991) and the screening version (PCL-SV; Hart, Cox, & Hare, 1995) have the largest research base. The PCL-R is considered a "robust predictor of future violent behavior" (Conroy, 2003). The PCL-R is a structured interview and file review that produces 20 scales loaded on two broad factors within the conceptual domain of psychopathy (Hare, Harpur, & Hakstian, 1990). The measure requires specialized training and is rather lengthy, but it is considered to have good interrater reliability (see Melton et al., 1997).

Webster, Douglas, Eaves, and Hart (1995) developed the HCR-20, which consists of 20 ratings of historical, clinical, and risk management factors. Douglas and Webster (1999) identified retrospectively that scores above the median increased the likelihood of past violence and antisocial behavior on average by a factor of 4. Douglas, Ogloff, Nicholls, and Grant (1999) found that scores above median increased the risk of violence by factors of 6 to 13 in a group of civilly committed patients during the 2 years after their hospital discharge.

The Violence Risk Appraisal Guide (VRAG; Harris, Rice, & Quinsey, 1993) was developed in Canada on a large number of men with serious criminal offenses housed in a maximum security hospital. Of 50 predictor variables, a series of regression equations identified 12 variables that became the VRAG. The VRAG is a somewhat time-consuming file review because it includes the PCL-R as one of its variables. This weakness not withstanding, it has demonstrated itself as a useful predictive tool (Rice & Harris, 1995).

The last risk assessment method reviewed here was developed from the MacArthur Violence Risk Assessment Study (Monahan et al., 2001). The MacArthur researchers developed an iterative classification tree "approach to violence risk assessment . . . predicated on an interactive and contingent model of violence, one that allows many different combinations of risk factors to classify a person as high or low risk" (Monahan, 2003, pp. 533–534). The goal was to incorporate the type of information reasonably available in clinical records in a manner that does not make the assessment of risk arduously long. The tree incorporates a sequence of questions that classify subjects as either high or low risk.

Monahan and colleagues (2001) evaluated the iterative classification tree in a multiple model approach that combined risk assessment methods. They classified all the civilly committed patients in to one of five categories of risk and followed their progress for 20 weeks after discharge. Results of this method were favorable. In Monahan's words (2003), "This combination of models produced results not only superior to those of any of its constituent models, but superior to any other actuarial violence risk assessment procedure reported in the literature to date" (p. 534).

Evaluating risk of violence has become increasingly sophisticated with the development of specific assessment methods. Each of these methods was developed with prisoners or psychiatric patients at risk for violence, and none has been validated with neurological patients. Logic would dictate a similar profile of risk-increasing variables between the two populations (particularly with the apparent prevalence rate for neurocognitive compromise in violent offenders; Martell, 1992), but ultimately this remains an empirical question. Until that research materializes, neuropsychologists who practice risk assessment in the criminal setting must rely on clinical judgment predicated on other, established nonneurological risk factors.

DEATH PENALTY ISSUES

Nowhere does the need for competent and ethical practice demonstrate itself greater than in the practice of capital cases. As with any criminal case, neuropsychologists can be called on to provide expertise at any phase of the process; nonetheless, there are unique issues in capital cases that go beyond the obvious life-or-death outcome. These issues include a priori ethical considerations, competency to be executed and to waive appeals, age requirements for imposing a death sentence, mental retardation, and death penalty mitigation.

A Priori Ethical Considerations

Before accepting the responsibility of practicing in capital cases, the neuropsychologist must consider his or her personal position on the death penalty in general. Ethical standards dictate that psychologists recognize when personal views have the potential to interfere with our professional work. As I reviewed in chapter 12, the roles of forensic evaluators are different from that of clinical providers. There are times when our decisions may have untoward implications for criminal defendants. Each neuropsychologist must objectively evaluate his or her feelings toward the death penalty and decide if he or she is capable of accepting the possibility of providing an opinion that, in some aspect, will pave the way for an execution of a human being (Denney, in press).

For example, forensic evaluators are occasionally requested to provide an opinion on whether a criminal defendant is competent to be executed. A neuropsychologist should not accept this role if unwilling to provide an affirmative opinion if the data support such a conclusion. As in any other forensic endeavor, forensic practitioners need to remain objective in their roles and remember the client in this instance is the court, not the defendant. In my opinion, clinicians who are strongly opposed to the death penalty have too great a possibility of inadvertent bias to participate in capital cases as nonpartisan evaluators.

Competence to Be Executed

In 1986, the U.S. Supreme Court ruled in a complicated and lengthy criminal due process and competency case called *Ford v. Wainwright*. Defendant Ford was convicted of a capital offense and sentenced to death. While on death row, the issue of his mental health and competency arose. The Florida state procedure at that time did not allow an adversarial or judicial determination of competency because it was determined by the governor with the assistance of a panel of mental health professionals. In ruling Florida's procedure unconstitutional, the U.S. Supreme Court also held that executing a person not competent because of mental illness is a violation of the 8th Amendment right to be free from cruel and unusual punishment. The Court concluded that doing so (a) has questionable retributive value, (b) has no deterrence value, and (c) simply affronts humanity. Fascinating quotations that give insight to the reasoning behind this decision include the need to protect the "condemned from fear and pain without the comfort of understanding" and the need to protect the "dignity of society from barbarity."

In deciding *Ford*, the U.S. Supreme Court did not address the specific aspects of competency to be executed much beyond the basic *Dusky* requirements (*Dusky v. United States*, 1960; see chapter 12). The Court referenced Florida's standard that the person must have the mental capacity to understand the nature of the death penalty and why it was imposed. Justice Powell, in the concurring opinion, pointed out that a person needs to understand the connection between the crime and the punishment. Most other jurisdictions that allow execution have more detailed standards. An example description is presented in Reisner and Slobogin (1990); the test of competency is whether the prisoner lacks, as a result of:

defects of his faculties, sufficient intelligence to understand the nature of the proceedings against him, what he was tried for, the purpose of his punishment, the impending fate which awaits him, a sufficient understanding to know any fact which might exist which would make his punishment unjust or unlawful, and the intelligence requisite to convey such information to his attorneys or the court. (p. 946)

This more detailed inquiry suggests the prisoner must have capacity to assist in any potential appeals in addition to an understanding of his current legal situation (as indicated in *Dusky*) and an appreciation of impending death. K. Heilbrun and colleagues (K. Heilbrun, 1987; K. Heilbrun & McClaren, 1988; K. Heilbrun, Radelet, & Dvoskin, 1992) suggested the ability to prepare for death spiritually and psychologically as a needed component of competency as well.

Related to the issue of evaluating competency for execution is the controversial concern over the ethical appropriateness of providing treatment for condemned prisoners for the purpose of restoring their competency to be executed. The issue has been debated at length (Ferris, 1997; Leong, Weinstock, Silva, & Eth, 1993). The American Medical Association (1995) put forth a statement that providing treatment for the restoration of competence for such reasons is ethically unacceptable unless it is to relieve extreme suffering. Bonnie (1990) outlined an analysis that revealed the issue as a complex one with no easy answers.

Much of the concern pertains to the greater harm in facilitating a person's death versus relieving suffering. There are instances when individuals would rather receive treatment and die a sane person than languish away on death row in a state of mental deterioration (see *Singleton v. Norris*, 1997, Heaney concurring; *Singleton v. Norris*, 2003). The issue could be resolved by adopting the recommendation of commuting a death row inmate's sentence to life without parole if the inmate is found incompetent for execution (Wexler & Winick, 1991). Of course, this decision could raise the potential for malingering to new heights.

Whether one should provide competency restoration treatment to death row inmates is an issue that will likely continue in debate for many years. Until some definitive guidance is provided in this thorny ethical area, it is doubly incumbent for neuropsychologists to be aware of their views and the potential impact these views can have on professional opinions in capital cases.

Competency to Waive Death Penalty Appeals

Individuals executed in the United States during 2001 spent an average of 11 years and 10 months on death row (U.S. Department of Justice, 2001). It is not uncommon under prolonged housing on the unique setting of death row for individuals to grow weary of the ongoing appeals process. In death penalty cases, prisoners receive legal representation even when they do not wish it; consequently, they can find themselves in a position to refuse appeals filed on their behalf. Refusing further appeal amounts to the prisoner "volunteering" for execution. Just over 12% of those executed between 1977 and 2001 chose to drop their appeals (Amnesty International, 2001). This situation becomes complicated because it is not uncommon for prisoners to develop mental health concerns while on death row (Cunningham & Goldstein, 2003). In fact, 2 of the 19 prisoners on death row in the United States during 2001 died as a result of suicide (U.S. Department of Justice). It is not surprising that appeals courts request mental health evaluation for prisoners wishing to waive their appeals.

There is no unique standard for waiving death penalty appeals beyond that generally spelled out in case law. It can be deduced from *Dusky v. United States* (1960), *Godinez v. Moran* (1993), and *North Carolina v. Alford* (1970) that individuals must have a factual and rational understanding of their situation and are waiving their appeal in a knowing, intelligent, and voluntary manner (see chapter 12 for a discussion of this aspect of competency). In addition to other possible mental health concerns, it is important for the mental health evaluator to rule out depression as the precipitating cause for such a waiver.

Death Penalty and Mental Retardation

In 2002, the U.S. Supreme Court decided the case of *Atkins v. Virginia*, a case spelling out that it is excessive to execute a mentally retarded individual. It is rare for the High Court to overturn its own previous decision, but it did just that in *Atkins*. The court previously addressed this issue in *Penry v. Lynaugh* (1989). In *Penry*, the court decided it was not necessarily "cruel and unusual punishment" to execute a mentally retarded individual based on an analysis of societal views at that time as evidenced by state laws. Societal views dictate the "evolving standards of decency" as it relates to cruel and unusual. Because very few states had prohibitions against executing the mentally retarded, the court concluded the prevailing societal thought suggested it was not so extreme as to be considered cruel and unusual. The court did spell out, however, that the cruel and unusual clause of the 8th Amendment requires a case-by-case analysis. In the case of mental retardation, the jury must be able to consider the impact of mental retardation evidence in its decision about sentencing. The *Penry* case was a controversial 5-to-4 decision, so it was not surprising to see the issue addressed again in *Atkins*.

During August 1996, Daryl Atkins and an accomplice abducted Eric Nesbitt, robbed him, forced him to withdraw an additional $200 from an ATM, and then drove him to an isolated location, where he was shot eight times and killed. Atkins was convicted of abduction, armed robbery, and capital murder. During the penalty phase of his trial, a psychologist for the defense testified that he had a full-scale IQ of 59 and concluded he was mildly mentally retarded. A rebuttal psychiatrist testified he was a psychopath and not mentally retarded. The jury, nonetheless, sentenced Atkins to death. The Supreme Court of Virginia affirmed the judgment of the trial court, and the case was appealed to the U.S. Supreme Court.

In July 2002, the U.S. Supreme Court reversed the judgment of the Virginia Supreme Court and remanded the case back to the sentencing court to consider sentencing other than the death penalty. In coming to this conclusion, the U.S. Supreme Court reevaluated society's perspective on the issue in a similar fashion as was done in *Penry*. The court outlined that a punishment is excessive and therefore prohibited by the 8th Amendment as cruel and unusual if it is not "graduated and proportioned to the offense." A claim that a judgment is excessive must be judged by the standards that currently prevail. Society's evolving standards of decency must allow for a proportionality review that is informed by "objective factors to the maximum possible extent."

As in *Penry*, the Court viewed legislation enacted by the country's legislatures to be the clearest and most reliable objective evidence of contemporary values. At the time of *Penry*, there were only two states with statutes against executing the mentally retarded. Although an additional 16 states enacted statutes prohibiting the execution of mentally retarded offenders since *Penry*, "It is not so much the number of these states that is significant, but the consistency of the direction of the change." The Court further concluded that mental retardation does not necessarily eliminate a person's ability to appreciate right from wrong, but the condition causes diminished capacities to understand and process information, communicate, abstract from mistakes and learn from experience, engage in logical reasoning, control impulses, and understand the reaction of others. The Court noted "their deficiencies do not warrant an exemption from criminal sanctions, but they do diminish their personal culpability" (p. 348).

The U.S. Supreme Court considered two additional reasons to agree with the legislative consensus. First, the Court maintained there is uncertainty as to whether either justification underpinning the death penalty—retribution and deterrence of capital crimes—applies to mentally retarded offenders. With respect to retribution, the severity of the appropriate punishment necessarily depends on the offender's culpability. If the culpability of the average murderer is insufficient to justify imposition of the death penalty, the reduced culpability of the mentally retarded criminal surely does not merit that form of retribution. Regarding deterrence, the same cognitive and behavioral deficits that lessen the culpability of mentally retarded defendants also make it less likely that they can control their conduct based on the possibility of execution. Second, mentally retarded offenders face an increased risk for wrongful execution because they may unwittingly provide false confessions, be less able to provide meaningful assistance to their counsel, are typically poorer witnesses, and may inadvertently foster the perception they lack remorse for their crimes based on their demeanor in court.

The *Atkins* (2002) decision makes the diagnostic aspect of forensic assessment in capital cases even more important. Although each state must follow the *Atkins* decision, the U.S. Supreme Court did not spell out the specifics of how mental retardation is defined or, for that matter, how much mental retardation is needed to obviate the death penalty. The Court left these details up to the states to decide. In addition to subaverage intelligence, the diagnosis requires impairments in adaptive functioning and evidence of the condition prior to age 18 years. It is not difficult to fathom a situation in which an individual is raised in an extremely rural setting with no access to special education assessments or classes. In this situation, there may be little evidence of subaverage intelligence prior to the age of 18 years. For individuals who have been incarcerated because they were young juveniles, adaptive functioning may be rather difficult to assess. Common measures of adaptive functioning have not been validated in the correctional environment and may not translate well.

Last, what is the evaluator to do with illegal aliens and those from other countries and cultures? These concerns place an additional burden on the evaluator and the profession's measurement tools. It is absolutely imperative that evaluations done in capital cases proceed with utmost care and consideration, *particularly* before empirically derived methods to address these concerns are developed.

Death Penalty Mitigation

In 1972, the U.S. Supreme Court considered the death penalty in the United States at that time to be cruel and unusual punishment because the manner in which capital sentences were decided in Georgia was capricious (*Furman v. Georgia*, 1972). This decision discontinued death penalty litigation in the United States at the time because none of the states had a system that was substantially different. The death penalty statutes were rewritten by 35 states to correct the problem (Latzer, 1998).

The Court accepted as constitutional Georgia's rewrite of their statute (*Gregg v. Georgia*, 1976). Georgia's capital sentencing process included the presentation before a judge or jury of *aggravating* and *mitigating* factors. With the exception of treason or aircraft hijacking, it required at least 1 of 10 specified aggravating circumstances to be established beyond reasonable doubt to impose the death penalty. In jury trials, the judge was bound by the jury's decision. The process also allowed the defense to introduce mitigating circumstances, but the jury was not bound to cite any particular mitigating fact to make the binding recommendation against the death penalty. The Court noted, "No longer can a jury wantonly and freakishly impose the death sentence; it is always circumscribed by the legislative guidelines" (*Gregg v. Georgia*, p. 893).

Regarding mitigating circumstances, the U.S. Supreme Court referenced the American Law Institute's *Model Penal Code* (Tent. Draft No. 9, 1959, comment 3, p. 71) list of potential facts:

(a) The defendant has no significant history of prior criminal activity.

(b) The murder was committed while the defendant was under the influence of extreme mental or emotional disturbance.

(c) The victim was a participant in the defendant's homicidal conduct or consented to the homicidal act.

(d) The murder was committed under circumstances which the defendant believed to provide a moral justification or extenuation for his conduct.

(e) The defendant was an accomplice in a murder committed by another person and his participation in the homicidal act was relatively minor.

(f) The defendant acted under duress or under the domination of another person.

(g) At the time of the murder, the capacity of the defendant to appreciate the criminality [wrongfulness] of his conduct or to conform his conduct to the requirements of law was impaired as a result of mental disease or defect or intoxication.

The defense is certainly not limited to this particular list of mitigating facts. In *Lockett v. Ohio* (1978), the U.S. Supreme Court held the judge or jury could "not be precluded from considering as a mitigating factor, any aspect of the defendant's character or record and any circumstances of the offense that the defendant proffers as a basis for a sentence of less than death" (p. 604). Regarding this decision, Cunningham and Goldstein (2003) noted these possibilities for mitigation:

Any information regarding the defendant's background, as a child or as an adult, could be considered relevant. Thus, factors such as a history of childhood trauma (e.g., physical or sexual abuse), verbal abuse, exposure to drugs and alcohol, neglect and abandonment, undiagnosed or misdiagnosed conditions (e.g., mental retardation, emotional disturbance, learning disability, attention deficit/hyperactivity disorder), gang or cult membership, witnessing a death of a family member or friend could be considered nonstatutory mitigation. In addition, any circumstances related to the crime could be considered mitigating. Such nonstatutory factors as the minor role played by the defendant in the crime, his or her suggestibility quiescence to authority, perceived coercion, a sense desperation based on real or imaginary beliefs, or a need for self-perceived moral retribution could be introduced as non-statutory mitigators. Lockett requires defense attorneys, forensic psychological and psychiatric experts to explore all avenues of mitigation because the factors that can be introduced are not limited to those specifically delineated by statute. (p. 412, emphasis in the original)

The neuropsychologist contemplating death penalty mitigation work is referred to the work of Cunningham and Goldstein (2003) and Reynolds, Price, and Niland (2003) for a thorough review of important aspects of this work. The time involvement in death penalty mitigation is certainly not consistent with common neuropsychological, or even forensic, work (see the survey of Sweet, Peck, Abramowitz, & Etzweiler, 2002, in which clinical interview and history time in minutes was $M = 57$, $SD = 27$). Cunningham and Goldstein noted, "Obtaining a history in this comprehensive detail routinely requires 8 to 20 hours of interview with the defendant, exclusive of any psychological testing" (p.

422). Further they noted neuropsychological and neurological assessments are "indicated" in most cases because, first, such findings could have a significant mitigating effect, and second, there is a growing body of research implicating neurocognitive compromise in violent offenders.

Neuropsychological assessment in death penalty litigation could also focus on aggravating factors, but in this regard it is likely limited to addressing increased risk of dangerousness. Other aggravating factors are uniquely not related to mental health (e.g., particularly heinous crime, killing in association with another crime, etc.). Neuropsychologists can evaluate capital defendants to demonstrate the absence of mitigating factors (i.e., rebut a defense expert). It is important for evaluators to remain objective regardless of who requests their services. Death penalty mitigation is truly a unique area of practice and one that requires the utmost competence, integrity, and ethical conduct. As Cunningham and Goldstein (2003) pointed out, "In no situation is professional competence more important than in death penalty cases . . . it is imperative to present findings in a thorough, objective fashion" (p. 416).

ETHICAL AND PROFESSIONAL ISSUES IN CRIMINAL FORENSICS

The unique aspect of practicing neuropsychology in the criminal forensic setting carries with it a unique set of ethical concerns. As this volume contains a chapter specifically covering ethical considerations in forensic neuropsychological practice, I focus on only those issues specific to the criminal forensic setting. In addition to familiarity with the new "Ethical Principles of Psychologists and Code of Conduct" (American Psychological Association, 2002), neuropsychologists need to be fluently aware of the "Specialty Guidelines for Forensic Psychologists" ("Guidelines" hereafter; Committee on Ethical Guidelines, 1991), issues of confidentiality, and 5th Amendment protections.

Specialty Guidelines for Forensic Psychologists

The "Guidelines" were jointly developed and adopted by Division 41 of the American Psychological Association (American Psychology–Law Society) and the American Academy of Forensic Psychology (AAFP; members of the forensic board affiliated with the American Board of Forensic Psychology) in 1991. The "Guidelines" were intended to be consistent with the 1990 American Psychological Association's "Ethical Principles," but they also provided more specific guidance for psychologists providing forensic services. The 1992 "Ethical Principles" included a small subsection on forensic activities; however, this subsection was eliminated, and much of its contents scattered throughout the code or subsumed under "9.01 Bases for Assessments" in the 2002 "Ethical Principles." The "Guidelines" are aspirational in nature, yet they outline appropriate professional conduct when providing psychological expertise to the judicial system. A joint committee from Division 41 and AAFP are currently rewriting the "Guidelines" (Randy Otto, personal communication, August 25, 2003).

The "Guidelines" define forensic psychology as:

all forms of professional psychological conduct when acting, with definable foreknowledge, as a psychological expert on explicitly psycholegal issues, in direct assistance to courts, parties to legal proceedings, correctional and forensic mental health facilities, and administrative, judicial, and legislative agencies acting in an adjudicative capacity. (p. 657)

The "Guidelines" were not written to apply to psychologists asked to provide professional psychological services when the psychologist was not aware at the time of the service that it would become forensic in nature. For these individuals, however, they may be helpful in preparing to communicate professional opinions in the forensic arena. See the work of Denney (in press) for an application of the "Guidelines" (as well as the new "Ethical Principles") to two neuropsychology cases completed in the criminal forensic setting. It is important for neuropsychologists practicing in the criminal forensic arena to be familiar with the "Guidelines." The "Guidelines" cover many more aspects of forensic practice, but I cover just two critical areas, confidentiality and protecting criminal defendant rights.

Confidentiality in Criminal Forensics

A correct understanding of confidentiality is imperative in the criminal setting. Some jurisdictions provide confidentiality between the evaluator and defendant under the "work product rule" as set out by case law (*United States v. Alvarez*, 1975). Other jurisdictions do not provide for mental health evaluation confidentiality; in other words, the fact of the evaluation and the evaluator's opinion are discoverable even if there was no report written and the requesting attorney does not wish testimony (*Edney v. Smith*, 1976). When providing evaluations as a result of a direct court order, confidentiality does not exist. It is imperative for the evaluator to understand the rule in use within that case jurisdiction. The evaluator must describe his or her understanding of the use of the information to the defendant. This difficulty arises when a clinician evaluates competency to stand trial, but the clinician's testimony is requested for issues of rebutting an insanity defense or, worse, to provide an opinion regarding potential aggravating issues prior to sentencing. Such an occurrence is not unusual in death penalty cases and has been the issue of U.S. Supreme Court rulings (e.g., *Estelle v. Smith*, 1981).

Estelle v. Smith (1981) is another case in which James Grigson, M.D., provided testimony. The difficulty in this case was that Dr. Grigson may have informed Smith that he was evaluating him on his competency to stand trial, but he said nothing about any future testimony on other potential issues. Subsequent to the evaluation, Smith was found competent to proceed and convicted of capital murder. Texas maintains a bifurcated capital trial process by which the defendant undergoes trial regarding guilt initially, and then he or she undergoes another trial by the same jury regarding whether to impose the death penalty. For the jury to impose a death penalty, the prosecution must demonstrate potential for future violence. During the sentencing phase of Smith's case, Dr. Grigson testified that the man was a psychopath and likely to kill again. The jury sentenced Smith to death. The ethical concern here is that Dr. Grigson did not provide Smith with a full disclosure of potential uses for the information gained in the competency evaluation. In addition to the clear admonition in the "Ethical Principles," the "Guidelines" address this issue at IV.E.3:

After a psychologist has advised the subject of a clinical forensic evaluation of the intended uses of the evaluation and its work product, the psychologist may not use the evaluation work product for other purposes without explicit waiver to do so by the client or the client's legal representative.

Neuropsychologists must be cognizant of criminal defendant's rights regarding limits of confidentiality and informed assent. Related to this specific event is the duty to watch out for the constitutional rights of criminal defendants.

Fifth Amendment Protections

In the example in the preceding section, the U.S. Supreme Court held that Smith's 5th Amendment right to be protected from self-incrimination was violated by allowing Dr. Grigson to testify on the issue of future dangerousness at the penalty phase of the proceedings. The High Court noted:

When Dr. Grigson went beyond simply reporting to the court on the issue of competence and testified for the prosecution at the penalty phase on the crucial issue of respondent's future dangerousness, his role changed and became essentially like that of an agent of the state recounting unwarned statements made in a postarrest custodial setting.

Even though he warned the defendant about the limits of confidentiality, Dr. Grigson provided him with no indication the information used in the competency evaluation could be used against him at a future penalty proceeding. Actions that cause an infringement on a defendant's constitutional rights, such as was done here, not only violate the "Ethical Principles" (Principle E as well as Informed Consent), but also are counter to that espoused in the "Guidelines" at IV.E:

Forensic psychologists have an obligation to ensure that prospective clients are informed of their legal rights with respect to the anticipated forensic service, of the purposes of any evaluation, of the nature of procedures to be employed, of the intended uses of any product of their services, and of the party who has employed the forensic psychologist.

The "Ethical Principles" also point out psychologists' responsibility to avoid harm. It is clear that, in the case of *Estelle v. Smith* (1981), Dr. Grigson did not avoid harm. One could argue that providing potentially damaging testimony in any capital case is tantamount to causing harm. By that reasoning, any unbiased ethical forensic work could be considered unethical. Clearly, this is not the case. There is a difference between providing an unfavorable opinion and violating a defendant's constitutional rights. It is important to keep this distinction clear (Denney, in press; Denney & Wynkoop, 2000; K. Heilbrun, 2001).

It is generally important for forensic examiners to limit the scope of their opinions to the referral questions and the related and supporting conclusions. In the example, Dr. Grigson did not limit his opinion to competency. When asked to testify at the sentencing phase, the safest course of action would have been to refuse to do so based on the fact he did not provide Smith with a warning that information derived from the evaluation could be used against him in a sentencing proceeding (Denney, in press). In addition, an evaluation regarding dangerousness is an entirely different endeavor with a potentially substantial difference in data sources and evaluative measures. Dr. Grigson should have recommended that the attorney requesting such testimony seek another evaluation from an independent examiner. Relatedly, it is important for examiners to limit their opinions in written reports to strictly the referral question and supporting conclusion as well. Additional nonrequested opinions in forensic reports can play havoc on the legal proceedings. Forensic examiners are asked to provide expert opinions about very specific issues; well-trained and competent forensic psychologists realize this fact.

Training and Certification in Criminal Forensics

It is hoped this chapter and chapter 12 have made it clear that performing neuropsychological evaluations in the criminal forensic arena is a unique endeavor that requires a unique knowledge domain. The "Ethical Principles" make it clear that psychologists do not perform activities for which they are not adequately trained. The amount of specialized forensic training required for ethical and competent practice is not clear. The issue was preliminarily addressed by Otto and Heilbrun (2002). Some states have developed minimal requirements for criminal forensic practice (Farkas, DeLeon, & Newman, 1997). Often, these requirements include a few hours attending state-sponsored educational events with varying amounts of mandated supervision.

Sullivan and Denney (2003) attempted to present basic and aspirational requirements for competent criminal forensic neuropsychological practice. No one really knows the exact point at which clinical neuropsychological practice ends

and criminal forensic practice begins. The "Guidelines" suggest criminal forensic work begins when one knowingly accepts such a case. In addition to Sullivan
and Denney, Heilbronner and Frumkin (2003) raised the issue of this "dividing
line" and make a recommendation for one potential model of practice. It is good
that these issues are beginning to be discussed in the professional literature.
Time will reveal how well such suggestions are accepted.

Neuropsychologists interested in developing criminal forensic practices can
begin acquiring knowledge content from texts and seminars. I strongly recommend *Psychological Evaluations for the Courts* (2nd ed., Melton et al., 1997).
It is an astounding text that covers nearly the entirety of forensic practice, both
civil and criminal. This endorsement is not intended to mean there are no other
good texts; there are. Most of the other texts are more specific in scope. At this
point, there are no texts geared solely to the application of neuropsychology to
criminal forensics.

Seminar training can be obtained from national workshops by the AAFP.
These workshops are uniformly strong in content and presented at various times
during the year and in various locations around the country. Supervision is also
a necessary component of training in criminal forensics. I recommend receiving
supervision from an individual who has proven competency to provide psychological services in the criminal forensic setting. Attainment of board certification
in forensic psychology by the American Board of Forensic Psychology is the
clearest example of this achievement. I admonish eager neuropsychologists to
be wary of board-certifying bodies that bestow "diplomate" status with the ease
of signing a credit card (so-called vanity boards and checkbook credentials).
These bodies have attempted to improve their appearance by including multiple
choice examinations, but still do not require face-to-face, oral examinations of
knowledge base and practice skill at the hands of documented experts in the
field. Otto and Heilbrun (2002) presented a clear discussion on this issue. Last,
the *National Benchbook on Psychiatric and Psychological Evidence and Testimony* (Parry, 1998), a judge's handbook, addresses the issue of board certification and vanity boards specifically:

> The court should be aware that while specialty board certification is prestigious within
> the various professions, witnesses who have not obtained this level of credentialing are
> not automatically presumed to be deficient by comparison, nor are they unsuited *per se*
> to provide expert testimony. Judges must also be wary of witnesses claiming certification
> by various "mail-order" boards, that do not require an oral examination or other indicia
> of a rigorous qualifying process. (p. 55)

Neuropsychologists entering the arena of forensic practice need to prepare
adequately for the heightened scrutiny that comes with the court of law (Sullivan
& Denney, 2003). Attempting to bypass this preparation by presenting oneself
as competent based on a vanity board is misrepresentation to the public. Al-

though the public, and many in the judicial system, will not recognize this ruse, misrepresentation nonetheless remains ethically inappropriate.

SUMMARY

In this chapter, I have built on chapter 12 by reviewing major areas of importance to neuropsychological practice in the criminal forensic arena. Covered were the nature of the forensic mental health evaluation in general, criminal responsibility, sentencing issues, risk assessment, competency to be executed, death penalty mitigation, and important professional and ethical concerns. The chapter dealt strictly with adult criminal proceedings. There is a host of other issues inherent in juvenile work. Although there is a considerable body of literature dealing with psychological evaluation of individuals in the juvenile justice system (see Grisso's work), the first step in application of clinical neuropsychology and neurodevelopmental issues to that population has only recently begun (Grisso et al., 2003; Wynkoop, 2003).

The application of clinical neuropsychology to assist parties in the criminal justice system is a unique practice opportunity. It requires a distinctly different knowledge base in addition to solid, empirically based, clinical neuropsychological knowledge and skill. Neuropsychologists interested in working in the criminal forensic setting are encouraged to acquire that knowledge base and skill in a manner sufficient for competent and ethical practice of an applied empirical science.

NOTES

Opinions expressed in this chapter are those of the author and do not necessarily represent the position of the Federal Bureau of Prisons or the U.S. Department of Justice.

1. There are several variants in spelling for M'Naghten. Moran (1981), in his 18-month period of research, found documents that appeared to indicate the man actually spelled his name "McNaughtan," but M'Naghten is used here because it was used in the original legal case.
2. Formally adopted by the ALI on May 24, 1962.
3. *Very loosely* drawn from *Texas v. Andrea Yates* case (2003).

REFERENCES

American Law Institute. (1955). *Model Penal Code* Section 4.01(1)(2), (Tent. Draft No. 4). Philadelphia: Author.

American Law Institute. (1959). *Model Penal Code* (Tent. Draft No. 9, comment 3). Philadelphia: Author.

American Medical Association Council on Ethical and Judicial Affairs. (1995). Physician participation in capital punishment: Evaluation of prisoner competence to be executed:

Treatment to restore competence to be executed. *CEJA Report 1995*, Section 6-A-95. Chicago: Author

American Psychological Association. (2002). Ethical principles of psychologists and code of conduct. *American Psychologist, 57*, 1060–1073.

Amnesty International. (2001, April). *The illusion of control.* Retrieved May 10, 2003, from www.amnestyusa.org/abolish/reports/amr510532001.html

Atkins v. Virginia, 153 L. Ed 2d 335 (2002).

Barefoot v. Estelle, 103 S.Ct. 3383 (1983).

Barnard, P. G. (1998). Diminished capacity and automatism as a defense. *American Journal of Forensic Psychology, 16*, 27–62.

Barratt, E. S., Kent, T. A., Bryant, S. G., & Felthous, A. R. (1991). A controlled trial of phenytoin in impulsive aggression. *Journal of Clinical Psychopharmacology, 11*, 388–389.

Barratt, E. S., Stanford, M. S., Dowdy, L., Liebman, M. J., & Kent, T. A. (1999). Impulsive and premeditated aggression: A factor analysis of self-reported acts. *Psychiatry Research, 86*, 163–173.

Barratt, E. S., Stanford, M. S., Felthous, A., & Kent, T. A. (1997). The effects of phenytoin on impulsive and premeditated aggression: A controlled study. *Journal of Clinical Psychopharmacology, 17*, 341–349.

Barratt, E. S., Stanford, M. S., Kent, T. A., & Felthous, A. (1997). Neuropsychological and cognitive psychophysiological substrates of impulsive aggression. *Biological Psychiatry, 41*, 1045–1047.

Bars, D. R., Heyrend, F. L., Simpson, C. D., & Munger, J. C. (2001). Use of visual evoked-potential studies and EEG data to classify aggressive, explosive behavior of youths. *Psychiatric Services, 52*, 81–86.

Benson, D. F., & Miller, B. L. (1997). Frontal lobes: Clinical and anatomic aspects. In T. E. Feinberg & M. J. Farah (Eds.), *Behavioral neurology and neuropsychology* (pp. 401–408). New York: McGraw–Hill.

Best, M., Williams, J. M., & Coccaro, E. F. (2002). Evidence for a dysfunctional prefrontal circuit in patient with an impulsive aggressive disorder. *Proceedings of the National Academy of Science, 99*, 8448–8453.

Bonnie, R. J. (1990). Dilemmas in administering the death penalty: Conscientious abstention, professional ethics, and the needs of the legal system. *Law and Human Behavior, 14*, 67–90.

Bonta, J., Law, M., & Hanson, R. K. (1998). The prediction of criminal and violent recidivism among mentally disordered offenders: A meta-analysis. *Psychological Bulletin, 123*, 123–142.

Borum, R., & Grisso, T. (1995). Psychological test use in criminal forensic evaluations. *Professional Psychology: Research and Practice, 26*, 465–473.

Brower, M. C., & Price, B. H. (2001). Neuropsychiatry of frontal lobe dysfunction in violent and criminal behaviour: A critical review. *Journal of Neurology, Neurosurgery, and Psychiatry, 71*, 720–726.

Clark, C. R. (1999). Specific intent and diminished capacity. In I. B. Weiner & A. K. Hess (Eds.), *Handbook of forensic psychology* (2nd ed., pp. 350–378). New York: Wiley.

Coccaro, E. F. (1992). Impulsive aggression and central serotonergic system function in humans: An example of a dimensional brain-behavior relationship. *International Clinical Psychopharmacology, 7*, 3–12.

Coccaro, E. F., & Kavoussi, R. J. (1997). Fluoxetine and impulsive aggressive behavior in personality-disordered subjects. *Archives of General Psychiatry, 54*, 1081–1088.

Coccaro, E. F., Siever, L. J., Klar, H., Maurer, G. M., Cochrane, K., Cooper, T. B., et al. (1989). Serotonergic studies in affective and personality disorder patients: Correlates with suicidal and impulsive aggression. *Archives of General Psychiatry, 43*, 587–599.

Cochrane, R. E., Grisso, T., & Frederick, R. I. (2001). The relationship between criminal charges, diagnoses, and psycholegal opinions among federal pretrial defendants. *Behavioral Sciences and the Law, 19*, 565–582.

Committee on Ethical Guidelines for Forensic Psychologists. (1991). Specialty guidelines for forensic psychologists. *Law and Human Behavior, 15*, 655–665. Retrieved August 2, 2004, from http://www.abfp.com/downloadable/foren.pdf

Conklin, S. M., & Stanford, M. S. (2002). Differences in the late positive potential during an affective picture task in impulsive aggressive individuals [abstract]. *Psychophysiology, 39*(Suppl.), S27.

Conroy, M. A. (2003). Evaluation of sexual predators. In I. B. Weiner (Series Ed.) & A. M. Goldstein (Vol. Ed.), *Handbook of psychology, Vol. 11: Forensic psychology* (pp. 463–484). Hoboken, NJ: Wiley.

Cunningham, M. D., & Goldstein, A. M. (2003). Sentencing determinations in death penalty cases. In I. B. Weiner (Series Ed.) & A. M. Goldstein (Vol. Ed.), *Handbook of psychology, Vol. 11: Forensic psychology* (pp. 407–436). Hoboken, NJ: Wiley

Damasio, A. R., & Anderson, S. W. (2003). The frontal lobes. In K. M. Heilman & E. Valenstein (Eds.), *Clinical neuropsychology* (4th ed., pp. 404–446). New York: Oxford University Press.

Davis v. United States, 160 U.S. 469 (1895).

Denney, R. L. (in press). Ethical challenges in forensic neuropsychology, section 1: Neuropsychology in the criminal forensic arena. In S. Bush (Ed.), *A casebook of ethical challenges in neuropsychology*. Lisse, The Netherlands: Swets and Zeitlinger.

Denney, R. L., & Wynkoop, T. F. (2000). Clinical neuropsychology in the criminal forensic setting. *Journal of Head Trauma Rehabilitation, 15*, 804–828.

Dolan, M., Deakin, W. J. F., Roberts, N., & Anderson, I. (2002). Serotonergic and cognitive impairment in impulsive aggressive personality disordered offenders: Are there implications for treatment? *Psychological Medicine, 32*, 105–117.

Douglas, K., Ogloff, J., Nicholls, T., & Grant, I. (1999). Assessing risk for violence among psychiatric patients: The HCR-20 Violence Risk Assessment Scheme and the Psychopathy Checklist: Screening Version. *Journal of Consulting and Clinical Psychology, 67*, 917–930.

Douglas, K., & Webster, C. (1999). The HCR-20 Violence Risk Assessment Scheme: Concurrent validity in a sample of incarcerated offenders. *Criminal Justice and Behavior, 26*, 3–19.

Drake, M. E., Hietter, S. A., & Pakalnis, A. (1992). EEG and evoked potentials in episodic-dyscontrol syndrome. *Neuropsychobiology, 26*, 125–128.

Drake, M. E., Pakalnis, A., Brown, M. E., & Hietter, S. A. (1988). Auditory event related potentials in violent and nonviolent prisoners. *European Archives of Psychiatry and Neurological Sciences, 238*, 7–10.

Durham v. United States, 214 F.2d 862 (D.C. Cir. 1954).

Dusky v. United States, 362 U.S. 402 (1960).

Edney v. Smith, 425 F. Supp. 1038 (E.D.N.Y. 1976).

Estelle v. Smith, 451 U.S. 454 (1981).

Evans, J. R. (1997). Quantitative EEG findings in a group of death row inmates. *Archives of Clinical Neurology, 12*, 315–316.

Farkas, G., DeLeon, P., & Newman, R. (1997). Sanity examiner certification: An evolving national agenda. *Professional Psychology: Research and Practice, 28*, 73–76.

Favole, R. J. (1983) Mental disability in the American criminal process: A four issue survey. In J. Monahan & H. Steadman (Eds.), *Mentally disordered offenders: Perspectives from law and social science* (pp. 281–295) New York: Plenum Press.

Ferris, R. (1997). Psychiatry and the death penalty. *Psychiatric Bulletin, 21*, 746–748.

Ford v. Wainwright, 477 U.S. 399 (1986).

Frick, P. J. (1995). Callous-unemotional traits and conduct problems: A two-factor model of psychopathy in children. *Issues in Criminological and Legal Psychology, 24*, 47–51.

Furman v. Georgia, 408 U.S. 238 (1972).

Gerstle, J. E., Mathias, C. W., & Stanford, M. S. (1998). Auditory P300 and self-reported impulsive aggression. *Progress in Neuro-Psychopharmoacological and Biological Psychiatry, 22*, 575–583.

Giancola, P. R., Moss, H. B., Martin, C. S., Kirisci, L., & Tarter, R. E. (1996). Executive cognitive functioning predicts reactive aggression in boys at high risk for substance abuse: A prospective study. *Alcoholism: Clinical and Experimental Research, 20*, 740–744.

Godinez v. Moran, 125 L. Ed. 2d, 509 U.S. 389 (1993).

Golden, C. J., Jackson, M. L., Peterson-Rohne, A., & Gontkovsky, S. T. (2002). Neuropsychological factors in violence and aggression. In V. B. Van Hasselt & M. Hersen (Eds.), *Aggression and violence: An introductory text* (pp. 40–53). Needham Heights, MA: Allyn and Bacon.

Golding, S., & Roesch, R. (1987). The assessment of criminal responsibility: Approach to a current controversy. In I. B. Weiner & A. K. Hess (Eds.), *Handbook of forensic psychology* (pp. 395–432).

Golding, S. L., Skeem, J. L., Roesch, R., & Zapf, P. A. (1999). The assessment of criminal responsibility: Current controversies. In A. K. Hess & I. B. Weiner (Eds.), *The handbook of forensic psychology* (2nd ed., pp. 379–408). Hoboken, NJ: Wiley.

Goldstein, A. M., Morse, S. J., & Shapiro, D. L. (2003). Evaluation of criminal responsibility. In I. B. Weiner (Series Ed.) & A. M. Goldstein (Vol. Ed.), *Handbook of psychology, Vol. 11: Forensic psychology* (pp. 381–406). Hoboken, NJ: Wiley.

Gregg v. Georgia, 49 L.Ed.2d 859 (1976).

Gregg, T. R., & Siegel, A. (2001). Brain structures and neurotransmitters regulating aggression in cats: Implications for human aggression. *Progress in Neuro-Psychopharmacology and Biological Psychiatry, 25*, 91–140.

Grisso, T. (1988). *Competency to stand trial evaluations: A manual for practice.* Sarasota, FL: Professional Resource Exchange.

Grisso, T., & Applebaum, P. S. (1992). Is it unethical to offer predictions of future violence? *Law and Human Behavior, 16*, 621–633.

Grisso, T., Steinberg, L., Woolard, J., Cauffman, E., Scott, E., Graham, S., et al. (2003). Juveniles' competence to stand trial: A comparison of adolescents' and adults' capacities as trial defendants. *Law and Human Behavior, 27*, 333–363.

Hare, R. D. (1991). *The Hare Psychopathy Checklist–Revised.* Toronto, Ontario, Canada: Multi-Health Systems.

Hare, R. D., Harpur, T. J., & Hakstian, A. R. (1990). The revised Psychopathy Checklist: Reliability and factor structure. *Psychological Assessment, 2*, 338–341.

Harris, G., Rice, M., & Quinsey, V. L. (1993). Violent recidivism of mentally disordered offenders: The development of a statistical prediction instrument. *Criminal Justice and Behavior, 20*, 315.

Hart, S., Cox, D., & Hare, R. (1995). *The Hare Psychopathy Checklist: Screening version.* Niagara, NY: Multi-Health Systems.

Heilbronner, R. L., & Frumkin, I. B. (2003). Neuropsychology and forensic psychology: Working collaboratively in criminal cases. *Journal of Forensic Neuropsychology, 3,* 5–12.

Heilbrun, A. B., Heilbrun, L. C., & Heilbrun, K. L. (1978). Impulsive and premeditated homicide: An analysis of subsequent parole risk of the murderer. *Journal of Criminal Law and Criminology, 69,* 108–114.

Heilbrun, K. (1987). The assessment of competency for execution: An overview. *Behavioral Sciences and the Law, 5,* 383–396.

Heilbrun, K. (2001). *Principles of forensic mental health assessment.* New York: Kluwer Academic/Plenum.

Heilbrun, K., & McClaren, H. (1988). Assessment of competency to execution? A guide for mental health professionals. *Bulletin of the American Academy of Psychiatry and the Law, 16,* 205–216.

Heilbrun, K., Radelet, M., & Dvoskin, J. (1992). The debate of treating individuals incompetent for execution. *American Journal of Psychiatry, 149,* 596–604.

Houston, R. J., & Stanford, M. S. (2001). Mid-latency evoked potentials in self-reported impulsive aggression. *International Journal of Psychophysiology, 40,* 1–15.

Houston, R. J., Stanford, M. S., Villemarette-Pittman, N. R., Conklin, S. M., & Helfritz, L. E. (2003). Neurobiological correlates and clinical implications of aggressive subtypes. *Journal of Forensic Neuropsychology, 3,* 67–87.

Hubbard, J. A., Smithmyer, C. M., Ramsden, S. R., Parker, E. H., Flanagan, K. D., Dearing, K. F., et al. (2002). Observational, physiological, and self-report measures of children's anger: Relations to reactive versus proactive aggression. *Child Development, 73,* 1101–1118.

Jewish Publication Society. (1982). *Tanakh: A new translation of the holy scriptures according to the traditional Hebrew texts.* Philadelphia: Author.

Kavoussi, R. J., Liu, J., & Coccaro, E. F. (1994). An open trial of sertraline in personality disordered patients with impulsive aggression. *Journal of Clinical Psychiatry, 55,* 137–141.

Kent, T. A., Brown, C. S., Bryant, S. G., Barratt, E. S. Felthous, A. R., & Rose, R. M. (1988). Blood platelet uptake of serotonin in episodic aggression: Correlation with red blood cell proton T_1 and impulsivity. *Psychopharmacology Bulletin, 24,* 454–457.

Kiehl, K. A., Hare, R. D., Liddle, P. F., & McDonald, J. J. (1999). Reduced P300 in criminal psychopaths during a visual oddball task. *Biological Psychiatry, 45,* 1498–1507.

Latzer, B. (1998). *Death penalty cases: Leading U.S. Supreme Court cases on capital punishment.* Boston: Butterworth-Heinemann.

Leong, G. B., Weinstock, R., Silva, J. A., & Eth, S. (1993). Psychiatry and the death penalty: The past decade. *Psychiatric Annals, 23,* 41–47.

Lewis, D. O., Lovely, R., Yeager, C., & Della Femina, D. (1989). Toward a theory of the genesis of violence: A follow-up study of delinquents. *Journal of the American Academy of Child and Adolescent Psychiatry, 28,* 431–436.

Lewis, D. O., Moy, E., Jackson, L. D., Aaronson, R., Restifo, N., Serra, S., et al. (1985). Biopsychological characteristics of children who later murder: A prospective study. *American Journal of Psychiatry, 142,* 1161–1167.

Linnoila, M., & Charney, D. S. (1999). The neurobiology of aggression. In D. S. Charney, E. J. Nestler, & B. S. Bunney (Eds.), *Neurobiology of mental illness* (pp. 855–871). New York: Oxford University Press.

Linnoila, M., Virkkunen, M., Scheinin, M., Nuutila, A., Rimon, R., & Goodwin, F. K.

462   FORENSIC NEUROPSYCHOLOGY

(1983). Low cerebrospinal fluid 5-hydroxyindoleacetic acid concentration differentiates impulsive from non-impulsive violent behavior. *Life Sciences, 33*, 2609–2614.

Lockett v. Ohio, 438 U.S. 586 (1978).

Macmillan, M. (2000). *An odd kind of fame: Stories of Phineas Gage.* Cambridge, MA:
MIT Press.

Malone, R. P., Bennett, D. S., Luebbert, J. F., Rowan, A. B., Biesecker, B. A., Blaney,
B. L., et al. (1998). Aggression classification and treatment response. *Psychopharmacology Bulletin, 34*, 41–45.

Marlowe, D. B., Lambert, J. B., & Thompson, R. G. (1999). Voluntary intoxication and
criminal responsibility. *Behavioral Sciences and the Law, 17*, 195–217.

Martell, D. A. (1992). Estimating the prevalence of organic brain dysfunction in maximum-security forensic psychiatric patients. *Journal of Forensic Science, 37*, 878–
893.

Mathias, C. W., & Stanford, M. S. (1999). P300 under standard and surprise condition
in self-reported impulsive aggression. *Progress in Neuro-Psychopharmacology and
Biological Psychiatry, 23*, 1037–1051.

McDonald v. United States, 312 F.2d 847 (DC Cir. 1962).

McLearen, A. M., Pietz, C. A., & Denney, R. L. (2004). Evaluation of psychological
damages. In W. O'Donohue & E. Levensky (Eds.), *Forensic psychology* (pp. 267–
299). New York: Academic.

Melton, G. B., Petrila, J., Poythress, N. G., & Slobogin, C. (1997). *Psychological evaluations for the courts* (2nd ed.). New York: Guilford Press.

Mesulam, M.-M. (2000). Behavioral neuroanatomy: Large-scale networks, association
cortex, frontal syndromes, the limbic system, and hemispheric specializations. In
M.-M. Mesulam (Ed.), *Principles of behavioral and cognitive neurology* (2nd ed., pp.
1–120). New York: Oxford University Press.

Miczek, K. A. (1987). The psychopharmacology of aggression. In L. L. Iverson, S. D.
Iverson, & S. H. Snyder (Eds.). *Handbook of psychopharmacology* (pp. 183–228).
New York: Plenum Press.

Mills, V. M., Cassidy, J. W., & Katz, D. I. (1997). *Neurological rehabilitation: A guide
to diagnosis, prognosis, and treatment planning.* Malden, MA: Blackwell Science.

Monahan, J. (1992). Mental disorder and violent behavior: Perceptions and evidence.
American Psychologist, 47, 511–521.

Monahan, J. (2003). Violence risk assessment. In I. B. Weiner (Series Ed.) & A. M.
Goldstein (Vol. Ed.), *Handbook of psychology, Vol. 11: Forensic psychology* (pp.
527–540). Hoboken, NJ: Wiley.

Monahan, J., & Steadman, H. J. (1994). Toward a rejuvenation of risk assessment research. In J. Monahan & H. J. Steadman (Eds.). *Violence and mental disorder: Developments in risk assessment.* Chicago: University of Chicago Press.

Monahan, J., Steadman, H. J., Silver, E., Applebaum, P. S., Robbins, P. C., Mulvey,
E. P., et al. (2001). *Rethinking risk assessment: The MacArthur Study of Mental Disorder and Violence.* New York: Oxford University Press.

Moran, Richard (1981). *Knowing right from wrong: The insanity defense of Daniel Mc-
Naughten.* New York: Free Press.

Mossman, D. (1994). Assessing predictions of violence: Being accurate about accuracy.
Journal of Consulting and Clinical Psychology, 62, 783–792.

Mrad, D. (1996, September). *Criminal responsibility evaluations.* Paper presented at Issues in Forensic Assessment Symposium, Federal Bureau of Prisons, Atlanta, GA.

Mungus, D. (1988). Psychometric correlates of episodic violent behavior: A multidimen-
sional neuropsychological approach. *British Journal of Psychiatry, 152*, 180–187.

Nestor, P. G., & Haycock, J. (1997). Not guilty by reason of insanity of murder: Clinical and neuropsychological characteristics. *Journal of the American Academy of Psychiatry and Law*, 25, 161–171.

New, A. S., Hazlett, E. A., Buchsbaum, M. S., Goodman, M., Reynolds, D., Mitropoulou, V., et al. (2002). Blunted prefrontal cortical [18]fluorodeoxyglucose positron emission tomography response to meta-chlorophenylpiperazine in impulsive aggression. *Archives of General Psychiatry*, 59, 621–629.

North Carolina v. Alford, 400 U.S. 25 (1970).

Otto, R. K., & Heilbrun, K. (2002). The practice of forensic psychology: A look toward the future in light of the past. *American Psychologist*, 57, 5–18.

Parry, J. W. (1998). *National benchbook on psychiatric and psychological evidence and testimony*. Washington, DC: American Bar Association Commission on Mental and Physical Disability Law.

Parsons v. State. 81 Ala. 577, 2 So. 854 (1887).

Paschall, M. J., & Fishbein, D. H. (2002). Executive cognitive functioning and aggression: A public health perspective. *Aggression and Violent Behavior*, 7, 215–235.

Penry v. Lynaugh, 492 U.S. 1 (1989).

People v. Schmidt, 216 N.Y. 324, 110 N.E., 945 (1915).

Perlin, M. L. (1992). *The law and persons with mental disability–Tape 6: The criminal law process*. Springfield, IL: Baxley Media Group. Retrieved August 2, 2004, from http://www.baxleymedia.com/catalog/legal/mental.htm

Pulkkinen, L. (1996). Proactive and reactive aggression in early adolescence as precursors to anti-and prosocial behavior in young adults. *Aggressive Behavior*, 22, 241–257.

Raine, A. (2002). Annotation: The role of prefrontal deficits, low autonomic arousal, and early health factors in the development of antisocial and aggressive behavior in children. *Journal of Child Psychology and Psychiatry and Allied Disciplines*, 43, 417–434.

Raine, A., Meloy, J. R., Bihrle, S., Stoddard, J., LaCasse, L., & Buchsbaum, M. S. (1998). Reduced prefrontal and increased subcortical brain functioning assessed using positron emission tomography in predatory and affective murderers. *Behavioral Sciences and the Law*, 16, 319–332.

Raine, A., & Venables, P. H. (1988). Enhanced P3 evoked potentials and longer P3 recovery time in psychopaths. *Psychophysiology*, 25, 30–38.

Raine, A., Venables, P. H., & Williams, M. (1990). Relationships between N1, P300, and contingent negative variation recorded at age 15 and criminal behavior at age 24. *Psychophysiology*, 27, 567–574.

Reisner, R., & Slobogin, C. (1990). *Law and the mental health system* (2nd ed.). St. Paul, MN: West.

Rex v. M'Naghten, 10 Cl. & F. 200, 8 Eng. Rep. 718 (H.L. 1843).

Reynolds, C., Price, J. R., & Niland, J. (2003). Applications of neuropsychology in capital felony (death penalty) defense. *Journal of Forensic Neuropsychology*, 3, 89–123.

Rice, M., & Harris, G. (1995). Violent recidivism: Assessing predictive validity. *Journal of Consulting and Clinical Psychology*, 63, 737–748.

Robinson, D. N. (1996). *Wild beasts and idle humours: The insanity defense from antiquity to the present*. Cambridge, MA: Harvard University Press.

Rogers, R. (1984). *Rogers Criminal Responsibility Assessment Scales (RCRAS) and test manual*. Odessa, FL: Psychological Assessment Resources.

Rogers, R., & Ewing, C. P. (1992). The measurement of insanity: Debating the merits of the R-CRAS and its alternatives. *International Journal of Law and Psychiatry*, 15, 113.

Scarpa, A., & Raine, A. (2000). Violence associated with anger and impulsivity. In J. C. Borod (Ed.), *The neuropsychology of emotion* (pp. 320–339). New York: Oxford University Press.

Shaikah, M. B., De Lanerolle, N. C., & Siegel, A. (1997). Serotonin 5-HT$_{1A}$ and 5-HT$_{2/1C}$ receptors in the midbrain periaqueductal gray differentially modulate defensive rage behavior elicited from the medial hypothalamus of the cat. *Brain Research, 765*, 198–207.

Shapiro, D. L. (1984). *Psychological evaluation and expert testimony*. New York: van Nostrand Reinhold.

Shapiro, D. L. (1991). *Forensic psychological assessment*. Boston: Allyn and Bacon.

Shapiro, D. L. (1999). *Criminal responsibility evaluations: A manual for practice*. Sarasota, FL: Professional Resource Press.

Siegel, A., and Shaikah, M. B. (1992). Neurotransmitters and aggressive behavior: Some new perspectives. In K. T. Strongman (Ed.). *International review of studies on emotion* (Vol. 2, pp. 5–22). Chichester, England: Wiley and Sons.

Silver, E., Cirincione, C., & Steadman, J. H. (1994). Demythologizing inaccurate perceptions of the insanity defense: Legal standards and clinical assessment. *Applied and Preventive Psychology, 2*, 163–178.

Singleton v. Norris, 108 F.3d 872 (8th Cir., 1997). See Judge Heaney concurring. Retrieved August 2, 2004, from http://caselaw.lp.findlaw.com/scripts/getcase.pl?court=8th&navby=case&no=953032p

Singleton v. Norris, No. 00–1492 (8th Cir., 2003). Retrieved August 2, 2004, from http://caselaw.lp.findlaw.com/data2/circs/8th/001492p.pdf

Smithmyer, C. M., Hubbard, J. A., & Simons, R. F. (2000). Proactive and reactive aggression in delinquent adolescents: Relations to aggression outcome expectancies. *Journal of Clinical Child Psychology, 29*, 86–93.

Stanford, M. S., Greve, K. W., & Gerstle, J. E. (1997). Neuropsychological correlates of self-reported impulsive aggression in a college sample. *Personality and Individual Differences, 23*, 961–966.

Stanford, M. S., Houston, R. J., Mathias, C. W., Greve, K. W., Villemarette-Pittman, N. R., & Adams, D. (2001). A double-blind placebo-controlled crossover study of phenytoin in individuals with impulsive aggression. *Psychiatry Research, 103*, 193–203.

State v. Jones, 50 N.J. 369 (1871).

Steadman, H. J., McGreevy, M. A., Morrissey, J. P., Callahan, L. A., Robbins, P. C., & Cirincione, C. (1993). *Before and after Hinckley: Evaluating insanity defense reform*. New York: Guilford Press.

Steadman, H. J., Rosenstein, M. J., MacAskiel, R. L., & Manderschied, R. W. (1988). A profile of mental disordered offenders admitted to inpatient psychiatric services in the United States. *Law and Human Behavior, 12*, 91–99.

Sullivan, J. P., & Denney, R. L. (2003). Constitutional and judicial foundations in criminal forensic neuropsychology. *Journal of Forensic Neuropsychology, 3*, 13–44.

Swanson, J. W., Holzer, C. E., Ganju, V., & Jono, R. T. (1990). Violence and psychiatric disorder in the community: Evidence from the epidemiologic catchment area surveys. *Hospital and Community Psychiatry, 41*, 761–770.

Sweet, J. J., Peck, E. A., Abramowitz, C., & Etzweiler, S. (2002). National Academy of Neuropsychology/Division 40 of the American Psychological Association practice survey of clinical neuropsychology in the United States, part I: Practitioner and practice characteristics, professional activities, and time requirements. *The Clinical Neuropsychologist, 16*, 109–127.

United States v. Alvarez, 519 F.2d 1036 (3rd Cir., 1975).

United States v. Brawner, 471 F.2d 969 (DC Cir., 1972).

United States Department of Justice. (2001, December). Capital punishment 2001. *Bureau of Justice Statistics Bulletin*, NCJ 197020. Retrieved May 10, 2003, from http://www.ojp.usdoj.gov/bjs/abstract/cp01.htm

United States v. Dubray, 854 F.2d 1099 (8th Cir., 1988).

United States v. Segna, 555 F.2d 226 (9th Cir., 1977).

United States v. Sullivan, 544 F.2d 1052 (9th Cir., 1976).

Villemarette-Pittman, N. R., Stanford, M. S., & Greve, K. W. (2003). Language and executive function in self-reported impulsive aggression. *Personality and Individual Differences, 34*, 1533.

Vitaro, F., Gendreau, P. L., Tremblay, R. E., & Oligny, P. (1998). Reactive and proactive aggression differentially predict later conduct problems. *Journal of Child Psychology and Psychiatry and Allied Disciplines, 39*, 377–385.

Volavka, J., Martell, D., & Convit, A. (1992). Psychobiology of the violent offender. *Journal of Forensic Sciences, 37*, 237–251.

Volkaw, N. D., Tancredi, L. R., Grant, C., Gillespie, H., Valentine, A., Mullani, N., et al. (1995). Brain glucose metabolism in violent psychiatric patients: A preliminary study. *Psychiatry Research: Neuroimaging, 61*, 243–253.

Wade v. United States, 426 F.2d (9th Cir., 1970).

Washington v. United States, 390 F.2d 444 (D.C. Cir., 1967).

Webster, C., Douglas, K., Eaves, D., & Hart, S. (1995). *HCR-20: Assessing risk for Violence* (version 2). Vancouver, British Columbia, Canada: Simon Fraser University.

Weinshenker, N. J., & Siegel, A. (2002). Bimodal classification of aggression: Affective defense and predatory attack. *Aggression and Violent Behavior, 7*, 327–250.

West Publishing. (1990). *Black's law dictionary* (6th ed). St. Paul, MN: Author.

Wexler, D., & Winick, B. (1991). Therapeutic jurisprudence as a new approach to mental health law policy analysis and research. *University of Miami Law Review, 45*, 992–997.

Wynkoop, T. F. (2003). Neuropsychology of juvenile adjudicative competence. *Journal of Forensic Neuropsychology, 3*, 45–65.

Index